Autism Spectrum Disorder

Autism Spectrum Disorder

Editor: Harvey Wilson

FOSTER ACADEMICS

www.fosteracademics.com

www.fosteracademics.com

FOSTER ACADEMICS

Cataloging-in-Publication Data

Autism spectrum disorder / edited by Harvey Wilson.
p. cm.
Includes bibliographical references and index.
ISBN 978-1-63242-527-0
1. Autism spectrum disorders. 2. Autism. 3. Developmental disabilities. I. Wilson, Harvey.
RC553.A88 A98 2018
616.858 82--dc23

Foster Academics,
118-35 Queens Blvd., Suite 400,
Forest Hills, NY 11375, USA

ISBN 978-1-63242-527-0 (Hardback)

Printed and bound in China.

Contents

Preface

Every book is initially just a concept; it takes months of research and hard work to give it the final shape in which the readers receive it. In its early stages, this book also went through rigorous reviewing. The notable contributions made by experts from across the globe were first molded into patterned chapters and then arranged in a sensibly sequential manner to bring out the best results.

Autism spectrum disorder is a disorder that causes difficulties in communication and interaction. Some of the characteristics of this disorder are repetitive behavior, sensory issues and cognitive issues. It is mainly diagnosed around the age of three to four. The main causes of autism are genetics, neuroanatomical abnormalities and environmental factors. The topics covered in this extensive book deal with the core aspects of autism spectrum disorder. It will prove to be immensely beneficial to students and researchers in this field.

It has been my immense pleasure to be a part of this project and to contribute my years of learning in such a meaningful form. I would like to take this opportunity to thank all the people who have been associated with the completion of this book at any step.

Editor

1

A Reciprocal Model of Face Recognition and Autistic Traits: Evidence from an Individual Differences Perspective

Drew W. R. Halliday[1,3], Stuart W. S. MacDonald[1], Suzanne K. Sherf[2], James W. Tanaka[1,3]*

1 University of Victoria, Victoria, British Columbia, Canada, **2** The Pennsylvania State University, State College, Pennsylvania, United States of America, **3** The Centre for Autism Research, Technology and Education, Victoria, British Columbia, Canada

Abstract

Although not a core symptom of the disorder, individuals with autism often exhibit selective impairments in their face processing abilities. Importantly, the reciprocal connection between autistic traits and face perception has rarely been examined within the typically developing population. In this study, university participants from the social sciences, physical sciences, and humanities completed a battery of measures that assessed face, object and emotion recognition abilities, general perceptual-cognitive style, and sub-clinical autistic traits (the Autism Quotient (AQ)). We employed separate hierarchical multiple regression analyses to evaluate which factors could predict face recognition scores and AQ scores. Gender, object recognition performance, and AQ scores predicted face recognition behaviour. Specifically, males, individuals with more autistic traits, and those with lower object recognition scores performed more poorly on the face recognition test. Conversely, university major, gender and face recognition performance reliably predicted AQ scores. Science majors, males, and individuals with poor face recognition skills showed more autistic-like traits. These results suggest that the broader autism phenotype is associated with lower face recognition abilities, even among typically developing individuals.

Editor: Christina Schmitz, Lyon Neuroscience Research Center, France

Funding: The funders had no role in study design, data collection and analysis, decision to publish, or preparation of the manuscript. This research was supported by grants from the Temporal Dynamics of Learning Center (NSF Grant #SBE-0542013), National Institute of Child Health and Human Development (NIH Grant HD-46526) and the Natural Sciences and Engineering Research.

Competing Interests: The authors have declared that no competing interests exist.

* E-mail: jtanaka@uvic.ca

Introduction

While repetitive behaviours, delayed language and impaired social function are the hallmarks of autism, many individuals on the autism spectrum experience problems recognizing faces [1–2] and interpreting facial expressions [3]. Despite the well-established link between autism and face recognition [2,4–7], it is less clear whether impaired face recognition is the consequence of, or a contributor to, the autistic condition. On one hand, a reluctance to socially engage with others and an aversion to making eye contact will invariably lead to less perceptual experience with faces, which in turn, could result in impaired face processing ability [4]. On the other hand, if impoverished face recognition skills are systemic to the autistic condition, a compromised face processing system might interfere with everyday social interactions, (e.g., social confusion and miscommunication) and further exacerbate the autistic condition.

In this study, we employ a hierarchical multiple regression method to examine the reciprocal relation between face recognition and autistic traits in a sub-clinical population. Our main findings are that whereas autistic-like tendencies reliably predict poor face recognition performance, the converse is also true, that impaired face processing predicts autistic-like tendencies.

Autism spectrum disorder (ASD) is characterized by deficits in communication and social interactions, displays of repetitive stereotypic behaviours, and expressions of restricted interests [8]. By definition, autism is a spectrum disorder with individuals presenting a range of symptoms that are classified as mild to extreme in their severity. As such, the autism continuum extends to people who may lie outside the formal autism diagnosis, but who nevertheless display autistic-like behaviours, [9–11]. The Autism Quotient (AQ) was developed as a self-assessment questionnaire, designed to measure a person's degree of autistic traits [11]. Participants rate their level of agreement on a four-point scale to statements indicative of ASD characteristics (e.g., When I talk, it isn't always easy for others to get a word in edgeways). The AQ measure has been used to identify group differences in the Broader Autism Phenotype [12]. For example, studies have shown that undergraduate science majors score significantly higher on the AQ measure than non-science majors [11,13]. By adopting an individual differences approach, our goal is to study a potential endophenotype of autism in the larger, subclinical ASD population, to yield important insights into the roots of the disorder.

In the autism literature, a clear link has been established between the autistic condition and impaired face processing abilities. Compared to their typically developing (TD) peers, individuals with ASD show less interest in faces [14–16] and perform worse on measures of face memory [e.g., 2,7,17]. Brain regions that are differentially activated by faces (i.e., fusiform gyrus) show reduced activation in groups of adults [4,18] and adolescents [19] with ASD. However, the level of fusiform activity exhibited by persons with ASD may depend on whether they are attending to the eyes of the face [20], viewing a familiar or unfamiliar face [21] or are socially anxious [22]. Within the TD population, individuals who report high degrees of autistic characteristics also exhibit functional and structural brain abnormalities in neural regions involved in social face processing [23]. Studies employing event-related-potential (ERP) methods indicate that the brain response to faces is delayed in individuals with ASD relative to TD control participants [24].

Although persons with autism display selective deficits in their face processing skills, it is less clear whether individuals with face deficits present autistic-like tendencies. Developmental prosopagnosia is a selective deficit in face recognition skills due to unspecified, congenital origins. Not surprisingly, persons with a life-long impairment in their ability to recognize familiar faces experience a great deal of anxiety that forces them to avoid social situations [25]. However, growing up with a severe face recognition deficit does not necessarily lead to the development of autistic-like behaviours. In one study, a sample of individuals with developmental prosopagnosia completed the AQ and other social cognition measures [26]. The questionnaire results indicated that these individuals were not prone to autistic behaviours nor were they impaired in their social interactions. As with ASD, individuals with prosopagnosia are impaired in their face recognition abilities, however unlike ASD individuals, they are motivated to be socially engaged and to develop compensatory strategies for person recognition (e.g., identification through clothing, voice or gait cues). Although face deficits do not predict autistic tendencies, it is possible that people with autistic tendencies are susceptible to face processing difficulties that further exacerbate the autistic condition.

In the current study, we explore the potential reciprocal relationship between face recognition abilities and the autistic phenotype in a large, non-clinical sample of university students. Related studies have shown that face recognition skills are correlated with measures of social cognition in the TD population. For example, individuals who perform worse on measures of face memory report low degrees of empathy [27] and extraversion [28]. Although these studies controlled for visuospatial and object recognition abilities, they used group differences to compare the high and low ends of their respective distributions (i.e., empathy or extraversion) to do so. By examining group differences (e.g., comparing face and object recognition abilities in individuals scoring high vs. low on a proxy of social cognition) rather than individual differences, the shared variance between face and object recognition is not properly accounted for (for a discussion, see [29]). Examining individual differences facilitates not only investigating the unique contributions of predictor variables (e.g., face and object recognition abilities), it also examines variance within the entire distribution of scores, rather than the high and low ends exclusively. Here, we employ a hierarchical multiple regression model to isolate the relationship between autistic traits and facial and emotion recognition abilities, while controlling for general visuospatial and object recognition abilities. We predict that a person's degree of self-reported autistic traits (i.e., their AQ score) will be uniquely associated with their ability to recognize facial identity and facial expression. Accordingly, individuals who report higher degrees of autistic traits will show a selective deficit in facial and emotion recognition.

Methods

Ethics Statement

The institutional review boards at both the University of Victoria and Carnegie Mellon University approved this study.

Participants

131 participants (85 females) aged 18–30 years ($m = 20.4$ years, $SD = 2.6$) were recruited to participate in this study. 26 participants from Carnegie Mellon University (20 males) were recruited from the Computer Science and Engineering departments. 105 participants from the University of Victoria (79 females) were recruited from various introductory Psychology classes. In total, participants identified 31 different majors.

Procedures

Participants gave written informed consent and were presented with the battery of measures in the following order: Immediate Memory Face task, Immediate Memory Bird task, Emotion Recognition task, Embedded Figures Test, and Autism Quotient (AQ). Participants completed the experiment individually in a quiet room, on computers equipped with Intel Pentium 4 processors and 15-inch Sony Trinitron E240 or LG Flatron F700P monitors, set at a screen resolution of 1024 by 768 pixels. Participants were compensated with bonus course credit or money ($10), and were debriefed immediately after completing the experiment.

Immediate Memory (IM) Face Task. This task measured participants' short-term memory for novel faces by requiring them to match identity, and was adapted from the original *Let's Face It!* skills battery [2]. A study face was shown in frontal view for 1,000 msec, followed by a noise mask for 500 msec, and finally three probe faces at the same 3/4 orientation for 3,000 msec. Participants chose the target face corresponding to the study face based on identity from the three alternative choices. Face stimuli included grey-scaled images from the Joe Stein Face Set with external features removed. Images subtended 5.28°×7.17° of

Table 1. Descriptive Characteristics.

	Mean	SD	Range	Skewness	Kurtosis	Cronbach's α
IM Face	0.68	0.11	.43–.93	−1.07	−1.16	.53*
IM Bird	0.63	0.09	.37–.80	−1.98	0.53	.62*
Emo Rec	0.68	0.09	.37–.93	−1.63	1.32	.45*
EFT	−2.37	6.70	−16–15	1.97	−0.79	
AQ	55.38	11.35	23–90	−0.14	1.34	

**Based on previous piloting.*

Table 2. Correlations between all measures.

	Major	IM Face	IM Bird	Emo Rec	EFT	AQ
Gender	r=.43**	r=.17*	r=.10	r=.24**	r=−.08	r=−.22**
Major		r=.07	r=−.07	r=.06	r=−.01	r=−.27**
IM Face			r=.22**	r=.19*	r=−.08	r=−.20*
IM Bird				r=.39**	r=.28**	r=−.10
Emo Rec					r=.15	r=−.03
EFT						r=−.05

*$p<.05$.
**$p<.01$.

visual angle in the horizontal and vertical dimensions, respectively. There were 30 trials in total presented in fixed sequential order.

Immediate Memory (IM) Bird Task. This task measured participants' short-term memory for birds, and served as a control measure for the IM Face task. As in the face identity task, a study image was shown for 1,000 msec, followed by a noise mask for 500 msec, and finally three probe images for 3,000 msec. The probe images were all from the same genus, with the correct image corresponding to the exact same species of bird as the study image. Sparrows, Warblers, Orioles, Tanagers, Blackbirds, Buntings and Flycatchers comprised the stimulus set. Images were grey-scaled and subtended visual angles of 5.65°×7.05° in the horizontal and vertical dimensions, respectively. There were 30 trials in total presented in fixed sequential order.

Emotion Recognition Task. This task measured participants' ability to recognize six basic emotions across different identities. As in the previous tasks, a study face was shown for 1,000 msec, followed by a noise mask for 500 msec, and finally three probe faces in frontal view for 3,000 msec, one of which depicted the same emotion as the study face. Faces were chosen from the Karolinska Face Set [30] and expressed the following emotions: sadness; anger; fear; happiness; disgust and surprise. Images were grey-scaled, contained external features, and subtended visual angles of 5.28°×7.17° in the horizontal and vertical dimensions, respectively. There were 30 trials in total presented in fixed sequential order.

Embedded Figures Test. This task involved disembedding simple shapes from complex visual scenes and was adapted from the original pencil-paper version [31]. This task served to measure participants' global ability for visuospatial perception; our ability to process information about where objects are in space. Participants viewed each scene separately and completed as many of the 16 trials as possible within a 12-minute time period by choosing from five basic shapes, the one that was hidden within the complex figure.

Autism Quotient. The Autism Quotient (AQ) is a 50-item self-report questionnaire based on five subscales (communication, social interaction, imagination, attention to detail, and attention switching) relating to the triad of impairments characterizing ASD [11]. It is designed for use with people of normal intelligence to quantify their degree of autistic traits. Participants rated each statement as either 'definitely agree,' 'slightly agree,' 'slightly disagree,' or 'definitely disagree.'

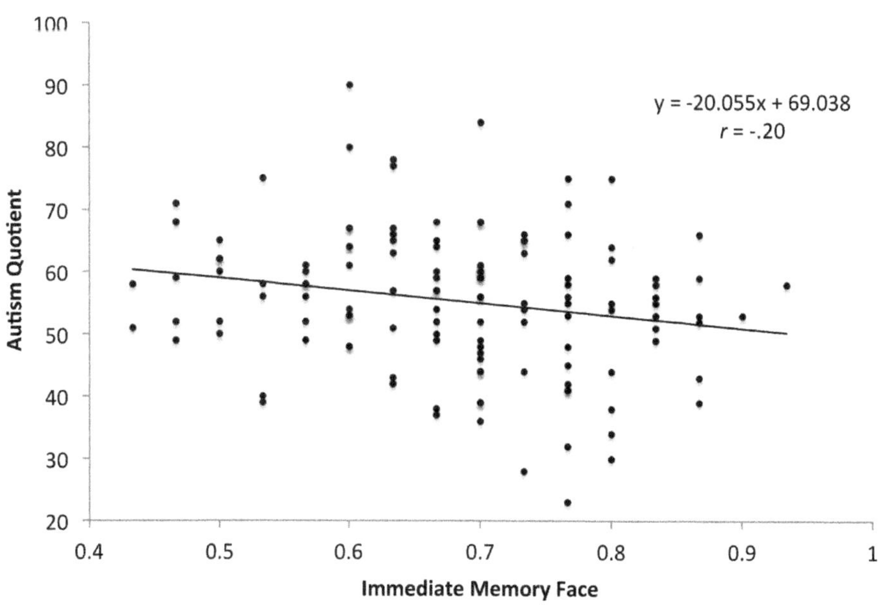

Figure 1. Autism Quotient scores as a function of Immediate Memory Face scores.

Table 3. Hierarchical regression on face recognition scores as a function of university major, gender, bird recognition and Autism Quotient.

Variables	B	SE B	β	semi-r	p
Stage 1					
Intercept	0.66	0.03			
Gender	0.04	0.02	0.17	0.15	0.05
Major	−0.00	0.02	−0.01	−0.01	0.40
Stage 2					
IM Bird	0.25	0.12	0.20	0.20	0.02
Stage 3					
AQ	−0.00	0.00	−0.16	−0.16	0.04

* *p* values are one-tailed.

Analyses. To test our primary hypotheses, we ran an initial correlation to examine the relationship between autistic traits (AQ) face identity recognition (IM Face), object recognition (IM Bird) emotion recognition, Embedded Figures, gender and major. Then, we employed hierarchical multiple regression in order to test the relative predictive contribution of variables entered in a blocked-entry order. Two hierarchical regression models were assessed, differing in terms of the dependent measure (AQ scores or IM Face scores). Given our strong, a priori hypotheses, we evoked one-tailed p-values for our regression analyses.

For the first block, gender and major were entered consistent with their robust associations to AQ scores reported in previous studies [e.g., 11]. The final stage of each model was reserved for AQ or identity recognition, in order to employ a conservative test of whether either variable remained a unique predictor after partialling out variance linked to the other theoretically motivated variables. We maintained a consistent order of variable entry across models to facilitate direct comparison, and report one-tailed p values in accordance with our a priori and directional hypotheses. Prior to these analyses, we examined skewness and kurtosis values (see Table 1) for each univariate distribution, as well as the scatterplots for each bivariate distribution. All data were univariate normal based on conventional standards (i.e., no values were greater than ±3.27). There were no multivariate outliers, based on visual inspection of residual plots, as well as Mahalanobis distances.

Results

Seven participants did not declare a major, and were not included in the analyses. Scores on the IM Face ($M = .68$, $SD = .11$) and the IM Bird ($M = .63$, $SD = .09$) measures were of comparable difficulty, and produced distributions with similar variability. Scores on the Embedded Figures Test were computed by subtracting incorrect responses from correct ones across trials attempted ($M = -2.37$, $SD = 6.70$), yielding a potential range of −16–16, where high scores correspond to superior featural processing. Table 1 summarizes the descriptive characteristics of each measure. Scores on the Autism Quotient ranged from 23–90 ($M = 55.38$, $SD = 11.35$). In keeping with recent studies that have used the AQ [e.g., 32–33] we used a 4-point scoring system rather than the original 2-point system in order to increase variability amongst scores to better examine individual differences. With the 2-point scoring system, a score of 32 is suggested to correspond with clinical cutoff [11]; with a 4 point scoring system, this translates to a score of 96. University majors were dichotomized into Science and non-Science majors, according to the criteria used by Baron-Cohen et al. [11].

Correlations among all measures

A Pearson product-moment correlation coefficient was computed to assess the relationship between scores on the Autism Quotient (AQ), and scores on the other four measures. Table 2 displays the correlations between all measures in the study. There was a significant negative correlation between AQ scores and scores on the IM Face, $r = -.20$, $p = .02$; a scatterplot summarizes these results (see Figure 1). The correlations between AQ scores, and scores on the IM bird, Emotion Recognition and Embedded Figures tasks were not significant ($p > .05$). These results suggest that there is a specific relationship between the magnitude of autistic traits and face recognition behaviour, and not a more general relationship between visual processing abilities and autistic traits. The correlations between AQ scores and gender ($r = -.22$, $p = .01$), and AQ scores and university major ($r = -.27$, $p = .002$)

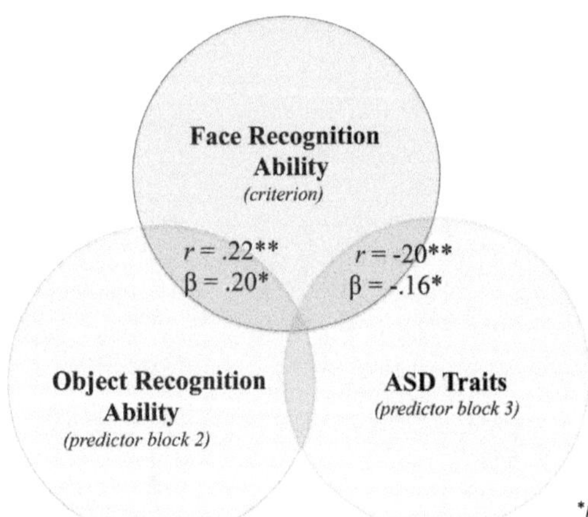

Figure 2. Venn representation of hierarchical regression analysis with face recognition ability (IM Face) as the criterion variable showing shared and unique variance with predictor variables. The variables presented are "selective" (i.e., gender and major are omitted from the diagram), however their effects are controlled for in the betas reported. Selected predictor variables include object recognition (IM Bird) and ASD traits (AQ) with β values reported at the stage the variable was entered. The overlap between predictors is not represented to scale and is for illustrative purposes.

Table 4. Hierarchical regression on Autism Quotient scores as a function of university major, gender, face recognition, and bird recognition.

Variables	B	SE B	β	semi-r	p
Stage 1					
Intercept	65.27	3.35			
Gender	−3.61	2.35	−0.15	−0.14	0.06
Major	−4.75	2.28	−0.20	−0.19	0.02
Stage 2					
IM Face	−17.69	8.93	−0.17	−0.18	0.03
Stage 3					
IM Bird	−10.38	11.68	−0.08	−0.08	0.20
Stage 2					
IM Bird	−10.38	11.67	−0.08	−0.08	0.18
Stage 3					
IM Face	−16.11	9.11	−0.16	−0.16	0.04

The order of the final two variables in the model (IM Bird and IM Face) was altered in two separate analyses to show that even when IM Face was entered last, it emerged as a significant predictor.
* *p* values are one-tailed.

were also significant. Given the lack of relation with AQ scores, the Emotion Recognition and EFT measures were not included in subsequent analyses. The IM Bird task was retained in subsequent analyses as some studies have found superior object recognition abilities in individuals with ASD [2]. Moreover, the IM Bird and Face tasks are identical in their presentation of stimuli, which affords a comparison of the relationship between autistic traits, and face and object recognition abilities.

Predicting Face Recognition Performance - Multiple Regression

A hierarchical multiple regression was performed modelling IM Face scores as a function of gender, major, IM bird scores, and AQ scores. Gender and major were entered in the first block of the model, followed by IM bird scores in the second stage, and AQ scores in the final stage. AQ was placed in the final block to determine whether it uniquely predicted IM Face scores independent of the other variables.

Table 3 displays the unstandardized regression coefficients, intercepts, βs (standardized coefficient), SE B, semi-r and *p* values for each stage of the hierarchical regression model. The overall regression model including all 4 predictors simultaneously was significant, $F(4,119) = 2.88$, $p = .03$, $R^2 = .09$. In the final model with all variables entered, block 2 object recognition ($\beta = .18$, $p = .03$, one-tailed) and block 3 AQ ($\beta = -.16$, $p = .04$, one-tailed) significantly predicted face recognition scores. Notably, AQ emerged as significant, despite being entered in the final stage of the regression analysis. Figure 2 depicts the shared and unique variance between selected predictor variables and IM Face scores.

Predicting AQ scores – Multiple Regression

A separate hierarchical multiple regression was performed modelling AQ scores as a function of gender, major, IM bird scores, and IM Face scores. Whilst zero-order bidirectional associations were established in the initial correlation analysis, in the hierarchical analysis we sought to examine the partial associations between key predictors of interest and AQ scores. In order to assess the unique predictive power of face recognition (stage 2) over object (bird) recognition (stage 3), as well as the converse, we performed two regression analyses that switched the entry order of stages 2 and 3. Table 4 displays the unstandardized regression coefficients, intercepts, βs (standardized coefficient), SE B, semi-r and *p* values for each stage of the hierarchical regression model. As expected, when entered in stage 1, major significantly predicted individual differences in AQ scores, with a near significant association with gender. Entering IM Face in stage 2 significantly predicted AQ scores after accounting for the stage 1 measures. This remained true even when IM Face was entered last in stage 3, following gender, major, and IM bird. In contrast, a notable dissociation was observed for IM bird, which failed to uniquely predict AQ scores in stage 2 or 3 (i.e., before or after IM Face). The overall regression model including all 4 predictors simultaneously was significant $F(4,119) = 4.33$, $p = .003$, $R^2 = .13$. In this final model, block 1 university major ($\beta = -.22$, $p = .02$, one-tailed) and block 3 face recognition ($\beta = -.16$, $p = .04$, one-tailed) uniquely predicted self-reported autistic traits. Figure 3 depicts the relationships between selected predictor variables and AQ scores.

Comparing AQ scores across Majors

To compare AQ scores across university major, we grouped majors into Sciences ($n = 52$), and non-Science majors (i.e., Social Sciences and Humanities; $n = 72$), and found significant differences between the two groups. Science majors ($m = 59.13$, $SD = 11.12$) scored higher on the AQ than non-Science majors ($m = 52.76$, $SD = 11.18$), $t(2,122) = 3.14$, $p = .002$. This finding is consistent with other studies [11,13,34], where Science majors have reported more autistic traits than non-Science majors.

Discussion

In this study, we investigated how sub-clinical autistic traits and face recognition in the TD population are related to the demographic variables of gender and university major as well as to cognitive abilities involved in visual perception, object and emotion recognition. The pairwise correlations showed reliable associations between self-reported autistic traits with gender and university major. These results are consistent with previous

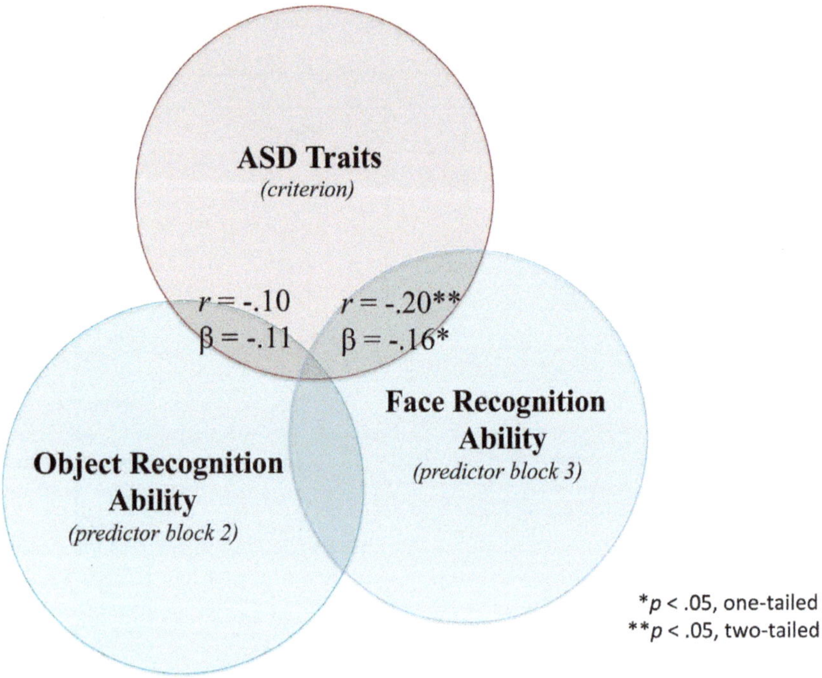

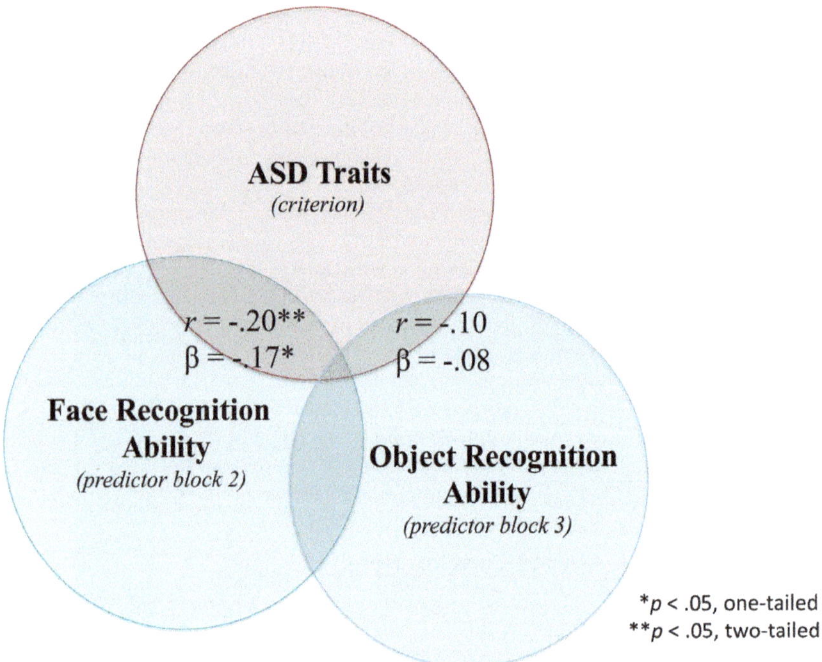

Figure 3. Venn representation of hierarchical regression analysis with Autism Quotient scores as the criterion variable showing shared and unique variance with predictor variables. The variables presented are "selective" (i.e., gender and major are omitted from the diagram), however their effects are controlled for in the betas reported. (*a*) Selected predictor variables include stage 2 face recognition (IM Face) and stage 3 object recognition (IM Bird) or (*b*) stage 2 object recognition (IM Bird) and stage 3 face recognition (IM Face); β values reported at the stage the variable was entered. The overlap between predictors is not represented to scale and is for illustrative purposes.

findings in which autism has been linked to gender [35–36], university major [11] and face processing skill [1–2]. Face recognition ability correlated with gender, object recognition, emotion recognition and AQ.

To better understand the unique contributions of the factors to face recognition and AQ, we performed two hierarchical regression analyses. In Model 1, we investigated whether gender, major, IM Bird recognition and AQ measures reliably predicted IM Face recognition performance. In Stage 1, gender and university major were simultaneously entered into the model (see Table 3). The analysis showed that gender reliably predicted face recognition abilities where women tended to perform better on the IM Face recognition measure than men, which is in keeping with previous findings [37–38]. In Stage 2 of the model, the IM Bird recognition measure reliably predicted IM Face recognition indicating that object recognition uniquely contributes to face recognition ability [39–40]. In Stage 3 of the model, the AQ measure reliably predicted scores on the IM Face measure. This result indicates that face recognition deficits predict autistic tendencies in a sub-clinical population similar to the face processing deficits observed in individuals who are formally diagnosed with autism [1–2].

In a second model, we investigated whether gender, major, IM Bird recognition and IM Face recognition measures reliably predicted AQ performance. In Stage 1, gender and university major were simultaneously entered as the first factors into the model (see Table 4). Consistent with previous results [11,13,34], the analysis revealed that major was significantly predictive of AQ score such that students who majored in the sciences (Engineering, Computer Sciences and Mathematics) tended to score higher on the AQ scale than non-Science students. In Stage 2, two versions of the model were tested in which either the object recognition measure (IM Bird) was entered in Stage 2 and the face recognition measure (IM Face) (Model 2A) in Stage 3 or the converse order in which face recognition measure was entered in Stage 2 and the object recognition measure in Stage 3 (Model 2B). In Model 2A, the analysis showed that the IM Face measure reliably predicted AQ scores, indicating that face recognition abilities uniquely contributed to autistic characteristics. The IM Bird measure did not capture any additional variance when it was entered as a predictor in Stage 3 of the model. When the order of entry was reversed in Model 2B, the IM Bird measure still failed to predict AQ scores in Stage 2 whereas the IM Face measure continued to be a reliable predictor of AQ when entered last in Stage 3. Although the shared variance between face and object recognition performance is reliable ($r = .22$, Table 2), only the face recognition measure uniquely predicted autistic characteristics as measured by the AQ scale.

Dawson et al. [41] note that there is a reciprocal relationship between impaired face perception and impaired social cognition in young individuals with ASD. They propose that neither faces nor social interactions elicit the same reward value that they do for typically developing children. The implications of this are twofold and not necessarily mutually exclusive. Firstly, a primary perceptual deficit such as impaired facial recognition can have broader implications for aspects of social cognition that rely on the face (e.g., engaging in joint attention, recognizing emotions). Conversely, facial recognition deficits may be a byproduct of a lack of social motivation (i.e., faces are not tagged with positive affect because the individual is not interested in social stimuli). Similarly, Schultz et al. [4] found that the level of fusiform gyrus activation correlated negatively with the social cognition subscale of Autism Diagnostic Observation Schedule. The developmental trajectories of face perception and social cognition appear to be intimately related, and they likely influence one another over time. Notably, gender appears to affect the direction of the relationship between face identity coding and social interactions, with males but not females showing a positive correlation [33].

Our findings show that a person's degree of autistic traits in the typically developing population can be predicted by their performance on an identity recognition measure, one with relatively few trials. This measure is sensitive to individual differences in face recognition, and provides an implicit insight to social cognition, which is a limiting factor for individuals with the autism condition. We propose that it is equally plausible for the relationship between impaired face perception and core ASD traits to work both ways. On one hand, our findings suggest that the autism condition can lead to a general disinterest or aversion to social stimuli, such as faces, and produce a decline in face recognition skill (see Figure 2). On the other hand, our results suggest that it is equally plausible that impaired face perception can exacerbate core ASD symptoms pertaining to the social and communicative aspects of the condition (see Figures 3a and 3b). The implications of these findings are important for developing intervention programs that focus on face training and creating reward systems that emphasize the importance of faces from an early age [42]. These findings provide a tractable treatment strategy for ameliorating the symptoms of autism through face training, which in turn, may improve the quality of social interactions for individuals with ASD. Effectively, intervention programs targeting the recognition of faces may not simply be targeting a symptom of ASD, but may instead be targeting a more fundamental deficit of the disorder.

Although we make no claims about the direction of causality, our results show that the relationship between impaired face perception and core ASD traits can work both ways, and suggest that the relationship is dynamic and mutually reinforcing. We note however, that additional research (e.g., using large-sample, longitudinal designs with lead-lag models to examine differences in the onset of deficits) will ultimately be required to address the circular nature of the relationship. We propose that a primary deficit in social interactions is possibly compounded by an impaired ability to recognize the human face, as it is a highly social stimulus from which we infer a great deal of information that contributes to our social functioning. Facial recognition deficits are not a causal factor to developing ASD; however, we suggest that they may exacerbate the autism condition.

Author Contributions

Conceived and designed the experiments: JT DH SS SM. Performed the experiments: JT DH SS SM. Analyzed the data: JT DH SS SM. Contributed reagents/materials/analysis tools: JT DH SS SM. Wrote the paper: JT DH SS SM.

References

1. Weigelt S, Koldewyn K, Kanwisher N (2012). Face identity recognition in autism spectrum disorders: A review of behavioral studies. Neurosci Biobehav Rev 36(3): 1060–84.
2. Wolf JM, Tanaka JW, Klaiman C, Cockburn J, Herlihy L, et al. (2008). Specific impairment of face-processing abilities in children with autism spectrum disorder using the Let's Face It! skills battery. Autism Res 1: 329–340.
3. Tanaka JW, Wolf JM, Klaiman C, Koenig K, Cockburn J, et al. (2012). The perception and identification of facial emotions in individuals with autism spectrum disorders using the Let's Face It! emotion skills battery. J Child Psychol Psychiatry 53(12): 1259–67.
4. Schultz RT, Gauthier I, Klin A, Fulbright R, Anderson A, et al. (2000). Abnormal ventral temporal cortical activity during face discrimination among individuals with autism and Asperger syndrome. Arch Gen Psychiatry 57: 331–340.
5. Dawson G, Carver L, Meltzoff AN, Panagiotides H, McPartland J, et al. (2002). Neural correlates of face and object recognition in young children with autism spectrum disorder, developmental delay, and typical development. Child Development 73(3): 700–717.
6. Joseph RM, Tanaka J (2002). Holistic and part-based face recognition in children with autism. J Child Psychol Psychiatry 43: 1–14.
7. Scherf KS, Behrmann M, Minshew N, Luna B (2008). Atypical development of face and greeble recognition in autism. J Child Psychol Psychiatry 49: 838–847.
8. American Psychiatric Association (2000). Diagnostic and Statistical Manual of Mental Disorders, 4th Edition, Text Revision (DSM-IVTR). Washington, DC: American Psychiatric Publishing.
9. Frith U (1991). Autism and Asperger's syndrome. Cambridge: Cambridge University Press.
10. Baron-Cohen S (1995). Mindblindness: An essay on autism and theory of mind. Boston: MIT Press/Bradford Books.

11. Baron-Cohen S, Wheelwright S, Skinner R, Martin J, Clubley E (2001). The autism-spectrum quotient: Evidence from Asperger syndrome/high-functioning autism, males and females, scientists and mathematicians. J Autism Dev Disord 31: 5–17.
12. Lainhard JE, Ozonoff S, Coon H, Kransy L, Dinh E, et al. (2002). Autism, regression, and the broader autism phenotype. Am J Med Genet 113: 231–237.
13. Austin EJ (2005) Personality correlates of the broader autism phenotype as assessed by the autism spectrum quotient (AQ). Pers Individ Dif 38: 451–460.
14. Osterling J, Dawson G (1994). Early recognition of children with autism: A study of first birthday home videotapes. J Autism Dev Disord 24: 247–257.
15. Mars AE, Mauk JE, Dowrick PW (1998). Symptoms of pervasive developmental disorders as observed in prediagnostic home videos of infants and toddlers. J Pediatr 132: 500–504.
16. Swettenham J, Baron-Cohen S, Charman T, Cox A, Baird G, et al. (1998). The frequency and distribution of spontaneous attention shifts between social and non social stimuli in autistic, typically developing, and nonautistic developmentally delayed infants. J Child Psychol Psychiatry 39: 747–753.
17. Serra M, Althaus M, de Sonneville LM, Stant AD, Jackson AE, et al. (2003). Face recognition in children with a pervasive developmental disorder not otherwise specified. J Autism Dev Disord 33: 303–317.
18. Schultz RT (2005). Developmental deficits in social perception in autism: The role of the amygdala and fusiform face area. Int J Dev Neurosci 23: 125–141.
19. Scherf KS, Luna B, Minshew N, Behrmann M (2010). Location, location, location: Alterations in the functional topography of face- but not object- or place-related cortex in adolescents with autism. Front Hum Neurosci 4: 1–16.
20. Hadjikhani N, Joseph RM, Snyder J, Chabris CF, Clark J, et al. (2004). Activation of the fusiform gyrus when individuals with autism spectrum disorder view faces. Neuroimage 22(3): 1141–1150.
21. Pierce K, Redcay E (2008). Fusiform function in children with an ASD is a matter of "who". Biol Psychiatry 64: 552–560.
22. Kleinhans NM, Richards T, Weaver K, Johnson LC, Greenson J, et al. (2010). Association between amygdala response to emotional faces and social anxiety in autism spectrum disorders. Neuropsychologia 48(12): 3665–70.
23. von dem Hagen EAH, Nummenmaa L, Yu R, Engell AD, Ewbank MP, et al. (2011). Autism spectrum traits in the typical population predict structure and function in the posterior superior temporal sulcus. Cereb Cortex 21: 493–500.
24. McPartland J, Dawson G, Webb SJ, Panagiotides H, Carver LJ (2004). Event-related brain potentials reveal anomalies in temporal processing of faces in autism spectrum disorder. J Child Psychol Psychiatry 45: 1235–1245.
25. Yardley L, McDermott L, Pisarski S, Duchaine B, Nakayama K (2008). Psychosocial consequences of developmental prosopagnosia: A problem of recognition. J Psychosocial Research 65: 445–451.
26. Duchaine B, Murray H, Turner M, White S, Garrido L (2009). Normal social cognition in developmental prosopagnosia. Cog Neuropsychol 26:7: 620–634.
27. Bate S, Parris B, Haslam C, Kay J (2010). Socio-emotional functioning and face recognition ability in the normal population. Pers Individ Dif 48: 239–242.
28. Li J, Tian M, Fang H, Xu M, Li H, et al. (2010). Extraversion predicts individual differences in face recognition. Commun Integr Biol 3: 295–298.
29. DeGutis J, Wilmer J, Mercado RJ, Cohan S (2013). Using regression to measure holistic face processing reveals a strong link with face recognition ability. Cognition 126: 87–100.
30. Lundqvist D, Flykt A, Öhman A (1998). The Karolinska Directed Emotional Faces-KDEF [CD-ROM]. Department of Clinical Neuroscience, Psychology section, Karolinska Institutet, Stockholm, Sweden.
31. Spreen O, Strauss E (1998). A compendium of neuropsychological tests: Administration, norms, and commentary. New York, New York: Oxford University Press.
32. Hoekstra RA, Bartels M, Cath DC, Boomsma DI (2008). Factor structure, reliability and criterion validity of the Autism-Spectrum Quotient (AQ): A study in Dutch population and patient groups. J Autism Dev Disord 38: 1555–1566.
33. Rhodes G, Jeffery L, Taylor L, Ewing L (2013). Autistic traits are linked to reduced adaptive coding of face identity and selective poorer face recognition in men but not women. Neuropsychologia 51: 2702–2708.
34. Baron-Cohen S, Bolton P, Wheelwright S, Scahill V, Short L, et al. (1998). Autism occurs more often in families of physicists, engineers, and mathematicians. Autism 2: 297–301.
35. Lord C, Schopler E, Revicki D (1982). Sex differences in autism. J Autism Dev Disord 12(4): 317–330. doi:10.1007/BF01538320
36. Werling DM, Geschwind DH (2013). Sex differences in autism spectrum disorders. Curr Opin Neurol 26(2): 146–53. doi:10.1097/WCO.0b013e32835ee548.
37. Herlitz A, Nilsson LG, Bäckman L (1997). Gender differences in episodic memory. Mem Cognit 25(6): 801–11.
38. Rehnman J, Herlitz A (2007). Women remember more faces than men do. Acta Psychologica 124(3): 344–55. doi:10.1016/j.actpsy.2006.04.004
39. Dennett HW, McKone E, Tavashmi R, Hall A, Pidcock M, et al. (2012). The Cambridge Car Memory Test: A task matched in format to the Cambridge Face Memory Test, with norms, reliability, sex differences, dissociations from face memory, and expertise effects. Behav Res Methods 44(2): 587–605. doi:10.3758/s13428-011-0160-2
40. McGugin RW, Richler JJ, Herzmann G, Speegle M, Gauthier I (2012). The Vanderbilt Expertise Test reveals domain-general and domain-specific sex effects in object recognition. Vision Res 69: 10–22. doi:10.1016/j.visres.2012.07.014
41. Dawson G, Webb SJ, Wijsman E, Schellenberg G, Estes A, et al. (2005). Neurocognitive and electrophysiological evidence of altered face processing in parents of children with autism: Implications for a model of abnormal developmental of social brain circuitry in autism. Dev Psychopathol 17: 679–697.
42. Tanaka JW, Wolf JM, Klaiman C, Koenig K, Cockburn J, et al. (2010). Using computerized games to teach face recognition skills to children with autism spectrum disorder: The Let's Face It! program. J Child Psychol Psychiatry 51: 944–95.

2

Brain Activity of Adolescents with High Functioning Autism in Response to Emotional Words and Facial Emoticons

Doug Hyun Han[1]*, Hee Jeong Yoo[2], Bung Nyun Kim[3], William McMahon[4], Perry F. Renshaw[5]

1 Department of Psychiatry, Chung Ang University Hospital, Seoul, South Korea, **2** Department of Psychiatry, Seoul National Bundang Hospital, Seoul, South Korea, **3** Department of Psychiatry, Seoul National Hospital, Seoul, South Korea, **4** Department of Psychiatry, University of Utah, Salt Lake City, Utah, United States of America, **5** The Brain Institute, University of Utah, Salt Lake City, Utah, United States of America

Abstract

Studies of social dysfunction in patients with autism spectrum disorder (ASD) have generally focused on the perception of emotional words and facial affect. Brain imaging studies have suggested that the fusiform gyrus is associated with both the comprehension of language and face recognition. We hypothesized that patients with ASD would have decreased ability to recognize affect via emotional words and facial emoticons, relative to healthy comparison subjects. In addition, we expected that this decreased ability would be associated with altered activity of the fusiform gyrus in patients with ASD. Ten male adolescents with ASDs and ten age and sex matched healthy comparison subjects were enrolled in this case-control study. The diagnosis of autism was further evaluated with the Autism Diagnostic Observation Schedule. Brain activity was assessed using functional magnetic resonance imaging (fMRI) in response to emotional words and facial emoticon presentation. Sixty emotional words (45 pleasant words +15 unpleasant words) were extracted from a report on Korean emotional terms and their underlying dimensions. Sixty emoticon faces (45 pleasant faces +15 unpleasant faces) were extracted and modified from on-line sites. Relative to healthy comparison subjects, patients with ASD have increased activation of fusiform gyrus in response to emotional aspects of words. In contrast, patients with ASD have decreased activation of fusiform gyrus in response to facial emoticons, relative to healthy comparison subjects. We suggest that patients with ASD are more familiar with word descriptions than facial expression as depictions of emotion.

Editor: Michelle Hampson, Yale University, United States of America

Funding: This work was supported by Korean Game Culture Foundation and a grant of the Korean Health Technology R&D Project, Ministry of Health & Welfare, Republic of Korea (A120013). The funders had no role in study design, data collection and analysis, decision to publish, or preparation of the manuscript.

Competing Interests: The authors have declared that no competing interests exist.

* E-mail: hduk@yahoo.com

Introduction

Language comprehension and facial affect recognition in patients with autism spectrum disorder

Autism is a developmental disorder characterized by deficits in three domains, including social reciprocity; early language and communication problems; and restrictive, repetitive and stereotyped behaviors [1]. Among these deficits, particular interest in social dysfunction has been focused on the perception of emotional words and facial affect in patients with autism spectrum disorder (ASD) [2–6]. Social dysfunction has also been associated with impairment of social perception and cognition, as demonstrated by observation of emotions, actions, body movements, hand gestures, and facial expressions [2]. In addition, social dysfunction has been related to early language and communication impairments in children with ASD [3,5]. In the domains of comprehension and use of pragmatic language, patients with ASD have been reported to demonstrate impairments in understanding non-literal meaning, such as emotion, humor, and metaphor [7,8].

Patients with ASD are also known to have impairments in their ability to recognize unfamiliar faces, compared to healthy subjects [9]. Moreover, defects in the perception of facial expression may be a core feature of social deficits in patients with ASD [4]. Patients with autism were impaired in their ability to recognize appropriate facial expressions in videotaped gestures, vocalizations and contexts [10]. Similarly, patients with Asperger's syndrome had difficulty in the comprehension and production of facial and language expressions of emotion [6].

Facial Emoticons: simplified facial emotion expression

The emoticon in computer-mediated communication may be used for the purpose of facilitating non-verbal emotional communication and for reinforcing the verbal parts of a message [11]. Although facial emoticons differ from facial expression, simplified text or cartoon facial expressions (emoticons) are frequently used in the context of social communication [11,12]. Lo [12] reported that emoticons, as "quasi-nonverbal cues", help most people perceive appropriate emotion, attitude, and intention during internet use. Based on these observations, there have also been several empirical results showing that the emoticon is associated with high levels of emotional abstraction [13] and non-verbal information recognition [14,15]. Interestingly, patients with ASD, relative to healthy comparison subjects, do not apply different strategies for perceiving cartoon faces, while they use different strategies during perception of real human faces [16,17]. While healthy comparison subjects used a configural strategy in assessing both real and cartoon faces, patients with ASD used a figural strategy in viewing cartoon faces and a local strategy in evaluating real faces [16]. In an assessment of attentional bias using saccade-related, event-related potentials (ERPs), patients with ASD showed a smaller interval in attentional time between faces and objects, relative to healthy comparison subjects [18]. Moreover, patients with ASD can fixate on cartoon characters longer than on real objects [17]. In an fMRI study of emoticon perception, the right inferior frontal gyrus of healthy volunteers, which has been associated with non-verbal communication, was activated in response to viewing facial emoticons [14].

Fusiform gyrus, language comprehension, and face recognition

Over the last decade, several neuroimaging studies have reported activation in focal brain areas in response to semantic comprehension of language and human facial affect recognition in healthy subjects. Bookheimer [19] reported that inferior frontal and temporal cortex play a crucial role in the comprehension of language in healthy subjects. Ghosh et al. [20] noted that contextual integration in lexical processing was associated with activation of the left fusiform gyrus. In a review of studies of the role of the fusiform gyrus in face recognition, Kanwisher and Yovel [21] suggested that the fusiform gyrus is specific for face recognition in terms of detecting and extracting the necessary perceptual information to recognize the face. Similarly, the fusiform gyrus is well known to be dysfunctional in prosopagnosia patients [22]. In a review of fMRI articles, Sabatinelli et al. [23] suggested that the early developmental failure of the ventral temporal area (amygdala-fusiform system) was associated with deficits in social perception and social cognition. However, in fMRI studies, there have been reports that the fusiform gyrus was not activated in response to viewing facial expressions of emotion in patients with ASD [24,25]. Also, while a healthy control group showed activation of right fusiform gyrus in response to a discrimination of facial expression task, patients with autism did not show activation [26].

Hypothesis

We hypothesized that patients with ASD would have decreased ability to recognize affect via emotional words and facial emoticons, relative to healthy comparison subjects. In addition, we expected that this decreased ability would be represented by altered activity of the fusiform gyrus in patients with ASD.

Method

Subjects

In response advertisements posted in Chung Ang University Hospital and other local hospitals, fifteen adolescents with autism spectrum disorders were screened. Inclusion criteria included: adolescents between the ages of 13 years to 18 years; diagnosed as having autism spectrum disorder; IQ≥70, ADOS score = 4–7 [27]. Exclusion criteria included: Comorbid Axis I Disorders, as determined by Korean Kiddie Schedule for Affective Disorders and Schizophrenia-Present and Life time version (K-SADS-PL) [28]; history of head trauma with loss of consciousness, seizure disorder, multiple sclerosis, brain tumor, claustrophobia, metal implantation or cerebrovascular accident; serious or chronic medical illness; IQ<70; and a history of substance abuse. Of these fifteen adolescents, three adolescents had IQ<70 and two adolescents were excluded due to co-morbid major depressive disorder and/or attention deficit hyperactivity disorder. Finally, 10 adolescents with ASD and 10 age and sex matched healthy comparison subjects have been recruited. The research protocol was approved by the Chung Ang University Hospital Institutional Review Board. Written informed assent was provided by adolescents and written informed consent was provided by parents.

Assessment

The diagnosis of autism was further evaluated with the ADOS [29] by social worker B.G.Y. who has both clinician and research certificates for ADOS and Autism Diagnostic Interview (ADI) based on training by supervisor Catherine Lord. The clinical symptoms were assessed by the child's mother using the Childhood Autism Rating Scale (CARS) parent version. IQ scores were obtained for all participants using the Korean Wechsler Adult Intelligence Scale (K-WAIS) [30]. Social communication was evaluated by the mother using the Social Communication Questionnaire (SCQ)-current form [31]. The inter-item consistency of SCQ Korean version has been reported to range from 0.84 to 0.93 [32].

Brain activity in both ASD patients and healthy subjects was assessed, in two separate scan sequences, in response to (1) emotional words and (2) scenes depicting emoticons in the scanner. All MR imaging was performed using 3 T blood oxygen level dependent (BOLD) functional magnetic resonance imaging (fMRI, Achieva 3.0, Philips, Eindhoven, the Netherlands). The stimulation was presented through an IFIS-SA^{TM} system (MRI Device Corporation, Waukesha, WI, USA) during a single fMRI scanning session. For the fMRI session, 180 echo planar images (EPI, 33 transverse slices, 4.0 mm thickness, voxel size of 1.8×1.8×4.0 mm, TE = 30 msec, TR = 3000 ms, Flip angle = 90°, in-plane resolution = 128×128 pixels, field of view (FOV) = 230×230 mm) were recorded at 3-second intervals. For anatomical imaging, 3D T1-weighted magnetization-prepared rapid gradient echo (MPRAGE) data were gathered with these parameters: TR = 2000 ms, TE = 4.00 ms, FOV = 256×256 mm, 340 slices, 0.9×0.9×1.0 mm voxel size, flip angle = 30°.

Tasks

Stimulation 1: Emotional words. Sixty emotional words (45 pleasant words +15 unpleasant words) were extracted from a report on Korean emotional terms and their underlying dimensions [33]. In ratings by forty young college students with a seven point analogue scale, the prototypicality and familiarity of these sixty words were 4.01–5.77 and 4.16–5.82, respectively [33]. Pleasant score of pleasant words was over 3.0 and the unpleasant score of unpleasant words was over 3.0. Both the pleasant score and unpleasant score in response to non-emotional words were less than 1.0 [33]. While in the scanner, each subject in patient group and healthy control group was asked to identify via microphone the one unpleasant emotional word presented among three pleasant words. Test-retest reliability for identification of emotional words was 0.82. The percentage of correct answers for emotional words in seventy healthy subjects was 81.2±10.3% (minimum = 56.6%, maximum = 96.7%). A video was constructed that was 450-seconds long and consisted of five continuous 90-second segments. Each 90-second segment consisted of three 30-second sub-segments. A white cross on a black background (B), a single non-emotional word (Match, M), and an emotional word stimulation (Stimulation, S) were included in these 90-second segments. The five segments were ordered as follows: B-M-S, B-S-M, M-B-S, S-B-M, and M-S-B. During the M sub-segment, three non-emotional words were presented every ten seconds. During

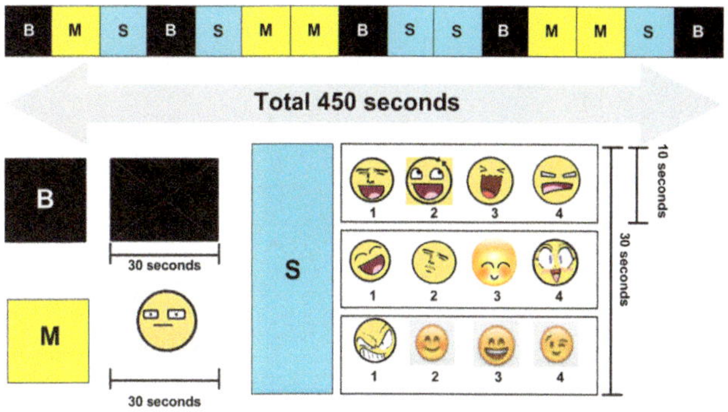

Figure 1. Facial emoticons.

the S sub-segment, three sets of four mixed emotional words were presented every ten seconds (Figure 1).

Stimulation2: Emoticon faces. Sixty emoticon faces (45 pleasant faces +15 unpleasant faces) were extracted and modified from on-line sites (http://image.search.naver.com/search.naver, http://forums.themavesite.com/index.php?topic = 6103.0)(Figure S3 in File S1). While in the scanner, each subject in patient group and healthy control group was asked to identify via microphone the number of unpleasant face emoticon among three other pleasant faced emotions. Test-retest reliability for facial emoticon identification is 0.84. The percentage of correct answers for facial emoticon identification in seventy healthy subjects was 86.6±9.2% (minimum = 66.7%, maximum = 100%). The sixty emotional words consisted of forty-five pleasant emotional words and fifteen unpleasant emotional words. The video used was 450-seconds long and consisted of five continuous 90-second segments. Each 90-second segment consisted of three 30-second sub-segments. A white cross on a black background (B), a single neutral face (Match, M), and an emoticon stimulation (Stimulation, S) were included in these 90-second segments. The five segments were ordered as follows: B-M-S, B-S-M, M-B-S, S-B-M, and M-S-B. During the M sub-segment, three neutral faces were presented every ten seconds. During the S sub-segment, three sets of four mixed emoticon faces were presented every ten seconds (Figure 1).

fMRI data analysis

Acquired fMRI data was analyzed by the Brain Voyager software package (BVQX 1.9, Brain Innovation, Maastricht, The Netherlands). In a multi-scale algorithm, each fMRI time series was registered to the MPRAGE 3D data set. The anatomic images were spatially normalized to standard Talairach space [34]. The time series data was also spatially normalized. Scan time correction and motion correction were applied during processing. Spatial smoothing using 6 mm FWHM Gaussian kernel and temporal smoothing using a 4 second Gaussian kernel were also applied. Head motion algorithms represent head movements by 6 parameters, three translation (displacement) parameters and three rotation parameters. Six parameters are estimated iteratively by analyzing how a source volume should be translated and rotated in order to better align with the reference volume. Head motion of less than 3.5 mm (translation) or 3.5° (rotation) relative to the target volume was considered to be acceptable. None of the ASD and healthy subjects was excluded due to excessive head movement in the present study. There was no difference in head motion between ASD patients and healthy comparison subjects (Table S1 and Figure S1 in File S1).

Statistical analysis

Differences in demographic data including age, IQ, CARS scores, SCQ scores, and percentage of correct answers in identifying emotional words/emoticons between ASD and healthy subjects were compared using the Mann-Whitney U test and ANCOVA test controlling for IQ. For the analysis of fMRI signal time-courses, the general linear model (GLM) and random effects analysis (RFX) were applied to construct individual and group statistical parametric maps of brain activation. Activations were computed by contrasting the S sub-segments (emotional words/emoticons) to their corresponding M sub-segments (neutral words/neutral emoticons). With that parametric maps, ANCOVA tests controlling for IQ were applied to identify clusters at a level of FDR<0.05, voxels >40. The Talairach code of clusters was identified by nearest coordinate in Talairach daemon [34].

As a second-level analysis in subjects with ASD, the correlations between mean β value in clusters and the mean SCQ scores were analyzed using partial correlations controlling for IQ, ADOS-communication score, and ADOS-social score. In order to account for multiple comparisons, we set significant p values = 0.0166 (0.05/3, CARS, SCQ, and correct response rates).

Results

Demographic characteristics

There were significant differences between ASD subjects and healthy comparison subjects in the IQ (U = 3.5, z = 3.5, p<0.01), CARS score (F = 15.5, df = 1, p<0.01), SCQ score (F = 53.4, df = 1, p<0.01), and the percentage of correct answers in identifying emotional words (F = 32.7, df = 1, p<0.01) and emoticon faces (F = 10.1, df = 1, p<0.01)(Table 1)(Figure S2 in File S1). The mean IQ values of the healthy subjects and the ASD subjects were 105.5±8.9 and 81.5±9.0, respectively. The correct response rates for emotional words in healthy subjects and ASD subjects were 86.4±8.4 and 40.3±11.6%, respectively. The correct response rates for facial emoticons in the healthy subjects and ASD subjects were 90.3±9.1 and 53.0±14.6%, respectively.

Correct responses to emoticon were positively correlated with the correct response to emotional words (r = 0.91, p<0.01). There were no significant correlations between IQ and correct response of emotional words or emoticon. Controlling for IQ, the mean SCQ score were negatively correlated with the correct response to emotional words (r = −0.77, p = 0.01) in ASD patients. Controlling for IQ, SCQ score was negatively correlated with the correct responses to emoticons at a trend level (r = −0.73, p = 0.02).

Clusters in the interaction between emotional words and subject factors at baseline

In an F test, interaction between group (ASD vs. Healthy subjects) and stimuli (Emotional words vs. Neutral words), two clusters of activity in patients with ASD were increased, compared to healthy subjects (FDR<0.05, p<0.00038); Cluster1 (CL1): Talairach x, y, z; 55, −39, −9, voxels = 242, right temporal lobe, fusiform gyrus, Brodmann area 20; Cluster2 (CL2): 32, −80, −17, voxels = 70, Right Occipital fusiform Gyrus, Brodmann area 19 (Figure 2)(Figure 3)(Table2). In an F test, interaction between group (ASD vs. Healthy subjects) and stimuli (Emotional words vs. Neutral words), there were no significant clusters of activity in patients with ASD that were decreased, compared to healthy subjects (FDR<0.05, p<0.00038).

Table 1. Demographic Characteristics.

Subjects	Age (Mo)	Sex	ADOS			CARS	SCQ	IQ		
			A	B	Diagnosis			FSIQ	VIQ	PIQ
Patients with ASD										
ASD 1	204	F	3	4	ASD	21	22	88	92	74
ASD 2	198	M	2	9	ASD	26.5	29	77	82	83
ASD 3	202	M	3	9	Autism	23	26	71	75	74
ASD 4	215	F	5	13	Autism	37.5	14	80	77	82
ASD 5	205	M	4	12	Autism	29	16	71	76	62
ASD 6	158	M	4	11	Autism	30.5	18	79	73	84
ASD 7	160	M	5	6	Autism	34.5	22	85	90	75
ASD 8	209	M	3	6	ASD	21	23	75	73	74
ASD 9	212	M	4	9	Autism	26.5	25	93	96	89
ASD 10	161	M	4	4	ASD	21.5	22	78	72	81
mean±SD[a]	192.4±23.1	8M/2F				27.1±5.8	21.7±4.6	81.5±8.9	80.6±8.9	77.8±7.6
Healthy Control Subjects										
HC1	191	M	-	-	Healthy	16	3	100	103	95
HC2	202	M	-	-	Healthy	15	2	110	110	107
HC3	216	M	-	-	Healthy	16.5	4	117	115	116
HC4	156	F	-	-	Healthy	15.5	3	116	125	99
HC5	155	M	-	-	Healthy	15	2	109	114	100
HC6	118	M	-	-	Healthy	15	1	109	108	109
HC7	158	M	-	-	Healthy	17	2	94	97	92
HC8	214	M	-	-	Healthy	15	1	94	90	102
HC9	178	M	-	-	Healthy	15.5	2	93	97	89
HC10	190	F	-	-	Healthy	15	3	120	119	116
mean±SD[b]	178.8±32.5	8M/2F				15.5±0.7	2.3±0.9	106.2±10.2	107.8±8.9	102.5±9.4
Statistics	U = 33.0, z = 1.3, p = 0.19					F = 15.5, df = 1, p<0.01	F = 53.4, df = 1, p<0.01	U = 3.50, z = 3.51, p<0.01	U = 2.50, z = 3.59, p<0.01	U = 03.50, z = 3.74, p<0.01
a vs b										

Mann-Whitney U test, SCQ: Social Communication Questionnaire, FSIQ: IQ total, VIQ: verbal IQ, PIQ: performance IQ, A: ADOS-A (Autism Diagnostic Observation Schedule-A): communication score, B: ADOS-B: social score, the threshold scores for a diagnosis of autism on the ADOS are 3 and 6 for communication and social symptoms, respectively. Threshold scores for a less severe diagnosis of ASD on the ADOS are 2 and 4 for communication and social symptoms, respectively. Mo: months, CARS: Child Autism Rating Scale, ASD: autism spectrum disorders, HC: healthy comparison subjects.

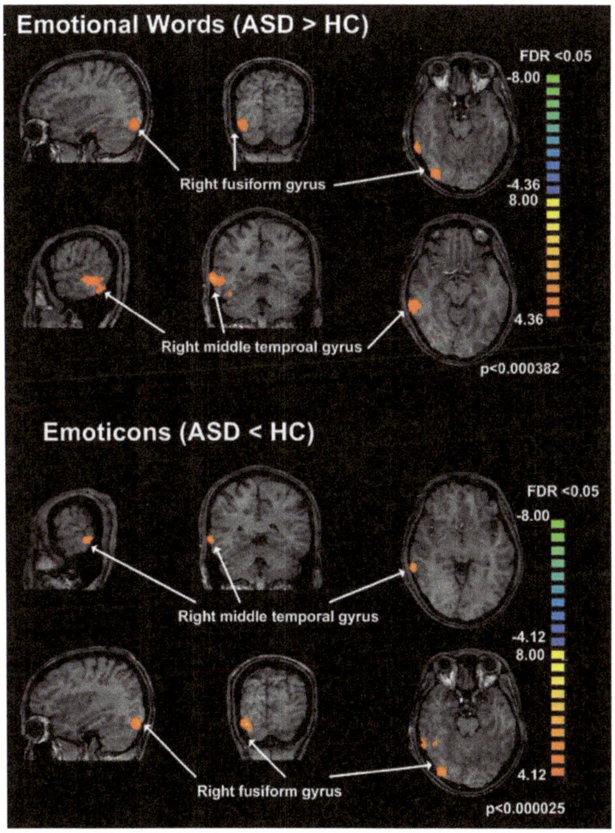

Figure 2. Brain activity in response to emotional words / facial emoticons. Brain activity in response to emotional words (ASD > healthy subjects), Cluster1 (CL1): right temporal lobe, fusiform gyrus, Brodmann area 20; Cluster2 (CL2): Right Cerebrum,Occipital Lobe,Fusiform Gyrus, Right Cerebrum, Occipital Lobe, Inferior Occipital Gyrus, Right Cerebellum, Posterior Lobe. Brain activity in response to emoticons (ASD < healthy subjects), Cluster3 (CL3): Right Cerebrum,-Temporal Lobe, Middle Temporal Gyrus, Cluster4 (CL4): Right Cerebellum, Posterior Lobe, Right Cerebrum,Occipital Lobe, Fusiform Gyrus.

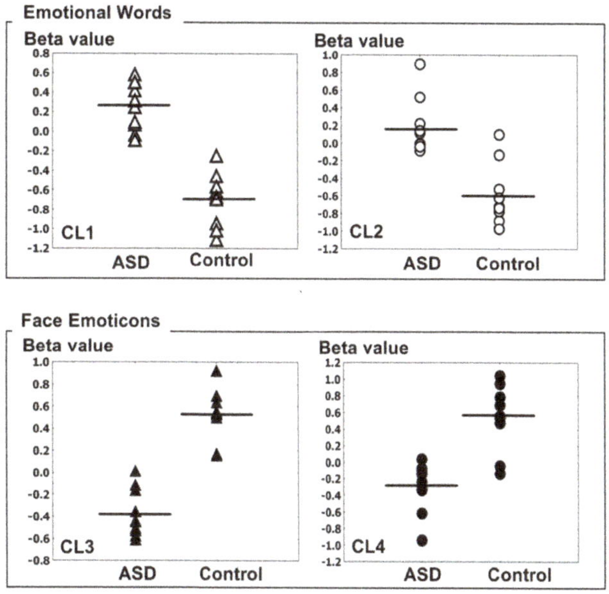

Figure 3. The beta values of brain activity in response to emotional words / facial emoticons. Cluster1 (CL1, unfilled triangle): right temporal lobe, fusiform gyrus, Brodmann area 20; Cluster2 (CL2, unfilled circle): Right Cerebrum,Occipital Lobe,Fusiform Gyrus, Right Cerebrum, Occipital Lobe, Inferior Occipital Gyrus, Right Cerebellum, Posterior Lobe, Cluster3 (CL3, filled triangle): Right Cerebrum,Temporal Lobe, Middle Temporal Gyrus, Cluster4 (CL4, filled circle): Right Cerebellum, Posterior Lobe, Right Cerebrum,Occipital Lobe, Fusiform Gyrus.

Clusters in the interaction between facial emoticons and subject factors at baseline

In an F test, interaction between group (ASD vs. Healthy subjects) and stimulus (Emoticons vs. Neutral faces), two clusters of activity in patients with ASD were decreased (FDR<0.05, p<0.000025); Cluster3 (CL3): Talairach x, y, z; 61, −39, −4, Right Cerebrum, Temporal Lobe, Middle Temporal Gyrus, Brodmann area 21, Cluster4 (CL4): Talairach x, y, z; 31, −82, −20, Right Cerebellum, Posterior Lobe, Right Occipital fusiform Gyrus, Brodmann area 18 (Figure 2)(Figure 3)(Table2). In an F test, interaction between group (ASD vs. Healthy subjects) and stimulus (Emoticon vs Neutral faces), there were no significant clusters of activity in patients with ASD that were increased, compared to healthy subjects (FDR<0.05, p<0.000025).

Correlations between Social Communication Questionnaire (SCQ) and brain activity

The mean SCQ score in ASD patients was negatively correlated with the mean beta value of right temporal fusiform gyrus in response to emotional words ($r = -0.82$, $p = 0.02$)(Figure 4). There were no significant correlations between SCQ scores, CARS scores, correct responses on emotional words/emoticon tests and the beta value of other clusters in response to emotional words. Similarly there were no significant correlations between SCQ scores, CARS scores, correct responses on emotional words/emoticon tests, and the beta value of other clusters in response to facial emoticons. There was no significant correlation between CARS score and other clusters.

Discussion

As expected, patients with ASD showed lower correct response rates for recognizing affect via emotional words and facial emoticons. However, there were divergent patterns of brain activation for emotional words and facial emoticons. The fusiform gyrus in the patients with ASD activated to a greater extent during emotional word tasks, relative to the healthy comparison subjects. Conversely, the activity of fusiform gyrus of patients with ASD was lower in response to facial emoticons, compared to healthy subjects.

Difficulty in recognizing emotional and non-verbal meanings in words and facial affect in patients with ASD has been reported in several studies [2–6]. Moreover, the decreased recognition of emotion and non-verbal meanings has been associated with increased activity of fusiform gyrus in patients with ASD [20,24,25]. In solving verbal and visual problems, the dissociation between verbal and visuo-spatial abilities in terms of reduced activation of fronto-temporal language areas and increased activation of occipito-parietal and ventral temporal circuits has been noted in patients with ASD [35,36]. In solving verbal problems, patients with ASD may use the right hemisphere as compensation for a dysfunctional left hemisphere [37–39]. In a study of speaker-incongruent sentences vs. speaker-congruent sentences, patients with ASD showed increased activation in right inferior frontal gyrus, compared to healthy controls [38]. During

Table 2. Clusters in the interaction between emotional words, emoticons and subject factors at baseline.

Talairach Code			voxels	t	p	regions
x	y	z				
Clusters in the interaction between emotional words and subject factors (ASD>healthy subjects)						
32	−80	−17	70	4.36	FDR <0.05, P<0.000382	Right Fusiform Gyrus, BA 19
55	−39	−9	242	4.36	FDR <0.05, P<0.000382	Right Middle Temporal Gyrus, BA 20
Clusters in the interaction between facial emoticons and subject factors (ASD<healthy subjects)						
61	−39	−4	40	5.62	FDR <0.05, P<0.000025	Right Middle Temporal Gyrus, BA 21
31	−82	−20	65	4.12	FDR <0.05, P<0.000643	Right fusiform Gyrus, BA 18

ASD: patients with autism spectrum disorder, FDR: false discovery rate, BA: Brodmann Area.

pragmatic language comprehension, increased activation in the right inferior frontal gyrus in patients with ASD has also been observed [37,39]. Taken together, we hypothesize that the fusiform gyrus in the patients with ASD may require greater activation in order to interpret to the meaning of emotional words, compared to healthy subjects. The increased activation within fusiform gyrus in response to emotional words in patients with ASD may be associated with a compensatory mechanism to control social information processing. Dichter et al. [40] have reported that patients with ASD showed greater activation within the anterior cingulate in response to the stimuli of social target detection, compared to healthy subjects. In addition, mean SCQ scores (higher SCQ scores are associated with greater deficits in social communication) were negatively correlated with brain activity within the fusiform gyrus in response to emotional words. However, mean SCQ scores had no correlation with brain activity within any other cluster in response to facial emotion. The observations suggest that patients with ASD may be more familiar with verbal expression than facial expression during emotional communication. Taken together, we hypothesize that the fusiform gyrus in the patients with ASD may require greater activation in order to interpret to the meaning of emotional words, compared to healthy subjects. In other words, that pattern was though as cortical inefficiency during social information processing [41].

As an explanation for the social deficits in patients with ASD, the disability in facial emoticon recognition is thought to be associated with emotional salience [9,26] or lack of social insight [42]. Simplified carton facial expressions (emoticons) are frequently used in the context of social communication, because emoticons can be used as a surrogate for nonverbal emotional expression [11,12]. In a study of the role of emoticons in computer-mediated communication, Derks et al. [11] suggested that emoticons are commonly used in a manner similar to facial behavior in face to face communication with respect to social context and interpersonal interaction. In the case of real facial experiments, Schultz et al. [26] reported that patients with ASD were hard put to differentiate even neutral face recognition. Among various social brain areas, the lateral fusiform gyrus or fusiform face area has been thought to be important for the rapid recognition of faces [43]. In face discrimination tasks, patients with ASD showed less activation of the fusiform gyrus, compared to healthy subjects [26]. Patients with ASD are thought to recognize faces in a different manner compared to healthy subjects. They focus more on feature-based than configural analyses [44] and the fusiform gyrus is known to be associated with configural processing [43]. The decreased activation within fusiform gyrus in response to emoticons in patients with ASD may be due to the use of different cognitive strategies to solve problems, relative to healthy subjects. Those differences may be caused by differences in programmed cell death, lack of functional specialization or deviant myelination during synaptogenesis and brain development [45,46]. Patients with ASD have difficulty with face discrimination, due not to the emotional valence, but to different patterns of facial recognition, compared to healthy subjects. We expect that ASD patients would

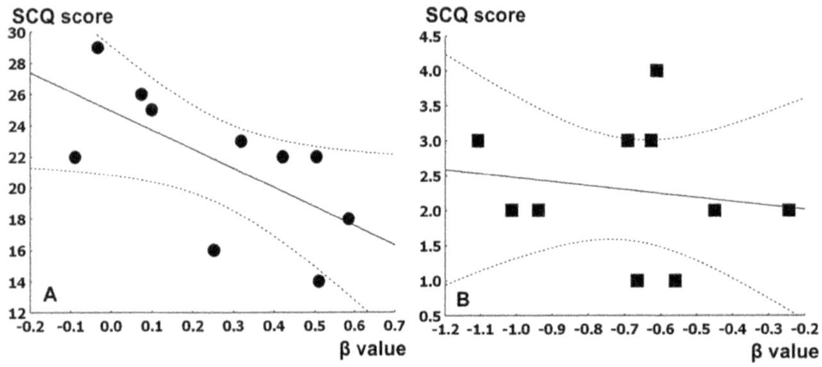

Figure 4. Correlation between mean SCQ score and the mean beta value within right temporal fusiform gyrus. A: The correlation between mean SCQ score in ASD patients and the mean beta value within right temporal fusiform gyrus in response to emotional words, with a partial correlation controlling for IQ, $r = -0.82$, $p = 0.015$. B: The correlation between mean SCQ score in healthy control subjects and the mean beta value within right temporal fusiform gyrus in response to emotional words, with a partial correlation controlling for IQ, $r = -0.16$, $p = 0.67$.

show a similar neural response following the presentation of one pleasant emoticon out of three unpleasant ones, compared to current paradigm (one unpleasant one out of three pleasant ones).

In response to the emoticon task, right middle temporal gyrus was less activated in ASD patients, compared to healthy subjects. This brain region has been implicated in the pathophysiology of ASD in several prior studies. Freitag et al. [47] have suggested that the interpretation of complex motion may be associated with gray matter volumes within the right medial temporal cortex. Alaerts et al. [48] reported that hypoactivity of posterior superior temporal sulcus might be linked with the social deficits characteristic of ASD patients. Herrington et al [49] reported that the detection of a point-light walking figure was associated with the activity within inferior frontal gyrus, fusiform gyrus, and amygdala. In an fMRI study with stimulation in response to a biological motion task, Koldewyn et al. [50] reported that ASD patients showed reduced posterior superior temporal sulcus, parietal, and frontal activity, relative to healthy comparison subjects. Taken together, these results may be associated with decreased bodily motion or gesture perception. ASD patients are thought to have decreased visual sensitivity to human movements and gesture comprehension [51].

There are several limitations in the current study. First, the number of participants was too small to allow generalization of the results. Second, spoken responses during scanning may have increased subject motion and altered apparent brain activity [52]. To address this issue, we monitored and corrected for possible motion artifacts. In addition, patients with ASD and healthy control subjects were asked to respond equally in the task (emotional word/emoticon) stimulation. However, the two subject groups performed this emoticon labeling the task with different degrees of accuracy, which is a limitation in terms of comparing the extent of BOLD activation across groups. Finally, we did not measure response times in this experiment.

Conclusions

The brain response to emotional words in patients with ASD, although requiring a greater degree of fusiform gyrus activation relative to healthy comparisons subjects, is similar to healthy comparison in the manner of activation. In contrast, the fusiform gyrus response to emoticon faces is different from healthy comparison subjects. Patients with ASD have great activation of the fusiform gyrus in response to emotional aspects of words, when compared to healthy subjects. However, relative to healthy comparison subjects, patients with ASD have lower activation of fusiform gyrus in response to emotional meaning in facial emoticons.

Supporting Information

File S1 This file contains Table S1 and Figure S1-Figure S3. Table S1,Translation and Rotation during scans. Figure S1, Head motion correction. Figure S2, Comparison of behavioral scores between ASD patients and healthy comparison subjects. Figure S3, Face emoticons.

Author Contributions

Conceived and designed the experiments: DHH HJY. Performed the experiments: DHH BNK . Analyzed the data: WM PFR. Contributed reagents/materials/analysis tools: WM PFR. Wrote the paper: DHH PFR.

References

1. American Psychiatric Association (1994) Diagnostic and statistical manual of mental disorders, fourth ed. (DSM-IV).Washington, DC: American Psychiatric Association.
2. Allison T, Puce A, McCarthy G (2000) Social perception from visual cues: role of the STS region. Trends Cogn Sci 4: 267–278.
3. Charman T (2003) Why is joint attention a pivotal skill in autism? Philos Trans R Soc Lond B Biol Sci 358: 315–324.
4. Hauck M, Fein D, Maltby N, Waterhouse L, Feinstein C (1998) Memory for faces in children with autism. Child Neuropsychol 4: 187–198.
5. Mundy P, Sigman M, Kasari C (1990) A longitudinal study of joint attention and language development in autistic children. J Autism Dev Disord 20: 115–128.
6. Scott DW (1985) Asperger's syndrome and non-verbal communication: a pilot study. Psychol Med 15: 683–687.
7. Happe FG (1993) Communicative competence and theory of mind in autism: a test of relevance theory. Cognition 48: 101–119.
8. Tager-Flusberg H, Joseph RM (2003) Identifying neurocognitive phenotypes in autism. Philos Trans R Soc Lond B Biol Sci 358: 303–314.
9. Grelotti DJ, Gauthier I, Schultz RT (2002) Social interest and the development of cortical face specialization: what autism teaches us about face processing. Dev Psychobiol 40: 213–225.
10. Hobson RP (1986) The autistic child's appraisal of expressions of emotion. J Child Psychol Psychiatry 27: 321–342.
11. Derks D, Bos AE, von Grumbkow J (2008) Emoticons in computer-mediated communication: social motives and social context. Cyberpsychol Behav 11: 99–101.
12. Lo SK (2008) The nonverbal communication functions of emoticons in computer-mediated communication. Cyberpsychol Behav 11: 595–597.
13. Yuasa M, Saito K, Mukawa N (2006) Emoticons convey emotions without cognition of faces: an fMRI study; Montreal, Canada.
14. Yuasa M, Keiichi S, Naoki M (2007) Brain Activity Associated with Emoticons: An fMRI Study. IEEJ Transactions on Electronics, Information and Systems 127: 1865–1870.
15. Yuasa M, Keiichi S, Naoki M (2011) Brain Activity When Reading Sentences and Emoticons: An fMRI Study of Verbal and Nonverbal Communication. Electronics and Communications in Japan, 94: 17–24.
16. Rosset DB, Rondan C, Da Fonseca D, Santos A, Assouline B, et al. (2008) Typical emotion processing for cartoon but not for real faces in children with autistic spectrum disorders. J Autism Dev Disord 38: 919–925.
17. van der Geest JN, Kemner C, Camfferman G, Verbaten MN, van Engeland H (2002) Looking at images with human figures: comparison between autistic and normal children. J Autism Dev Disord 32: 69–75.
18. Kikuchi Y, Senju A, Akechi H, Tojo Y, Osanai H, et al. (2011) Atypical disengagement from faces and its modulation by the control of eye fixation in children with autism spectrum disorder. J Autism Dev Disord 41: 629–645.
19. Bookheimer S (2002) Functional MRI of language: new approaches to understanding the cortical organization of semantic processing. Annu Rev Neurosci 25: 151–188.
20. Ghosh S, Basu A, Kumaran SS, Khushu S (2010) Functional mapping of language networks in the normal brain using a word-association task. Indian J Radiol Imaging 20: 182–187.
21. Kanwisher N, Yovel G (2006) The fusiform face area: a cortical region specialized for the perception of faces. Philos Trans R Soc Lond B Biol Sci 361: 2109–2128.
22. Barton JJ, Press DZ, Keenan JP, O'Connor M (2002) Lesions of the fusiform face area impair perception of facial configuration in prosopagnosia. Neurology 58: 71–78.
23. Sabatinelli D, Fortune EE, Li Q, Siddiqui A, Krafft C, et al. (2011) Emotional perception: meta-analyses of face and natural scene processing. Neuroimage 54: 2524–2533.
24. Critchley HD, Daly EM, Bullmore ET, Williams SC, Van Amelsvoort T, et al. (2000) The functional neuroanatomy of social behaviour: changes in cerebral blood flow when people with autistic disorder process facial expressions. Brain 123 (Pt 11): 2203–2212.
25. Pierce K, Muller RA, Ambrose J, Allen G, Courchesne E (2001) Face processing occurs outside the fusiform 'face area' in autism: evidence from functional MRI. Brain 124: 2059–2073.
26. Schultz RT, Gauthier I, Klin A, Fulbright RK, Anderson AW, et al. (2000) Abnormal ventral temporal cortical activity during face discrimination among individuals with autism and Asperger syndrome. Arch Gen Psychiatry 57: 331–340.
27. Suzuki K, Matsuzaki H, Iwata K, Kameno Y, Shimmura C, et al. (2011) Plasma cytokine profiles in subjects with high-functioning autism spectrum disorders. PLoS One 6: e20470.
28. Kim YS, Cheon KA, Kim BN, Chang SA, Yoo HJ, et al. (2004) The reliability and validity of Kiddie-Schedule for Affective Disorders and Schizophrenia-Present and Lifetime Version- Korean version (K-SADS-PL-K). Yonsei Med J 45: 81–89.

29. Lord C, Risi S, Lambrecht L, Cook EH Jr., Leventhal BL, et al. (2000) The autism diagnostic observation schedule-generic: a standard measure of social and communication deficits associated with the spectrum of autism. J Autism Dev Disord 30: 205–223.
30. Yeom TH, Park YS, Oh KJ, Lee YH (1992) Korean version Wechsler adult intelligence scale. Seoul: Korean Guidance.
31. Berument SK, Rutter M, Lord C, Pickles A, Bailey A (1999) Autism screening questionnaire: diagnostic validity. Br J Psychiatry 175: 444–451.
32. Yoo HJ (2008) The Social CommunicationQuestionnaire. Seoul: Hakjisa Publisher.
33. Park IJ, Min KH (2005) Making a list of Korean Emotion Terms and Exploring Dimensions Underlying Them. Korean Journal of Social and Personality Psychology 19: 109–129.
34. Talairach J, Tournoux P (1988) Co-Planar Stereotactic Atlas of the Human Brain. New York: Thieme Medical Publishers, Inc.
35. Minshew NJ, Keller TA (2010) The nature of brain dysfunction in autism: functional brain imaging studies. Curr Opin Neurol 23: 124–130.
36. Sahyoun CP, Belliveau JW, Soulieres I, Schwartz S, Mody M (2010) Neuroimaging of the functional and structural networks underlying visuospatial vs. linguistic reasoning in high-functioning autism. Neuropsychologia 48: 86–95.
37. Mason RA, Williams DL, Kana RK, Minshew N, Just MA (2008) Theory of Mind disruption and recruitment of the right hemisphere during narrative comprehension in autism. Neuropsychologia 46: 269–280.
38. Tesink CM, Buitelaar JK, Petersson KM, van der Gaag RJ, Kan CC, et al. (2009) Neural correlates of pragmatic language comprehension in autism spectrum disorders. Brain 132: 1941–1952.
39. Wang AT, Lee SS, Sigman M, Dapretto M (2006) Neural basis of irony comprehension in children with autism: the role of prosody and context. Brain 129: 932–943.
40. Dichter GS, Felder JN, Bodfish JW (2009) Autism is characterized by dorsal anterior cingulate hyperactivation during social target detection. Soc Cogn Affect Neurosci 4: 215–226.
41. Buchsbaum MS, Buchsbaum BR, Hazlett EA, Haznedar MM, Newmark R, et al. (2007) Relative glucose metabolic rate higher in white matter in patients with schizophrenia. Am J Psychiatry 164: 1072–1081.
42. Baron-Cohen S, Leslie AM, Frith U (1985) Does the autistic child have a "theory of mind"? Cognition 21: 37–46.
43. Kanwisher N, McDermott J, Chun MM (1997) The fusiform face area: a module in human extrastriate cortex specialized for face perception. J Neurosci 17: 4302–4311.
44. Hobson RP, Ouston J, Lee A (1988) What's in a face? The case of autism. Br J Psychol 79 (Pt 4): 441–453.
45. Carper RA, Courchesne E (2005) Localized enlargement of the frontal cortex in early autism. Biol Psychiatry 57: 126–133.
46. Chugani DC, Muzik O, Rothermel R, Behen M, Chakraborty P, et al. (1997) Altered serotonin synthesis in the dentatothalamocortical pathway in autistic boys. Ann Neurol 42: 666–669.
47. Freitag CM, Konrad C, Haberlen M, Kleser C, von Gontard A, et al. (2008) Perception of biological motion in autism spectrum disorders. Neuropsychologia 46: 1480–1494.
48. Alaerts K, Woolley DG, Steyaert J, Di Martino A, Swinnen SP, et al. (2013) Underconnectivity of the superior temporal sulcus predicts emotion recognition deficits in autism. Soc Cogn Affect Neurosci.
49. Herrington JD, Nymberg C, Schultz RT (2011) Biological motion task performance predicts superior temporal sulcus activity. Brain Cogn 77: 372–381.
50. Koldewyn K, Whitney D, Rivera SM (2011) Neural correlates of coherent and biological motion perception in autism. Dev Sci 14: 1075–1088.
51. Kaiser MD, Delmolino L, Tanaka JW, Shiffrar M (2010) Comparison of visual sensitivity to human and object motion in autism spectrum disorder. Autism Res 3: 191–195.
52. Huang J, Francis AP, Carr TH (2008) Studying overt word reading and speech production with event-related fMRI: a method for detecting, assessing, and correcting articulation-induced signal changes and for measuring onset time and duration of articulation. Brain Lang 104: 10–23.

3

Social Attention, Affective Arousal and Empathy in Men with Klinefelter Syndrome (47,XXY): Evidence from Eyetracking and Skin Conductance

Sophie van Rijn[1,2]*, Marjolein Barendse[1], Stephanie van Goozen[1,3], Hanna Swaab[1,2]

1 Clinical Child and Adolescent Studies, Leiden University, Leiden, The Netherlands, **2** Leiden Institute for Brain and Cognition, Leiden, The Netherlands, **3** School of Psychology, Cardiff University, Cardiff, United Kingdom

Abstract

Individuals with an extra X chromosome (Klinefelter syndrome) are at risk for problems in social functioning and have an increased vulnerability for autism traits. In the search for underlying mechanisms driving this increased risk, this study focused on social attention, affective arousal and empathy. Seventeen adults with XXY and 20 non-clinical controls participated in this study. Eyetracking was used to investigate social attention, as expressed in visual scanning patterns in response to the viewing of empathy evoking video clips. Skin conductance levels, reflecting affective arousal, were recorded continuously during the clips as well. Empathic skills, i.e. participants' understanding of own and others' emotions in response to the clips was also assessed. Results showed reduced empathic understanding, decreased visual fixation to the eye region, but increased affective arousal in individuals with Klinefelter syndrome. We conclude that individuals with XXY tend to avoid the eye region. Considering the increased affective arousal, we speculate that this attentional deployment strategy may not be sufficient to successfully downregulate affective hyper-responsivity. As increased affective arousal was related to reduced empathic ability, we hypothesize that own affective responses to social cues play an important role in difficulties in understanding the feelings and intentions of others. This knowledge may help in the identification of risk factors for psychopathology and targets for treatment.

Editor: Kun Guo, University of Lincoln, United Kingdom

Funding: This work was supported by a Veni grant (grant number 016.095.060 to SVR) from the Netherlands Organization for Scientific Research (www.NWO.nl). The funders had no role in study design, data collection and analysis, decision to publish, or preparation of the manuscript.

Competing Interests: The authors have declared that no competing interests exist.

* E-mail: srijn@fsw.leidenuniv.nl

Introduction

Klinefelter syndrome (KS) is a chromosome aneuploidy characterized by an additional X chromosome in boys and men (47, XXY), with a prevalence of 1:500 to 1:1000 male births [1]. The presence of an exceptional high density of genes on X chromosome that are essential for neural development [2], warrants the study of cognitive functioning in individuals with an extra X chromosome. Intellectual level of boys and men with KS is typically in the normal range, although on average somewhat lower, specifically with regard to verbal IQ [3,4]. However, there is an increased risk for specific cognitive dysfunctions in areas of language, executive functioning and social cognition [3–8].

Social and emotional functioning of individuals with KS has recently received increased attention. Although the behavioural phenotype may be variable, on average boys and men with KS are at risk for difficulties with social interactions and social adjustment. These social difficulties include shyness, social withdrawal, social anxiety, difficulties in peer-relationships, social impulsivity, communication difficulties, depressed adaptive skills, and reduced social assertiveness [9–16]. Also, recent studies have suggested that boys and men with Klinefelter syndrome are at increased risk for autism traits and symptoms [13,17–20].

Traditionally, it has been thought that social dysfunction arises from the language deficits typically seen in males with KS or it has been considered a consequence of daily life struggles associated with the condition. However, recent studies have shown that impairments in social cognitive processing may also play an important role. Social cognitive processing, i.e. the ability to perceive, understand and express social signals, has a contribution to social functioning that is independent of other cognitive abilities such as intelligence, language and attention [21]. There is evidence showing that Klinefelter syndrome can be associated with increased risk for difficulties in the identification of emotions of others based on facial expressions [7], difficulties with recognizing affective tone of voice (emotional prosody) [22], and reduced sensitivity to gaze direction [8]. Interstingly, there are also data suggesting that Klinefelter syndrome can be associated with abnormalities in emotional reactivity. In earlier studies using self-report measures, men with KS reported to be more easily affectively aroused than controls in response to emotion inducing events [7], and reported to experience higher levels of distress than controls during social interactions, for example when dealing with criticism or when starting a conversation with others [13]. These studies on social and emotional processing call for further investigation, particularly considering social dysfunctioning and vulnerability for autism symptoms in individuals with Klinefelter syndrome. The present study aims to provide in this by examining to what degree Klinefelter syndrome is associated with abnormalities in a) empathy in response to social stimuli, b) attention towards social stimuli and c) affective (physiological) arousal in response to social stimuli.

Empathy has been defined as 'the capacity to (*a*) be affected by and share the emotional state of another, (*b*) assess the reasons for the other's state, and (*c*) identify with the other, adopting his or her perspective' [23]. Baron-Cohen emphasized that empathic responses entail appropriate emotions, that are triggered by someone else's emotional state [24].Empathy is essential for the regulation of social interactions, as it allows one to automatically and quickly relate to the emotional states of others [23]. Because empathy allows one to understand the feelings and intentions of others, it helps in predicting their behavior [24]. It has been proposed that limited empathy is one of the neurocognitive constructs underlying the social and communicative difficulties observed in individuals with ASD [25]. Empathy has not yet been studied in individuals with Klinefelter syndrome.

Social attention involves an spontaneous and automatic visual orientation towards objects with social importance, namely individuals, their faces, and especially their eyes [26]. Due to the extensive amount of information that can be extracted, the eye region represents a crucial area of the face. More than other facial features, the eyes are central to all aspects of social communication such as identity, emotional state as well as direction of attention and related potential targets for intentions. This is also illustrated by studies showing that scanning of the face always starts with the eyes regardless of its emotion [27,28]. A review by Itier [29] demonstrated that of all facial features the eye region is the most attended to and the source of information most utilized, independent of the task, whether it concerns gaze, head orientation, identity, gender, facial expression or age. Considering that individuals with autism spectrum disorders (ASD) often show a reduced tendency to focus on the eyes of others, which has been related to impairments in understanding the emotions of others and increased social anxiety [30,31], a study on attention to such social cues in individuals with Klinefelter syndrome is warranted.

Affective arousal is an indicator of emotional reactivity. An emotion is 'a complex psychological state that involves three distinct components: a physiological response, a subjective experience (feeling), and a behavioral or expressive response' [32]. For social adaptation, the regulation of emotions plays an important role. Emotion regulation refers to the ability to monitor, evaluate, and modify the intensity and temporal dynamics of emotional reactions through extrinsic means (managing overt behaviors and social situations) and intrinsic means (recruiting cognitive and psychophysiological systems) [33,34]. Emotions help facilitate behaviors that are adaptive to the social environment [33]. However, emotions can also negatively impact social functioning of an individual when emotions occur at the wrong time, in the wrong place and at the wrong intensity level. Studies on ASD suggest abnormalities in the intensity level of affective arousal to social stimuli [35], which may result from emotion regulation impairments [36]. Interestingly, Dalton, et al [37] showed that in individuals with ASD increased affective arousal, as reflected in increased neural activation in the amygdala, is associated with reduced gaze fixation. They proposed that reduced fixation towards eyes of others as seen in individuals with ASD, may help downregulate this overarousal to social cues.

So far, studies on emotional reactivity in individuals with Klinefelter syndrome primarily included behavioural measures and self-report data; no research has been done on psychophysiological indices of affective arousal, i.e. implicit, objective arousal responses that may or may not match with explicit, subjective experience of emotion. One of the psychophysiological indices of affective arousal is skin conductance (SC). SC changes are mainly dependent on the activity of sweat glands innervated by the sympathetic branch of the autonomic nervous system (ANS), which is involved in up- and down-regulation of many homeostatic mechanisms in the body, preparing organisms for 'flight or fight' responses. The most frequently used measures of ANS activity, reflected in changes in the electrical properties of the skin, are the number of fluctuations in skin conductance (skin conductance responses, SCRs), the amplitude of these fluctuations, and the overall tonic level of the skin conductance. Skin conductance is a sensitive and objective index of implicit emotional responses that may occur without conscious awareness or are beyond cognitive intent [38,39]. In the general population, the presentation of affective faces or scenes typically leads to a short increase in skin conductance, reflecting an affective response [40,41]. Emotional video clips typically also induce physiological reactions, such as an increase in skin conductance level and in amount and amplitude of SCRs, reflecting affective arousal [42]. The strength of skin conductance responses varies from person to person.

To summarize, individuals with KS often have problems in social and emotional functioning, and are at higher risk for autism traits. In the search for underlying mechanisms driving this increased risk we propose that the study of social cognition and emotion processing, in addition to language and other cognitive domains, may help in the identification of risk factors and targets for treatment. In this study we focused on social attention and emotion processing in KS using a neurocognitive approach. To this end, we investigated physiological arousal (i.e., skin conductance level) and visual scanning patterns whilst viewing empathy evoking video clips. These implicit measures of social attention (fixation patterns) and emotional reactivity (arousal) were related to more explicit measures, i.e. the understanding of emotions of others and one's own emotions in response to the video clips.

Methods

Ethics statement

The study was approved by the Ethics Committee of Leiden University. Written informed consent, according to the declaration of Helsinki, was obtained from all participants.

Participants

Seventeen (young) adults with Klinefelter syndrome (mean age 37.91 years, SD 12.02) were included in this study, as well as 20 non-clinical controls (mean age 32.64 years, SD 12.23). Mean age did not differ between groups, but the mean education level was higher for the control group ($F(1,35) = 26.72$, $p < 0.001$). Participants with KS were recruited with help of the Dutch Klinefelter support group (NKV) or were attending the outpatient clinic at the department of Child and Adolescent Studies at Leiden University. Seven of the men with XXY were using testosterone supplements. Control participants were recruited by the researchers, with help of information brochures that were distributed in public areas outside university campus. All participants had normal or corrected-to-normal vision. In the XXY group, mean IQ was 94.21 (SD 14.81). Written informed consent, according to the declaration of Helsinki, was obtained from all participants.

Intellectual functioning

All participants completed the subtests Blockdesign (perceptual organization skills) and Vocabulary (verbal skills) of the of the Dutch adaptations of theWAIS-III (WechslerAdult Intelligence

Scales) [43,44], i.e. V-BD short form. This short form can be used to estimate full scale IQ (FSIQ) according to the algorithm (2.9*(sum of normed scores)+42) [45]. The V-BD short form correlates high with full scale IQ (r = .88) [46] and the V-BD short form has been found valid for the estimation of intelligence, with a good reliability (r = .91) and validity (.82) [45].

Eye tracking during affective clips

After a 5 point calibration procedure four affective, empathy evoking video clips of approximately 90 seconds each [47] were presented in randomized order on a LCD screen 65 cm away from the participant. Total fixation duration within specific areas of interest was measured with the Tobii T120 eye tracker (Tobii Technology, Sweden), which records the X and Y coordinates of participant's eye position at 120 Hz by using corneal reflection techniques. Gaze data were processed using Tobii Studio (3.0), using the Tobii I-VT fixation filter. The 'Dynamic AOI (Area of Interest)' tool, using freeform shapes, was used to draw AOI's. Dynamic AOIs were grouped into the following categories: *facial features (without mouth and eyes), eyes, mouth, body, objects* and *other (i.e. on the screen, outside other AOI's).*

The primary emotions of the main character in the video clip were pain/surprise, sadness/upset, fear/anxiety or happy/cheerful, based on ratings obtained in a pilot study aimed at identifying the two most reported emotions for each video clip. The four video clips were scenes selected from t.v. broadcasted movies. The 'pain/surprise' clip concerned a man getting stuck between rocks while climbing, and showed his face while amputating his own arm (not shown) in order to survive. The 'sad/upset' clip showed the reaction of a boy who is told his father has just died. The 'fear/anxiety' clip showed a child in a rowing boat at sea, while faced with a shark attack. The 'happy/cheerful' clip showed the ecstatic reaction of a horse racer en his team while winning the race. In all clips, auditory input was included, as vocal responses (including sounds of pain and crying as well as affective prosody, i.e. emotional tone of voice) are part of social cues in social situations. The clips were English spoken.

There was a fixed time interval between presentation of the video clips during which the explicit empathy test was performed. Eyetracking data from the four emotional video clips were collapsed for data analysis as total duration of the AOI's within each emotional video was not explicitly controlled for.

Physiological arousal during affective clips

Physiological data were collected continuously during the entire video presentation with a sample rate of 500 samples/s using Acqknowledge software (Biopac System Inc.). Measurements were acquired through a Galvanic skin response amplifier (GSR100C) and a Biopac data acquisition system (mp150-Windows). The physiological monitoring equipment was synchronized with Tobii software by event markers representing the beginning and ending of each video. In Acqknowledge, a 0.5–2 Hz band-pass filter was applied. A skin conductance response was defined as an increase in Skin conductance level (SCL) with a minimum of 0.05 µS within a timeframe of 3 seconds (considering the typical rise time for a skin conductance response of 1 to 3 seconds). SCL (µS) and number of skin conductance responses (SCRs) per minute were examined. Skin conductance measurements were done during a rest condition and during the four emotional video clips. During the non-emotional, rest measurement participants watched a relaxing video clip of an aquarium, lasting three minutes.

Explicit empathy test

After each clip participants completed two questionnaires, one concerning the emotions of the main character and the other concerning their own emotions while viewing the clip. By placing a cross on a continuous line of 10 cm they indicated how strong they or the main character felt on a range of 10 emotions (anger, sad, pain, upset, fearful, happy, scared, cheerful, surprised and hurt). Participants were also asked to explain the reason for the emotion they rated that they felt most strongly. A total empathy score was calculated, based on three components: recognizing the most important emotion of the main character (there were two emotions for each clip that were considered 'correct' based on a pilot study at Cardiff University), feeling emotions concurrent with the emotions of the main character and giving an empathic reason for one's own emotion(s), similar to Braaten, et al. [48], although they computed separate scores for matching of emotions and interpretation of emotions. Total empathy score in this study was calculated as follows. If participants gave the two 'correct' emotions of the main character a higher score (i.e. stronger intensity) than the other emotions on the list, they received two points (one point per emotion). Furthermore, they received two points if the emotions they indicated as strongest and second strongest for themselves, were the same emotions as those which they indicated as strongest and second strongest for the main character (one point for each emotion). Finally, they received a point if the reason they gave for their own emotion(s) was empathic, defined as 'The participant provided an explanation that included a direct reference to the character's feelings or experience'. In addition, explanations for own emotions should fit the content of the video clip, in order to count as an empathic response. For example, an empathic response would be when participants stated they wondered what it would be like for him/her to experience that. An example of a non-empathic reason would be "I was surprised to see this movie". This leads to a maximum score of 20 points, 5 for each video. The reasons participants gave were coded afterwards by the experimenter and a second coder who was (in contrast to the experimenter) blind to the clinical status of the participants. Interrater agreement was 92.6%.

Procedure

Before electrodes were attached, participants cleaned their hands. Skin conductance electrodes were placed on the middle phalanges of the ring and middle fingers of the participant's non-dominant hand. A non-affective (baseline) video clip was shown first, after which the 4 emotional video clips were presented in counterbalanced order. Before the start of the non-affective clip participants were instructed to sit quietly, watch the video and try to relax. Before the start of the empathy evoking video clips, participants were instructed to watch the four short clips, sit quietly and minimize their movements, and answer the questions subsequently.

Statistical analyses

Total empathy scores in the two groups (control, XXY) were compared using ANVOCA, controlling for verbal skills. For groupwise (XXY, control) comparisons in specific empathic scores (3 subscales) and fixation duration (6 AOI's), MANCOVA and ANCOVA was used respectively. To exclude that verbal skills had an effect in the performance test, normscore on the Vocabulary subtest of the WAIS-III was included as a covariate in analyses of the explicit empathy test. Repeated measures analysis was used to assess group differences in changes in SCL and SCRs from rest to the emotional video clips (4 clips). Only those variables that showed significant group differences (control, XXY) were included in correlational analyses. For correlational analyses, spearman's rho was used. Level of significance was set at $p<0.05$.

Results

Intellectual functioning

Mean IQ was 94.22 (SD 14.81) in the XXY group and 108.14 (SD 10.33) in the control group, which was significantly different ($F(1,35)=11.21$, $p=0{,}002$, but within the normal range for all participants. Mean normscore for the subtest Vocabulary was 8.03 (SD 2.12) for the XXY group and 12.42 (SD 2.01) for the control group, which was significantly different ($F(1,35)=42.02$, $p<0.001$. Mean normscore for the subtest Blockdesign was 10.05 (SD 3.64) for the XXY group and 10.44 (SD 2.65) for the control group, which was not significantly different ($F(1,35)=0.11$, $p=0.74$.

Explicit empathy test

The total empathy score was 13.01 (*SD* 2.45) in the control group and 9.44 (*SD* 2.83) in the XXY group, which was significantly different ($t(1,34)=9.31$, $p=0.004$, Cohen's $d=1.44$) as indicated by ANCOVA (controlling for verbal skills).

MANCOVA with the three empathy scores showed a main multivariate effect of group (control, XXY), $F(3,32)=4.94$, $p=0.006$, but no main multivariate effect on the covariate verbal skills ($p=0.70$). Univariate effects of group were present for correctly labelling the emotions of the main characters in the affective clips ($F(1,34)=4.32$, $p=0.04$, Cohen's $d=0.73$), and empathic explanations for their own emotions ($F(1,34)=12{,}02$, $p=0.001$ Cohen's $d=1.70$), with lower scores in the XXY group. However, there was no significant effect of group for correspondence between their own reported emotions and the emotions of the main characters ($p=0.17$). In the XXY group there were no systematic confusions in terms of mislabeling emotions. Data are presented in figure 1.

Social attention during empathy clips: Eyetracking

ANOVA indicated a significant group effect on total fixation duration in the AOI 'eyes' ($F(1,35)=4.50$, $p=0.04$. The XXY group spend less time fixating on eyes as compared to the control group, with an effect size of 1.23 (Cohen's *d*). This appeared to be a specific effect, as other AOI's did not show significant group effects. Covarying for level of education did not change the significance of the results. Furthermore, within the XXY group, there were no significant differences in fixation duration between those who were using and not using testosterone supplements. For mean total fixation durations in each AOI, see figure 2. An illustration of eyegaze patterns in both groups is presented in figure 3.

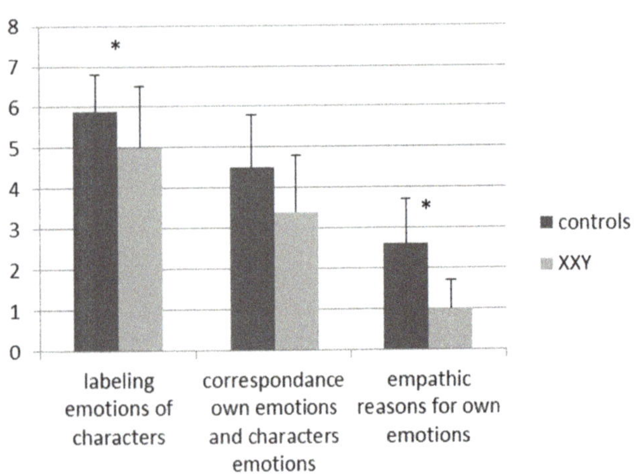

Figure 1. Empathy scores (mean, SD) in the XXY group versus the control group. *significant at $p=0.05$.

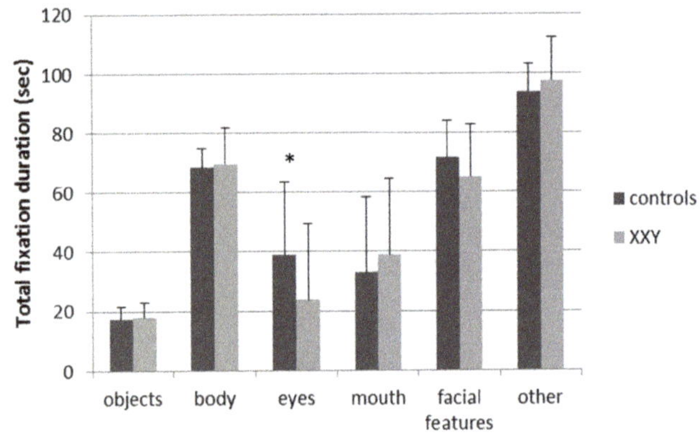

Figure 2. Total fixation duration (mean, SD) within specific areas of interest (AOI) while watching emotional video clips for the XXY group and control group separately. *significant at $p=0.05$.

Relation between visual scanning patterns and self-reported empathy

Within the XXY group and the control group, there were no significant correlations between total fixation duration to the eyes and the empathy scores.

Physiological arousal during affective clips: Skin conductance

One outlier, with a *Z* score of 3.84 for skin conductance level during rest, was removed from the control group. We analyzed both skin conductance level (SCL) and the number of skin conductance responses per minute (SCRs). During the rest condition, while viewing the non-emotional video clip, there was a significant difference between the control group and XXY group in SCL ($F(1,34)=7.82$, $p=0.008$) and SCR ($F(1,34)=10.71$, $p=0.002$), with lower skin conductance levels and a lower number of SCRs in the XXY group. Considering that many factors influence absolute levels of skin conductance, our main interest was in a relative measure, i.e. group differences in affective responsivity. For this, we used repeated measures analyses to

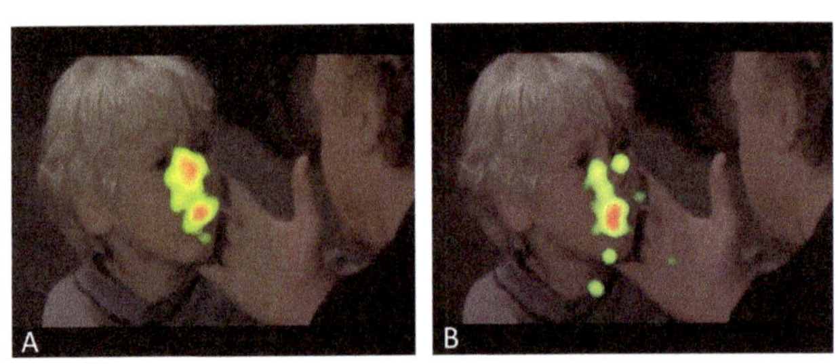

Figure 3. Heat maps of the control group (A) en XXY group (B) reflecting total fixation duration in a scene involving a boy being told his father has died, illustrating the group differences in visual fixation on the eyes.

compare the increase in arousal from rest to the emotional clips in both groups. All repeated measures analyses showed a significant main effect of condition (at $p<0.01$), indicating that arousal (expressed in SCL and SCRs) was overall higher during the affective clips as compared to rest (irrespective of group membership). For SCRs, a significant group (control, XXY) by condition (rest, emotion) interaction was found for 'fear/anxiety' ($F(1,34) = 5.82$, $p = 0.02$) and 'pain/surprise' ($F(1,34) = 4.43$, $p = 0.04$). The increase in arousal from rest to the affective clips (i.e. affective responsivity) was larger in the XXY group as compared to the control group. The differences in SCRs between rest and the affective clips are presented for both groups in figure 4. For SCL, no significant group (control, XXY) by condition (rest, emotion) interactions were observed.

Relation between physiological arousal and self-reported empathy

Within the XXY group, the number of SCRs during the fear/anxiety video clip was significantly inversely correlated with the total empathy score ($r = -0.53$, $p = 0.02$). In others words, higher levels of arousal during the fear/anxiety video clip were related to lower levels of empathy. Importantly, the number of SCRs during rest was not correlated with total empathy score ($r = 0.01$, $p = 0.94$), indicating that the effect was specific for the emotional video clip. In the control group, there was no significant correlation.

Discussion

In this study we investigated empathy, social attention, and affective arousal in response to social stimuli in individuals with Klinefelter syndrome (KS). Social attention (eye gaze patterns) and emotional reactivity (physiological arousal) were measured and related to more explicit, behavioral measures, i.e. the understanding of own and others' emotions.

The behavioral measures showed that individuals with KS compared to controls had more difficulty responding in an empathic way to the emotional video clips, as reflected in an overall lower empathy score, which was driven by a reduced ability to identify the emotions of the main character and in showing less empathic reasons they reported for their own emotion(s). There were no significant group differences in rating own emotions in concordance with the main character's emotions. The empathy deficits were independent of verbal skills, as this was controlled for in the analyses, and which showed no significant effect of verbal skills on empathy scores. In the XXY group, mean total empathy score was 1.44 standard deviations below that of controls.

Objective measures of social attention revealed atypical eyegaze patterns in the XXY group. Eyetracking during viewing of the emotional video clips showed that individuals with KS spent less time looking at the eyes of the video characters as compared to the control group (i.e. displayed a shorter fixation duration). The effect size (Cohen's *d*) indicated that mean fixation duration in the XXY group was 1.23 standard deviations below that of controls. This effect was specific for the eye region, as looking times for other type of stimuli such as 'face', 'body', 'object' and 'mouth' were similar for the KS and control groups. Looking time outside these areas but on screen was also similar, indicating that there was no overall difference in attention to the video clip. Taken together, considering that in social communication the most crucial information comes from the eyes, a reduced tendency to focus on the eyes of others in individuals with KS can have profound effects on adaptive social functioning. The related deficits in empathic understanding in KS support this interpretation.

Support for the link between social attention impairments and social dysfunction largely comes from studies in the field of autism. For example, when looking at video clips of social situations, individuals with autism spectrum disorder (ASD) spend less time focusing on eyes and more time focusing on mouths, bodies and objects [49]. Differences in eyegaze patterns have also been found

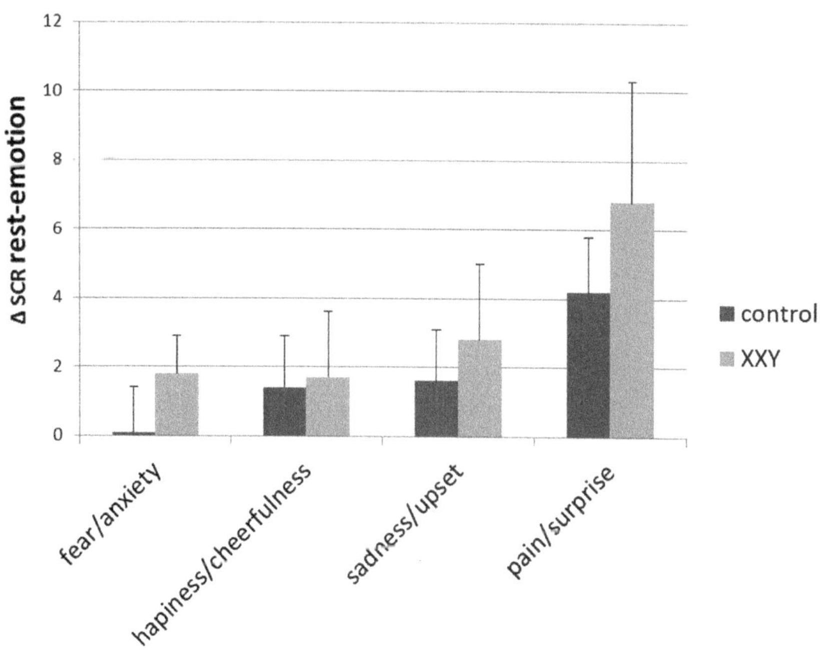

Figure 4. Increase in number of SCRs (mean, SD) per minute from rest to the affective clips in the control group and XXY group.
* significant at $p<0.05$.

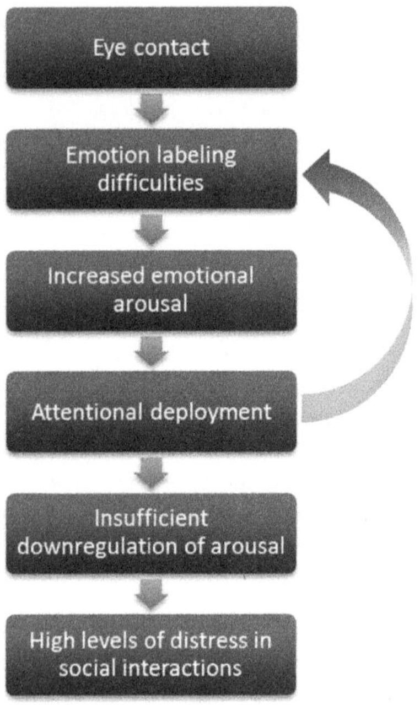

Figure 5. The emotion regulation hypothesis of social dysfunction in Klinefelter syndrome.

when individuals with and without ASD view pictures of faces [37,50], with reduced attention to the eye region in those with ASD. Several studies have found that in individuals with autism less attention to the eye region of faces is associated with more impaired emotion recognition skills [30,31] and higher levels of social anxiety [31]. Another study found similar relations in children with ASD and typically developing controls: emotion recognition accuracy was positively related to fixation time on the eye region and negatively to fixation time on the mouth region [51]. We speculate that reduced attention to the eye region, and related difficulties in empathy and emotion understanding, might in part drive the increased vulnerability for social difficulties and autism traits in individuals with KS.

Besides difficulties in processing of emotions of others, we also observed abnormalities with regard to own emotions in adults with KS. To study emotional reactivity, we used an objective measure of affective arousal as expressed in psychophysiological responses, i.e. skin conductance, during the emotional video clips. This showed that in comparison to the control group, individuals with KS showed a stronger increase in arousal response to emotional video clips compared to controls. This was specifically observed for the clips in which the main character was experiencing fear/anxiety or pain/surprise. This finding of increased affective responsivity matches up with earlier behavioural studies. Using a behavioural questionnaire, Ratcliffe, et al [14] found that a group of 14 boys with KS were on average 'more affected by feelings' than the control group. In a study on emotion processing using self-report questionnaires, men with KS reported to be more easily emotionally aroused by emotion inducing events ('emotionality') as compared to the control group [7]. Also, increased experience of distress during social interaction was reported (using questionnaires) by adults with KS in a study on social functioning and autism traits [13].

Interestingly, higher levels of affective arousal in the XXY group were associated with lower overall levels of empathic ability, as reflected in a reduced ability to identify the emotions of the main character, their own emotions being less concordant with the main character's emotions and in showing less empathic reasons they reported for their own emotion(s). A decreased ability to identify and label emotions was not only evident in this study, but also observed in an earlier behavioural study [7] showing that men with KS reported a reduced ability to identify, experience, verbally describe and reflect on one's own affective arousal states, which also been conceptualized as 'alexithymia' (literally translated 'lacking words for feelings') [52,53]. Such a mismatch between reduced (subjective) labeling of emotion versus increased (objective) affective arousal is shown to be associated with deficient emotion regulation [54]. Although speculative, the degree of affective arousal in response to social cues may (in part) reflect emotion regulation deficiencies as has been suggested for individuals with ASD [36].

The emotion regulation model by Gross [34] distinguishes antecedent focused emotion regulation mechanisms and response focused emotion regulation mechanisms, with some more adaptive than others. Response-focused regulation occurs after the emotional responses are generated. It includes response modulation, which refers to efforts to suppress the experience or expression of emotion. Antecedent regulation is obtained by (1) altering the interpretation of a situation to change its emotional impact, i.e. cognitive change or (2) directing attention towards or away from specific aspects of the situation, i.e. attentional deployment. The two key attentional deployment mechanisms described by the process model are *concentration* and *distraction*. Distraction involves changing the focus of attention to different aspects of the situation or moving attention away from the situation altogether. It may also involve a change in internal focus, such as invoking memories or thoughts that are inconsistent with the undesirable emotional state. Based on our finding of less attentional focus to the eye region in individuals with KS (interpreted as avoidance), we speculate that individuals with KS use attentional deployment, specifically distraction, as an emotion regulation mechanisms. However, as participants were not instructed to exert effortful regulation of their emotions, our findings may largely reflect implicit and automatic attentional deployment. In contrast to explicit use of emotion regulation strategies, requiring conscious effort, monitoring, and some level of insight or awareness, emotion regulation mechanisms can also be triggered automatically by the stimulus itself and can take place without monitoring, insight or awareness [55].

A recent meta-analysis has shown that strategies involving attentional deployment prove to be less effective (effect size 0.0) than strategies involving cognitive change, i.e. reappraisal, which had a small-to-medium sized effect (effect size 0.36) on emotional responses [56]. Although speculative, the use of a less effective emotion regulation strategy does line up with the finding of increased emotional arousal in the XXY group. Interestingly, Bebko, et al. [57] using eyetracking found that irrespective of emotion regulation strategy, individuals who looked less at emotional areas of presented pictures, were less likely to experience emotion regulation success.

Although picking up emotional signals of others is important for successful social interactions [58,59], one's own emotions seem to play an equally important role in social adaptive behavior [60,61]. Poor emotion regulation has been associated with lower quality of friendships, reduced interpersonal sensitivity, less prosocial tendencies and more social conflicts in young adults [60–62] as well as reduced social adaptation and low peer friendship nominations in children and adolescents [63–65]. In line with our findings, deficiencies in affective reactivity and identification and labeling of affect have also been reported in the field of autism.

High levels of alexithymia, including difficulties in adequately assessing and labeling own affective arousal states, have been observed in individuals with ASD [66–71]. Interestingly, children and adolescents with ASD have also been found to show a stronger skin conductance reaction to faces with direct and averted gaze compared to typically developing children [35]. However, findings are inconsistent as other studies have found that children and adults with ASD show similar skin conductance responses to objects and faces, in contrast to individuals without ASD who show a stronger reaction to faces than to objects [72,73].

This study also had several limitations, which should be addressed. First, the XXY group may not be representative for KS individuals at large, considering that inclusion was done in a subgroup who was seeking information about their condition or seeking help for psychological problems. Nonetheless, findings in this article are applicable and relevant for those individuals with KS who have social difficulties. Second, the sample sizes were relatively small, based on which one should be cautious in interpreting and generalizing the results. Especially for the correlational analyses, our findings need replication in a larger sample. Third, we were not able to compare visual fixation duration across emotions, as exposure times of the areas of interest were not explicitly controlled for across the video clips. Finally, participants were not explicitly instructed to regulate their emotions during viewing of the video clips, so we were not able to assess explicit emotion regulation skills.

Taken together, our data suggest a profile of increased emotional arousal, together with decreased attention to and difficulties with labeling of emotional information, in individuals with Klinefelter syndrome. These findings tentatively suggest impairments in emotion regulation and social attention. As increased affective responsivity was related to reduced empathic ability, we hypothesize that emotional responsivity plays an important role in difficulties in understanding the feelings and intentions of others. Although speculative, focussing on the eyes of others might evoke increased emotional arousal in individuals with KS, because of the difficulties in emotion labelling. As a result, attention may be automatically diverted away from the eyes. However, as attentional deployment has proven to be less effective in the regulation of emotions than reappraisal strategies, this may not be sufficient to successfully downregulate this increased arousal, resulting in high levels of distress in social interactions. By diverting attention away from the eyes, individuals with KS may also miss out on crucial information with regard to the feelings and intentions of others, which may further add to the emotion labelling difficulties. For an overview of this theoretical model, see figure 5.

Our interpretation is supported by findings in autism, showing that individuals with ASD often show a reduced tendency to focus on the eyes of others, which has been related to impairments in understanding the emotions of others [30]. Also, difficulties in processing own emotions, as expressed in high levels of alexithymia, are related to deficits in joint-attention (i.e. shared eye contact), theory of mind and empathic ability [74,75] in individuals with ASD. Interestingly, although Theory of Mind is typically considered as the ability to assess other people's mental states, there is compelling evidence that the processes of assessing other's mental states and one's own mental states are closely related [76]. As argued by Samson, et al. [77], this may not only hold for cognitive states, but also for emotional states. Future studies are needed to address the relationship between the processing of own emotions and Theory of Mind skills. It would also be interesting to further study the role of language deficits in relation to empathy impairments and more thoroughly study systematic biases in emotion labeling. Although biases were not observed in the current study, it would be interesting to assess such biases more rigorously, using reaction time paradigms and facial stimuli varying in degree of emotional expression as well as blended emotional expressions.

Understanding the relation between cognition and emotion, and their impact on social adaptation, may help the diagnosis and treatment of individuals with KS. The findings in this study may also contribute to the identification of cognitive and emotional mechanisms that can be targeted in treatment and are aimed at improving social functioning. For example, we speculate that interventions focusing on improving emotion awareness and emotion regulation might also have positive effects on social cognition, as more socially relevant information will be available when adequate emotional responsivity allows for more thorough visual scanning of eyes and other crucial facial features. In turn, any improvements in labeling of social cues that may arise from more thorough visual scanning, might contribute to more adaptive levels affective arousal. Interestingly, it has already been shown that coherence between subjective and objective (psychophysiological) aspects of emotion is greater in those who have specialized training involving the promotion of greater body awareness [78]. Considering the increased vulnerability for psychopathology in KS, further research is needed on the predictive value of emotion regulation deficits and deviant social attention in relation to risk for autism symptoms, as well as other psychopathology such as psychotic symptoms, depression and anxiety. Insight in such underlying mechanisms of behavior, and opportunities to positive influence these mechanisms over the course of development, might also contribute to new insights into etiology and treatment of developmental psychopathology. Future, preferably longitudinal, studies including childhood populations may help in meeting this aim. Such studies may also help in unfolding the developmental course of emotion regulation impairments and assessing the contribution of social cognitive deficits, language impairments as well as executive dysfunctioning.

Acknowledgments

We would like to thank Thijs Schrama at Leiden University for help with the experimental paradigm and data-analysis, and Kelly Main at School of Psychology in Cardiff, UK, for the affective video clips. We thank Francien Martin for help with participant recruitment.

Author Contributions

Conceived and designed the experiments: SvR MB SvG HS. Performed the experiments: SvR MB. Analyzed the data: SvR MB. Contributed reagents/materials/analysis tools: SvR SvG HS. Wrote the paper: SvR MB SvG HS.

References

1. Bojesen A, Juul S, Gravholt CH (2003) Prenatal and postnatal prevalence of Klinefelter syndrome: a national registry study. The Journal of Clinical Endocrinology and Metabolism 88: 622–626.
2. Zechner U, Wilda M, Kehrer-Sawatzki H, Vogel W, Fundele R, et al. (2001) A high density of X-linked genes for general cognitive ability: a run-away process shaping human evolution? Trends Genet 17: 697–701.
3. Boada R, Janusz J, Hutaff-Lee C, Tartaglia N (2009) The cognitive phenotype in Klinefelter syndrome: A review of the literature including genetic and hormonal factors. Developmental Disabilities Research Reviews 15: 284–294.
4. Leggett V, Jacobs P, Nation K, Scerif G, Bishop DVM (2010) Neurocognitive outcomes of individuals with a sex chromosome trisomy: XXX, XYY, or XXY:

a systematic review. Developmental Medicine and Child Neurology 52: 119–129.
5. Lee NR, Wallace GL, Clasen LS, Lenroot RK, Blumenthal JD, et al. (2011) Executive Function in Young Males with Klinefelter (XXY) Syndrome with and without Comorbid Attention-Deficit/Hyperactivity Disorder. Journal of the International Neuropsychological Society 17: 522–530.
6. van Rijn S, Aleman A, Swaab H, Krijn T, Vingerhoets G, et al. (2007) What it is said versus how it is said: comprehension of affective prosody in men with Klinefelter (47,XXY) syndrome. Journal of the International Neuropsychological Society 13: 1065–1070.
7. van Rijn S, Swaab H, Aleman A, Kahn RS (2006) X Chromosomal effects on social cognitive processing and emotion regulation: A study with Klinefelter men (47,XXY). Schizophrenia Research 84: 194–203.
8. van't Wout M, van Rijn S, Jellema T, Kahn RS, Aleman A (2009) Deficits in implicit attention to social signals in schizophrenia and high risk groups: behavioural evidence from a new illusion. PloS one 4: e5581.
9. Ratcliffe S (1999) Long-term outcome in children of sex chromosome abnormalities. Archives of Disease in Childhood 80: 192–195.
10. Geschwind DH, Dykens E (2004) Neurobehavioral and psychosocial issues in Klinefelter syndrome. Learning Disabilities Research & Practice 19: 166–173.
11. Boone KB, Swerdloff RS, Miller BL, Geschwind DH, Razani J, et al. (2001) Neuropsychological profiles of adults with Klinefelter syndrome. Journal of the International Neuropsychological Society 7: 446–456.
12. Visootsak J, Graham JM (2009) Social function in multiple X and Y chromosome disorders: XXY, XYY, XXYY, XXXY. Developmental Disabilities Research Reviews 15: 328–332.
13. van Rijn S, Swaab H, Aleman A, Kahn RS (2008) Social behavior and autism traits in a sex chromosomal disorder: Klinefelter (47XXY) syndrome. Journal of Autism and Developmental Disorders 38: 1634–1641.
14. Ratcliffe S, Butler GE, Jones M (1991) Edinburgh study of growth and development of children with sex chromosome abnormalities- IV. Birth Defects: Original Articles Series 26: 1–44.
15. Robinson A, Bender B, Linden M, Salbenblatt J (1991) Sex chromosome aneuploidy: The Denver prospective study. Birth Defects: Original Articles Series 26: 59–115.
16. Stewart D, Bailey J, Netley C, Park E (1991) Growth, development and behavioral outcome from mid-adolescence to adulthood in subjects with chromosome aneuploidy: the Toronto study. Birth Defects: Original Articles Series 26: 131–188.
17. Tartaglia N, Cordeiro L, Howell S, Wilson R, Janusz J (2010) The spectrum of the behavioral phenotype in boys and adolescents 47,XXY (Klinefelter syndrome). Pediatr Endocrinol Rev 8 Suppl 1: 151–159.
18. Bruining H, Swaab H, Kas M, Van Engeland H (2009) Psychiatric characteristics in a self-selected sample of boys with klinefelter syndrome. Pediatrics 123: e865–e870.
19. Bishop DV, Jacobs PA, Lachlan K, Wellesley D, Barnicoat A, et al. (2011) Autism, language and communication in children with sex chromosome trisomies. Archives of Disease in Childhood 10: 954–959.
20. van Rijn S, Stockmann L, Borghgraef M, Bruining H, van Raavenswaaij-Arts C, et al. (in press) The social behavioral phenotype in boys and girls with an extra X chromosome: a comparison with autism spectrum disorder. Journal of Autism and Developmental Disorders.
21. Pinkham AE, Penn DL, Perkins DO, Lieberman J (2003) Implications for the Neural Basis of Social Cognition for the Study of Schizophrenia. American Journal of Psychiatry 160: 815–824.
22. Van Rijn S, Aleman A, Swaab H, Krijn T, Vingerhoets G, et al. (2007) What is said versus how it is said: Comprehension of affective prosody in men with Klinefelter (47,XXY) syndrome. Journal of the International Neuropsychological Society (JINS): 1065–1070.
23. de Waal FB (2008) Putting the altruism back into altruism: the evolution of empathy. Annual Review of Psychology 59: 279–300.
24. Baron-Cohen S (2010) Empathizing, systemizing, and the extreme male brain theory of autism. In: Savic I, editor. Sex Differences in the Human Brain, Their Underpinnings and Implications. pp. 167–175.
25. Baron-Cohen S (2002) The extreme male brain theory of autism. Trends in Cognitive Sciences 6: 248.
26. Klein JT, Shepherd SV, Platt ML (2009) Social Attention and the Brain. Current Biology 19: R958–R962.
27. Schyns PG, Petro LS, Smith ML (2007) Dynamics of visual information integration in the brain for categorizing facial expressions. Current Biology 17: 1580–1585.
28. Vinette C, Gosselin F, Schyns PG (2004) Spatio-temporal dynamics of face recognition in a flash: it's in the eyes. Cognitive Science 28: 289–301.
29. Itier RJ, Batty M (2009) Neural bases of eye and gaze processing: The core of social cognition. Neuroscience and Biobehavioral Reviews 33: 843–863.
30. Kirchner JC, Hatri A, Heekeren HR, Dziobek I (2011) Autistic Symptomatology, Face Processing Abilities, and Eye Fixation Patterns. Journal of Autism and Developmental Disorders 41: 158–167.
31. Corden B, Chilvers R, Skuse D (2008) Avoidance of emotionally arousing stimuli predicts social-perceptual impairment in Asperger's syndrome. Neuropsychologia 46: 137–147.
32. Myers DG (2004) Theories of Emotion. New York, NY: Worth Publishers.
33. Gross JJ (2002) Emotion regulation: Affective, cognitive, and social consequences. Psychophysiology 39: 281–291.
34. Gross JJ, Thompson RA (2007) Emotion regulation: Conceptual foundations. In: Gross JJ, editor. Handbook of emotion regulation. New York, NY: Guilford Press. pp. 3–24.
35. Joseph RM, Ehrman K, McNally R, Keehn B (2008) Affective response to eye contact and face recognition ability in children with ASD. Journal of the International Neuropsychological Society 14: 947–955.
36. Mazefsky CA, Herrington J, Siegel M, Scarpa A, Maddox BB, et al. (2013) The Role of Emotion Regulation in Autism Spectrum Disorder. Journal of the American Academy of Child and Adolescent Psychiatry 52: 679–688.
37. Dalton KM, Nacewicz BM, Johnstone T, Schaefer HS, Gernsbacher MA, et al. (2005) Gaze fixation and the neural circuitry of face processing in autism. Nature Neuroscience 8: 519–526.
38. Boucsein W (2012) Electrodermal activity. New York: Springer.
39. Dawson ME, Schell AM, Filion DL (2007) The electrodermal system. In: Cacioppo JT, Tassinary LG, Berntson GG, editors. Handbook of Psychophysiology. New York: Cambridge University Press. pp. 159–181.
40. Fusar-Poli P, Landi P, O'Connor C (2009) Neurophysiological response to emotional faces with increasing intensity of fear: A skin conductance response study. Journal of Clinical Neuroscience 16: 981–982.
41. Jonsson P, Sonnby-Borgstrom M (2003) The effects of pictures of emotional faces on tonic and phasic autonomic cardiac control in women and men. Biological Psychology 62: 157–173.
42. Kreibig SD, Wilhelm FH, Roth WT, Gross JJ (2007) Cardiovascular, electrodermal, and respiratory response patterns to fear- and sadness-inducing films. Psychophysiology 44: 787–806.
43. Wechsler D (1997) Wechsler Adult Intelligence Scale-Third Edition (WAIS-III). San Antonio, TX, USA: The Psychological Corporation.
44. Wechsler D (2005) WAIS-III NL. Wechsler Adult Intelligence Scale WAIS-III. Third edition, Dutch version. Manual. Amsterdam: Harcourt Test Publishers.
45. Campbell JM (1998) Internal and external validity of seven Wechsler Intelligence Scale for Children - Third Edition short forms in a sample of psychiatric inpatients. Psychological Assessment 10: 431–434.
46. HerreraGraf M, Dipert ZJ, Hinton RN (1996) Exploring the effective use of the vocabulary/block design short form with a special school population. Educational and Psychological Measurement 56: 522–528.
47. Main K (2012) Developing a new empathy paradigm: are gender differences consistent accross self-reported and psychophysiological measures?: Cardiff University, UK.
48. Braaten EB, Rosen LA (2000) Self-regulation of affect in attention deficit-hyperactivity disorder (ADHD) and non-ADHD boys: Differences in empathic responding. Journal of Consulting and Clinical Psychology 68: 313–321.
49. Klin A, Jones W, Schultz R, Volkmar F, Cohen D (2002) Visual fixation patterns during viewing of naturalistic social situations as predictors of social competence in individuals with autism. Archives of General Psychiatry 59: 809–816.
50. Pelphrey KA, Sasson NJ, Reznick JS, Paul G, Goldman BD, et al. (2002) Visual scanning of faces in autism. Journal of Autism and Developmental Disorders 32: 249–261.
51. Bal E, Harden E, Lamb D, Van Hecke AV, Denver JW, et al. (2010) Emotion Recognition in Children with Autism Spectrum Disorders: Relations to Eye Gaze and Autonomic State. Journal of Autism and Developmental Disorders 40: 358–370.
52. Sifneos PE (1973) The prevalence of 'alexithymic' characteristics in psychosomatic patients. Psychotherapy and Psychosomatics 22: 255–262.
53. Booth-Butterfield M, Booth-Butterfield S (1990) Conceptualizing affect as information in communication production. Human Communication Research 16: 451–476.
54. Connelly M, Denney DR (2007) Regulation of emotions during experimental stress in alexithymia. Journal of Psychosomatic Research 62: 649–656.
55. Gyurak A, Gross JJ, Etkin A (2011) Explicit and implicit emotion regulation: A dual-process framework. Cognition & Emotion 25: 400–412.
56. Webb TL, Miles E, Sheeran P (2012) Dealing With Feeling: A Meta-Analysis of the Effectiveness of Strategies Derived From the Process Model of Emotion Regulation. Psychological Bulletin 138: 775–808.
57. Bebko GM, Franconeri SL, Ochsner KN, Chiao JY (2011) Look Before You Regulate: Differential Perceptual Strategies Underlying Expressive Suppression and Cognitive Reappraisal. Emotion 11: 732–742.
58. Hooker C, Park S (2002) Emotion processing and its relationship to social functioning in schizophrenia patients. Psychiatry Research 112: 41–50.
59. Pinkham AE, Penn DL (2006) Neurocognitive and social cognitive predictors of interpersonal skill in schizophrenia. Psychiatry Research 143: 167–178.
60. Lopes PN, Brackett MA, Nezlek JB, Schatz A, Sellin I, et al. (2004) Emotional intelligence and social interaction. Personality and Social Psychology Bulletin 30: 1018–1034.
61. Lopes PN, Salovey P, Cata S, Beers M (2005) Emotion regulation abilities and the quality of social interaction. Emotion 5: 113–118.
62. Lopes PN, Salovey P, Straus R (2003) Emotional intelligence, personality, and the perceived quality of social relationships. Personality and Individual Differences 35: 641–658.
63. Eisenberg N, Fabes RA, Guthrie IK, Reiser M (2000) Dispositional emotionality and regulation: Their role in predicting quality of social functioning. Journal of Personality and Social Psychology 78: 136–157.
64. Halberstadt AG, Denham SA, Dunsmore JC (2001) Affective social competence. Social Development 10: 79–119.

65. Mestre JM, Guil R, Lopes PN, Salovey P, Gil-Olarte P (2006) Emotional intelligence and social and academic adaptation to school. Psicothema 18: 112–117.
66. Konstantareas MM, Stewart K (2006) Affect regulation and temperament in children with autism spectrum disorder. Journal of Autism and Developmental Disorders 36: 143–154.
67. Hill E, Berthoz S, Frith U (2004) Brief report: Cognitive processing of own emotions in individuals with autistic spectrum disorder and in their relatives. Journal of Autism and Developmental Disorders 34: 229.
68. Fitzgerald M, Bellgrove MA (2006) The overlap between alexithymia and asperger's syndrome [1]. Journal of Autism and Developmental Disorders 36: 573–576.
69. Bird G, Silani G, Brindley R, Singer T, Frith C, et al. (2006) Alexithymia in autism spectrum disorders. Human Brain Mapping.
70. Berthoz S, Hill EL (2005) The validity of using self-reports to assess emotion regulation abilities in adults with autism spectrum disorder. Eur Psychiatry 20: 291–298.
71. Tani P, Lindberg N, Joukamaa M, Nieminen-von Wendt T, von Wendt L, et al. (2004) Asperger syndrome, alexithymia and perception of sleep. Neuropsychobiology 49: 64–70.
72. Hirstein W, Iversen P, Ramachandran VS (2001) Autonomic responses of autistic children to people and objects. Proceedings of the Royal Society of London Series B-Biological Sciences 268: 1883–1888.
73. Hubert BE, Wicker B, Monfardini E, Deruelle C (2009) Electrodermal reactivity to emotion processing in adults with autistic spectrum disorders. Autism 13: 9–19.
74. Bird G, Press C, Richardson DC (2011) The Role of Alexithymia in Reduced Eye-Fixation in Autism Spectrum Conditions. Journal of Autism and Developmental Disorders 41: 1556–1564.
75. Bird G, Silani G, Brindley R, White S, Frith U, et al. (2010) Empathic brain responses in insula are modulated by levels of alexithymia but not autism. Brain 133: 1515–1525.
76. Frith U, Frith CD (2003) Development and neurophysiology of mentalizing. Philosophical Transactions of the Royal Society B: Biological Sciences V358: 459.
77. Samson AC, Huber O, Gross JJ (2012) Emotion Regulation in Asperger's Syndrome and High-Functioning Autism. Emotion 12: 659–665.
78. Sze JA, Gyurak A, Yuan JW, Levenson RW (2010) Coherence Between Emotional Experience and Physiology: Does Body Awareness Training Have an Impact? Emotion 10: 803–814.

4

The Relationship between Child Maltreatment and Emotion Recognition

Michiko Koizumi[1,2], Haruto Takagishi[3]*

1 Graduate School of Education, Hokkaido University, Sapporo, Japan, 2 Japan Society for the Promotion of Science, Tokyo, Japan, 3 Tamagawa University Brain Science Institute, Tokyo, Japan

Abstract

Child abuse and neglect affect the development of social cognition in children and inhibit social adjustment. The purpose of this study was to compare the ability to identify the emotional states of others between abused and non-abused children. The participants, 129 children (44 abused and 85 non-abused children), completed a children's version of the Reading the Mind in the Eyes Test (RMET). Results showed that the mean accuracy rate on the RMET for abused children was significantly lower than the rate of the non-abused children. In addition, the accuracy rates for positive emotion items (e.g., hoping, interested, happy) were significantly lower for the abused children, but negative emotion and neutral items were not different across the groups. This study found a negative relationship between child abuse and the ability to understand others' emotions, especially positive emotions.

Editor: Marina Pavlova, University of Tuebingen Medical School, Germany

Funding: This work was supported by JSPS KAKENHI Grant Number 11J02666. The funders had no role in study design, data collection and analysis, decision to publish, or preparation of the manuscript.

Competing Interests: The authors have declared that no competing interests exist.

* E-mail: takagishi@lab.tamagawa.ac.jp

Introduction

Child abuse and neglect are critical issues worldwide. The Japanese Ministry of Health, Labor and Welfare reported 56,384 cases of child abuse and neglect in 2010; this number has been increasing annually [1]. Child abuse and neglect can be classified into four categories: physical abuse, psychological abuse, sexual abuse, and neglect [2]. Child abuse and neglect affects children physically and psychologically, as well as inhibiting social adjustment. Previous studies in Japan have shown that about 50% of juveniles who turn to delinquency were abused by their parents [3,4], and most parents who abuse their children were also abused by their parents during childhood [5,6]. It is well known that being abused is one of several significant risk factors for mental disorders (e.g., borderline personality disorder, mood disorder), sex crime victimization, and domestic violence, among others [7–9]. Furthermore, the experience of being abused affects children's social cognition, especially the ability to understand others.

Some studies have examined the impact of abuse on the understanding of others' emotions and beliefs [10–14]. Cicchetti et al. [13] reported that 3- to 8-year-old abused children had difficulty passing a false belief task, which measures the development of Theory of Mind, an ability to represent others' beliefs [15,16]. Pears and Fisher [11] found that abused children who lived with foster parents performed poorer on an affective perspective-taking test [17] than those who were not abused and lived with their biological parents. These two studies suggest that the family environment plays a critical role in the ability to develop an understanding of others' beliefs and emotions. Moreover, abused children show abnormal patterns in their recognition of the facial expressions of other people. Employing the photographs of facial expressions [18], Pollak et al. [14] found that physically abused children were more likely to perceive others' emotions as anger, while neglected children were more likely to perceive them as sad. In addition, physically abused children were sensitive to the expression of anger [10,12]; they reacted to an angry face faster than non-abused children and had difficulty directing attention away from the angry face.

A number of studies have reported that abused children have difficulty getting along with other people [19,20]. The reason for this may stem from a deficit in the ability to recognize the facial expressions of others and infer their beliefs and emotions from these expressions. Thus, it is important to examine the impact of being abused on the ability to understand others through facial expressions. Previous studies have employed puppet play [11] or Ekman's photographs of facial expressions and morphing movies made from these photos [12–14]. However, tests using Ekman's photographs were limited by the ease at which participants identified the emotional expressions, which may have led to a ceiling effect. Furthermore, photos of standard emotional expressions such as "angry," "happy," or "sad" are not suitable for measuring the ability to understand the more complex or subtle expressions seen in daily life; thus, we believe that, to identify the full impact of abuse on the ability to understand others' emotions and infer intentions, photos with a wider variety of expressions, for example, "joking," "bored," and "interested," were necessary. For these reasons, we selected the "Reading the Mind in the Eyes" Test (RMET) [20,21] to measure more accurately the ability to understand complex or subtle expressions. The RMET was developed by research wherein people were asked to identify the emotion expressed in a photograph that showed only the eyes, and the most frequent response was considered the correct answer. Therefore, the RMET is the most suitable test to measure the level of participant's social recognition in real social situations. Our prediction was that the accuracy of abused children on the RMET would be lower than that of non-abused children.

Materials and Methods

Ethics Statement

This study was approved by the ethical committee at the Department of Education, Hokkaido University, Japan. The parents of the control group participants and the agent of parental authority for the abused children signed informed consent forms in advance.

Participants

Participants were 129 Japanese children in two groups: abused and non-abused (control). There were 44 children (male = 27, female = 17) in the abused group and 85 children (male = 50, female = 35) in the control group. There was no significant difference in gender proportion between the groups (χ^2 (1) = 0.078, p = .78). The demographic characteristics of the two groups are shown in Table 1. The child guidance center confirmed that children in the abused group had been victims of child abuse and neglect. Children in the abused group were 6 to 17 years old (M = 11.7, SD = 2.8) and the control group children were aged 10 to 18 (M = 11.7, SD = 2.2). There was no significant difference of age between two groups (t(72) = 0.03, p = .98). We did not test for the presence of development disorder due to child welfare system regulations in Japan. The abused children lived in a child welfare institution; foster care is not common in Japan. The institution's mission is to care for children with social adaptation or mental health problems. The children in the control group lived with their families.

In the public child welfare system in Japan, specific categories of maltreatment (e.g., physical abuse, psychological abuse, sexual abuse, and neglect) experienced by a child are protected, along with the identity of the abuser, socioeconomic status, and home environment, so we could not access this information even though our purpose was academic and the children's identities would be protected. Therefore, it was not possible to examine the impact of these variables on RMET performance without the assistance of the child welfare institution.

Reading the Mind in the Eyes Test

All participants completed the child version of the RMET [20]. This version of the RMET has 28 items and measures the ability to understand the emotional states of others. Participants are asked to look at pictures of human eyes and to choose the emotion that best fits the picture from four possibilities. Previous studies have found that adults with Asperger syndrome or high functional autism were less accurate than adult participants without autism spectrum disorder [21]. In the child version of the RMET, adults read the four choices aloud and children circled the answer they chose.

Table 1. Participant characteristics.

	Abused Group		Control Group		p-value[b]
	M	SD	M	SD	
N (Male/Female)	44 (27/17)		85 (50/35)		0.78
Age	11.7	2.8	11.7	2.2	0.98
AQ [a] total	22.5	7.9	15.1	6.2	<.0001

Notes: [a]AQ: Autism Quotient, Japanese version;
[b]χ^2 test for gender, t-tests for all others.

Autism Spectrum Quotient (AQ)

The AQ measures the symptoms of autism spectrum disorder. This scale has 50 items and is divided into 5 subscales: social skills, attention switching, attention to detail, communication, and imagination. Higher scores are associated with more autism-spectrum symptoms. The adult version of this test is a self-reported questionnaire; for the child version, the child's guardian reads the questions and the child responds. In this study, we used the Japanese version of the AQ [23]. This test is a low stress situation for the child, which is particularly important when working with abused children, because it is administered by a parent or guardian. As the child participants in this study may have a developmental disorder, we used the child version of the AQ to control for the effect of Pervasive Development Disorder (PDD) on RMET performance.

Data Analysis

In line with the previous studies using the RMET, the 28 items were classified by their emotional valence: positive (7 items), negative (10 items), or neutral (11 items) [21]. The classification of these items is summarized in Table 2. Because the number of items in each valence was different, we used the accuracy rate in the analyses.

First, we compared the mean level of AQ score between the abused and non-abused groups. Second, we compared the mean accuracy rate for each emotion valence (positive, negative, and neutral) between the abused and non-abused groups. Finally, using a multiple regression analysis, controlling for age, gender, and the AQ score, we tested the effect of being abused on emotion recognition.

Results

The mean AQ score of the abused group was significantly higher than that of the control group (abused group: M = 22.5, SD = 7.9; control: M = 15.1, SD = 6.2; t(70) = 5.3, p<.001, d = 1.08) (Table 1). The performance scores on the RMET are shown in Figure 1. The mean accuracy rate on the RMET of the abused group was significantly lower than was the control group accuracy (abused group: M = 0.60, SD = 0.15; control: M = 0.65, SD = 0.09; t(60) = 2.19, p = .032, d = 0.44). The score for positive emotional valence in the abused group was lower than that in the control group (t(127) = 3.12, p = .002, d = 0.61), but the difference in scores for negative and neutral emotional valences was not significant (negative: t(127) = 1.20, p = .23, d = 0.21, neutral: t(63) = 1.16, p = .25, d = 0.24).

Finally, a regression analysis revealed that there was a significant positive effect of age (β = .23, p = .008) and negative effect of group (control = 0; abused group = 1) (β = −.22, p = .022) on position emotion RMET score, but the effects of gender (female = 0, male = 1) (β = .07, p = .41) and AQ score (β = −.08, p = .39) were not significant.

Discussion

Our findings revealed that the accuracy of the abused children on the RMET was significant lower than the accuracy of the control group. Interestingly, this pattern was observed in only the

Table 2. Classification of RMET items by emotional valence.

Positive (7 items)		Negative (10 items)		Neutral (11 items)	
Item No.		Item No.		Item No.	
1	Kind	2	Sad	5	Making somebody do something
3	Friendly	4	Upset	8	Remembering
7, 19, 21	Interested	6, 25	Worried	9, 13, 14, 22	Thinking about something
11	Hoping	10, 15, 27	Not believing	12, 24	Serious
28	Happy	17	A bit worried	16	Made up her mind
		18	Thinking about something sad	23	Sure about something
		20	Not pleased	26	Nervous

identification of positive emotions. Furthermore, the impact of being abused on the ability to recognize positive emotion remained low after the effects of age, gender, and AQ score were removed. These results indicated that abused children were less able to recognize positive emotional expressions. Why did abused children have difficulty inferring positive emotions from facial expressions? One explanation may be that the abused children had less exposure to positive emotions from their parents than did non-abused children and may have seen their parents' negative emotional expression more often, perhaps even excessively. Therefore, abused children could identify negative expressions as well as non-abused children, but they could not identify positive expression. Indeed, Pollak et al. [14] suggested that fewer learning opportunities might affect a neglected child's ability to discern or discriminate others' emotions. According to embodied cognition theory [22], people understand others' emotion using their own sensorimotor experiences. Therefore, poor emotion recognition in abused children may stem from less experience with positive emotions.

A second possible explanation is based on the inconsistency between a parent's facial expression and future outcomes, such as the abuse that a child is subject to in an abusive family. In interpersonal situations, adults and children anticipate future outcomes from the cues found in others' facial expressions. If others look like happy, positive outcomes are anticipated. If others look angry, negative outcomes are anticipated. According to a

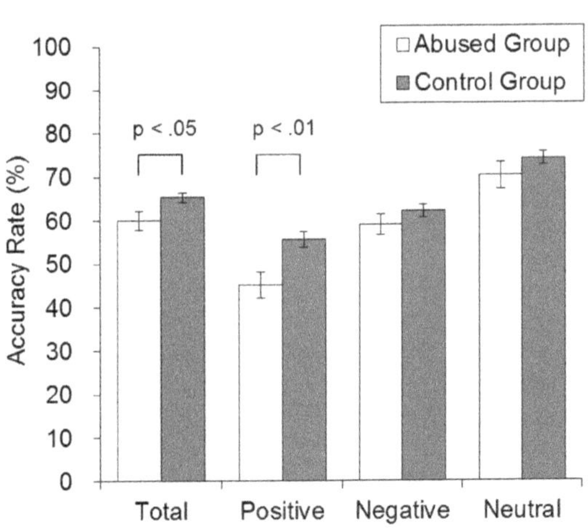

Figure 1. Mean accuracy rate for each emotional valence by group. Error bars represent standard errors.

classic psychological experiment, infants estimate their own safety from a parent's facial expression [23]. Negative facial expressions, such as angry or sad, from their parents make children upset, and positive facial expressions, such as joy and happiness, put children at ease. However, parents' positive facial expressions are not always a sign of a positive future outcome in abusive families. As abusive parents sometimes harm their children while smiling, children may not associate a positive expression with a positive outcome, and they may have trouble learning to recognize positive expressions as a result. On the other hand, a strong association between negative expressions and violence has been observed in abusive families, so children may become more sensitive to negative expressions to protect themselves. Previous studies have shown that physically abused children were sensitive to angry facial expressions [24]. Thus, the deficits in social cognition observed in abused children may be the result of adaptations engendered by living in an abusive family.

A third possible explanation comes from cognitive neuroscience. Using MRIs, recent research has demonstrated that the experience of being abused affects some areas of a child's brain [25,26]. Tomoda and colleagues [25] showed that the experience of witnessing domestic violence reduced children's gray matter volume and the thickness of the visual cortex. Other studies have found a reduction of gray matter volume in the hippocampus in adults participants who were abused by their parents in childhood [27], and in the medial orbitofrontal cortex and middle temporal cortex in abused children [28]. As the medial orbitofrontal cortex is the area of the brain that processes emotion recognition [29,30], and a recent functional MRI study demonstrated that the orbitofrontal cortex area is activated when participants identified positive emotions on the RMET [31], the RMET performance of abused children might be affected by a deficit in the medial orbitofrontal cortex.

There are some limitations to the present study. Unfortunately, we could not obtain permission to use restricted information about the abused children (e.g., the type of child abuse, the age at which abuse occurred, the identity of the abuser, and treatment information). In Japan, it is difficult to obtain such information for use in academic research. As previous research has shown differential impacts of the type of child maltreatment on a child's cognition and brain [26,27], we need to examine the impact of the type of abuse and the child's age when abused on the ability of understanding the emotions of others in Japanese children.

Conclusions

Further research is needed to better understand the impact of child abuse on social cognition; we should use fMRIs to examine the relationship between the reduction of gray matter volume in child's brain or dysfunction in the area of social brain (e.g., amygdala, medial prefrontal cortex, superior temporal sulcus, and other areas) and the performance on emotional recognition tasks. Longitudinal research, which could conduct fMRIs and emotion recognition tasks in the same samples repeatedly, could assess the impact of abuse on children properly. Thus, we could address the question of whether a child's brain was damaged by being abused. By doing so, more specific therapeutic interventions can be developed to improve abused children's interpersonal communications.

Author Contributions

Conceived and designed the experiments: MK. Performed the experiments: MK. Analyzed the data: MK HT. Contributed reagents/materials/analysis tools: MK. Wrote the paper: MK HT.

References

1. Ministry of Health LaW (2012) Annual Report on Health, Labor and Welfare the book of materials. 186 p.
2. Herrenkohl RC (2005) The definition of child maltreatment: from case study to construct. Child Abuse Negl 29: 413–424.
3. Okada R (2002) Violence to Children and from Children. Japanese Journal of Clinical Psychology 2: 169–174.
4. Justice RaTIotMo (2001) Report by research division 11- The study of child maltreatment.
5. Yagi A, Yoshino K, Karino M (2007) Influence from parents' violence on domestic violence assailant and child abuse: Men and women comparison by citizen inquiry. Japanese Journal of Child Abuse and Neglect 9: 46–54.
6. Oliver JE (1993) Intergenerational transmission of child abuse: rates, research, and clinical implications. American Journal of Psychiatry 150: 1315–1324.
7. Nishizawa S (2010) Child Abuse. Tokyo: Kodansha.
8. Daigneault I, Hebert M, McDuff P (2009) Men's and women's childhood sexual abuse and victimization in adult partner relationships: a study of risk factors. Child Abuse & Neglect 33: 638–647.
9. MacMillan HL, Fleming JE, Streiner DL, Lin E, Boyle MH, et al. (2001) Childhood abuse and lifetime psychopathology in a community sample. American Journal of Psychiatry 158: 1878–1883.
10. Masten CL, Guyer AE, Hodgdon HB, McClure EB, Charney DS, et al. (2008) Recognition of facial emotions among maltreated children with high rates of post-traumatic stress disorder. Child Abuse & Neglect 32: 139–153.
11. Pears KC, Fisher PA (2005) Emotion understanding and theory of mind among maltreated children in foster care: Evidence of deficits. Development and Psychopathology 17: 47–65.
12. Pollak SD, Tolley-Schell SA (2003) Selective attention to facial emotion in physically abused children. Journal of Abnormal Psychology 112: 323–338.
13. Cicchetti D, Rogosch FA, Maughan A, Toth SL, Bruce J (2003) False belief understanding in maltreated children. Development and Psychopathology 15: 1067–1091.
14. Pollak SD, Cicchetti D, Hornung K, Reed A (2000) Recognizing emotion in faces: Developmental effects of child abuse and neglect. Developmental Psychology 36: 679–688.
15. Wimmer H, Perner J (1983) Beliefs about beliefs: Representation and constraining function of wrong beliefs in young children's understanding of deception. Cognition 13: 103–128.
16. Premack D, Woodruff G (1978) Does the chimpanzee have a theory of mind? Behavioral and Brain Sciences 1: 515–526.
17. Denham SA (1986) Social cognition, prosocial behavior, and emotion in preschoolers: Contextual validation. Child Development 57: 194–201.
18. Ekman P, Friesen WV (1976) Pictures of facial affect. CA: Consulting Psychologists Press.
19. Elliott GC, Cunningham SM, Linder M, Colangelo M, Gross M (2005) Child physical abuse and self-perceived social isolation among adolescents. Journal of Interpersonal Violence 20: 1663–1684.
20. Price JM, Glad K (2003) Hostile attributional tendencies in maltreated children. Journal of Abnormal Child Psychology 31: 329–343.
21. Fertuck EA, Jekal A, Song I, Wyman B, Morris MC, et al. (2009) Enhanced 'Reading the Mind in the Eyes' in borderline personality disorder compared to healthy controls. Psychological Medicine 39: 1979–1988.
22. Wilson M (2002) Six views of embodied cognition. Psychonomic Bulletin & Review 9: 625–636.
23. Sorce JF, Emde RN, Campos J, Klinnert MD (1985) Maternal emotional signaling–its effect on the visual-cliff behavior of 1-year-olds. Developmental Psychology 21: 195–200.
24. Pollak SD, Kistler DJ (2002) Early experience is associated with the development of categorical representations for facial expressions of emotion. Proceedings of the National Academy of Sciences 99: 9072–9076.
25. Teicher MH (2002) Scars that won't heal: The neurobiology of child abuse. Scientific American 286: 54–61.
26. Tomoda A, Polcari A, Anderson CM, Teicher MH (2012) Reduced visual cortex gray matter volume and thickness in young adults who witnessed domestic violence during childhood. PLoS ONE 7: e52528.
27. Teicher MH, Anderson CM, Polcari A (2012) Childhood maltreatment is associated with reduced volume in the hippocampal subfields CA3, dentate gyrus, and subiculum. Proceedings of the National Academy of Sciences.
28. De Brito SA, Viding E, Sebastian CL, Kelly PA, Mechelli A, et al. (2013) Reduced orbitofrontal and temporal grey matter in a community sample of maltreated children. Journal of Child Psychology and Psychiatry 54: 105–112.
29. Shamay-Tsoory SG, Tibi-Elhanany Y, Aharon-Peretz J (2006) The ventromedial prefrontal cortex is involved in understanding affective but not cognitive theory of mind stories. Social Neuroscience 1: 149–166.
30. Leopold A, Krueger F, dal Monte O, Pardini M, Pulaski SJ, et al. (2012) Damage to the left ventromedial prefrontal cortex impacts affective theory of mind. Social Cognition and Affective Neuroscience 7: 871–880.
31. Frick C, Lang S, Kotchoubey B, Sieswerda S, Dinu-Biringer R, et al. (2012) Hypersensitivity in borderline personality disorder during mindreading. PLoS ONE 7: 8.

5

Sexuality and Gender Role in Autism Spectrum Disorder: A Case Control Study

Susanne Bejerot*, Jonna M. Eriksson

Department of Clinical Neuroscience, Karolinska Institutet, Stockholm, Sweden

Abstract

The 'extreme male brain theory of autism' describes an extreme male pattern of cognitive traits defined as strong systemising abilities paired with empathising weaknesses in autism spectrum disorder. However, beyond these cognitive traits, clinical observations have suggested an ambiguous gender-typed pattern regarding several sexually dimorphic traits. The aim of the present study was to investigate if patterns of non-cognitive sexually dimorphic traits differed between the autism spectrum disorder and control groups. Fifty adults with autism spectrum disorder and intelligence within the normal range, and 53 neurotypical controls responded to questions on gender role, self-perceived gender typicality and gender identity, as well as sexuality. Measures used were a Swedish modification of the Bem Sex Role Inventory and questions on sexuality and gender designed for the purpose of this study. Our results showed that one common gender role emerged in the autism spectrum disorder group. Masculinity (e.g. assertiveness, leadership and competitiveness) was weaker in the autism spectrum disorder group than in the controls, across men and women. Self-perceived gender typicality did not differ between the groups but tomboyism and bisexuality were overrepresented amongst women with autism spectrum disorder. Lower libido was reported amongst both male and female participants with autism spectrum disorder compared with controls. We conclude that the extreme male patterns of cognitive functions in the autistic brain do not seem to extend to gender role and sexuality. A gender-atypical pattern for these types of characteristics is suggested in autism spectrum disorder.

Editor: Christina Schmitz, Lyon Neuroscience Research Center, France

Funding: This study was founded through the Swedish Medical Research Council (Grant No 523-2011-3646) the St. Göran Foundation, the Swedish Society of Medicine and the Thuring Foundation. The funders had no role in study design, data collection and analysis, decision to publish, or preparation of the manuscript.

Competing Interests: The authors have declared that no competing interests exist.

* E-mail: susanne.bejerot@gmail.com

Introduction

The extreme male brain theory of autism describes an autistic personality characterised by extremes of typical male personality traits [1] in terms of systemising skills and weaknesses in empathy [2,3]. This connection to sex-related differences might be an important clue to the aetiology of autism spectrum disorder (ASD). Previous studies have shown that elevated levels of testosterone in amnion fluid predict autistic cognitive traits in childhood [4,5]. In both sexes, prenatal exposure to testosterone affects the foetal brain resulting in masculinised future personality and behaviours [6,7]. This is illustrated by an increased rate of tomboyism and masculinisation in women with congenital adrenal hyperplasia (CAH), an enzymatic defect resulting in highly elevated prenatal testosterone levels [8]. Although most women with CAH are heterosexual, rates of bisexual and homosexual orientation are elevated amongst this population [9]. Similarly, neural masculinisation [10] and tomboyism [11,12] have also been reported in females with ASD. In addition, ASD has been shown to be overrepresented in men as well as women with gender identity disorder [13]. It has also been implied that gender identity disorder is overrepresented in ASD [14,15]. Further, bisexuality and homosexuality are suggested to be more common in men with ASD than in men in the general population [16], while data on women with ASD is lacking.

Animal studies have indicated that abnormal prenatal testosterone levels may also affect sexual behaviour and desire in the adult animal [17,18], but whether this relationship also applies to humans is unknown. Exposure to prenatal androgens seems to be one factor in the multifaceted aetiology of autism, in line with the extreme male brain theory of autism. A study of differences between ASD and typically developed individuals regarding other sexually dimorphic traits (presumably related to prenatal masculinisation or defeminisation) may add to the knowledge of the development of an androgen dependent form of ASD. To date, no studies have examined if the extreme male cognitive pattern and the lack of gender differences in systemising-empathising dimensions extend to other sexually dimorphic traits, such as gender role and sexuality in individuals with ASD. Clinical experience, however, suggests that masculinity, expressed as male typical territorial or sexual behaviour [19,20], is attenuated in ASD of both sexes.

The current study constitutes the second half of a larger case control study on sexuality, androgen levels and anthropometric measures [21]. We found that the women with ASD had elevated testosterone levels and several physical masculinised characteristics, whereas the men with ASD displayed several physical feminised characteristics. However, the testosterone levels in the men with ASD did not differ significantly from the controls'. The current study further investigated how ASD relates to a set of non-physical attributes including gender role, gender identity, self-perceived gender typicality, androgynous behaviour in childhood, and sexuality. Gender role was assessed as adherence to a set of stereotypically male or female skills, while other aspects were self-reported. We hypothesized that male typical behaviour and perception would be weakened in ASD of both sexes, and that gender identity would be less pronounced than amongst controls.

Methods

Ethics statement

The study design was discussed in depth and approved by the local empowerment board within the Swedish Autism Society (Autism & Aspergerförbundet). The Regional Ethic committee in Stockholm approved the study protocol (Dnr 2005/644-31/3) and the investigation was conducted according to the principles expressed in the Declaration of Helsinki. All participants provided written consent and reimbursement was offered for participation (approximately £95). All participants who declined to participate or did not otherwise participate were not disadvantaged in any way by not participating in the study.

Individuals with ASD were recruited through a website for adults with ASD or through a requests sent to outpatients at a tertiary psychiatric unit for adults with ASD as well as to a community-based information centre. This centre offers information about legal aspects on the ASD diagnosis, social services etc., and is mainly serving adults diagnosed with ASD in teens or adulthood. The written request concerning the study included a brief information and the participant themselves either responded on e-mail or by post if they were interested in participating. Thereafter a brief telephone interview was conducted to ensure that the subject had attended mainstream schooling and had not been diagnosed with intellectual disability. The participants' ability to consent to the study was further confirmed in the interview by the first author, a senior psychiatrist with extensive training and experience with adult ASD. A total of three individuals were deemed not to have the capacity to consent and were subsequently excluded; two of these had a comorbid psychosis and the third had epilepsy and brain damage. None of the included participants had a caretaker or a guardian. Moreover, half of the ASD sample had a university degree and eight were parents themselves suggesting a relatively high level of functioning. For a capable group of adults with ASD – such as the participants in the present study – a requirement of consent from next of kin would presumably be perceived as humiliating, and the local empowerment board within the Swedish Autism Society did not support such a requirement.

Participants and procedure

The study involved 103 Swedish adults, including 50 adults (26 men, 24 women) diagnosed with ASD and 53 neurotypical controls (28 men, 25 women) matched on gender and age, demographics are shown in **Table** 1. Individuals with ASD were recruited through an outpatient tertiary psychiatric unit for adult ASD, a community-based centre for adults with ASD, and through a website for adults with ASD, see flowchart (**Figure** 1). Controls were recruited after the ASD group in order to be matched for gender and age. Sources for recruitment were a non-profit keep-fit organization, university, student residences, private companies, dentists and vaccination centres, employment agencies and through word-of-mouth recommendations. Inclusion criteria for both groups were Swedish/Caucasian descent and age between 20 and 47 years. Exclusion criteria were any disease or medication affecting androgen status, congenital syndrome, neurological or genetic syndrome, psychosis, diagnosed malformations, intellectual disability or having attended special education in primary or secondary school. Additional exclusion criteria in the control group were ASD or ASD in a first-degree family member. All participants denied any use of anabolic steroids and other androgen treatments other than hormonal contraceptives, used by 7 women with ASD and 14 women in the control group.

Participants in the ASD group had all been diagnosed with ASD prior to this study and their medical records were reviewed. Local diagnostic procedures require that each patient is assessed rigorously by a psychiatrist and psychologist experienced with ASD over approximately 12–20 hours before receiving the diagnosis. The assessment includes neuropsychological tests, including Wechsler Adult Intelligence Scale, and interviews with parents to obtain a developmental history. For inclusion in the current study, a senior psychiatrist with extensive training and experience with adult ASD confirmed all diagnoses through an independent diagnostic interview using the Autism Diagnostic Observation Schedule [22] and also assessed general functioning [23]. Participants were interviewed for background information and gender typical behaviour in childhood. The questionnaires regarding gender role, gender identity and sexuality were completed by the participants.

Assessment

Gender role. Gender role was measured using the MF scale [24,25], a validated Swedish modification of the Bem Sex Role Inventory, measuring stereotypical masculine and feminine traits [26]. In contrast to the Bem Sex Role Inventory which presents a single adjective (e.g. 'competitive') the MF scale provide full statements (e.g. 'I am competitive'). The MF scale consists of 43 items rated on a four-point Likert scale (1 = "I totally disagree", 2 = "I slightly disagree", 3 = "I slightly agree" and 4 = "I fully agree"). The male and female stereotypes (subscales labelled MF_M and MF_F, respectively) are assessed with 17 items each, and a further 9 items are gender neutral. The MF_M subscale contains statements regarding power, assertiveness, leadership abilities and competitiveness, while the MF_F subscale mainly measures how tender, caring and submissive a person is. In order to estimate current masculine and feminine gender roles, we performed a pilot validation study of the MF scale in a large non-clinical Caucasian and Swedish born adult population sample (N = 637, 46% men and 54% women; age range 19–65 years) (un-published). This showed mean MF_M scores of 48.6 (6.3) for men and 45.3 (5.8) for women, and mean MF_F scores of 42.4 (4.8) for men and 46.4 (4.4) for women.

Gender perception, sexual debut and behaviours. Gender identity, androgynous behaviour, gender typicality and sexuality were examined through 10 self-rated items constructed for the purpose of this study. Each item had explicit wording and straightforward response alternatives. *Gender identity* was defined as to what gender the person feels he/she belongs to; *androgynous behaviour in childhood* was characterised as being sissy/tomboyish in childhood, and *gender typicality* was defined as how gender typical the person assessed him-/herself in adulthood, in relation to other people of the same sex. Regarding sexuality, we focused on areas that possibly – but certainly not exclusively – could be related to foetal testosterone levels: libido, taking sexual initiatives, sexual interest, orgasms and sexual orientation [8,27]. Additionally two items on sexual debut were included. The items and their response options are presented in **Table 2**.

Measures of cognitive autistic traits and functioning. To describe the groups, two measures of cognitive traits, commonly used in ASD evaluations were included, The Autism Spectrum

Table 1. Demographic data of the study samples.

		ASD group		Control group	
		Males (n = 26)	**Females (n = 24)**	**Males (n = 28)**	**Females (n = 25)**
Age, years: mean (s.d.)		31.8 (7.8)	28.1 (6.3)	32.9 (7.4)	27.7 (6.7)
Education, n					
	≤9 years	5	3	1	0
	≤12 years	9	9	2	5
	University level	12	12	25	20
Cohabiting with partner, *n* (%)		3 (11.5)	6 (25)	14 (50)	12 (48)
Having children, *n* (%)		5 (19.2)	3 (12.5)	8 (28.6)	3 (12.0)
The Autism-Spectrum Quotient: mean (s.d.)		28.0 (9.4)	31.9 (7.9)	11.7 (5.4)	10.4 (4.2)
Reading the Mind in the Eyes: mean (s.d.)		25 (5)	24 (4)	27 (3)	29.5 (2.5)
GAF, current (past month): mean (s.d.)					
	Symptoms	54 (13)	52 (12)	98 (4)	97 (5)
	Functioning	57 (13)	56.5 (13)	98 (3)	97 (5)

ASD; autism spectrum disorder.

Quotient (AQ) [28] and "The Reading the Mind in the Eyes test" [29]. The AQ is a 50 item self-evaluation questionnaire, assessing personal preferences and habits, and "The Reading the Mind in the Eyes test" is a measure of mentalising skills through testing the ability to decipher emotions in photos of expressive sets of eyes. Both instruments have shown gender-variations in neurotypical people. General functioning was quantified using the Global

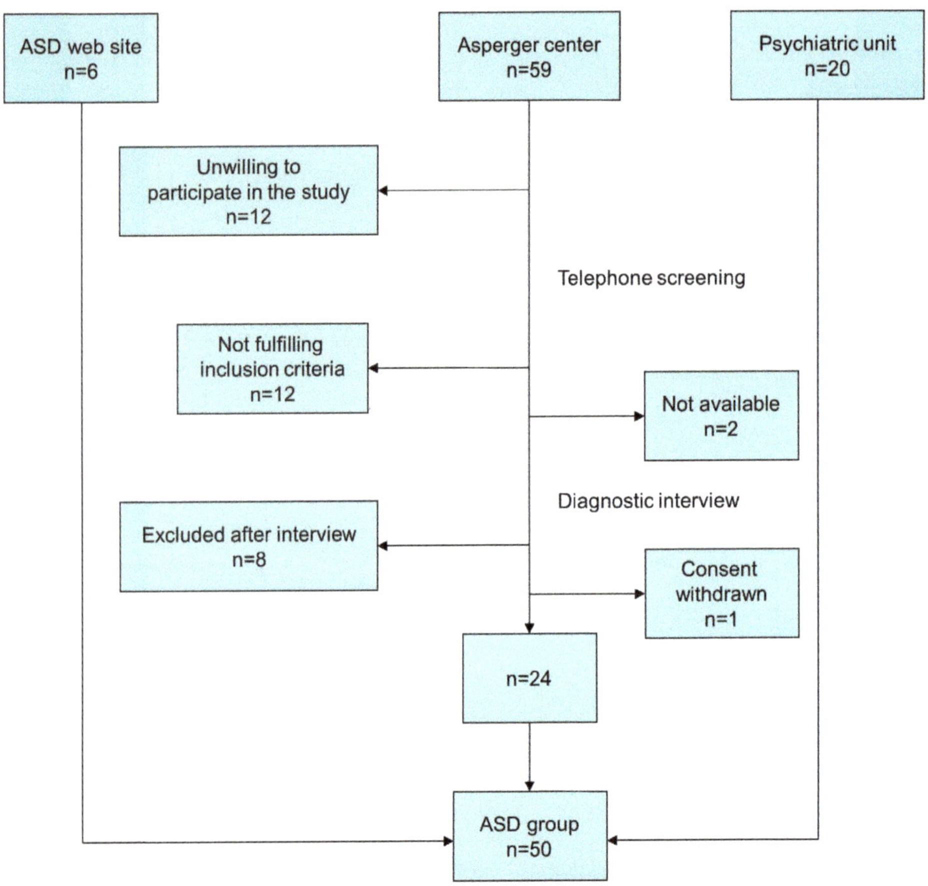

Figure 1. Flow chart for recruitment of participants with autism spectrum disorder.

Table 2. Gender perception, sexual debut and behaviour items.

Measure	Item	Response alternatives	Dichotomized responses	Interpretation
Gender perception				**as a gender-atypical pattern**
Gender identity	What is your gender identity?	"Woman", "In-between man and woman", "man", "transsexual"		
			In between man and woman, transsexual, opposite sex	Yes
			Biological sex	No
Androgynous behaviour in childhood	Were you a 'sissy'/tomboy during childhood?	"Yes"/"No"/"Don't know"		
			Yes	Yes
			No	No
Gender typicality	Do you perceive yourself as typical for your gender?	"Yes, absolutely" "Yes, to some extent" "No, not at all" "Don't know"		Reversed item, i.e. "No" indicates gender atypicality and "Yes, to some extent" some gender atypicality.
Sexual debut				
Intercourse	Have you had sexual intercourse?	"Yes"/"No"	Yes/No	
Debut age	Age for sexual debut?	Age in years		
Sexual behaviour				**as a masculinised pattern**
Libido	Have you been sexually aroused past month?	"No", "1–3 times", "4–6 times", "7–15 times", "every day"		
			Higher ≥4 times	Yes
			Lower <4 times	No
Sexual initiative	Who takes initiative to have sex?	"I", "both", "partner", "no one"		
			Initiator: I, both	Yes
			Not initiator: partner, no one	No
Sexual interest	Are you interested in sex?	"No, not at all", "Not very much", "Yes, quite", "very interested"		
			"Yes, quite", "very interested"	Yes
			"No, not at all", "Not very much	No
Orgasm frequency	Have you had an orgasm during the past month?	"No", "1–3 times", "4–6 times", "7–15 times", "every day"		
			Higher ≥4 times	Yes
			Lower <4 times	No
Sexual orientation	Whom are you attracted to?	"Men", "women", "both men and women", "neither", "other"		
			Attracted to females	Yes
			Not attracted to females	No

Note. Response alternatives "don't know" were treated as missing data.

Assessment of Functioning (GAF) [23]. Symptoms and functioning are assessed separately, each with scores ranging from 0 to 100.

Statistical analysis

Comparisons between participants with ASD and controls were made using Student's t-test for normally distributed data, the Mann-Whitney U test for non-parametrical data and χ^2-test for categorical variables. Missing data on the MF_M and MF_F subscales (0.06%) and the AQ (0.4%) was substituted using the mean value of all the items in the respective scale. A two tailed P value of <0.05 was considered significant. The gender identity was dichotomised into either biological sex or not (in-between man and woman, transsexual and non-biological sex). Sexual behaviour items were dichotomised for more straight forward interpretation of masculine dimensions of sexuality (**Table** 2).

Results

Gender role, gender identity and androgynous behaviour in childhood

As shown in **Table** 3, both men and women with ASD rated themselves as having a less masculine gender role than the controls, according to the MF_M subscale. More individuals with ASD than controls reported an atypical gender identity ($\chi^2(1, N=103)=10.1$, $\varphi=0.31$, $P=0.001$). When separated by sex, this reached significance only for the woman. Although no difference was found between men with ASD and controls on being 'a sissy in childhood', women with ASD rated themselves as being more tomboyish in childhood compared with the female controls. However, regarding self-perceived gender typicality, no significant difference was shown between the ASD group and controls for either sex (Men: MWU = 335, P = 0.98; Women: MWU = 235, P = 0.34). **Table** 4 shows the correlations between the gender role and gender perception measures in ASD males and females respectively. Additional correlations as well as frequencies and percentages of non-dichotomised gender perception data are presented in **Table** S1–S5 in File S1.

Sexuality measures

Results for the sexuality measures are presented in **Table 5** and correlations between the measures in **Table 6**. Four men and four women (16%) in the ASD group had never had intercourse at the time of the interview, significantly more than reported by the controls ($\chi^2 = 9.39$; $P = 0.002$). Amongst the participants that had experienced their sexual debut, this occurred later for the men-women combined ASD group (mean age: ASD males = 22.1(5.9), ASD females = 18.7(4.7); Control males = 17.4(4), Control females = 16.5(2.7); $MWU_{combined} = 844$, $N_{ASD} = 43$, $N_C = 53$, $P = 0.03$, $r = 0.13$). The combined ASD group reported fewer moments of sexual arousal ($\chi^2(1, N = 102) = 12.0$, $P = 0.0005$, $\varphi = 0.34$), less sexual interest ($\chi^2(1, N = 103) = 10.0$, $P = 0.002$, $\varphi = 0.31$) and less inclination to initiate sex compared with the controls ($\chi^2(1, N = 95) = 18.0$, $P = 0.00002$, $\varphi = 0.44$). **Figure** 2 shows frequencies of sexual arousal in men and women with and without ASD. Fewer men and women with ASD fell into the high frequency of orgasms group (≥4 times monthly). Notably, ten women (44%) with ASD had not had any orgasm the previous month, compared to 4 women (16%) in the control group. Homosexuality or bisexuality were equally common in the male groups (homosexual, $n_{ASD} = 2$; $n_C = 2$; bisexual, $n_{ASD} = 1$; $n_C = 2$). However, amongst the women, sexual attraction towards other females was reported more frequently in the ASD group (homosexual, $n_{ASD} = 1$; $n_C = 0$; bisexual, $n_{ASD} = 13$; $n_C = 4$). One woman and one man with ASD reported asexuality. Frequencies and percentages of non-dichotomised sexuality data as well as correlations within the male and female ASD groups respectively are presented in **Table** S6–S11 in File S2.

Discussion

In this study we have compared a set of sexually dimorphic characteristics between men and women with ASD and age matched controls. Differences in gender role, gender identity, gender behaviour in childhood and sexual behaviour and orientation were observed between individuals with ASD and neurotypical controls. Furthermore, gender differences across almost all measures were less pronounced in the ASD group than in the control group.

As foetal exposure to androgens also affects other aspects of the adult personality such as gender role, gender identity, gender behaviour and sexual orientation [30], it is reasonable to expect these traits to be similarly affected, that is, masculinised in women with ASD. This effect was partly supported in the present study. Women with ASD reported gender behaviour in childhood, adult gender identity and sexual orientation towards a masculine profile, whereas no significant differences in these characteristics were observed amongst the men. In contrast however, other measures pointed towards a de-masculinisation across gender. Both men and women with ASD reported an almost a-masculine gender role. Compared with controls, they reported lower libido, less likelihood to take sexual initiatives in romantic relationships and lower frequencies of both sexual arousal and orgasms. Although asexuality was reported in ASD, it was not reported amongst the controls. Taken together this suggests a reduced (or absent) sexual drive and de-masculinised sexual behaviour amongst the ASD participants. These findings align with the observations of attenuated masculine physical features previously reported in the ASD men, but contrast to the enhanced androgynous physical features (and elevated testosterone levels) observed in the ASD women [21].

Table 3. Gender role and gender identity measures in 50 individuals with autism spectrum disorder (ASD) and 53 neurotypical controls.

		ASD group			Control group					Effect size	
MF Gender role	**Sex**	**N**	**Mean(s.d.)**	**z-score**	**N**	**Mean(s.d.)**	**z-score**	**t(df)**	**P**	**r**	
MF_M subscale score	M	26	41.7(6.2)	−1.09 (0.99)	28	47.9(6.0)	−0.1 (0.96)	−3.7(52)	0.0005	0.46	↓
	F	24	40.0(6.6)	−0.91 (1.13)	25	47.2(5.8)	0.33 (0.99)	−4.1(47)	0.0002	0.51	↓
MF_F subscale score	M	26	44.6(6.1)	0.45 (1.28)	28	42.2(4.2)	−0.04 (0.87)	1.7(52)	0.1	0.22	±
	F	24	45.8(6.2)	−0.15 (1.41)	25	46.9(4.3)	0.11 (0.98)	−0.8(47)	0.4	0.11	±
Gender identity and gender behaviour			n(%)			n(%)		χ^2(df)	P	Φ	
Gender-atypical identity in adulthood	M	26	3(11.5)		28	1(3.6)		1.3(1)	0.3		±
	F	24	8(33)		25	0(0)		10.0(2)	0.002	0.45	↑
†Androgynous behaviour in childhood	M	22	5(23)		28	7(25)		0.04(1)	0.8	-	±
	F	19	12(67)		24	8(33)		3.9(1)	0.05	0.31	↑

MF_M and MF_F scales' z-scores normalised for gender by data from the MF validation study. ↑ denotes an increase and ↓ a decrease in masculinity.
M = Males; F = Females;
MF_M = The Masculine subscale score for self-rated masculine gender role;
MF_F = The Feminine subscale score for self-rated feminine gender role; MWU = Mann-Whitney U test.
†2 men and 4 women with ASD and 1 woman in the control group responded "I don't know" and thus excluded in the analyses; in addition to missing data in 2 men and 1 woman with ASD.

Table 4. Spearman correlations of gender perception measures in autism spectrum disorder.

	Gender identity	Androgynous in childhood	Gender typicality	MF_M	MF_F
Gender identity	-	0.10	0.35	−0.41*	0.49*
Androgynous in childhood	0.13	-	0	−0.04	0.23
Gender typicality	0.43*	0.22	-	−0.47*	0.06
MF_M	0.19	0.22	0.37	-	−0.08
MF_F	−0.43*	−0.17	−0.03	0.03	-

Showing the men above the diagonal and the women below the diagonal.
Note. Due to missing data N varies between 19 and 26.
*P<0.05.

Gender role

The ASD group reported to have a gender role characterised by weak masculinity according to the MF scale. Intriguingly, for both men and women, the control group and the validation study sample reported higher scores on masculine gender role scale than both women and men with ASD. Moreover, the gender role in ASD participants was similar for men and women. An absence of sex differences in cognition regarding empathising and systemising skills which typically are dimorphic for sex, has been previously reported in ASD [1,2]. Similarly, the current findings suggest a gender role independent of sex in ASD – a gender defiant gender role.

Gender identity and typicality

Contradictory to the non-masculine gender role, ASD women reported greater masculinised gender behaviour in childhood as well as masculinised adult gender identity than control women. Two thirds stated that they were tomboys in childhood, compared with only one third of the female controls. The finding is congruent with earlier reports of increased tomboyism in female ASD [11,12]. Although the men with ASD did not differ from the male controls in regard to gender identity or gender behaviour in childhood, a genetic male diagnosed with gender identity disorder and ASD was initially included in this study, but withdrew (data not included). Another participant with ASD, genetic female, was similarly diagnosed with gender identity disorder. ASD is suggested to be overrepresented amongst people with gender identity disorder of both sexes [13]. In addition, a study of people with gender identity disorder found that the genetic females (but not the males) reported high scores on the AQ [31]. Only the genetic males that were either asexual or heterosexual in relation to birth sex scored similarly as high as the genetic females on the AQ [32]. Consistent with those findings, the three participants in the current study with asexuality or gender identity disorder scored above the median on the AQ. Whether asexuality, gender identity disorder and ASD share similar pathophysiology should be further investigated.

Self-perceived gender typicality did not differ significantly between the ASD females and the female controls. However, as gender typicality and gender identity correlated in ASD females, it is plausible that an effect would emerge in a larger sample.

Delayed sexual debut

In the current study the ASD group was less prone to initiate sex in a romantic relationship than the controls. Moreover 16% in the ASD group had never experienced intercourse. People with ASD are typically unsuccessful in forming social relationships and the majority are victimised by peers in childhood [33]. Plausibly, a history of rejection will result in low self-esteem and social withdrawal. In order to approach another person with sexual intent, initiative, as well as assertiveness and flirting abilities are critical; abilities that are poorly developed in ASD. As a result, sexual debut may be postponed or never occur.

Libido

Another reason for a delayed sexual debut could be low libido. In this study the participants with ASD reported a lower libido and orgasm frequency than the controls. In addition, asexuality was reported by two of the ASD participants. Several reports by people with ASD suggest that asexuality is not rare in this population [15,34,35]. The individual's level of sexual desire is the result of a complex interplay between many physiological and psychosocial factors [36]. Although prenatal levels of androgens affect sexual orientation and behaviours throughout life, the relationship to sexual drive in adults is as yet unknown. Adult levels of sex hormones however, do play an important role in sexuality, but variation in testosterone levels within normal ranges has not been shown to correlate with level of sexual desire [37]. Thus, the low libido reported by our participants with ASD cannot be explained by low testosterone levels as these were not lower than in the controls [21].

Sexual preferences

Although homosexuality was equally common in ASD and controls, bisexuality was acknowledged four times more frequently amongst women with ASD than amongst female controls. In the male ASD group, only one reported bisexuality compared with two amongst the male controls. Our sample was too small to reliably identify any small variations in sexual orientation. However the observed prevalence for the control men (14%) and for the ASD men (11%) both seem high, compared with estimates in British and American populations (4.6%, 5.4%) [38,39]. Although our results neither support, nor oppose the hypothesis of an increased rate of homo- and bisexuality in men with ASD, other studies lend support for this hypothesis. Aston interviewed 28 men with Asperger syndrome who previously or currently lived with a woman [10]. Although they stated to be heterosexual, three of them reported sexual relationships with other men. In another cohort of 24 men with ASD living in residential care, 17% were bisexual or homosexual [16]. Taken together, this suggests an elevated rate of homo- and bisexuality amongst the male ASD population similar to the female.

There are a number of possible explanations for increased bisexuality in ASD. Bisexuality could reflect independence towards social norms in the society, a standpoint that is common in the ASD population. Another plausible explanation is "gender

Table 5. Sexuality parameters; ↑ denotes an increase and ↓ a decrease in masculine sexuality in autism spectrum disorder (ASD) compared with controls.

		ASD group		Control group			Effect size	
	Sex	N	*n* (%)	N	*n* (%)	χ^2(df)	P	Φ	
Sexual intercourse	M	26	22(85)	28	28(100)	4.6(1)	0.05	0.29	↓
	F	23	19(83)	25	25(100)	4.7(1)	0.05	0.31	↓
Libido	M	26	20(77)	28	28(100)	7.3(1)	0.007	0.37	↓
	F	22	13(59)	25	20(80)	6.8(1)	0.009	0.38	↓
Sexual initiatives	M	22	15(68)	28	28(100)	4.6(1)	0.05	0.29	↓
	F	19	9(47)	25	23(92)	8.9(1)	0.005	0.45	↓
Sexual interest	M	26	20(77)	28	25(89)	1.5(1)	0.3	0.17	±
	F	24	11(46)	25	22(88)	9.9(1)	0.002	0.45	↓
Orgasm frequency ≥4 times monthly	M	26	17(65)	28	25(89)	4.4 (1)	0.03	0.29	↓
	F	23	7(30)	25	15(60)	4.2 (1)	0.04	0.30	↓
Sexual attraction towards females or both males and females	M	25	23(92)	28	26(93)	1.1 (2)	0.6	0.14	±
	F	22	14(64)	25	4(16)	11.2 (2)	0.0008	0.49	↑

M = Males; F = Females; Libido dichotomised into sexual arousal ≥4 times monthly (y/n), sexual initiative were dichotomized into 'takes initiative' (y/n); sexual interest (y/n); orgasm dichotomised into ≥4 times monthly (y/n).

blindness" that leads to an appraisal of a potential partner's qualities rather than the persons' specific gender. Alternatively, increased rates of bisexuality and male-type behaviour in women could be a delayed consequence of elevated levels of androgens in foetal life.

Limitations

A study of the current size addressing sexuality is likely to be affected by selection bias. Compared to an age equivalent clinical sample of adults with ASD [41], parenthood and university education were more common in the present study, but equivalent to participants in a study on sexual wellbeing in ASD [42]. This suggests that the presently studied ASD group was relatively resourceful and could possibly be considered more "neurotypical" than ASD subjects in general. Conversely, the male controls reported higher rates of non-heterosexuality than what could be expected in the general population and 25% stated being a sissy in childhood. In sum, our male controls are presumably less gender typical than the general population, which in fact strengthens our hypothesis on ASD as being a gender-atypical disorder. Furthermore, this may explain the non-significant findings in some of the analyses.

More women in the control group than in the ASD group used contraceptive pills. Although contraceptive pills may affect sexual interest, orgasm frequency and libido there are no conclusive data on which direction these functions are affected [43]. Also, fewer participants with ASD than controls had a partner. In this study, which also included assessment of hormonal and physical measures, we only matched the participants for age, sex and absence of tattoos in order to avoid selection bias. In a future study a preferable option would be to match controls for partnership and hormonal contraception.

For this particular study we constructed self-report items on gender behaviour in childhood, gender identity and sexuality in adulthood (Table 2). The use of a non-validated instrument could be viewed as a limitation but this was a necessary procedure in order to cover areas of interest, while keeping the number of items to a minimum. Long questionnaires have resulted in high dropout rates when applied to a comparable ASD population [42], something we wanted to avoid. It would have been preferable

Table 6. Spearman correlations of sexual measures.

	Libido	Sexual initiative	Sexual interest	Orgasm frequency
Libido	-	0.228	0.603***	0.718***
Sexual initiative	0.171	-	0.452**	0.249
Sexual interest	0.347*	−0.091	-	0.440**
Orgasm frequency	0.629***	0.295*	0.329*	-

Showing the autism spectrum disorder group above the diagonal and control group below.
Note. Due to missing data N varies between 42 and 53.
*P<0.05,
**P<0.01,
***P<0.001.

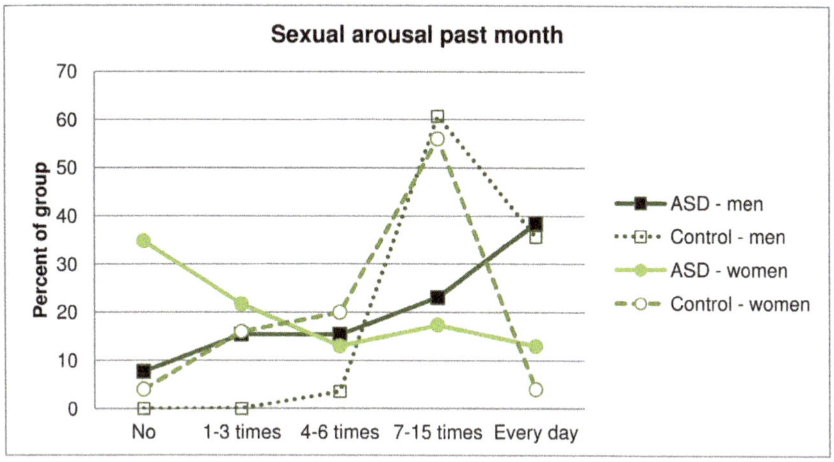

Figure 2. Frequencies of sexual arousal in men and women with and without autism spectrum disorder.

for a parent to confirm gender role behaviour in childhood. However, a prerequisite for a parent interview may create selection bias by excluding adults who reject parental interference (this applies to both subjects with ASD and controls). The validity of our findings is supported by the fact that responses on gender role and sexuality both suggested a weak masculine gender role and low libido in ASD. In addition, a number of case reports provide testimonies on gender-atypical life styles in the ASD population [15,44–49]. However, considering the small sample size in this study, current tests need replication in a larger sample.

Conclusion

This study lends support to a de-masculinised gender role independent of sex in the ASD population. The typical gender role characteristics associated with masculinised sexuality are rarely expressed in ASD, nor are ASD groups particularly feminine, with tomboyism common among women. People with ASD appear to have a lower sexual drive and minority sexual status is overrepresented compared with the non-clinical population.

While exhibiting an extreme male pattern of systemising and empathising skills across gender, men and women with ASD display a similarly gender defiant, however androgynous, gender identity. Concerning sexual behaviours and gender role a conspicuously de-masculinised pattern emerged. The extreme male brain theory of autism makes no claims about masculinity, thus not contradicting our findings. Whether prenatal androgen levels or other factors cause gender atypicality remain to be studied.

Supporting Information

File S1 Contains Tables S1–S5.

File S2 Contains Tables S6–S11.

Acknowledgments

Technical support was provided by Christina Arlinde and Ann Lindgren. Stephanie Plenty edited the manuscript. The authors want to express their gratitude towards all participants who agreed to sign up for the study and to Dr Sabina Bonde who assisted in some of the assessments.

Author Contributions

Conceived and designed the experiments: SB. Performed the experiments: SB JME. Analyzed the data: SB JME. Contributed reagents/materials/analysis tools: SB JME. Wrote the paper: SB JME.

References

1. Asperger H (1944) Die "Autistischen Psychopathen" im Kindesalter. Arch Psychiatr Nervenkr 117: 76–136.
2. Baron-Cohen S (2002) The extreme male brain theory of autism. Trends Cogn Sci 6: 248–254.
3. Baron-Cohen S, Hammer J (1997) Is autism an extreme form of the "male brain"? Adv Infancy Res 11: 193–217.
4. Auyeung B, Baron-Cohen S, Ashwin E, Knickmeyer R, Taylor K, et al. (2009) Fetal testosterone and autistic traits. Br J Psychol 100: 1–22.
5. Auyeung B, Taylor K, Hackett G, Baron-Cohen S (2010) Foetal testosterone and autistic traits in 18 to 24-month-old children. Mol Autism 1: 11.
6. Bao A-M, Swaab DF (2011) Sexual differentiation of the human brain: relation to gender identity, sexual orientation and neuropsychiatric disorders. Front Neuroendocrinol 32: 214–226. doi:10.1016/j.yfrne.2011.02.007
7. Savic I, Garcia-Falgueras A, Swaab DF (2010) Sexual differentiation of the human brain in relation to gender identity and sexual orientation. Prog Brain Res 186: 41–62.
8. Hines M (2011) Gender development and the human brain. Annu Rev Neurosci 34: 69–88.
9. Meyer-Bahlburg HFL, Dolezal C, Baker SW, New MI (2008) Sexual orientation in women with classical or non-classical congenital adrenal hyperplasia as a function of degree of prenatal androgen excess. Arch Sex Behav 37: 85–99.
10. Lai M-C, Lombardo MV, Suckling J, Ruigrok ANV, Chakrabarti B, et al. (2013) Biological sex affects the neurobiology of autism. Brain.
11. Knickmeyer RC, Wheelwright S, Baron-Cohen SB (2008) Sex-typical play: masculinization/defeminization in girls with an autism spectrum condition. J Autism Dev Disord 38: 1028–1035.
12. Ingudomnukul E, Baron-Cohen S, Wheelwright S, Knickmeyer R (2007) Elevated rates of testosterone-related disorders in women with autism spectrum conditions. Horm Behav 51: 597–604.
13. De Vries ALC, Noens ILJ, Cohen-Kettenis PT, van Berckelaer-Onnes IA, Doreleijers TA (2010) Autism spectrum disorders in gender dysphoric children and adolescents. J Autism Dev Disord 40: 930–936.
14. Tateno M, Ikeda H, Saito T (2011) [Gender dysphoria in pervasive developmental disorders]. Seishin Shinkeigaku Zasshi 113: 1173–1183.
15. Gerland G (2004) Autism: relationer och sexualitet. Stockholm, Sweden: Cura.
16. Hellemans H, Colson K, Verbraeken C, Vermeiren R, Deboutte D (2007) Sexual behavior in high-functioning male adolescents and young adults with autism spectrum disorder. J Autism Dev Disord 37: 260–269.
17. Henley CL, Nunez AA, Clemens LG (2010) Exogenous androgen during development alters adult partner preference and mating behavior in gonadally intact male rats. Horm Behav 57: 488–495.

18. Dela Cruz C, Pereira OCM (2012) Prenatal testosterone supplementation alters puberty onset, aggressive behavior, and partner preference in adult male rats. J Physiol Sci 62: 123–131.
19. Benenson JF, Markovits H, Muller I, Challen A, Carder HP (2007) Explaining sex differences in infants' preferences for groups. Infant Behav Dev 30: 587–595.
20. Markovits H, Benenson JF (2010) Males outperform females in translating social relations into spatial positions. Cognition 117: 332–340.
21. Bejerot S, Eriksson JM, Bonde S, Carlström K, Humble MB, et al. (2012) The extreme male brain revisited: gender coherence in adults with autism spectrum disorder. Br J Psychiatry 201: 116–123.
22. Lord C, Rutter M, DiLavore P, Risi S (2002) Autism Diagnostic Observation Schedule. ADOS Manual. Los Angeles.: Western Psychological Services.
23. American Psychiatric Association (1994) Diagnostic and statistical manual of mental disorders. 4th ed. Washington, DC: American Psychiatric Association.
24. Bergman H, Bergman I, Engelbrektsson K, Holm L, Johannesson K, et al. (1988) Handbook for Psychologists, part 1. Stockholm, Sweden: Karolinska Hospital.
25. Baghaei F, Rosmond R, Landén M, Westberg L, Hellstrand M, et al. (2003) Phenotypic and genotypic characteristics of women in relation to personality traits. Int J Behav Med 10: 365–378.
26. Bem SL (1974) The measurement of psychological androgyny. J Consult Clin Psychol 42: 155–162.
27. Wallen K (2005) Hormonal influences on sexually differentiated behavior in nonhuman primates. Front Neuroendocrinol 26: 7–26.
28. Baron-Cohen S, Wheelwright S, Skinner R, Martin J, Clubley E (2001) The autism-spectrum quotient (AQ): evidence from Asperger syndrome/high-functioning autism, males and females, scientists and mathematicians. J Autism Dev Disord 31: 5–17.
29. Baron-Cohen S, Wheelwright S, Hill J, Raste Y, Plumb I (2001) The "Reading the Mind in the Eyes" Test revised version: a study with normal adults, and adults with Asperger syndrome or high-functioning autism. J Child Psychol Psychiatry 42: 241–251.
30. Hines M (2010) Sex-related variation in human behavior and the brain. Trends Cogn Sci 14: 448–456.
31. Baron-Cohen S, Knickmeyer RC, Belmonte MK (2005) Sex differences in the brain: implications for explaining autism. Science 310: 819–823.
32. Jones RM, Wheelwright S, Farrell K, Martin E, Green R, et al. (2012) Brief report: female-to-male transsexual people and autistic traits. J Autism Dev Disord 42: 301–306.
33. Bejerot S, Humble MB (2013) Childhood clumsiness and peer victimization: a case-control study of psychiatric patients. BMC Psychiatry 13: 68.
34. Sinclare J (1995) Cognitive, Communication, and Interpersonal Deficits of Non-Autistic People.
35. Williams D (1994) Somebody Somewhere: Breaking Free from the World of Autism. New York: Three Rivers Press.
36. Pfaus JG (2009) Pathways of sexual desire. J Sex Med 6: 1506–1533.
37. Van Anders SM (2012) Testosterone and sexual desire in healthy women and men. Arch Sex Behav 41: 1471–1484.
38. Chandra A, Mosher WD, Copen C, Sionean C (2011) Sexual behavior, sexual attraction, and sexual identity in the United States: data from the 2006–2008 National Survey of Family Growth. Natl Health Stat Report 19: 1–36.
39. Johnson AM, Mercer CH, Erens B, Copas AJ, McManus S, et al. (2001) Sexual behaviour in Britain: partnerships, practices, and HIV risk behaviours. Lancet 358: 1835–1842.
40. Aston M (2003) Aspergers in love. London: Jessica Kingsley Publishers.
41. Rydén E, Bejerot S (2008) Autism spectrum disorders in an adult psychiatric population. A naturalistic cross-sectional controlled study. Clin Neuropsychiatry 5: 13–21.
42. Byers ES, Nichols S, Voyer SD, Reilly G (2013) Sexual well-being of a community sample of high-functioning adults on the autism spectrum who have been in a romantic relationship. Autism Int J Res Pract 17: 418–433.
43. Pastor Z, Holla K, Chmel R (2013) The influence of combined oral contraceptives on female sexual desire: a systematic review. Eur J Contracept Reprod Health Care 18: 27–43.
44. Landén M, Rasmussen P (1997) Gender identity disorder in a girl with autism–a case report. Eur Child Adolesc Psychiatry 6: 170–173.
45. Mukaddes NM (2002) Gender identity problems in autistic children Case histories. Child Care, Heal Dev 28: 529–532.
46. Williams PG, Allard AM, Sears L (1996) Case study: cross-gender preoccupations with two male children with autism. J Autism Dev Disord 26: 635–642.
47. Perera H, Gadambanathan T, Weerasiri S (2003) Gender identity disorder presenting in a girl with Asperger's disorder and obsessive compulsive disorder. Ceylon Med J 48: 57–58.
48. Kraemer B, Delsignore A, Gundelfinger R, Schnyder U, Hepp U (2005) Comorbidity of Asperger syndrome and gender identity disorder. Eur Child Adolesc Psychiatry 14: 292–296.
49. Tateno M, Tateno Y, Saito T (2008) Comorbid childhood gender identity disorder in a boy with Asperger syndrome. Psychiatry Clin Neurosci 62: 238.

6

Axonal Localization of Ca^{2+}-Dependent Activator Protein for Secretion 2 Is Critical for Subcellular Locality of Brain-Derived Neurotrophic Factor and Neurotrophin-3 Release Affecting Proper Development of Postnatal Mouse Cerebellum

Tetsushi Sadakata[1,2]*, Wataru Kakegawa[3], Yo Shinoda[2,4], Mayu Hosono[1], Ritsuko Katoh-Semba[4], Yukiko Sekine[4], Yumi Sato[4], Chihiro Saruta[4], Yasuki Ishizaki[5], Michisuke Yuzaki[3], Masami Kojima[2,6], Teiichi Furuichi[2,4]*

1 Advanced Scientific Research Leaders Development Unit, Gunma University, Maebashi, Gunma, Japan, **2** JST/CREST, Kawaguchi, Saitama, Japan, **3** Department of Physiology, School of Medicine, Keio University, Tokyo, Japan, **4** Department of Applied Biological Science, Tokyo University of Science, Noda, Chiba, Japan, **5** Department of Molecular and Cellular Neurobiology, Gunma University Graduate School of Medicine, Maebashi, Gunma, Japan, **6** Biointerface Research group, Health Research Institute, National Institute of Advanced Industrial Science and Technology (AIST), Ikeda, Osaka, Japan

Abstract

Ca^{2+}-dependent activator protein for secretion 2 (CAPS2) is a protein that is essential for enhanced release of brain-derived neurotrophic factor (BDNF) and neurotrophin-3 (NT-3) from cerebellar granule cells. We previously identified dex3, a rare alternative splice variant of CAPS2, which is overrepresented in patients with autism and is missing an exon 3 critical for axonal localization. We recently reported that a mouse model $CAPS2^{\Delta ex3/\Delta ex3}$ expressing dex3 showed autistic-like behavioral phenotypes including impaired social interaction and cognition and increased anxiety in an unfamiliar environment. Here, we verified impairment in axonal, but not somato-dendritic, localization of dex3 protein in cerebellar granule cells and demonstrated cellular and physiological phenotypes in postnatal cerebellum of $CAPS2^{\Delta ex3/\Delta ex3}$ mice. Interestingly, both BDNF and NT-3 were markedly reduced in axons of cerebellar granule cells, resulting in a significant decrease in their release. As a result, dex3 mice showed developmental deficits in dendritic arborization of Purkinje cells, vermian lobulation and fissurization, and granule cell precursor proliferation. Paired-pulse facilitation at parallel fiber-Purkinje cell synapses was also impaired. Together, our results indicate that CAPS2 plays an important role in subcellular locality (axonal vs. somato-dendritic) of enhanced BDNF and NT-3 release, which is indispensable for proper development of postnatal cerebellum.

Editor: Jean-Luc Gaiarsa, Institut National de la Santé et de la Recherche Médicale (INSERM U901), France

Funding: This study was supported by Grants-in-Aid for Scientific Research from the Japan Foundation for Neuroscience and Mental Health, the Uehara Memorial Foundation, the Takeda Science Foundation, the Nakajima Foundation, the Yamada Science Foundation, the Mother and Child Health Foundation, the NOVARTIS Foundation for the Promotion of Science, the Inamori Foundation, Scientific Research on Innovative Areas "Foundation of Synapse and Neurocircuit Pathology", the Japan Science and Technology Agency, the Japanese Ministry of Education, Culture, Sports, Science and Technology (MEXT; grant number 25110707), the Japan Society for the Promotion of Science (JSPS; grant numbers 25430061), the Institute of Physical and Chemical Research (RIKEN), and the Program to Disseminate Tenure Tracking System of MEXT granted to Gunma University. The funders had no role in study design, data collection and analysis, decision to publish, or preparation of the manuscript.

Competing Interests: The authors have declared that no competing interests exist.

* E-mail: sadakata-1024@umin.ac.jp (TS); tfuruichi@rs.tus.ac.jp (TF)

Introduction

Ca^{2+}-dependent activator protein for secretion 2 (CAPS2) is a member of the CAPS/CADPS protein family that regulates the trafficking of dense-core vesicles by binding both phosphoinositides and dense-core vesicles [1–5]. The human *CAPS2* gene locus (7q31.32) is located within the autism susceptibility locus 1 (AUTS1) [6] on chromosome 7q31–q33, one of several susceptibility loci for autism [7]. Mouse CAPS2 protein is associated with secretory vesicles containing brain-derived neurotrophic factor (BDNF) and is involved in promoting the activity-dependent release of BDNF [8,9]. BDNF plays a key role in many aspects of brain development and function, including the formation of synapses and circuits [10,11]. It has been shown that the decreased level of BDNF expression in methyl CpG-binding protein 2 (*Mecp2*)-mutant mice, a model of Rett syndrome [12], affects disease progression [13].

We previously showed that the expression of an exon 3-skipped (or -spliced out) form of CAPS2 (designated CAPS2-dex3) [14], which is now known as a rare alternative splicing variant [15,16], is increased in a subgroup of patients with autism and is not properly transported into axons [14]. Moreover, we demonstrated that neurons with increased expression of dex3 fail to properly coordinate local BDNF release from axons [14,15]. In addition, the association of CAPS2 with autism has been suggested not only by the presence of copy number variations in the CAPS2 gene in autistic patients [17–19], but also by decreased transcription of CAPS2 in the brains of people with autism [20]. Recently, it was also reported that *CAPS2* deletion and missense mutations of maternal origin contribute to onset [21].

We previously generated a mouse model CAPS2$^{\Delta ex3/\Delta ex3}$ that expressed autism-associated CAPS2 isoform dex3 and revealed that dex3 mice showed the autistic-like behavioral phenotypes [22]. In this report, we analyzed the cellular and physiological phenotypes of CAPS2$^{\Delta ex3/\Delta ex3}$ mice by focusing on the cerebellum and found that exon 3 skipping of CAPS2 influence subcellular locality (axon vs. somato-dendrite) of BDNF and NT-3 release, resulting in aberrant development of postnatal cerebellum.

Materials and Methods

Animals

CAPS2-exon3 skipped mice (deletion of exon 3, dex3) mice (CAPS2$^{\Delta ex3/\Delta ex3}$) were used as described in a previous study [22]. All experimental protocols were approved by the Institutional Animal Care and Use Committee of RIKEN, Gumma University, Keio University, and Tokyo University of Science. Mice were housed on a 12:12 h light dark cycle, with the dark cycle occurring from 20:00 to 8:00.

Antibodies

The following primary antibodies were used for immunohistochemistry: guinea pig polyclonal anti-CAPS2 (1:4,000 dilution) [9], rabbit polyclonal anti-BDNF (1:100 dilution) (Katoh-Semba et al., 1997), rabbit polyclonal anti-NT-3 (1:150 dilution) [23], rabbit polyclonal anti-calbindin (1:1,000 dilution; cat. no. AB1778, Millipore, Billerica, MA, USA), mouse monoclonal anti-tau (1:300 dilution; cat. no. 610672; BD Biosciences, San Jose, CA), and anti-phosphorylated Trk (Tyr490) (1:10 dilution; cat. no. 9141; Cell Signaling Technology, Beverly, MA).

Immunohistochemistry

C57BL/6J male mice were used after being sacrificed by anesthesia with diethyl ether. Mice were transcardially perfused, initially with PBS and then with 4% PFA in PBS. Tissues were dissected out, postfixed in 4% PFA at 4°C for 5 h, and cryoprotected by immersion in 15% sucrose in PBS overnight at 4°C. After embedding in Tissue-Tek OCT compound (Sakura Finetechnical, Tokyo, Japan), tissues were frozen in dry ice powder, and sectioned at a thickness of 15 µm using a cryostat (CM1850; Leica Microsystems, Frankfurt, Germany) at −18°C. Sections were air-dried for 1 h, and rinsed three times in PBS. After blocking with 5% donkey normal serum (Vector, Burlingame, CA, USA) in PBS, sections were reacted with specific primary antibodies at 4°C overnight, rinsed in PBS, reacted with the appropriate secondary antibody at room temperature for 1 h, and again rinsed in PBS. Immunoreacted sections were mounted with Vectorshield (Vector) mounting medium, and observed using a microscope (BX51, Olympus, Tokyo, Japan) equipped with a CCD camera (VB-7000, Keyence, Osaka, Japan). Digital images were processed using Adobe Photoshop 6.0 software.

Cerebellar primary cultures

Cerebellar primary cultures were prepared as described in a previous study [24] with minor modification. In brief, after rapid decapitation the cerebella of P0 mice were dissected out, digested for 13 minutes at 37°C with 0.1% Trypsin (Sigma-Aldrich, St. Louis, MO, USA) and 0.05% DNase I (Boehringer Mannheim, Indianapolis, IN, USA) in Ca^{2+}/Mg^{2+}-free Hanks' balanced salt solution [HBSS-CaMg(−); Sigma], and washed with HBSS-CaMg(−). They were then triturated by repeated passage through a 1-ml plastic micropipette tip in HBSS-CaMg(−) containing 0.05% DNase I and 12 mM $MgSO_4$, and washed with a serum-free Eagle minimal essential medium-based chemical-conditioned medium supplemented with 0.25% (w/v) glucose (Nacalai Tesque, Kyoto, Japan), 10 µg/ml insulin (Sigma-Aldrich), 0.1 nM L-thyroxine (Sigma-Aldrich), 0.1 mg/ml apotransferrin (Sigma-Aldrich), 1 mg/ml bovine serum albumin (BSA; Sigma-Aldrich), 2 mM L-glutamine (Nacalai Tesque), 1 µg/ml aprotinin (Sigma-Aldrich), 30 nM sodium selenite (Merck, Darmstadt, Germany), 100 U/ml penicillin (Banyu Pharmaceutical, Tokyo, Japan), and 135 µg/ml streptomycin (Meiji Seika K.K., Tokyo, Japan). The dissociated cells were plated at 5×10^5 cells per glass coverslip (12 mm in diameter; Matsunami, Tokyo, Japan), coated with poly-L-lysine (Sigma-Aldrich) and then cultured in the serum-free Eagle's minimal essential medium-based chemical-conditioned medium described above at 37 °C under a humidified 5% CO_2 atmosphere.

NT-3 release assay

The culture media were collected at 7 days *in vitro* (DIV). The quantity of NT-3 released into the media was measured using a highly sensitive two-site enzyme immunoassay as previously described [9,25].

Immunocytochemistry

Transfection was carried out using Lipofectamine 2000 Reagent (Invitrogen, Carlsbad, CA, USA). Forty-eight hours after transfection, cells were fixed with Zamboni's fixative (2% PFA in 0.1 M phosphate buffer, pH 7.4, containing 0.2% picric acid) at room temperature for 15 min. After washing three times with PBS, cells were permeabilized in PBS containing 0.02% Triton X-100 at room temperature for 5 min. After blocking with 5% normal donkey serum in PBS at room temperature for 60 min, cells were incubated with specific primary antibodies at 4°C overnight, rinsed in PBS, then incubated with Alexa-conjugated secondary antibodies (1:1,000 dilution; Invitrogen) at room temperature for 1 h, and again rinsed in PBS. Immunoreacted cells were mounted with Vectashield (Vector) mounting medium. Images were acquired with a microscope (BX51, Olympus) equipped with a CCD camera (VB-7000, Keyence). Digital images were processed using Adobe Photoshop 6.0 software. To quantify immunoreactivity, the region of interest was analyzed using NIH ImageJ software (National Institutes of Health, Bethesda, MD).

Electron microscopy

Under deep Nembutal anesthesia (250 mg/Kg, i.p.), P21 mice were transcardially perfused with 2 ml of saline followed by 25 ml of a mixture of 2.5% glutaraldehyde and 2% paraformaldehyde in 0.1 M PB. Brains were dissected and immersed in the same fixative at 4°C overnight. The cerebellum was cut into 300 mm transverse slices on a microslicer (VT1000S, Leica Microsystems) and post-fixed in cold 1% OsO_4 solution for 1 h. After dehydration in a graded series of alcohol solutions, slices were embedded in epoxy resin (EPON 812, Taab Laboratories, Reading, UK). Serial ultrathin 70 nm sections were cut on an ultramicrotome (EM UC6, Leica Microsystems), mounted on 200 mesh uncoated copper grids, and metal stained with uranyl acetate/lead citrate. The grids were examined with a transmission electron microscope (1200EX, JEOL) at 80 kV.

Electrophysiology

Parasagittal cerebellar slices (200 μm thick) were prepared from CAPS2$^{\Delta ex3/\Delta ex3}$ mice and wild-type littermates (P25–35) in accordance with the institution's guidelines of Keio University, as previously reported [26]. Whole-cell voltage-clamp recordings were made from visually identified Purkinje cells (PCs) with an Axopatch 200B amplifier (Axon Instruments, Foster City, CA), and the pCLAMP system (version 9.2, Axon Instruments) was used for data acquisition and analysis. Patch pipettes were pulled from borosilicate glass capillaries to achieve a resistance of 2 to 4 MΩ when filled with a solution containing (65 mM K-gluconate, 65 mM Cs-methanesulfonate, 10 mM KCl, 1 mM $MgCl_2$, 4 mM Na_2ATP, 1 mM Na_2GTP, 20 mM HEPES, 5 mM sucrose, and 0.4 mM EGTA (pH 7.3, 295 mOsm/kg). The external Ringer's solution contained 125 mM NaCl, 2.5 mM KCl, 2 mM $CaCl_2$, 1 mM $MgCl_2$, 26 mM $NaHCO_3$, 1.25 mM NaH_2PO_4, 10 mM D-glucose, and 0.1 mM picrotoxin (to inhibit GABAergic synapses) and was bubbled with 95% O_2 and 5% CO_2 at room temperature (24°C). To evoke parallel fiber-evoked excitatory postsynaptic currents (PF-EPSCs), a stimulating electrode was placed in the molecular layer (stimulus intensity, 0 to 200 μA, 10 μs duration), and selective stimulation of parallel fibers (PFs) was confirmed by the paired-pulse facilitation (PPF) of PF-EPSC amplitudes with a 50 ms interstimulus interval. The current traces were filtered at 1 kHz and digitized at 4 kHz.

Results

CAPS2 exon 3-skipped homozygote mice (CAPS2$^{\Delta ex3/\Delta ex3}$) were born and exhibited no obvious difference in life expectancy compared to control mice [22]. However, the body weight of CAPS2$^{\Delta ex3/\Delta ex3}$ male mice was lower than that of their wild-type littermates (34.21±0.97 g in wild types *vs.* 28.12±0.4 g in CAPS2$^{\Delta ex3/\Delta ex3}$ mice at 4 months old, mean ± s.e.m., $P<0.01$, by Student's *t*-test).

CAPS2-dex3 protein fails to accumulate in parallel fibers, axons of cerebellar granule cells, in the molecular layer of the cerebellar cortex

At first, we examined the subcellular localization of CAPS2-deletion of exon3 (dex3) expressed in CAPS2$^{\Delta ex3/\Delta ex3}$ mice. Development of the cerebellar cortex includes dynamic changes in the laminar architecture. The external granular layer (EGL), the site at which robust proliferation of granule cell precursors occurs, thickens progressively until a peak is reached at approximately the first postnatal week; the EGL then gradually thins as the proliferation of these precursors decline, disappearing by the weaning stage, which occurs around the third postnatal week. In the P7 cerebellum, wild-type CAPS2 protein was mostly localized in the granule cell axons (parallel fibers) extending into the molecular layer (ML) (Fig. 1A), whereas dex3 protein was not localized in the axons in the ML and instead accumulated densely in the cell soma in the internal granule cell layer (IGL) and sparsely in the EGL (Fig. 1B). This symmetric localization pattern was more drastic in the P21 cerebellum: wild-type CAPS2 protein was localized in the ML, axon of cerebellar granule cells (Fig. 1C), whereas dex3 protein was not in the ML but accumulated in the IGL, soma and/or dendrites of cerebellar granule cells (Fig. 1D).

We further analyzed the subcellular localization of CAPS2-dex3 protein using cerebellar primary cultures at 21 days *in vitro* (DIV) (Fig. 1E–M). In wild-type cultures, punctate immunoreactivity for CAPS2 was largely concentrated near Purkinje cells innervated by many granule cell axons, demonstrating the presynaptic localization of CAPS2 in parallel fibers (PFs) (Fig. 1E–G). In contrast, in CAPS2$^{\Delta ex3/\Delta ex3}$ cultures, CAPS2-immunoreactive signal was hardly detected around calbindin-immunopositive dendrites of Purkinje cells and predominated in soma of granule cells instead (Fig. 1K–M). In heterozygote CAPS2$^{+/\Delta ex3}$ cultures, CAPS2-immunoreactive signal was localized in granule cell soma as well as around the dendrites of Purkinje cells (Fig. 1H–J).

Taken together, the results obtained using an animal model showed that the exon 3-skipped alternative splicing affects the subcellular localization of CAPS2 protein in the axonal compartment.

CAPS2-dex3 affects axonal localization and release of BDNF and NT-3 in cerebellar granule cells

CAPS2 is found associated with secretory vesicles containing BDNF and NT-3, and it promotes release of these two neurotrophins from cerebellar granule cells [9]. TrkB, the BDNF receptor, is expressed in postsynaptic Purkinje cells as well as in presynaptic granule cells. BDNF is released from the PF terminals of granule cells, which innervate the distal dendrites of Purkinje cells, and is thought to function in autocrine and anterograde signaling [27,28]. BDNF is also known to be released from climbing fibers that innervate the proximal dendrites of Purkinje cells, and the trafficking of BDNF along climbing fibers is dependent on another family member, CAPS1 [29]. We examined the subcellular localization of endogenous BDNF in CAPS2$^{\Delta ex3/\Delta ex3}$ mice. In the P7 wild-type cerebellum, BDNF immunoreactivity was localized in the ML, IGL, and the soma and distal and proximal dendrites of Purkinje cells (Fig. 2A). In contrast, in the CAPS2$^{\Delta ex3/\Delta ex3}$ cerebellum, BDNF immunoreactivity was detected in the proximal dendrites of Purkinje cells, but seemed to be reduced in the ML (PF terminals) (Fig. 2C).

Secreted neurotrophins activate their Trk receptors on target cells, leading to the autophosphorylation of Trk receptors. To localize Trk receptors activated by neurotrophins released from granule cells, we next immunostained the cerebellar cortex of P7 wild-type and CAPS2$^{\Delta ex3/\Delta ex3}$ mice with an anti-phosphorylated Trk (pTrk) antibody (Fig. 2E and G). In the wild-type, intense pTrk immunoreactivity was observed in the ML and the Purkinje cell layer (Fig. 2E). The immunoreactivity in the wild-type ML was observed around both distal and proximal dendrites of Purkinje cells (reflecting Trk activation by anterograde signaling), although a part of this labeling was probably derived from the parallel fiber terminals (reflecting Trk activation by autocrine signaling). In comparison, in CAPS2$^{\Delta ex3/\Delta ex3}$ mice, pTrk immunoreactivity was decreased in the ML, but detectable at a similar level in the soma, compared with wild-type (Fig. 2G). These results suggest that, in the cerebellar cortex of P7 CAPS2$^{\Delta ex3/\Delta ex3}$ mice, there is a reduction in autocrine and paracrine activation of Trk by BDNF released from parallel fibers. It is probable that Trk activation in the Purkinje cell soma was dependent on BDNF released from climbing fiber terminals.

We next examined subcellular localization of NT-3 and quantified amounts of released NT-3 and cellular NT-3 in primary cultured cerebellar granule cells at 7DIV. In wild-type cerebellar sections at P7, the CAPS2 protein produced in granule cells is localized in both the internal granule layer and the molecular layer, in which soma and axons of granule cells, respectively, are localized (Fig. 1A). In contrast, at P21, the protein is almost exclusively localized in the molecular layer, in which the axon terminals of granule cells innervate the dendrites of Purkinje cells (Fig. 1C). Similarly, in wild-type cerebellar cultures at 7 DIV, CAPS2 immunoreactivity was localized not only in axons, but in soma of granule cells as well (Fig. 3A). NT-3 immunoreactivities were also localized in neurite meshwork as well as soma

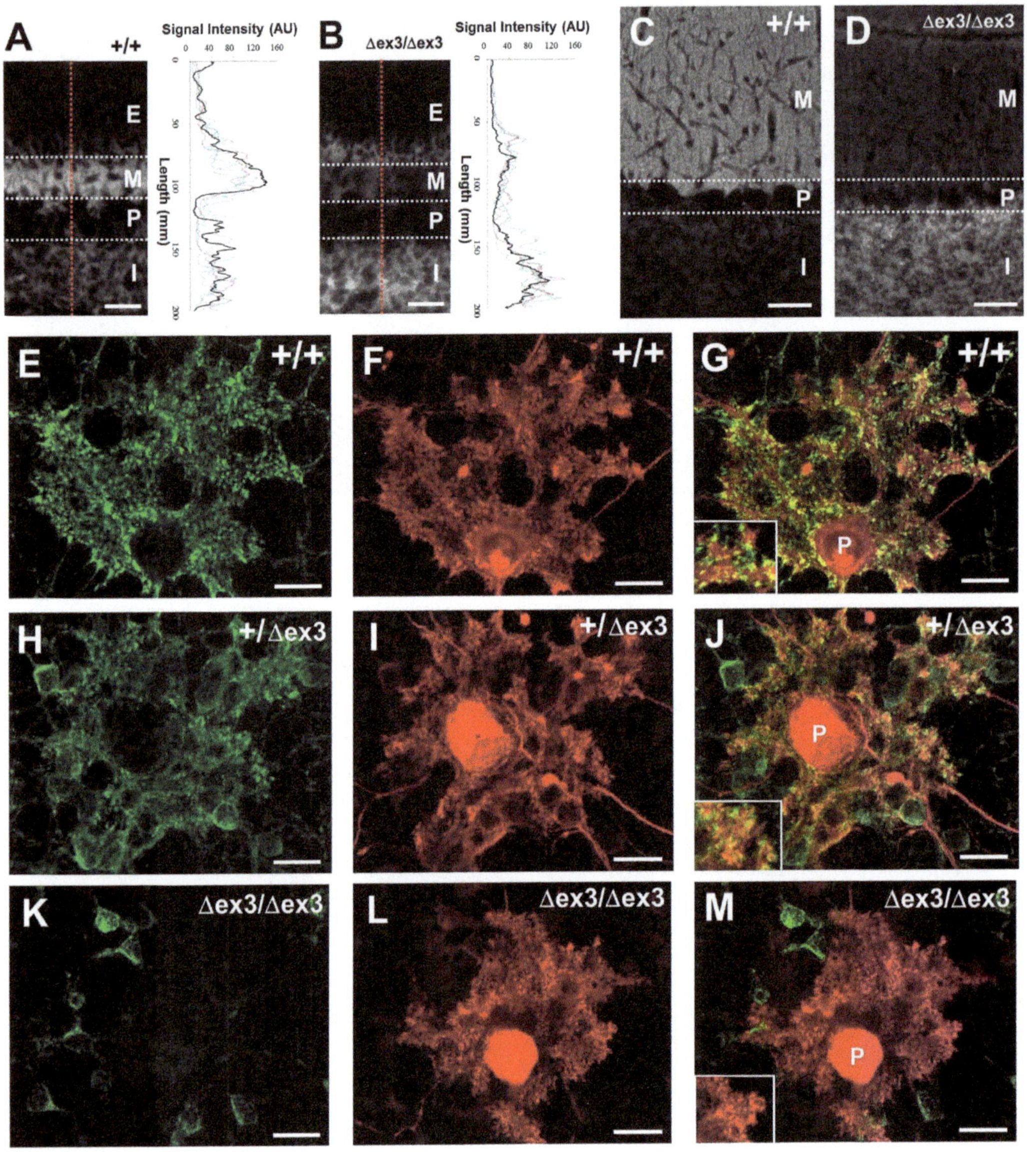

Figure 1. Distribution of CAPS2 protein in the CAPS2$^{\Delta ex3/\Delta ex3}$ mouse cerebellum and cerebellar culture. (A, B) Sagittal sections of P7 wild-type (A) and CAPS2$^{\Delta ex3/\Delta ex3}$ (B) cerebellum were immunolabeled with anti-CAPS2 antibody. Immunosignal intensity of red dotted lines is shown by black lines in the graphs. Signal intensity from the other three images is shown in colored lines. Scale bars, 30 μm. (C, D) Sagittal sections of P21 wild-type (C) and CAPS2$^{\Delta ex3/\Delta ex3}$ (D) cerebellum were immunolabeled with an anti-CAPS2 antibody. E, external granular layer; M, molecular layer; P, Purkinje cell layer; I, internal granular layer. Scale bars, 20 μm. (E–M) Subcellular localization of CAPS2 (green; E, H, K) and calbindin (red; F, I, L) in wild-type (E–G), CAPS2$^{+/\Delta ex3}$ (H–J) and CAPS2$^{\Delta ex3/\Delta ex3}$ (K–M) cerebellar primary cultures at 14 days *in vitro* (DIV). A merged image is shown in (G, J, M). Insets: higher magnification. P, Purkinje cell. Scale bars, 20 μm.

throughout the wild-type cell cultures (Fig. 3A–C). On the other hand, such meshwork-like neurite immunoreactivities for CAPS2 and NT-3 were decreased in CAPS2$^{\Delta ex3/\Delta ex3}$ cell cultures (Fig. 3D–F) compared with wild-type cultures. There was a significant difference in NT-3 immunolabeling intensity along the axon between wild-type and dex3 neurons (Fig. 3G). In addition, NT-3 immunolabeling intensity was increased in the somata of dex3 neurons compared with wild-type neurons (Fig. 3H).

We next analyzed the amounts of NT-3 released into cerebellar culture media. Endogenous NT-3, activity-dependently released into the media, was barely detectable in cultures by enzyme-linked immunoabsorbent assay [9]. We compared the total amount of NT-3 released into the culture media over a period of 7 days, during which a fraction of the NT-3 is likely released by spontaneous activity, between wild-type and mutant mouse cultures. As shown in Fig. 3I, the amount of NT-3 in the media was significantly reduced in CAPS2$^{\Delta ex3/\Delta ex3}$ cultures compared with wild-type cultures. On the contrary, the amount of NT-3 in the cell lysate was increased in CAPS2$^{+/\Delta ex3}$ and CAPS2$^{\Delta ex3/\Delta ex3}$ cultures as compared with wild-type cultures (Fig. 3J). Thus, it might be assumed that release of NT-3 was decreased and intracellular accumulation of NT-3 was increased instead in CAPS2$^{\Delta ex3/\Delta ex3}$.

Next, we tested subcellular localization of HA-tagged BDNF (BDNF-HA) that was exogenously overexpressed in cerebellar granule cell cultures. HA immunoreactivity was localized to axons

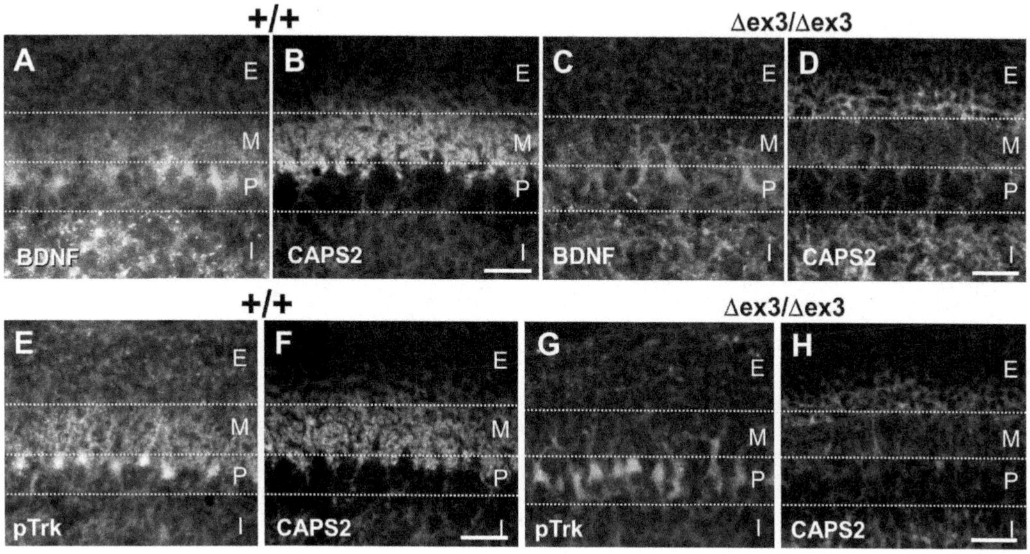

Figure 2. Decreased immunoreactivity of BDNF and phosphorylated Trk (Tyr490) in the molecular layer of CAPS2$^{\Delta ex3/\Delta ex3}$ cerebellum. (A–D) Sagittal sections of P7 wild-type (A, B) and CAPS2$^{\Delta ex3/\Delta ex3}$ (C, D) cerebellum were immunolabeled with an anti-BDNF (A, C) and an anti-CAPS2 (B, D) antibody. (E–H) Sagittal sections of P7 wild-type (E, F) and CAPS2$^{\Delta ex3/\Delta ex3}$ (G, H) cerebellum were immunolabeled with an anti-pTrk (E, G) and an anti-CAPS2 (F, H) antibody. E, external granular layer; M, molecular layer; P, Purkinje cell layer; I, internal granular layer. Scale bars, 40 μm.

with tau immunoreactivity in wild-type granule cells (Fig. 4A–C) but was yet very little in axons of CAPS2$^{\Delta ex3/\Delta ex3}$ granule cells (Fig. 4D–F). The amount of BDNF released into the culture media was hardly detected, even if BDNF was exogenously transfected as previously described [9,24]. Therefore, to compare BDNF release levels between wild-type and CAPS2$^{\Delta ex3/\Delta ex3}$ cultures, we evaluated immuno-intensity of endogenous BDNF incorporated into target Purkinje cell bodies after released from granule cell axons using confocal microscopy (Fig. 4G). The result showed that internalization of BDNF into the Purkinje cell soma was significantly reduced in CAPS2$^{\Delta ex3/\Delta ex3}$ granule cells compared with wild-type cells. On the other hand, amount of cellular BDNF contents was higher in CAPS2$^{\Delta ex3/\Delta ex3}$ cell lysates than wild-type cell lysates (Fig. 4H). Together, these data suggest that BDNF is accumulated in the cell soma and its release might be affected, when expression of exon 3-skipped CAPS2 is increased.

Developmental deficits in the postnatal cerebellum of CAPS2$^{\Delta ex3/\Delta ex3}$ mice

We analyzed morphological development of CAPS2$^{\Delta ex3/\Delta ex3}$ cerebellum. In terms of Purkinje cells, there was no significant difference in the cell density among three genotypes wild-type, CAPS2$^{+/\Delta ex3}$, and CAPS2$^{\Delta ex3/\Delta ex3}$ at P7 (Fig. 5A) and P21 (Fig. 5B). Moreover, there was no difference of Purkinje cell dendrite length among three genotypes at P7 and P21 (Fig. 5C and D). In terms of cerebellar lobulation, the area of vermian lobules VI-VII was decreased in CAPS2$^{\Delta ex3/\Delta ex3}$ cerebellum at P17 (Fig. 5E) but not P21 (Fig. 5F) as compared with wild-type. The depth of the intercrural fissure which divides the lobule VI and VII was decreased in CAPS2$^{\Delta ex3/\Delta ex3}$ cerebellum as compared with wild-type and CAPS2$^{+/\Delta ex3}$ (Fig. 5G). In terms of the EGL in which granule cell precursors robustly proliferate by the second postnatal period, CAPS2$^{+/\Delta ex3}$ and CAPS2$^{\Delta ex3/\Delta ex3}$ cerebella had thicker EGL than wild-type even at P17 (Fig. 5H). But, the EGL was no longer detectable in the CAPS2$^{\Delta ex3/\Delta ex3}$ cerebellum by P28 (data not shown). Taken together, these data suggest that postnatal CAPS2$^{\Delta ex3/\Delta ex3}$ cerebellum appears to have a developmental delay similarly to CAPS2 knockout (KO) cerebellum [24].

Next, we analyzed the fine structure of PF-Purkinje cell (PC) synapses at P21. In the wild-type cerebellum, synaptic vesicles within the PF terminals connecting Purkinje cell spines were concentrated near the active zones and were fully distributed over the presynaptic boutons of PFs (Fig. 6A). Overall synaptic cytoarchitecture regarding clear synaptic vesicles, active zone and postsynaptic density appeared to be similar between wild-type (Fig. 6A) and CAPS2$^{\Delta ex3/\Delta ex3}$ (Fig. 6B). Quantification of presynaptic vesicle distribution from the active zone showed that number of synaptic vesicle 300–600 nm far from the active zone tended to be larger in CAPS2$^{\Delta ex3/\Delta ex3}$ than wild-type (Fig. 6C), although there was no statistical difference between these two genotypes.

Impairment of short-term plasticity at CAPS2$^{\Delta ex3/\Delta ex3}$ PF-PC synapses

We investigated the synaptic function of PF-PC synapses at P25–35. Little difference was found to exist between wild-type and CAPS2$^{\Delta ex3/\Delta ex3}$ mice in terms of the peak amplitudes of PF-evoked excitatory postsynaptic currents (PF-EPSCs) (Fig. 7A), thus indicating that the basic synaptic transmission function in CAPS2$^{\Delta ex3/\Delta ex3}$ mice was unimpaired.

Paired-pulse facilitation (PPF) of the PF-EPSC (defined as the ratio of the amplitude of the second EPSC to that of the first EPSC) is thought to reflect changes in presynaptic function and is considered to be a kind of short-term synaptic plasticity [30]. We performed PPF analysis at PF-PC synapses in the anterior lobe (lobules II–V), central lobe (lobules VI–VII), and posterior lobe (lobule IX) at P25–35 (Fig. 7B). The results revealed that, for brief interstimulus intervals (<100 ms), the degree of PPF at PF-PC synapses was markedly lower in CAPS2$^{\Delta ex3/\Delta ex3}$ mice than in wild-type mice. Impairment of this presynaptic function was observed in all three lobes examined. However, synaptic plasticity at PF-PC synapses, such as a long-term depression (LTD), a molecular basis of the motor learning and memory [31], was

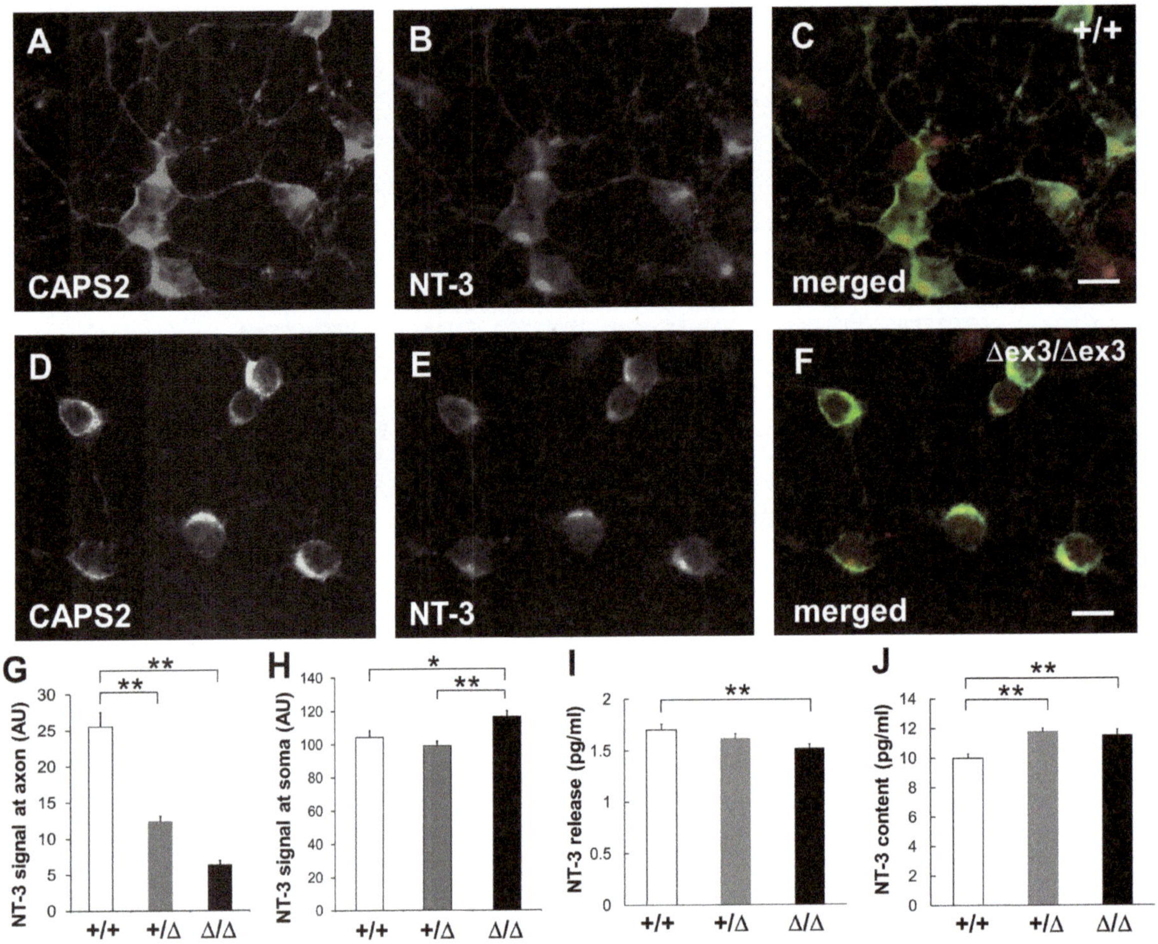

Figure 3. Decreased trafficking and release of NT-3 in the CAPS2$^{\Delta ex3/\Delta ex3}$ primary cerebellar culture. (A–F) Subcellular localization of CAPS2 (A, D) and NT-3 (B, E) in wild-type (A–C) and CAPS2$^{\Delta ex3/\Delta ex3}$ (D–F) cerebellar primary cultures at 7 DIV. A merged image of CAPS2 (*green*) and NT-3 (*red*) is shown in (C, F). Scale bars, 10 μm. (G) Immunolabeling intensities of NT-3 along the axons of wild-type (white bar, $n = 27$), CAPS2$^{+/\Delta ex3}$ (gray bar, $n = 23$) and CAPS2$^{\Delta ex3/\Delta ex3}$ (black bar, $n = 21$) cells are shown. Axons were identified by tau immunostaining and by their characteristic thin and long processes. Signal intensities were quantified with NIH ImageJ per unit length (arbitrary unit). (H) Immunolabeling intensities of NT-3 on the somata of wild-type (white bar, $n = 23$), CAPS2$^{+/\Delta ex3}$ (gray bar, $n = 23$) and CAPS2$^{\Delta ex3/\Delta ex3}$ (black bar, $n = 22$) cells are shown. Signal intensities were quantified per unit area (arbitrary unit). *$P<0.05$; **$P<0.01$, by Student's *t*-test. (I) NT-3 release activity in the wild-type (white bar, $n = 16$), CAPS2$^{+/\Delta ex3}$ (gray bar, $n = 21$) and CAPS2$^{\Delta ex3/\Delta ex3}$ (black bar, $n = 27$) cerebellar cultures was evaluated by measuring the levels of NT-3 spontaneously secreted into the culture medium by primary dissociation cultures at 7 DIV with an enzyme immunoassay. $P<0.05$, one-factor ANOVA. **$P<0.01$, by post-hoc *t*-test. (J) The amount of NT-3 in the cell lysates of wild-type (white bar, $n = 7$), CAPS2$^{+/\Delta ex3}$ (gray bar, $n = 13$) and CAPS2$^{\Delta ex3/\Delta ex3}$ (black bar, $n = 7$) cultures was evaluated as indicated in (I). $P<0.01$, one-factor ANOVA. **$P<0.01$, by post-hoc *t*-test. The error bars indicate the s.e.m.

normally observed in CAPS2$^{\Delta ex3/\Delta ex3}$ mice as well as wild-type littermates (data not shown). The results suggest that expression of dex3 disturbs the presynaptic properties of PF-PC synapses.

Discussion

In this report, we focused on the cellular and physiological phenotype in the cerebellum of a mouse line CAPS2$^{\Delta ex3/\Delta ex3}$ expressing dex3, the same as a rare alternatively-spliced variant of human CAPS2 that was identified in some individuals with autism [14]. We verified a deficit in axonal localization of dex3 protein in cerebellar granule cells in *in vitro* cultures as well as *in vivo*. Thus, we assume that CAPS2$^{\Delta ex3/\Delta ex3}$ mice have disturbance in CAPS2-mediated promotion of the secretory vesicle secretion pathway: probably decreased axonal promotion but normal somato-dendritic promotion. Interestingly, CAPS2$^{\Delta ex3/\Delta ex3}$ mice also displayed a decrease in axonal localization of BDNF and NT-3. Release of BDNF and NT-3 from cerebellar granule cells was decreased in CAPS2$^{\Delta ex3/\Delta ex3}$ mice. In connection with the indispensable role of these two neurotrophins in cerebellar postnatal development, CAPS2$^{\Delta ex3/\Delta ex3}$ mice showed several developmental deficits including decreased area of vermian lobules VI and VII, shallow intercrural fissures, delayed proliferation of granule cell precursors in the EGL, and delayed migration of post-mitotic granule cells. At PF-PC synapses, paired-pulse facilitation was also impaired in CAPS2$^{\Delta ex3/\Delta ex3}$ mice. CAPS2 is thought to promote BDNF and NT-3 release [9,24]. Our results suggest subcellular locality in CAPS2-mediated enhancement of BDNF and NT-3 release is associated with the proper development and function of the cerebellum.

Specific lobule hypoplasia and neurotrophin

We showed that the area of lobules VI-VII and the depth of intercrural fissure which divide lobule VI and VII were decreased in the CAPS2$^{\Delta ex3/\Delta ex3}$ cerebellum. BDNF and NT-3 KO mice

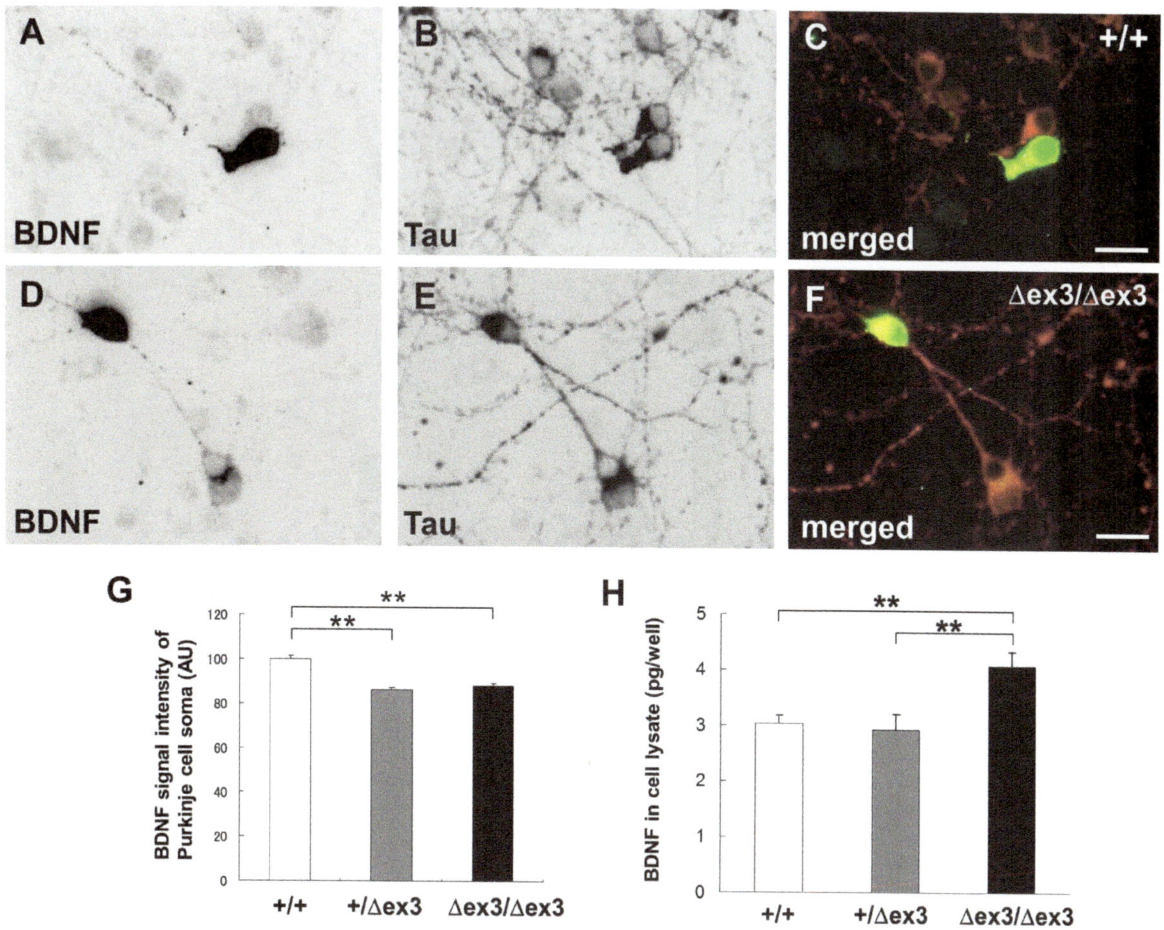

Figure 4. Aberrant distribution of BDNF and decreased BDNF immunoreactivity in the cerebellum. (A–F) Subcellular localization of exogenously expressed C-terminal HA-tagged BDNF (A, D) and tau protein (B, E) in wild-type (A–C) and CAPS2$^{\Delta ex3/\Delta ex3}$ (D–F) cerebellar primary cultures immunostained for HA and tau at 8 DIV. A merged image of HA (*green*) and tau (*red*) is shown in (C, F). Scale bars, 20 μm. (G) The intensity of BDNF immunoreactivity in the Purkinje cells of wild-type (white bar, $n=226$), CAPS2$^{+/\Delta ex3}$ (gray bar, $n=215$) and CAPS2$^{\Delta ex3/\Delta ex3}$ (black bar, $n=215$) cultures was quantified using confocal microscopy. $P<0.01$, one-factor ANOVA. $^{**}P<0.01$, by post-hoc *t*-test. (H) The amount of BDNF in the cell lysates of wild-type (white bar, $n=6$), CAPS2$^{+/\Delta ex3}$ (gray bar, $n=8$) and CAPS2$^{\Delta ex3/\Delta ex3}$ (black bar, $n=6$) cultures was evaluated at 7 DIV with an enzyme immunoassay. $P<0.01$, one-factor ANOVA. $^{**}P<0.01$, by post-hoc *t*-test. The error bars indicate the s.e.m.

also show a lobulation deficit between lobules VI and VII [27,32]. Katoh-Semba and her colleagues showed a higher concentration of NT-3 in posterior lobules than in anterior lobules, and that depletion of NT-3 from the mouse brain causes an increase in granule cell apoptosis within lobules VI-VII [25], suggesting that the requirement of neurotrophins for granule cell survival seems to be different between cerebellar lobules. In this regard, it is noteworthy that there are localized high BDNF protein levels in lobules VI-VII and localized high NT-3 mRNA levels in lobules VI-VII during development [24]. Taken together, these results suggest that lobules VI-VII express more BDNF and NT-3 than do the other cerebellar compartments during development; thus, these lobules are more susceptible to the effects of depletion of these neurotrophins.

PF-PC synapse function of CAPS2$^{\Delta ex3/\Delta ex3}$ cerebellum

We found the degree of PPF at PF-PC synapses was lower in CAPS2$^{\Delta ex3/\Delta ex3}$ mice, which seemed to be consistent in understanding a role of CAPS2 in PFs, because similar results were obtained in CAPS2 KO mice (Sadakata et al., 2007a). In addition, a concomitant decrease in PPF during enhancement of evoked EPSCs is generally accepted to be a strong indication for presynaptic modifications of synaptic transmission. BDNF KO mice is known to show impaired PPF at PF-PC synapses together with increased vesicle number per synapse [33]. In this regard, it is interesting the number of synaptic vesicle far from the active zone tended to be larger in CAPS2$^{\Delta ex3/\Delta ex3}$ PF terminal. It is probable that decrease PPF of CAPS2$^{\Delta ex3/\Delta ex3}$ mice depends on the change of synaptic vesicle distribution by decreased BDNF release.

The possible effect of CAPS2-dex3 copy number

The amount of BDNF released into the culture media was barely detectable, even when BDNF was exogenously transfected. Therefore, to compare BDNF release levels between wild-type and CAPS2$^{\Delta ex3/\Delta ex3}$ cultures, we evaluated the immunolabeling intensities of endogenous BDNF incorporated into target Purkinje cell bodies using confocal microscopy. In Fig. 4G, CAPS2$^{\Delta ex3/\Delta ex3}$ cultures showed a decrease in endogenous BDNF uptake into Purkinje neurons. Correspondingly, as shown in Fig. 4H, there was an increase in BDNF levels in their lysates, where most of the BDNF was likely derived from granule cells. In comparison, CAPS2$^{+/\Delta ex3}$ cultures showed a decrease in endogenous BDNF

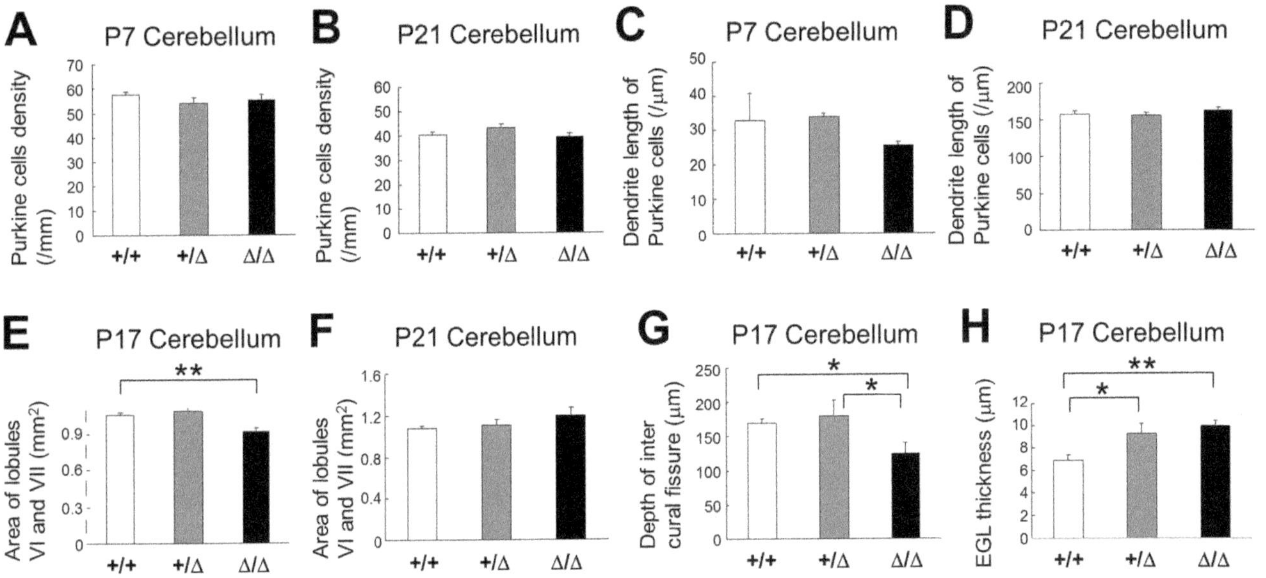

Figure 5. Abnormal immunohistochemistry in the CAPS2$^{\Delta ex3/\Delta ex3}$ cerebellum. (A) The cell densities of calbindin-positive Purkinje cells for wild-type (white, $n = 8$), CAPS2$^{+/\Delta ex3}$ (gray, $n = 9$), and CAPS2$^{\Delta ex3/\Delta ex3}$ (black, $n = 10$) mice at P7. (B) The cell densities of calbindin-positive Purkinje cells for wild-type (white, $n = 8$), CAPS2$^{+/\Delta ex3}$ (gray, $n = 10$), and CAPS2$^{\Delta ex3/\Delta ex3}$ (black, $n = 10$) mice at P21. (C) The dendrite length of calbindin-positive Purkinje cells for wild-type (white, $n = 24$), CAPS2$^{+/\Delta ex3}$ (gray, $n = 30$), and CAPS2$^{\Delta ex3/\Delta ex3}$ (black, $n = 30$) mice at P7. (D) The dendrite length of calbindin-positive Purkinje cells for wild-type (white, $n = 9$), CAPS2$^{+/\Delta ex3}$ (gray, $n = 10$), and CAPS2$^{\Delta ex3/\Delta ex3}$ (black, $n = 9$) mice at P21. (E) The area of lobules VI and VII of wild-type (white, $n = 10$), CAPS2$^{+/\Delta ex3}$ (gray, $n = 8$), and CAPS2$^{\Delta ex3/\Delta ex3}$ (black, $n = 12$) mice at P17. $P<0.01$, one-factor ANOVA. (F) The area of lobules VI and VII of wild-type (white, $n = 8$), CAPS2$^{+/\Delta ex3}$ (gray, $n = 8$), and CAPS2$^{\Delta ex3/\Delta ex3}$ (black, $n = 8$) mice at P21. (G) The depth of intercrural fissure between lobules VI and VII of wild-type (white, $n = 10$), CAPS2$^{+/\Delta ex3}$ (gray, $n = 6$), and CAPS2$^{\Delta ex3/\Delta ex3}$ (black, $n = 9$) mice at P17. $P<0.05$, one-factor ANOVA. (H) The thickness of the EGL of wild-type (white, $n = 12$), CAPS2$^{+/\Delta ex3}$ (gray, $n = 7$), and CAPS2$^{\Delta ex3/\Delta ex3}$ (black, $n = 15$) mice at P17. $P<0.05$, one-factor ANOVA. The error bars indicate the s.e.m. *$P<0.05$; **$P<0.01$, by post-hoc *t*-test.

uptake into Purkinje neurons, while there was no difference in BDNF levels in their lysates. With the available data, it is difficult to make definitive statements on BDNF dynamics in the different cultures, because one must consider multiple factors; i.e., BDNF produced and transported in granule cells, that released from granule cells, and that internalized by endocytosis into Purkinje cells via binding to TrkB receptors. In addition, a change in BDNF-TrkB signaling may affect the normal development and function of Purkinje cells and granule cells, even in CAPS2$^{+/\Delta ex3}$ animals. It is possible that there is a decrease in BDNF receptors in CAPS2$^{+/\Delta ex3}$ Purkinje cells compared with wild-type Purkinje cells. The effect of CAPS2-dex3 copy number on BDNF production, trafficking, release and endocytosis remain to be elucidated in future studies.

CAPS2 gene disruption and autistic phenotypes

In this report, we focused on the cerebellar phenotypes of CAPS2$^{\Delta ex3/\Delta ex3}$ mice and found that CAPS2$^{\Delta ex3/\Delta ex3}$ mice show the cerebellar phenotypes described above. Some of these phenotypes are similar with those observed in autistic patients.

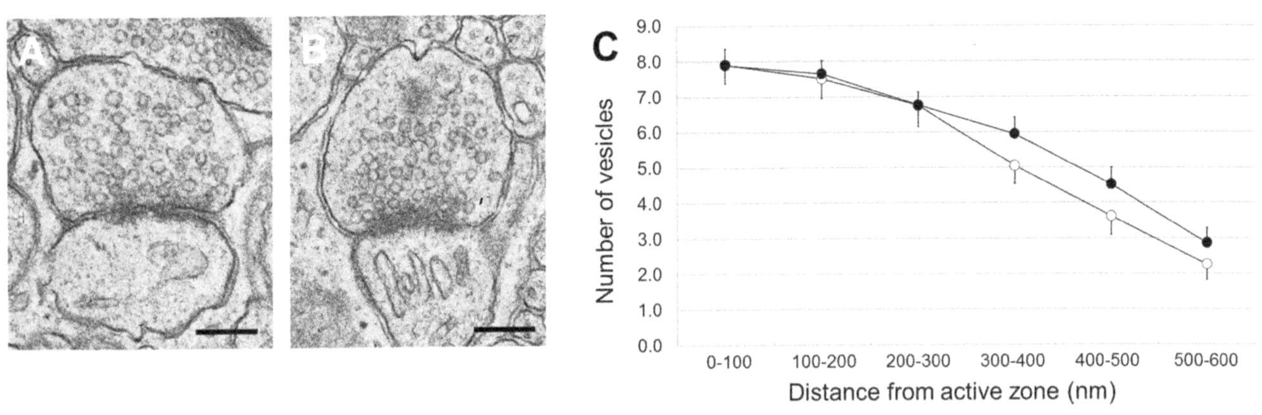

Figure 6. Distribution of vesicles within PF terminals. (A, B) Electron micrographs of a PF-PC synapse in the P21 wild-type cerebellum (A) and another in the CAPS2$^{\Delta ex3/\Delta ex3}$ cerebellum (B). Scale bars, 400 nm. (C) Quantification of vesicle distribution on the electron micrographs. The distance between vesicles and the active zone is indicated on the x-axis; numbers of vesicles of wild-type (open circles; $n = 51$) and CAPS2$^{\Delta ex3/\Delta ex3}$ (closed circles; $n = 54$) are represented on the y-axis. The error bars indicate the s.e.m.

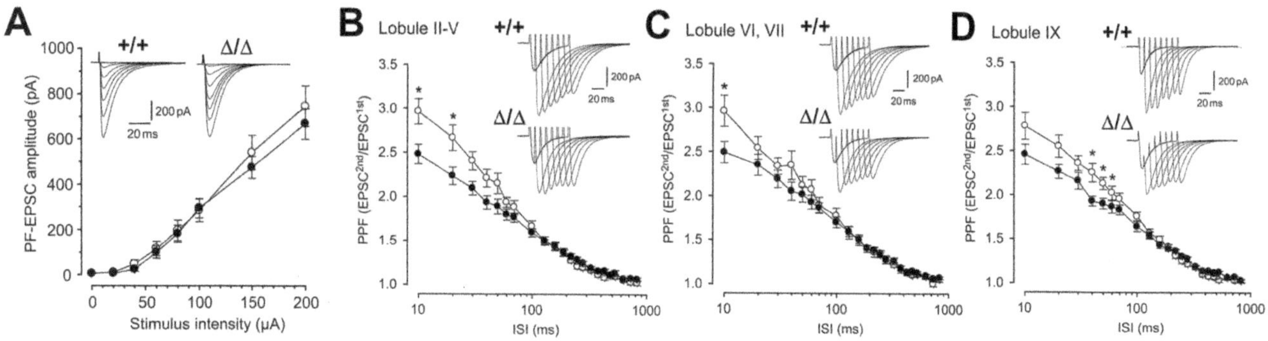

Figure 7. Impairment of short-term synaptic plasticity at PF-PC synapses in the CAPS2$^{\Delta ex3/\Delta ex3}$ mouse cerebellum. (A) Plots showing the relationship between the PF-EPSC amplitude and stimulus intensity applied to PFs in CAPS2$^{\Delta ex3/\Delta ex3}$ mice (closed circles; $n = 12$) and wild-type littermates (open circles; $n = 12$), at P25–35. Insets show representative EPSC traces evoked by PF stimuli of different intensities. (B–D) The mean paired-pulse ratios recorded from each lobule of P19–20 cerebellar slices were plotted against various interstimulus intervals. Recordings from lobules II–V (wild-type, $n = 14$; CAPS2$^{\Delta ex3/\Delta ex3}$, $n = 14$), VI–VII (wild-type, $n = 12$; CAPS2$^{\Delta ex3/\Delta ex3}$, $n = 16$), and IX (wild-type, $n = 13$; CAPS2$^{\Delta ex3/\Delta ex3}$, $n = 13$) are shown in (B), (C), and (D), respectively. Insets show representative traces obtained from CAPS2$^{\Delta ex3/\Delta ex3}$ mice and wild-type littermates. $V_h = -80$ mV. The error bars indicate the s.e.m. *$P < 0.05$, by the Mann–Whitney *U* test.

Abnormal reduction in lobules VI and VII of the cerebellar vermis is a characteristic morphological deficit reported in the brains of autistic patients [34], and hypoplasia of these lobules was also suggested to relate the abnormal exploratory behavior of autism [35]. It is of interest that decreased PPF was also shown in a mouse model of Rett syndrome [36], which is considered to be an autistic spectrum disorder. Taken together, our findings are suggestive of an association of the increased exon 3 splicing of CAPS2 in the cerebellar deficits of autistic patients.

Author Contributions

Conceived and designed the experiments: TS TF. Performed the experiments: TS WK Y. Shinoda MH RKS Y. Sekine Y. Sato CS. Analyzed the data: TS WK Y. Shinoda RKS Y. Sato YI MY MK. Wrote the paper: TS WK TF.

References

1. Binda AV, Kabbani N, Levenson R (2005) Regulation of dense core vesicle release from PC12 cells by interaction between the D2 dopamine receptor and calcium-dependent activator protein for secretion (CAPS). Biochem Pharmacol 69: 1451–1461.
2. Speidel D, Bruederle CE, Enk C, Voets T, Varoqueaux F, et al. (2005) CAPS1 regulates catecholamine loading of large dense-core vesicles. Neuron 46: 75–88.
3. Tandon A, Bannykh S, Kowalchyk JA, Banerjee A, Martin TF, et al. (1998) Differential regulation of exocytosis by calcium and CAPS in semi-intact synaptosomes. Neuron 21: 147–154.
4. Grishanin RN, Kowalchyk JA, Klenchin VA, Ann K, Earles CA, et al. (2004) CAPS acts at a prefusion step in dense-core vesicle exocytosis as a PIP_2 binding protein. Neuron 43: 551–562.
5. Sadakata T, Shinoda Y, Sekine Y, Saruta C, Itakura M, et al. (2010) Interaction of calcium-dependent activator protein for secretion 1 (CAPS1) with the class II ADP-ribosylation factor small GTPases is required for dense-core vesicle trafficking in the trans-Golgi network. J Biol Chem 285: 38710–38719.
6. IMGSAC (2001) Further characterization of the autism susceptibility locus AUTS1 on chromosome 7q. Hum Mol Genet 10: 973–982.
7. Cisternas FA, Vincent JB, Scherer SW, Ray PN (2003) Cloning and characterization of human *CADPS* and *CADPS2*, new members of the Ca^{2+}-dependent activator for secretion protein family. Genomics 81: 279–291.
8. Shinoda Y, Sadakata T, Nakao K, Katoh-Semba R, Kinameri E, et al. (2010) Calcium-dependent activator protein for secretion 2 (CAPS2) promotes BDNF secretion and is critical for the development of GABAergic interneuron network. Proc Natl Acad Sci U S A 108: 373–378.
9. Sadakata T, Mizoguchi A, Sato Y, Katoh-Semba R, Fukuda M, et al. (2004) The secretory granule-associated protein CAPS2 regulates neurotrophin release and cell survival. J Neurosci 24: 43–52.
10. Bibel M, Barde YA (2000) Neurotrophins: key regulators of cell fate and cell shape in the vertebrate nervous system. Genes Dev 14: 2919–2937.
11. Lu B (2003) BDNF and activity-dependent synaptic modulation. Learn Mem 10: 86–98.
12. Amir RE, Van den Veyver IB, Wan M, Tran CQ, Francke U, et al. (1999) Rett syndrome is caused by mutations in X-linked *MECP2*, encoding methyl-CpG-binding protein 2. Nat Genet 23: 185–188.
13. Chang Q, Khare G, Dani V, Nelson S, Jaenisch R (2006) The disease progression of *Mecp2* mutant mice is affected by the level of BDNF expression. Neuron 49: 341–348.
14. Sadakata T, Washida M, Iwayama Y, Shoji S, Sato Y, et al. (2007) Autistic-like phenotypes in *Cadps2*-knockout mice and aberrant *CADPS2* splicing in autistic patients. J Clin Invest 117: 931–943.
15. Sadakata T, Furuichi T (2009) Developmentally regulated Ca^{2+}-dependent activator protein for secretion 2 (CAPS2) is involved in BDNF secretion and is associated with autism susceptibility. Cerebellum 8: 312–322.
16. Eran A, Graham KR, Vatalaro K, McCarthy J, Collins C, et al. (2009) Comment on "Autistic-like phenotypes in *Cadps2*-knockout mice and aberrant *CADPS2* splicing in autistic patients". J Clin Invest 119: 679-680; author reply 680–671.
17. Okamoto N, Hatsukawa Y, Shimojima K, Yamamoto T (2011) Submicroscopic deletion in 7q31 encompassing *CADPS2* and *TSPAN12* in a child with autism spectrum disorder and PHPV. Am J Med Genet A 155A: 1568–1573.
18. Christian SL, Brune CW, Sudi J, Kumar RA, Liu S, et al. (2008) Novel submicroscopic chromosomal abnormalities detected in autism spectrum disorder. Biol Psychiatry 63: 1111–1117.
19. Szatmari P, Paterson AD, Zwaigenbaum L, Roberts W, Brian J, et al. (2007) Mapping autism risk loci using genetic linkage and chromosomal rearrangements. Nat Genet 39: 319–328.
20. Voineagu I, Wang X, Johnston P, Lowe JK, Tian Y, et al. (2011) Transcriptomic analysis of autistic brain reveals convergent molecular pathology. Nature 474: 380–384.
21. Bonora E, Graziano C, Minopoli F, Bacchelli E, Magini P, et al. (2014) Maternally inherited genetic variants of *CADPS2* are present in Autism Spectrum Disorders and Intellectual Disability patients. EMBO Mol Med.
22. Sadakata T, Shinoda Y, Oka M, Sekine Y, Sato Y, et al. (2012) Reduced axonal localization of a CAPS2 splice variant impairs axonal release of BDNF and causes autistic-like behavior in mice. Proc Natl Acad Sci U S A 109: 21104–21109.
23. Katoh-Semba R, Kaisho Y, Shintani A, Nagahama M, Kato K (1996) Tissue distribution and immunocytochemical localization of neurotrophin-3 in the brain and peripheral tissues of rats. J Neurochem 66: 330–337.
24. Sadakata T, Kakegawa W, Mizoguchi A, Washida M, Katoh-Semba R, et al. (2007) Impaired cerebellar development and function in mice lacking CAPS2, a protein involved in neurotrophin release. J Neurosci 27: 2472–2482.
25. Katoh-Semba R, Takeuchi IK, Semba R, Kato K (2000) Neurotrophin-3 controls proliferation of granular precursors as well as survival of mature granule neurons in the developing rat cerebellum. J Neurochem 74: 1923–1930.

26. Kakegawa W, Miyazaki T, Emi K, Matsuda K, Kohda K, et al. (2008) Differential regulation of synaptic plasticity and cerebellar motor learning by the C-terminal PDZ-binding motif of GluRδ2. J Neurosci 28: 1460–1468.
27. Bates B, Rios M, Trumpp A, Chen C, Fan G, et al. (1999) Neurotrophin-3 is required for proper cerebellar development. Nat Neurosci 2: 115–117.
28. Schwartz PM, Borghesani PR, Levy RL, Pomeroy SL, Segal RA (1997) Abnormal cerebellar development and foliation in BDNF$^{-/-}$ mice reveals a role for neurotrophins in CNS patterning. Neuron 19: 269–281.
29. Sadakata T, Kakegawa W, Shinoda Y, Hosono M, Katoh-Semba R, et al. (2013) CAPS1 deficiency perturbs dense-core vesicle trafficking and Golgi structure and reduces presynaptic release probability in the mouse brain. J Neurosci 33: 17326–17334.
30. Atluri PP, Regehr WG (1998) Delayed release of neurotransmitter from cerebellar granule cells. J Neurosci 18: 8214–8227.
31. Ito M (2001) Cerebellar long-term depression: characterization, signal transduction, and functional roles. Physiol Rev 81: 1143–1195.
32. Bangash MA, Park JM, Melnikova T, Wang D, Jeon SK, et al. (2011) Enhanced polyubiquitination of Shank3 and NMDA receptor in a mouse model of autism. Cell 145: 758–772.
33. Carter AR, Chen C, Schwartz PM, Segal RA (2002) Brain-derived neurotrophic factor modulates cerebellar plasticity and synaptic ultrastructure. J Neurosci 22: 1316–1327.
34. Courchesne E, Yeung-Courchesne R, Press GA, Hesselink JR, Jernigan TL (1988) Hypoplasia of cerebellar vermal lobules VI and VII in autism. N Engl J Med 318: 1349–1354.
35. Pierce K, Courchesne E (2001) Evidence for a cerebellar role in reduced exploration and stereotyped behavior in autism. Biol Psychiatry 49: 655–664.
36. Moretti P, Levenson JM, Battaglia F, Atkinson R, Teague R, et al. (2006) Learning and memory and synaptic plasticity are impaired in a mouse model of Rett syndrome. J Neurosci 26: 319–327.

7

Preserved Coupling between the Reader's Voice and the Listener's Cortical Activity in Autism Spectrum Disorders

Catherine Clumeck[1,2], Sarah Suarez Garcia[1], Mathieu Bourguignon[1], Vincent Wens[1], Marc Op de Beeck[1], Brice Marty[1], Nicolas Deconinck[3], Marie-Vincianne Soncarrieu[3], Serge Goldman[1], Veikko Jousmäki[4], Patrick Van Bogaert[1], Xavier De Tiège[1]*

1 Laboratoire de Cartographie fonctionnelle du Cerveau, UNI – ULB Neuroscience Institute, Université libre de Bruxelles (ULB), Brussels, Belgium, **2** Laboratoire de Recherches Psychiatriques, UNI – ULB Neuroscience Institute, Université libre de Bruxelles (ULB), Brussels, Belgium, **3** Centre de référence des troubles envahissants du développement et des troubles autistiques, Hôpital Universitaire des Enfants Reine Fabiola (HUDERF), Brussels, Belgium, **4** Brain Research Unit, O.V. Lounasmaa Laboratory and MEG Core, Aalto NeuroImaging, Aalto University, Espoo, Finland

Abstract

Purpose: Investigating the steadiness of the phase-coupling between the time-course of the reader's voice and brain signals of subjects with autism spectrum disorder (ASD) passively listening to connected speech using magnetoencephalography (MEG). In typically developed subjects, such coupling occurs at the right posterior temporal sulcus (pSTS) for frequencies below 1 Hz, and reflects the neural processing of sentence-level rhythmic prosody at the prelexical level.

Methods: Cortical neuromagnetic signals were recorded with MEG (Elekta Oy, Finland) while seven right-handed and native French-speaking ASD subjects (six males, one female, range: 13–20 years) listened to live (*Live*) or recorded (*Recorded*) voices continuously reading a text in French for five minutes. Coherence was computed between the reader's voice time-course and ASD subjects' MEG signals. Coherent neural sources were subsequently reconstructed using a beamformer.

Key findings: Significant coupling was found at 0.5 Hz in all ASD subjects in *Live* and in six subjects in *Recorded*. Coherent sources were located close to the right pSTS in both conditions. No significant difference was found in coherence levels between *Live* and *Recorded*, and between ASD subjects and ten typically developed subjects (right-handed, native French-speaking adults, 5 males, 5 females, age range: 21–38 years) included in a previous study.

Significance: This study discloses a preserved coupling between the reader's voice and ASD subjects' cortical activity at the right pSTS. These findings support the existence of preserved neural processing of sentence-level rhythmic prosody in ASD. The preservation of early cortical processing of prosodic elements in verbal language might be exploited in therapeutic interventions in ASD.

Editor: Gareth Robert Barnes, University College of London - Institute of Neurology, United Kingdom

Funding: Catherine Clumeck (Research Fellow) and Xavier De Tiège (Postdoctorate Clinical Master Specialist) benefit of a research grant form the Fonds de la Recherche Scientifique (FRS-FNRS, Belgium). This study was supported by a research grant from the FRS-FNRS (research project: J.0021.13). The funders had no role in study design, data collection and analysis, decision to publish, or preparation of the manuscript.

Competing Interests: The authors have declared that no competing interests exist.

* E-mail: xdetiege@ulb.ac.be

These authors contributed equally to this work.

Introduction

Autism spectrum disorders (ASD) represent an heterogeneous group of neurodevelopmental disorders of variable severity characterized by clinical features that can be classified into two main groups: social/communication disorders and narrow interest/stereotyped-repetitive behaviors (for a review, see [1]). While other neuropsychiatric disorders can share some of these symptoms, the precocity and the pervasive characteristic of social and communication impairments are highly specific of ASD (for a review, see [2]).

Based on structural and functional neuroimaging studies, several brain areas seem to play a major pathophysiological role in ASD social and communication impairments (for a review, see [3]). Among them, the cortical structures around the posterior superior temporal sulcus (pSTS) are of particular interest as they play a key functional role in social cognition, and are structurally and functionally abnormal in ASD subjects (for a review, see [4]). Indeed, several studies pointed out the involvement of the pSTS in the visual analysis of social cues such as gaze orientation or body movements (for a review, see [5]). Accumulating evidence also reveals that the pSTS is implicated in social perception through the auditory analysis of vocal and non-vocal sounds (for reviews, see [4,6]). Functional neuroimaging studies have actually demonstrated the existence of voice-selective regions in both pSTS [7]. Based on these data, some authors suggest that a major functional role of the pSTS is to parse auditory or visual inputs into discrete units in order to extract their meaning [6]. Finally, this brain area was also identified as being part of cortical networks supporting theory of mind (for a review, see [8]) and mirror neuron (for reviews, see [9–11]) processes; such processes being impaired in ASD subjects [12–15]. In addition, several structural and functional neuroimaging studies have shown pSTS abnormalities in ASD such as decreased gray matter concentration in the cortex around the pSTS [16–18], rest hypoperfusion [4,19], and abnormal activation during social tasks or vocal sound processing [20–22]. Taken together, these data suggest that the pSTS plays a key role in the pathophysiology of social and communication impairments found in ASD. Several authors thus hypothesize that anomalies involving the pSTS region during early brain development could represent the first step in the cascade of neural dysfunctions underlying ASD [4].

In humans, successful speech comprehension involves segmentation of speech signals into various timescales or temporal windows (TW), so that the spectrotemporal information is concurrently extracted within separate neural streams for speech perception and then integrated in brain regions involved in subsequent lexical computations for speech comprehension (for a review, see [23]). Up to now, two timescales have been investigated in depth in the context of speech perception: the 20–50 ms TW corresponding to the duration of phonemes, and the 150–300 ms TW corresponding to the duration of syllables and some prosodic phenomena (for a review, see [24]). Longer TWs, at the level of the second(s), are involved in sentence-level information [24]. In the context of an ecological continuous listening condition, we recently identified a novel coupling phenomenon at the sentence level, referred to as cortico-vocal coherence (CVC), between the time-course of the reader's voice and the listener's brain signals [25]. Significant coherence or phase coupling below 1 Hz was observed in all subjects within right pSTS and posterior superior temporal gyrus (pSTG) for the speech conditions, and within supra-temporal auditory cortices only for the non-speech vocal condition. In addition, significant coupling at 4–6 Hz (syllable level) was observed in 40% of the subjects at the supratemporal auditory cortex bilaterally. The coupling observed below 1 Hz corresponded to the neural integration of rhythmic prosody at the sentence level within right temporal voice sensitive areas; rhythmic prosody corresponding here to natural pauses occurring in the text in relation to punctuation marks or pauses associated with reader's breathing. These data suggested that right, non dominant, temporal voice sensitive areas contain neurons preferentially integrating sentence rhythmic prosody (TW>1 second) during natural speech perception reflected in rhythmic neuronal activity fluctuations below 1 Hz. Considering the key role of the right pSTS in inter-individual communicative behaviors and the importance of pauses or silences to guide successful verbal conversation [26], the strong reader–listener coupling at the right pSTS observed in this listening setting, was also interpreted as potentially corresponding to the neural processes involved in the recognition of relevant transitions in the speaker's discourse. These neural processes might serve as cues to drive the listener to initiate speech during interactional verbal communication or turn-taking transitions. Interestingly, turn-taking ability is known to be impaired in ASD with reasonable speech development (for a review, see [27]). This impairment is considered to be associated with pragmatic language deficits such as difficulties in sustaining conversation and turn-taking transitions, or in prosody perception [27]. Prosody, which is defined by the suprasegmental features of speech (variation in pitch, intonation, stress, rate, rhythm, duration, pausing, and loudness), facilitates speech comprehension and interindividual verbal communication (for a review, see [28]). While deficits in prosody appear not to be universal in ASD, atypical use of prosody is considered as a hallmark of speakers with such disorders [29]. Furthermore, several behavioral, neurophysiological and neuroimaging data have reported impairments in the production and the perception of prosody in ASD (for reviews, see [28,30]).

Therefore, considering the putative dysfunction of the pSTS in ASD and the impairments in prosodic perception and pragmatic language in subjects with this disorder, this study aims at investigating the steadiness of the coupling between the time-course of the reader's voice and ASD subjects' brain signals using magnetoencephalography (MEG) and the CVC approach. We predict that pSTS dysfunction in ASD might be reflected in a weaker coupling in ASD subjects, or that the location of coherent brain areas will differ from that observed in typically developed subjects. Conversely, if coupling is unaffected in ASD, it might represent a theoretical support for therapeutic interventions based on low-frequency prosodic content of language to foster social communication in this disorder.

Methods

Participants

ASD subjects' clinical details are summarized in Table 1.

Seven right-handed and native French-speaking subjects (6 males and 1 female, age range: 13–20 years, mean age: 16, normal audition) diagnosed with Asperger Syndrome (2 patients) or autistic disorder (5 patients) were included in the study. The handedness was assessed with the Edinburgh handedness Inventory [31]. The intellectual functioning was assessed by an abbreviated version of the Wechsler Intelligence scale for Children (Fourth Edition) [32] or the Wechsler Adult Intelligence Scale (Third Edition) [33]. The ASD was diagnosed according to DSM-IV criteria [34] and subsequently confirmed by the Autism Diagnostic Observation Schedule-Generic (ADOS) [35]. Based on ADOS, all subjects had weak (2 subjects) or clear (5 subjects) expressive prosodic disorder. To complete the assessment of the expressive language already explored with the ADOS, a brief assessment of the ASD subjects' lexical level was conducted with the *Test de Langage Oral Complexe pour Collégiens* (TLOCC) [36]. Subjects with neurological comorbidities or taking psychotropic treatment were excluded from the study except for one subject who was taking quetiapine (200 mg) for sleep disorder.

The study had the prior approval by the ULB-Hôpital Erasme Ethics Committee. The ASD subjects and their parents gave written informed consent before participating to the study.

Data obtained in the ten right-handed and native French-speaking typically developed healthy adult subjects (range 21–38 years; mean age: 25 years; 5 females and 5 males) included in the seminal CVC study [25] were used for statistical comparisons. This study had the prior approval by the ULB-Hôpital Erasme Ethics Committee. The subjects gave written informed consent before participating to the study.

Experimental paradigm

The experimental paradigms used in this study were adapted from [25]. Subjects' cortical neuromagnetic signals were recorded while they were listening to live (*Live*) or recorded (*Recorded*) voices continuously reading a text in French during 5 min. Both texts were chosen for their emotional neutrality in order to reduce the effect of affective prosody, and for the absence of any dialog in order to minimize prosody modulations. As in the seminal study, the first condition (*Live*) consisted in the passive listening of a text (http://www.eodi.org/la_revolution_francaise.html) read by a native French-speaking male (XDT, same as Exp1m in [25])

Table 1. Patients' clinical details.

								Mean
Subjects	1	2	3	4	5	6	7	
Age	18	20	19	15	14	13	15	16
Sex	M	M	M	M	M	F	M	
Diagnosis	AD	AD	AD	ASD	AD	ASD	AD	
Weschler Scales (mean = 10, SD = 3)								
Block design	13	12	3	4	9	12	7	8,5
Similarities	8	9	11	14	8	19	5	10,5
Matrix reasoning	13	12	8	5	10	8	8	9,1
Comprehension	6	5	6	9	1	14	3	6,2
TLOCC								
Comprehension (mean = 57,8; SD = 12,1)	48	58	38	62	22	68	44	48,5
Expression (mean = 46,1; SD = 14,4)	20	42	27	58	14	68	24	36,1
ADOS								
Communication (cut-off for autism = 3)	4	6	5	5	5	5	6	5,1
Social interaction (cut-off for autism = 6)	11	14	9	11	9	7	12	10,4
Total C+SI (cut-off for autism = 10)	15	20	14	16	14	12	18	15,5
Speech abnormalities* (0 = normal, 2 = speech clearly abnormal)	2	2	2	1	2	1	2	1,7

(M: male; F: female; AD: autistic disorder; ASD: Asperger syndrome; SD: standard deviation; TLOCC: test de langage oral complexe pour collégiens; ADOS: autism diagnostic observation schedule; C: communication; SI: social interaction;
*: speech abnormalities associated with autism, coded item 2 of the ADOS Language and Communication domain).

sitting 2 m in front of the subject inside the magnetically shielded room (MSR). The reader's vocal activity was recorded, time-locked to MEG signals, with a three-axis accelerometer attached to the left side of the reader's throat (ADXL330 *i*MEMS Accelerometer, Analog Devices, Inc., Norwood, MA, USA). Subjects were asked to fixate the gaze at a point in the MSR to avoid any gaze contact with the reader. In a second condition (*Recorded*), subjects passively listened to a recording of a native French-speaking female reading a French text (http://www.litteratureaudio.com/livre-audio-gratuit-mp3/zola-emile-la-terre.html) during 5 min. This condition was designed to test the influence of human interactional factors (e.g., human presence) on the CVC phenomenon. A loudspeaker (Panphonics Oy, Espoo, Finland) was positioned 2 m in front of the subjects inside the MSR. Signals of the recorded voice were recorded time-locked to MEG signals. In a third 5-min session (*Rest*), subjects were asked, as in the two previous conditions, to relax, fixate the gaze at a point in the MSR and not to move. The three experimental conditions (*Live*, *Recorded*, and *Rest*) were randomized across subjects.

Data acquisition, preprocessing, and analyses

The methods used for data acquisition, preprocessing, and analyses have been extensively detailed in [25] and will therefore be briefly described below.

Data Acquisition. MEG signals were recorded at the ULB-Hôpital Erasme with a whole-scalp-covering neuromagnetometer (Vectorview & Maxshield™; Elekta Oy, Helsinki, Finland). Head position inside the MEG helmet was continuously monitored using four head-tracking coils. The locations of the coils and at least 150 head-surface (on scalp, nose and face) points with respect to anatomical fiducials were determined with an electromagnetic tracker (Fastrak, Polhemus, Colchester, VT, USA). The recording passband was 0.1–330 Hz for MEG signals and 0–330 Hz for accelerometer and recorded voice signals; all signals were sampled at 1 kHz.

Data preprocessing. Continuous MEG data were preprocessed off-line using the signal-space-separation method to suppress external interferences and to correct for head movements [37]. In one subject, MEG signals in *Live* were preprocessed off-line using the spatio-temporal signal-space-separation (coefficient correlation: 0.95, window length: 4 s) to subtract system artefacts. Then, for frequency and coherence analyses, 2048 ms epochs were extracted with 1638 ms overlap, leading to a frequency resolution of 0.5 Hz. Epochs where MEG signals exceeded 3 pT (magnetometers) or 0.7 pT/cm (gradiometers) were rejected to avoid contamination of the data by eye movements, muscle activity, or artefacts of the MEG sensors. This yielded more than 590 artifact-free epochs for each subject and condition.

Coherence analysis in sensor space. Subsequently, voice signals were band-passed around voice fundamental frequency (f0; 100–200 Hz, *Live*; 130–300 Hz, *Recorded*) and rectified in order to compute for each epoch the coherence between the f0 time-course and MEG signals. In both conditions, the analyses were based on the voice fundamental frequency (f0) as this parameter is a highly relevant feature for speech processing (see [25] for more details). The coherence is an extension of Pearson correlation coefficient to the frequency domain, quantifying the degree of coupling between two signals, providing a number between 0 (no linear dependency) and 1 (perfect linear dependency) for each frequency [38]. The degree of coupling between MEG signals (frequency band: 0.1–330 Hz) and the f0 time-course were first determined by computing coherence spectra in the sensor space. Frequencies that displayed significant coupling in the sensor space in most subjects were identified and used as frequencies of interest for coherent source analyses.

Coherence analysis in source space. Coherence analyses were then performed in the source space using the Montreal Neurological Institute (MNI) template. Notwithstanding the risk of decrease in spatial accuracy, the MNI template was used rather than individual structural magnetic resonance imaging (MRI) in order to facilitate ASD subjects' recruitment as some of them refused to undergo MRI. For each subject, MEG and segmented MNI coordinate systems were coregistered using the three anatomical fiducial points for initial estimation and the head-surface points to manually refine the surface coregistration. The MEG forward model was then computed using the MNE suite (Martinos Center for Biomedical Imaging, Massachusetts, USA). Cortical sources coherent with the f0 time-course were identified using dynamic imaging of coherent sources (DICS) [39] and subsequently visualized on the MNI template. Separate coherence maps were computed for each possible combination of frequencies of interest, subjects, and conditions. Both planar gradiometers and magnetometers were simultaneously used for inverse modeling.

Finally, to produce coherence maps at the group level, we computed the generalized f-mean across subjects of normalized maps, according to $f(\bullet) = \operatorname{arctanh}(\sqrt{(\bullet)})$, namely, the Fisher z-transform of the square root.

Statistical analyses. The statistical significance of sensor-space individual-level coherence was assessed using surrogate data-based statistics, based on coherence computed between surrogate f0 time-courses and original MEG data [40] (for more details, see also [41,42]).

The statistical significance of source-space group-level coherence was assessed using a non-parametric permutation test based on coherence between vocal signals and rest condition MEG data [43] (for more details, see also [44]).

Non-parametric Wilcoxon and Mann-Whitney test were used to assess the difference between conditions and between ASD and typically developped subjects from the seminal CVC study [25]. Finally, correlations were computed to establish relations between coherence levels and age, and behavioural data reflecting autistic symptoms severity.

Results

Coherence at the sensor level

Figure 1 and Table 2 summarize the results obtained at the sensor level.

In line with the seminal CVC study carried out in a group of healthy adult subjects [25], coherence between voice and MEG signals consistently peaked at ~0.5 Hz in all ASD subjects. Right-hemisphere-dominant coherence levels were statistically significant at ~0.5 Hz in all subjects in *Live* (coherence values from 0.04 to 0.28; $p<0.05$; see Figure 1 and Table 2) and in six subjects in *Recorded* (coherence values from 0.06 to 0.29; $p<0.05$; see Figure 1 and Table 2). No difference in sensor-space coherence levels at 0.5 Hz was found between *Live* and *Recorded* ($p = 0.87$), nor between ASD subjects and the typically developed healthy adult subjects investigated in the seminal CVC study (*Live*, $p = 0.28$; *Recorded*, $p = 0.31$).

No other peak in coherence was found at the sensor level, and particularly at 4–6 Hz. The 0.5-Hz coherent frequency was therefore considered as the only frequency of interest to compute individual and group-level coherence maps.

Coherence at the source level

Figure 2 illustrates the location of the coherence local maxima on the MNI template in both conditions.

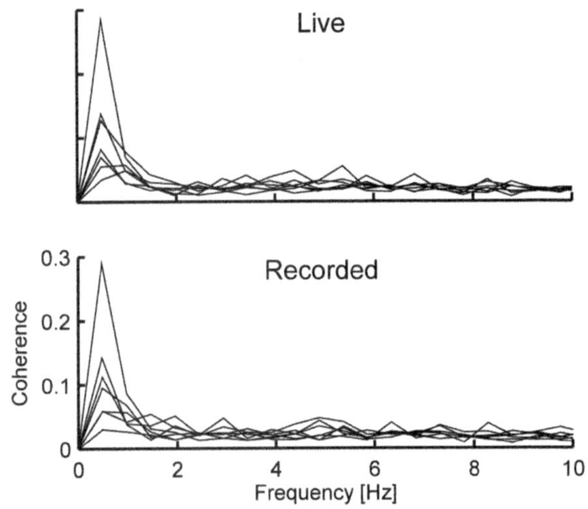

Figure 1. Individual coherence spectra in ASD subjects. Individual coherence spectra obtained in each condition for the right-hemisphere MEG sensor showing the maximum coherence level. Significant coherence at 0.5 Hz was observed in all ASD subjects in *Live* and in 6 out of 7 subjects in *Recorded*. Y-axis values are identical on both plots.

Group-level analysis revealed maximum coherence at the right STS (MNI coordinates: [64 –15 –11] mm; coherence value: 0.07, $p<0.05$) in *Live* and at the middle temporal gyrus (MTG) (MNI coordinates: [64 –18 –18] mm; coherence value: 0.07, $p<0.05$) in *Recorded*. Considering the limited spatial resolution afforded by the coregistration procedure used in this study, these coherence local maxima can be considered very close to the one reported in the seminal CVC study (Exp1m, pSTS, [66 -26 -1] mm) [25].

No local coherence maximum was observed at supratemporal auditory cortex bilaterally. At a lower threshold, a local coherence maximum was also observed at the left parietal operculum in both listening conditions, in accordance with the seminal CVC study [25].

Correlations between sensor-space coherence level and behavioural data

Correlation analyses did not disclose any association between sensor-space coherence levels and age or behavioural scores (age, IQ, ADOS and TLOCC: $p>0.05$).

Discussion

Despite scientific evidences of right pSTS dysfunction in ASD, this study demonstrates significant coupling in ASD subjects between neural activity at this cortical structure and the slow fluctuations of a heard voice during continuous connected speech listening, a phenomenon previously demonstrated in healthy subjects. Indeed, the coupling between the reader's voice f0 time-course and listener's cortical MEG signals was similar at 0.5 Hz in terms of coherence levels and location of coherence local maxima between ASD subjects and the typically developed healthy adult subjects investigated in the seminal CVC study [25]. This study also suggests that CVC levels at 0.5 Hz do not vary according to age or autistic symptom severity in ASD subjects. No coupling was found at 4–6 Hz between the reader's voice f0 time-course and listener's cortical MEG signals in ASD subjects, in accordance with the scarcity of such coupling in typically developed subjects using our experimental setting [25].

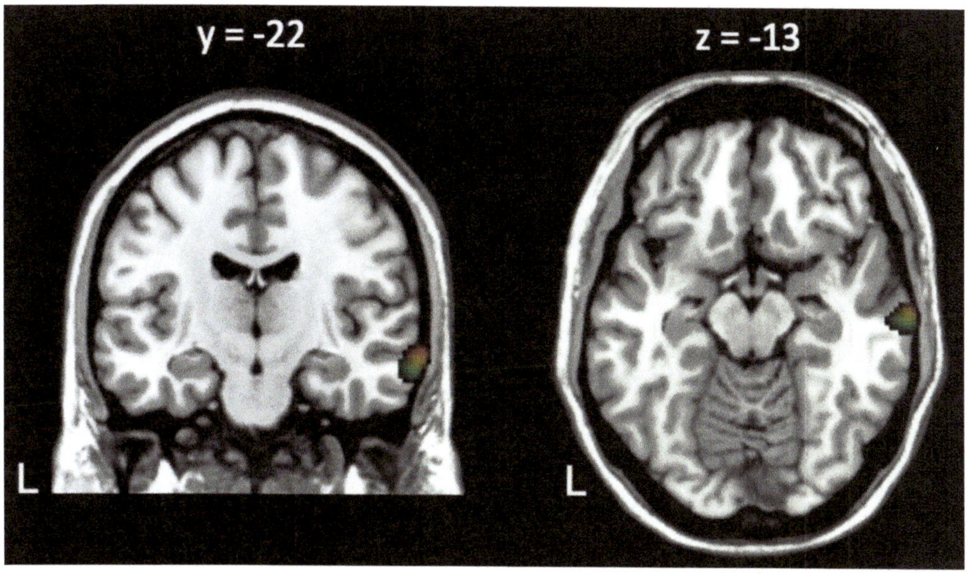

Figure 2. Group-level coherence maps in ASD subjects. Group level coherence maps computed at 0.5 Hz in each condition (*Live*, red; *Recorded*, green; intersection between *Live* and *Recorded*, yellow). In *Live*, the maximum coherence occured at the right superior temporal sulcus and in *Recorded*, at the upper bank of the middle temporal gyrus. Coherence maps were thresholded at the maximum of coherence to isolate the local coherence maxima (*Live*, coherence threshold: 0.64–0.71; *Recorded*, coherence threshold: 0.60–0.67).

Preserved coupling between the reader's voice and listener's MEG signals in ASD

The preserved coupling between the reader's voice and listener's MEG signals observed in the ASD subjects investigated in this study may be explained by several factors. In line with the neural complexity hypothesis [45,46] and the enhanced perceptual theory (for a review, see [47]), the cortico-vocal coupling might be preserved in ASD subjects because of the low-level neural processing engaged in this coupling phenomenon. Indeed, the CVC experimental paradigm consists in unimodal (auditory) stimulation. Moreover, this coupling phenomenon occurring at the right pSTS is considered to involve prelexical processing levels in speech perception as it was also observed when typically developed subjects listened to a totally incomprehensible language (native French-speaking subjects listening to Finnish) [25]. Interestingly, accumulating data suggest that ASD subjects perform normally, or even better than typically developed subjects, in tasks that require low-level processing or involve simple material [48], whereas they underperform in tasks that engage high-level neural processing such as multimodal sensory processing [49,50] or complex cognitive or social tasks [13,51]. Electrophysiological and neuroimaging data support this particular perceptive profile (for reviews, see [28,46,47]), which seems to be explained by an association of local over-connectivity and long-range under/dys-connectivity [52,53]. Still, some authors consider that speech perception is complex *per se* and numerous studies have suggested more severe impairments or cerebral dysfunctions for speech than for non-speech stimuli in ASD subjects [28,46]. However, albeit speech signals are indeed highly complex auditory stimuli, it might be hypothesized that the prelexical speech perception processes subtending the CVC phenomenon involve low-level neural processes that would not be impaired in ASD subjects.

It could be hypothesized that the preserved coupling observed in our ASD subjects might have been favored by the slow rate at which the suprasegmental pauses or silences occur in speech (typically, for sentence rhythmic prosody, below 1 Hz). Indeed, it has been proposed that the temporality of the sensory stimulations, apart from their multimodal character, plays a key role in the pathophysiological basis of some behavioural impairments characterizing ASD [53]. Indeed, although altered temporal integration in the auditory modality as well as impaired spatio-temporal integration in the visual modality have been repeatedly observed in this population, slowing down the speed of sensory stimulations has been shown to improve imitative, verbal and cognitive performances [53]. It might therefore be of interest to determine if the coupling observed for shorter timescales (4–7 Hz, a TW corresponding to syllables and some prosodic phenomena)

Table 2. Sensor-space coherence levels at 0.5 Hz.

Participants	Live	Recorded	Controls
1	0.1266	0.1130	0.0818
2	0.0692	0.0295*	0.0804
3	0.0804	0.0577	0.1302
4	0.0482	0.0953	0.0518
5	0.2846	0.2904	0.1647
6	0.0564	0.0582	0.1862
7	0.1377	0.1427	0.1255
8	—	—	0.0960
9	—	—	0.3072
10	—	—	0.1802
min	0.0482	0.0295	0.0518
max	0.2846	0.2904	0.3072
mean	0.1126	0.1121	0.1404

*$p > 0.05$.
Live and Recorded: sensor-space coherence levels obtained in ASD patients.
Controls: sensor-space coherence levels obtained in Exp1m in the seminal CVC study (see Table 1, Bourguignon et al. 2013).

between neural and vocal activities during speech are preserved or not in ASD subjects [54].

Finally, a functional MRI study investigating the neural basis of prosodic speech deficits (linguistic and emotional prosody) in subjects with high functioning autism failed to find any clear deficit in pSTS recruitment compared with typically developed healthy subjects [55]. But and more interestingly, apart from an increased recruitment of the left supramarginal gyrus, ASD subjects were characterized by an absence of deactivation in key nodes of the default mode network (DMN) such as the precuneus, the anterior cingulate cortex and the left middle frontal gyrus; DMN deactivation correlating with prosodic skills in that study [55]. The DMN is a set of brain regions characterized by a high level of metabolic activity at rest and a low level of activity during goal-directed or externally focused cognitive tasks (for a review, see [56]). Several lines of evidence suggest that DMN suppression during goal-directed tasks is functionally relevant, particularly in terms of cognitive performance (i.e., the more the DMN activity is suppressed, the better is the cognitive performance) (for a review, see [57]). DMN suppression possibly reflects adaptive disengagement of "goal-irrelevant" brain functions (e.g., mind-wandering), which would be required to get properly engaged in goal-directed tasks [57]. So, the inability of deactivating DMN nodes while processing prosodic connected speech observed in ASD subjects could account for the existence of a less efficient processing of the relevant information, i.e. the prosodic dimension of speech, in ASD subjects [55]. Whether the deficits in DMN deactivation are related to altered functional integration between task-dependent networks and the DMN, or to a DMN dysfunction per se remains an open issue. Still, these fMRI data are congruent with the results of the present study suggesting preserved neural processing of suprasegmental rhythmic prosody at the right pSTS. Taken together, these data suggest that alterations in functional integration beyond the pSTS might therefore account for the rhythmic prosodic impairments described in the ASD population. This latter hypothesis is supported by MEG data obtained in subjects with Asperger syndrome that investigated another sensory modality, i.e. social visual cues processing [58]. In that study, neural activations were normal in strength and timing at the early stage of the cortical activation sequence (i.e., visual, STS and inferior parietal lobule activations) but were abnormal for the later stage (i.e., inferior frontal and primary motor cortex activations). This finding was interpreted as the absence of any significant deficit of high-level visual stimuli processing at the STS level in Asperger syndrome [58].

Importantly, the preservation of early cortical processing of prosodic elements in verbal language might potentially be exploited in therapeutic interventions in ASD. An anecdotic report already suggests in 1979 that the stress put on the melodic content of language has been helpful in the language therapy of an autistic boy [59]. The benefit of music therapy for verbal communication reported in ASD might also stem from the low frequency variations of auditory (music) stimuli carrying pertinent information potentially exploitable for social communication improvements [60,61]. Also, it is important to consider that disruption of interactional synchrony is an important feature of ASD that has recently attracted some attention [62]. Since interpersonal synchrony is the dynamic and reciprocal adaptation of the temporal structure of behaviors between interactive partners [63], preservation of coherent activity at the pSTS suggests that a neural substrate is present in ASD for interactional synchrony based on auditory inputs during dyadic oral communication. This represents a neurophysiological support for early therapeutic interventions based on prosody, including those building on the typical prosodic characteristics of the so-called "parentese", a special type of speech directed towards infants typically used by adults (higher pitch, slower tempo, and exaggerated intonation contours [62].

Limitations of the study

First, ASD subjects were compared with the typically developed healthy subjects investigated in the seminal CVC study [25] and were therefore not matched for age and sex. Still, as all ASD subjects (except for one subject in *Recorded*) obtained significant sensor-space coherence levels with values similar to those observed in the seminal CVC study, we consider that the conclusions of this study are not affected by this limitation.

Second, the use of the MNI template for the source space coherence analyses in ASD subjects limits the accuracy of the coherent source localization (as compared with the use of individual MRI) [64]. Still, in the absence of an individual MRI, using a template head model results in a fairly precise head model for source space modelling [65]. This is further supported by the fact that, even with this lower spatial resolution approach, the localization of the right STS maximum coherence was very close to the one described in the seminal CVC study. This finding highly suggests that similar brain areas are involved in the CVC phenomenon in ASD and typically developed subjects.

Finally, we did not test behaviourally the rhythmic prosody perception skills of our ASD subjects, which limits the interpretation of the functional relevance of the preserved CVC phenomenon in this population. Indeed, even if our result highly suggest a normal neural processing of the suprasegmental speech rhythmic prosody at the prelexical level, we cannot determine if this preserved coupling gives rise to normal prosody perception at the behavioural level. The ASD subjects included in this study had weak to clear expressive prosodic disorder. This highlights the importance to investigate in future studies the correlation between CVC levels and prosody perception skills.

Conclusions

This study discloses a preserved coupling between the reader's voice and the listener's cortical activity in ASD subjects at the right pSTS. These findings support the existence of preserved neural processing of sentence-level rhythmic prosody in ASD. The preservation of early cortical processing of prosodic elements in verbal language might be exploited in therapeutic interventions in ASD.

Acknowledgments

The authors would like to thank Professor Riitta Hari (Brain Research Unit, O.V. Lounasmaa Laboratory and MEG Core, Finland), Professor Véronique Delvenne (Centre de référence des troubles envahissants du développement et des troubles autistiques, HUDERF, Belgium), and Professor Paul Linkowski (Laboratoire de Recherches Psychiatriques, UNI – ULB Neuroscience Institute, Belgium) for their support and fruitful discussions.

Author Contributions

Conceived and designed the experiments: CC SSG MB VJ PVB SG XDT. Performed the experiments: CC SSG MB ND M-VS VW BM MOdB XDT. Analyzed the data: CC SSG MB VW BM MOdB VJ XDT. Contributed reagents/materials/analysis tools: CC SSG MB VW BM MOdB VJ XDT. Wrote the paper: CC SSG MB VJ PVB SG XDT. Amended: VW BM MOdB ND M-VS.

References

1. Baron-Cohen S, Belmonte MK (2005) Autism: a window onto the development of the social and the analytic brain. Annu Rev Neurosci 28: 109–126.
2. Schultz RT (2005) Developmental deficits in social perception in autism: the role of the amygdala and fusiform face area. Int J Dev Neurosci 23: 125–141.
3. Schroeder JH, Desrocher M, Bebko JM, Cappadocia MC (2010) The neurobiology of autism: Theoretical implications. Research in Autism Spectrum Disorders 4: 555–564.
4. Zilbovicius M, Meresse I, Chabane N, Brunelle F, Samson Y, et al. (2006) Autism, the superior temporal sulcus and social perception. Trends Neurosci 29: 359–366.
5. Allison T, Puce A, McCarthy G (2000) Social perception from visual cues: role of the STS region. Trends Cogn Sci 4: 267–278.
6. Redcay E (2008) The superior temporal sulcus performs a common function for social and speech perception: implications for the emergence of autism. Neurosci Biobehav Rev 32: 123–142.
7. Belin P, Zatorre RJ, Lafaille P, Ahad P, Pike B (2000) Voice-selective areas in human auditory cortex. Nature 403: 309–312.
8. Frith CD, Frith U (2006) The neural basis of mentalizing. Neuron 50: 531–534.
9. Hari R, Kujala MV (2009) Brain basis of human social interaction: from concepts to brain imaging. Physiol Rev 89: 453–479.
10. Kilner JM (2011) More than one pathway to action understanding. Trends Cogn Sci 15: 352–357.
11. Rizzolatti G, Sinigaglia C (2010) The functional role of the parieto-frontal mirror circuit: interpretations and misinterpretations. Nat Rev Neurosci 11: 264–274.
12. Happe FG (1994) An advanced test of theory of mind: understanding of story characters' thoughts and feelings by able autistic, mentally handicapped, and normal children and adults. J Autism Dev Disord 24: 129–154.
13. Kaland N, Callesen K, Moller-Nielsen A, Mortensen EL, Smith L (2008) Performance of children and adolescents with Asperger syndrome or high-functioning autism on advanced theory of mind tasks. J Autism Dev Disord 38: 1112–1123.
14. Rizzolatti G, Fabbri-Destro M, Cattaneo L (2009) Mirror neurons and their clinical relevance. Nat Clin Pract Neurol 5: 24–34.
15. Williams JH, Whiten A, Suddendorf T, Perrett DI (2001) Imitation, mirror neurons and autism. Neurosci Biobehav Rev 25: 287–295.
16. Boddaert N, Chabane N, Gervais H, Good CD, Bourgeois M, et al. (2004) Superior temporal sulcus anatomical abnormalities in childhood autism: a voxel-based morphometry MRI study. Neuroimage 23: 364–369.
17. Hadjikhani N, Joseph RM, Snyder J, Tager-Flusberg H (2006) Anatomical differences in the mirror neuron system and social cognition network in autism. Cereb Cortex 16: 1276–1282.
18. von dem Hagen EA, Nummenmaa L, Yu R, Engell AD, Ewbank MP, et al. (2011) Autism spectrum traits in the typical population predict structure and function in the posterior superior temporal sulcus. Cereb Cortex 21: 493–500.
19. Ohnishi T, Matsuda H, Hashimoto T, Kunihiro T, Nishikawa M, et al. (2000) bhAbnormal regional cerebral blood flow in childhood autism. Brain 123 (Pt 9): 1838–1844.
20. Castelli F, Frith C, Happe F, Frith U (2002) Autism, Asperger syndrome and brain mechanisms for the attribution of mental states to animated shapes. Brain 125: 1839–1849.
21. Gervais H, Belin P, Boddaert N, Leboyer M, Coez A, et al. (2004) Abnormal cortical voice processing in autism. Nat Neurosci 7: 801–802.
22. Wang AT, Lee SS, Sigman M, Dapretto M (2007) Reading affect in the face and voice: neural correlates of interpreting communicative intent in children and adolescents with autism spectrum disorders. Arch Gen Psychiatry 64: 698–708.
23. Hickok G, Poeppel D (2004) Dorsal and ventral streams: a framework for understanding aspects of the functional anatomy of language. Cognition 92: 67–99.
24. Poeppel D, Idsardi WJ, van Wassenhove V (2008) Speech perception at the interface of neurobiology and linguistics. Philos Trans R Soc Lond B Biol Sci 363: 1071–1086.
25. Bourguignon M, De Tiège X, Op de Beeck M, Ligot N, Paquier P, et al. (2013) The pace of prosodic phrasing couples the listener's cortex to the reader's voice. Hum Brain Mapp 34: 314–326.
26. Wilson M, Wilson TP (2005) An oscillator model of the timing of turn-taking. Psychon Bull Rev 12: 957–968.
27. Rapin I, Dunn M (2003) Update on the language disorders of individuals on the autistic spectrum. Brain Dev 25: 166–172.
28. O'Connor K (2012) Auditory processing in autism spectrum disorder: a review. Neurosci Biobehav Rev 36: 836–854.
29. Jarvinen-Pasley A, Peppe S, King-Smith G, Heaton P (2008) The relationship between form and function level receptive prosodic abilities in autism. J Autism Dev Disord 38: 1328–1340.
30. Groen WB, Zwiers MP, van der Gaag RJ, Buitelaar JK (2008) The phenotype and neural correlates of language in autism: an integrative review. Neurosci Biobehav Rev 32: 1416–1425.
31. Oldfield RC (1971) The assessment and analysis of handedness: the Edinburgh inventory. Neuropsychologia 9: 97–113.
32. Wechsler D (2003) Wechsler Intelligence Scale for Children - Fourth Edition Administration and scoring manual. San Antonio, Texas: Harcourt Assessment, Inc.
33. Wechsler D (1997) Wechsler Adult Intelligence Scale - Third Edition. San Antonio, Texas: The Psychological Corporation.
34. American Psychiatric Association (1994) DSM-IV Diagnostic and Statistical Manual of Mental Disorders. Washington DC.
35. Lord C, Risi S, Lambrecht L, Cook EH Jr, Leventhal BL, et al. (2000) The autism diagnostic observation schedule-generic: a standard measure of social and communication deficits associated with the spectrum of autism. J Autism Dev Disord 30: 205–223.
36. Maurin N (2006) Test de Langage Oral Complexe pour Collégiens (TLOCC). In: Ortho-Edition, editor editors. Isbergues.
37. Taulu S, Simola J, Kajola M (2005) Applications of the Signal Space Separation Method. IEEE Trans Sign Proc 53: 3359–3372.
38. Halliday DM, Rosenberg JR, Amjad AM, Breeze P, Conway BA, et al. (1995) A framework for the analysis of mixed time series/point process data–theory and application to the study of physiological tremor, single motor unit discharges and electromyograms. Prog Biophys Mol Biol 64: 237–278.
39. Gross J, Kujala J, Hämäläinen M, Timmermann L, Schnitzler A, et al. (2001) Dynamic imaging of coherent sources: Studying neural interactions in the human brain. Proc Natl Acad Sci U S A 98: 694–699.
40. Faes L, Pinna GD, Porta A, Maestri R, Nollo G (2004) Surrogate data analysis for assessing the significance of the coherence function. IEEE Trans Biomed Eng 51: 1156–1166.
41. Bourguignon M, Jousmäki V, Op de Beeck M, Van Bogaert P, Goldman S, et al. (2012) Neuronal network coherent with hand kinematics during fast repetitive hand movements. Neuroimage 59: 1684–1691.
42. Piitulainen H, Bourguignon M, De Tiège X, Hari R, Jousmäki V (2013) Coherence between magnetoencephalography and hand-action-related acceleration, force, pressure, and electromyogram. Neuroimage 72: 83–90.
43. Nichols TE, Holmes AP (2002) Nonparametric permutation tests for functional neuroimaging: a primer with examples. Hum Brain Mapp 15: 1–25.
44. Bourguignon M, De Tiège X, Op de Beeck M, Van Bogaert P, Goldman S, et al. (2012) Primary motor cortex and cerebellum are coupled with the kinematics of observed hand movements. Neuroimage 66C: 500–507.
45. Bertone A, Mottron L, Jelenic P, Faubert J (2005) Enhanced and diminished visuo-spatial information processing in autism depends on stimulus complexity. Brain 128: 2430–2441.
46. Samson F, Mottron L, Jemel B, Belin P, Ciocca V (2006) Can spectro-temporal complexity explain the autistic pattern of performance on auditory tasks? J Autism Dev Disord 36: 65–76.
47. Mottron L, Dawson M, Soulieres I, Hubert B, Burack J (2006) Enhanced perceptual functioning in autism: an update, and eight principles of autistic perception. J Autism Dev Disord 36: 27–43.
48. Bonnel A, Mottron L, Peretz I, Trudel M, Gallun E, et al. (2003) Enhanced pitch sensitivity in individuals with autism: a signal detection analysis. J Cogn Neurosci 15: 226–235.
49. Brandwein AB, Foxe JJ, Butler JS, Russo NN, Altschuler TS, et al. (2013) The development of multisensory integration in high-functioning autism: high-density electrical mapping and psychophysical measures reveal impairments in the processing of audiovisual inputs. Cereb Cortex 23: 1329–1341.
50. Collignon O, Charbonneau G, Peters F, Nassim M, Lassonde M, et al. (2013) Reduced multisensory facilitation in persons with autism. Cortex 49: 1704–1710.
51. Golan O, Baron-Cohen S, Golan Y (2008) The 'Reading the Mind in Films' Task [child version]: complex emotion and mental state recognition in children with and without autism spectrum conditions. J Autism Dev Disord 38: 1534–1541.
52. Belmonte MK, Allen G, Beckel-Mitchener A, Boulanger LM, Carper RA, et al. (2004) Autism and abnormal development of brain connectivity. J Neurosci 24: 9228–9231.
53. Gepner B and Feron F (2009) Autism: a world changing too fast for a mis-wired brain? Neurosci Biobehav Rev 33: 1227–1242.
54. Peelle JE, Gross J, Davis MH (2013) Phase-locked responses to speech in human auditory cortex are enhanced during comprehension. Cereb Cortex 23: 1378–1387.
55. Hesling I, Dilharreguy B, Peppe S, Amirault M, Bouvard M, et al. (2010) The integration of prosodic speech in high functioning autism: a preliminary FMRI study. PLoS One 5: e11571.
56. Gusnard DA, Raichle ME (2001) Searching for a baseline: functional imaging and the resting human brain. Nat Rev Neurosci 2: 685–694.
57. Anticevic A, Cole MW, Murray JD, Corlett PR, Wang XJ, et al. (2012) The role of default network deactivation in cognition and disease. Trends Cogn Sci 16: 584–592.
58. Nishitani N, Avikainen S, Hari R (2004) Abnormal imitation-related cortical activation sequences in Asperger's syndrome. Ann Neurol 55: 558–562.
59. Miller SB, Toca JM (1979) Adapted melodic intonation therapy: a case study of an experimental language program for an autistic child. J Clin Psychiatry 40: 201–203.

60. Lim HA, Draper E (2011) The effects of music therapy incorporated with applied behavior analysis verbal behavior approach for children with autism spectrum disorders. J Music Ther 48: 532–550.
61. Lim HA (2010) Effect of "developmental speech and language training through music" on speech production in children with autism spectrum disorders. J Music Ther 47: 2–26.
62. Cohen D, Cassel RS, Saint-Georges C, Mahdhaoui A, Laznik MC, et al. (2013) Do parentese prosody and fathers' involvement in interacting facilitate social interaction in infants who later develop autism? PLoS One 8: e61402.
63. Delaherche E, Chetouani M, Mahdhaoui A, Saint-Georges C, Viaux S, et al. (2012) Interpersonal Synchrony: A Survey of Evaluation Methods across Disciplines. IEEE Trans Affect Comput 3: 349–365.
64. Henson RN, Mattout J, Phillips C, Friston KJ (2009) Selecting forward models for MEG source-reconstruction using model-evidence. Neuroimage 46: 168–176.
65. Litvak V, Mattout J, Kiebel S, Phillips C, Henson R, et al. (2011) EEG and MEG data analysis in SPM8. Comput Intell Neurosci 2011: 852961.

8

Autism Associated Gene, *ENGRAILED2*, and Flanking Gene Levels Are Altered in Post-Mortem Cerebellum

Jiyeon Choi[1], Myka R. Ababon[1], Mai Soliman[1], Yong Lin[2], Linda M. Brzustowicz[4], Paul G. Matteson[1], James H. Millonig[1,3,4]*

1 Center for Advanced Biotechnology and Medicine, Piscataway, New Jersey, United States of America, 2 Cancer Institute of New Jersey, Piscataway, New Jersey, United States of America, 3 Department of Neuroscience and Cell Biology, Robert Wood Johnson Medical School, Piscataway, New Jersey, United States of America, 4 Department of Genetics, Rutgers University, Piscataway, New Jersey, United States of America

Abstract

Background: Previous genetic studies demonstrated association between the transcription factor *ENGRAILED2* (*EN2*) and Autism Spectrum Disorder (ASD). Subsequent molecular analysis determined that the *EN2* ASD-associated haplotype (*rs1861972-rs1861973* A-C) functions as a transcriptional activator to increase gene expression. *EN2* is flanked by 5 genes, *SEROTONIN RECEPTOR5A (HTR5A), INSULIN INDUCED GENE1 (INSIG1), CANOPY1 HOMOLOG (CNPY1), RNA BINDING MOTIF PROTEIN33 (RBM33)*, and *SONIC HEDGEHOG (SHH)*. These flanking genes are co-expressed with *EN2* during development and coordinate similar developmental processes. To investigate if mRNA levels for these genes are altered in individuals with autism, post-mortem analysis was performed.

Methods: qRT-PCR quantified mRNA levels for *EN2* and the 5 flanking genes in 78 post-mortem cerebellar samples. mRNA levels were correlated with both affection status and *rs1861972-rs1861973* genotype. Molecular analysis investigated whether *EN2* regulates flanking gene expression.

Results: *EN2* levels are increased in affected A-C/G-T individuals ($p = .0077$). Affected individuals also display a significant increase in *SHH* and a decrease in *INSIG1* levels. *Rs1861972-rs1861973* genotype is correlated with significant increases for *SHH* (A-C/G-T) and *CNPY1* (G-T/G-T) levels. Human cell line over-expression and knock-down as well as mouse knock-out analysis are consistent with *EN2* and *SHH* being co-regulated, which provides a possible mechanism for increased *SHH* post-mortem levels.

Conclusions: *EN2* levels are increased in affected individuals with an A-C/G-T genotype, supporting *EN2* as an ASD susceptibility gene. *SHH, CNPY1*, and *INSIG1* levels are also significantly altered depending upon affection status or *rs1861972-rs1861973* genotype. Increased *EN2* levels likely contribute to elevated *SHH* expression observed in the post-mortem samples

Editor: Christopher Beh, Simon Fraser University, Canada

Funding: This work was supported by National Institutes of Health (R01 MH076624), New Jersey Governor's Council on Autism Research, National Alliance for Autism Research, Autism Speaks, and National Alliance for Research on Schizophrenia and Depression Young Investigator Award to JHM; National Institutes of Health (R01 MH076435, RC1 MH088288) to LMB. The funders had no role in study design, data collection and analysis, decision to publish, or preparation of the manuscript.

Competing Interests: The authors have declared that no competing interests exist.

* E-mail: Millonig@CABM.rutgers.edu

Introduction

Autism Spectrum Disorder (ASD) causes deficits in language and social skills along with increased repetitive interests and behaviors. ASD includes autism, Asperger Syndrome (AS), and Pervasive Developmental Disorder-Not Otherwise Specified (PDD-NOS). Individuals with autism display the most severe phenotypes while individuals with AS and PDD-NOS typically exhibit milder symptoms.

Genetic studies have implicated the homeobox transcription factor *ENGRAILED2 (EN2)* as an ASD susceptibility gene. We determined previously that the *EN2* intronic *rs1861972-rs1861973* haplotype is associated with ASD, with the A-C haplotype being over-transmitted to affected individuals while the other common haplotype (G-T) is over-represented in unaffected siblings [1,2]. Six other groups have also reported *EN2* association with ASD [3–8].

Our molecular genetic and biochemical studies demonstrated that the ASD-associated A-C haplotype functions as a transcriptional activator [9]. Luciferase assays determined that ASD-associated A-C haplotype is both sufficient and necessary for this activator function. A protein complex specifically binds to the A-C haplotype. These proteins were partially purified and two transcription factors, CUX1 and NFIB, were identified. Subsequent electromobility shift assays (EMSAs), over-expression and knock-down studies indicate that CUX1 and NFIB bind the A-C haplotype at the same time and both proteins are required to mediate the activator function. These data demonstrate that the

ASD-associated A-C haplotype is a functional *cis*-regulatory element, and suggest that increased *EN2* levels contribute to ASD risk [9]. Consistent with this possibility, recent study demonstrated that human *EN2* is epigenetically regulated and increased levels are observed in individuals with autism but these results were not correlated with the *rs1861972-rs1861973* haplotype [10].

EN2 also regulates developmental processes relevant to ASD. Numerous groups have demonstrated that *En2* is essential for the topographic mapping of axons in both the tectum and cerebellum [11–15]. A recent study suggests that *En2* is also important for maintaining excitatory/inhibitory balance [16]. Finally several groups have demonstrated that *En2* is required for the development of ventral mid-hindbrain neurotransmitter systems [17–23].

EN2 maps to a gene poor region of the genome but the five genes within 1Mb of *EN2* are co-expressed during brain development and perform similar biological functions. These genes are: *SONIC HEDGEHOG* (*SHH*), *INSULIN INDUCED GENE1* (*INSIG1*), *CANOPY1 HOMOLOG* (*CNPY1*), *SEROTONIN RECEPTOR5A* (*HTR5A*), and *RNA BINDING MOTIF PROTEIN33* (*RBM33*).

SHH is a morphogen that coordinates many aspects of CNS development including patterning, proliferation, and connectivity. *Shh* and *En2* are co-expressed in the embryonic mid-hindbrain as well as the post-natal and adult cerebellum. During embryogenesis Shh and En2 play important roles in the development of ventral mid-hindbrain neurotransmitter systems [24–26]. In the cerebellum Shh promotes granule cell neurogenesis while En2 inhibits proliferation [27,28].

INSIG1 regulates cholesterol biosynthesis, and cholesterol modification is needed for Shh activity [29,30]. *Insig1*, *Shh*, and *En2* are co-expressed in the embryonic mid-hindbrain as well as the adult cerebellum. Interestingly, Smith-Lemli-Opitz Syndrome (SLOS) is a mono-genic disorder with defects in cholesterol biosynthesis. 50-86% of individuals with SLOS are diagnosed with ASD, suggesting an involvement of cholesterol metabolism in the disorder [31].

CNPY1 is a positive regulator of Fgf signaling and Cnpy1 induces *En2* expression in the developing mid-hindbrain [32,33]. The Fgf pathway is necessary for neurogenesis, survival, and connectivity, all of which have been implicated in ASD [34]. *Cnpy1* and *En2* are also co-expressed in the adult cerebellum.

HTR5A is a 5HT receptor and abnormalities in the serotonin pathway have been consistently implicated in ASD [35]. *Htr5a* is co-expressed with *En2* throughout development and in the adult cerebellum. Finally, *RBM33* contains homology to a predicted RNA binding domain. RNA binding proteins regulate multiple aspects of RNA processing including splicing, translation, and in neurons transport mRNAs to the synapse for local translation [36]. *Rbm33* expression has not been analyzed developmentally but is detected with the other flanking genes in the adult cerebellum. Together these results indicate En2 and the flanking genes regulate similar developmental processes and are co-expressed during development, suggesting they may be co-regulated.

Given the ASD-associated A–C haplotype functions as a transcriptional activator in cultured mouse neurons and human cell lines [9], the next important question is whether the A–C haplotype and affection status are correlated with altered *EN2* expression in individuals with autism. To investigate this possibility, post-mortem analysis was performed. We asked if affection status and *rs1861972-rs1861973* genotype are correlated with *EN2* levels. Because the flanking genes regulate ASD relevant developmental functions and are co-expressed with *EN2*, their levels were also examined and correlated with affection status and *rs1861972-rs1861973* genotype.

Results

EN2 levels are elevated in post-mortem cerebellum

To investigate if *EN2* levels are altered in individuals affected with autism, 90 age and sex matched cerebellar post-mortem samples (35 autism and 55 control) were obtained from NICHD Brain and Tissue Bank for Developmental Disorders, and Harvard Brain Tissue Resource Center (Tables S1 and S2 in File S1). The adult cerebellum was chosen as a structure to analyze because *EN2* and all the flanking genes are expressed in the cerebellum, and our previous molecular analysis demonstrated that the ASD-associated A–C haplotype is functional in mouse cerebellar neurons. To assess genotype effects on *EN2* levels, genomic DNA was isolated and each sample was genotyped for *rs1861972* and *rs1861973*. The three genotypes (A-C/A-C, A-C/G-T, and G-T/G-T) were equally distributed between autism and control groups (Table S3 in File S1). To measure *EN2* mRNA levels, total RNA was also isolated and quality was assessed using RNA integrity number (RIN). 78 samples (29 autism and 49 control) with RIN values greater than 3 were used for the final analysis (Table S1 in File S1). cDNA was then generated and Taqman qRT-PCR was performed in triplicate for each sample and normalized to *GAPDH*.

Post-mortem analysis results can be significantly affected by covariates including: affection, genotype, age, sex, post-mortem interval (PMI), RNA integrity number (RIN), as well as interaction between affection, genotype, and sex (affection*genotype, affection*sex, genotype*sex, and affection*genotype*sex). To take this into account all statistical analysis was adjusted for these covariates. For each gene expression level, insignificant covariates were removed and then a statistical model was established to correct for any significant covariates (see methods for details). Prescription drug use and comorbidity information is also available for a subset of affected individuals but matching information is mostly absent for control individuals rendering covariate analysis impossible. If no drug use or comorbidity in control group is assumed, autism affection status was positively correlated with both prescription drug use and comorbid disorders like epilepsy ($P<.0001$).

While *EN2* was expressed at higher levels in the post-mortem samples from individuals with autism (Figure S1 in File S1), analysis of covariance for *EN2* levels demonstrated a significant interaction between affection and genotype ($p = 0.0006$) (Table S4 in File S1). This result indicates the effect of the *rs1861972-rs1861973* haplotype is significantly different between the autism and control groups. Based on this finding, *rs1861972-rs1861973* genotype effects on *EN2* levels were compared separately for the affected and control groups.

For individuals with autism, *EN2* levels exhibited significant differences among three genotypes ($p = 0.0225$)(Fig 1). Affected A-C/G-T heterozygotes displayed significantly higher *EN2* levels than two other genotypes (54% higher than the A-C/A-C, $p = 0.0077$ and 45% higher than the G-T/G-T, $p = 0.0243$) (Table 1 and Fig 1). For control individuals, *EN2* levels also exhibited significant differences among three genotypes ($p<0.0001$) (data not shown). However, G-T/G-T homozygotes displayed the highest *EN2* levels in control individuals (29% higher than the A-C/A-C, $p<.0001$, and 47% higher than the A-C/G-T, $p = 0.0001$) while A-C/G-T is the lowest (Table 1 and Fig 1). In other words, individuals with autism display 74% higher *EN2* levels than controls within A-C/G-T group ($p = 0.0005$) (Table 1

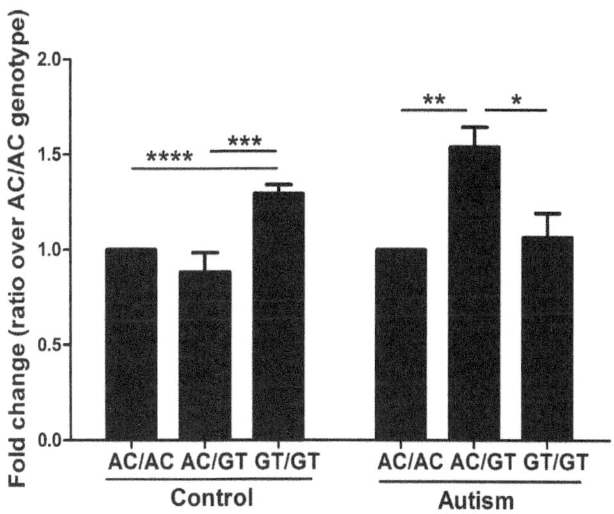

Figure 1. *EN2* levels are elevated in individuals with autism and an A-C/G-T genotype. *EN2* mRNA levels were measured in 29 autism and 49 control cerebellar samples using Taqman qRT-PCR. Based on the interaction between genotype and affection status, *EN2* levels were compared between genotypes (A-C/A-C, A-C/G-T, G-T/G-T) in control and autism groups separately. In each group *EN2* levels are normalized to 1 for A-C/A-C genotype and presented as fold change for the other genotypes (*EN2* levels are similar between control A-C/A-C and autism A-C/A-C group (<0.5% difference). Fold difference was calculated based on ΔΔCt values. Type 3 tests of fixed effects, *P<.05, **P<.01, ***P<.001, ****P<.0001. AC/AC – individuals homozygous for the *rs1861972-rs1861973* A-C haplotype, GT/GT – individuals homozygous for the G-T haplotype, AC/GT – individuals heterozygous for the A-C/G-T haplotype.

and Figure S2 in File S1). Although the effect of RIN is already taken into account in our statistical model, we performed the same analyses using samples of RIN>5(N = 59). The results displayed a similar pattern of changes albeit with slightly compromised significance due to the decreased number of samples.

These data demonstrate that *EN2* levels are elevated in A-C/G-T affected individuals. In addition, different *rs1861972-rs1861973* genotypes are correlated with increased *EN2* levels in affected (A-C/G-T) and control (G-T/G-T) individuals.

Mediators of A-C haplotype function are not increased in post-mortem cerebellum

Since the transcription factors, CUX1 and NFIB bind the A-C haplotype and mediate its function, their mRNA levels were also measured in the post-mortem samples. No significant interaction between affection status and genotype was observed for either gene. In addition, no significant difference in mRNA level was observed between affected and control groups or between the three genotype groups for either gene (Figure S3, Tables S5 and S6 in File S1). These data determined *CUX1* and *NFIB* transcript levels are not altered by affection status or *rs1861972-rs1861973* genotype in post-mortem cerebellum.

Post-mortem expression analysis for five flanking genes of *EN2*

Five genes flank *EN2* in a 1Mb region: *HTR5A* and *INSIG1* 5′ of *EN2* while *CNPY1*, *RBM33*, and *SHH* map 3′ of *EN2* (Fig 2). Animal studies indicate that *En2* and these 5 flanking genes are co-expressed (www.brain-map.org; genome.ucsc.edu/cgi-bin/hgVisiGene) and coordinate similar neurodevelopmental processes. These data led us to hypothesize that levels of the flanking genes may also be altered in the cerebellar post-mortem samples.

To examine this possibility, normalized mRNA levels were measured in the same 29 affected and 49 control individuals by Taqman qRT-PCR. Analysis of covariance resulted in slightly different final models for each gene (Tables S7-9 in File S1). Unlike *EN2*, no significant interaction between affection and genotype was observed for any of the five genes. Thus *EN2* is the only gene in the 1Mb area, whose expression levels display an interaction between affection status and *rs1861972-rs1861973* genotype. Based on this finding, comparisons for the five flanking genes were made separately for affection status and genotype.

SHH and *INSIG1* levels are altered in autism

After adjusting for covariates, *SHH* levels exhibited a significant increase in the affected group compared to control (26% increase, p = 0.0327) (Fig 3A, Table S10 in File S1). *INSIG1*, on the other

Table 1. *EN2* levels comparisons between affection and genotype groups.

Genotype	Affection	Least squared mean[a]	Standard errors[b]	P-value[c]	Fold change[d]	Standard errors[e]
AC/AC	Autism vs. Control	0.007615	0.1462	0.9586	0.9947	0.1015
AC/GT		−0.7963	0.2188	**0.0005**	1.7366	0.2678
GT/GT		0.2897	0.1599	0.0744	0.8180	0.0915
Affection	Genotype	Least squared mean[a]	Standard errors[b]	P-value[c]	Fold change[d]	Standard errors[e]
Autism	AC/AC vs. AC/GT	0.6236	0.2273	**0.0077**	0.6490	0.1041
	AC/AC vs. GT/GT	0.09040	0.1940	0.6426	0.9393	0.1280
	AC/GT vs. GT/GT	−0.5332	0.2315	**0.0243**	1.4471	0.2366
Control	AC/AC vs. AC/GT	−0.1803	0.1300	0.1699	1.1331	0.1027
	AC/AC vs. GT/GT	0.3725	0.08992	**<.0001**	0.7724	0.0483
	AC/GT vs. GT/GT	0.5527	0.1373	**0.0001**	0.6817	0.0653

[a]Least squared means were calculated from ΔΔCt values ($\Delta Ct^{autism}-\Delta Ct^{control}$ or $\Delta Ct^{1st\ genotype}-\Delta Ct^{2nd\ genotype}$) after adjusting for significant covariates.
[b]Standard error for least squared mean.
[c]Type 3 tests of fixed effects were performed considering all the significant covariates. Significant values (5% cut-off) are in bold.
[d]Fold change of each first group versus the second is calculated as $2^{-(\text{least squared mean})}$.
[e]Standard error of fold change.

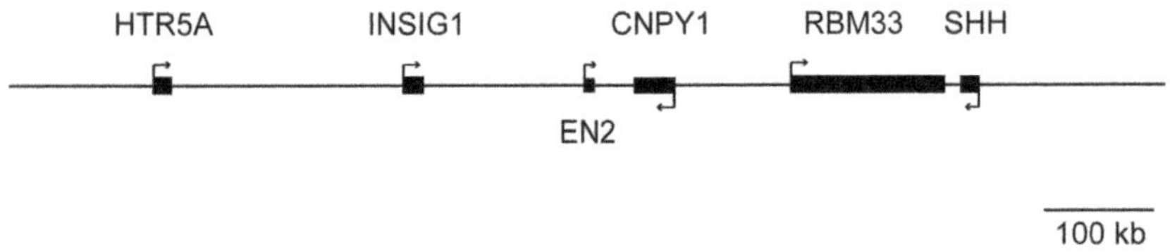

Figure 2. Genomic map of *EN2* and five flanking genes. Genomic region encompassing 500 kb upstream and 500 kb downstream of *EN2* gene is illustrated and drawn to scale. Solid boxes represent each gene and arrows indicate the transcribed DNA strand. Gene symbols for each gene are shown.

hand, displayed decreased levels in affected individuals compared to control (13% decrease, p = 0.0352) (Fig 3A, Table S11 in File S1). None of the other genes displayed a significant difference. These data demonstrate *SHH* and *INSIG1* levels are altered in these individuals with autism (Table 2 for summary).

SHH and *CNPY1* levels are correlated with *rs1861972-rs1861973* genotypes

Differences between the three genotypes were then compared regardless of affection status. *SHH* levels displayed a significant increase in A-C/G-T heterozygotes compared to A-C/A-C homozygotes (30% increase, p = 0.0297) (Fig 3B, Table S10 in File S1). *CNPY1* exhibited increased levels in G-T/G-T homozygotes compared to A-C/A-C and A-C/G-T individuals (50%, p = 0.0037 and 57% increase, p = 0.0013, respectively) (Fig 3B, Table S12 in File S1). None of the other genes displayed a significant difference. These data demonstrate that the *rs1861972-rs1861973* genotype is correlated with altered *SHH* and *CNPY1* levels (Table 2 for summary).

EN2 and *SHH* co-regulation

To investigate if increased levels of *EN2* could contribute to the altered expression of these flanking genes, *EN2* was over-expressed in non-neuronal (HEK293T) and neuronal (PFSK-1) cell lines, Flanking mRNA levels were measured by Taqman qRT-PCR, normalized to *GAPDH*, and compared to cells transfected with a non-silencing or empty vector. For *EN2* over-expression, average *SHH* mRNA levels are increased 5.72 fold in HEK293T cells and 5.5 fold in PFSK-1 cells (Fig 4a, b). We then examined the effect of *EN2* knock-down on flanking gene expression in both cell lines. 72% and 78% knock-down of *EN2* mRNA was observed in HEK293T and PFSK-1 cells respectivelly. Average *SHH* levels are significantly decreased by ~45% in both HEK293T and PFSK-1 cells (Fig 4c, d).

Next we examined the effect of stable CUX1 and NFIB single and double knock-downs generated in HEK293T cells. CUX1 and NFIB bind the ASD-associated A-C haplotype and mediate its activator function. Previous analysis demonstrated that endogenous *EN2* expression is decreased significantly by 60% only in the double knock-downs. The single knock-downs had no effect on *EN2* levels [9]. In the double knock-down, average *SHH* levels are significantly decreased (Fig 4e).

Finally we investigated the effect of the *En2* knock-out on flanking gene expression. Dopaminergic, noradrenergic and serotonergic neurons are generated from the ventral mid-hindbrain at E10.5. Previous studies indicate that Shh signaling

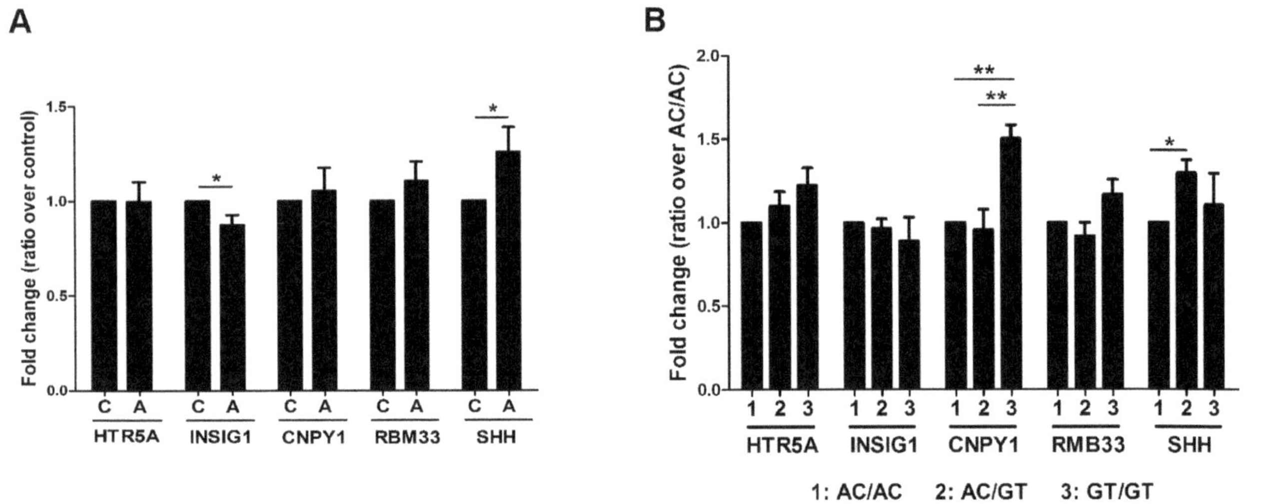

Figure 3. *SHH,INSIG1*, and *CNPY1* levels are correlated with affection status or *rs1861972-rs1861973* genotype. mRNA levels of the five flanking genes were measured using Taqman qRT-PCR. No interaction between affection status and genotype was observed, so comparisions between autism and control group were made regardless of genotype (A) and between the three genotypes regardless of affection status (B). (A) For each gene control levels are normalized to 1,and transcript levels are presented as fold change in autism using ΔΔCt values. Type 3 tests of fixed effects, *p<0.05. Note that *SHH* and *INSIG1* levels are significantly altered in affected individuals. C – control, A – autism group. (B) Each transcript level is normalized to 1 for the genotype with the lowest quantity (AC/AC for *HTR5A*; GT/GT for *INSIG1*; AC/GT for *CNPY1*; AC/GT for *RBM33*; AC/AC for *SHH*). Levels for other genotypes are presented as fold change using ΔΔCt values. Type 3 tests of fixed effects, *p<0.05, **p<0.01. *CNPY1* and *SHH* levels are correlated with *rs1861972-rs1861973* genotype.

Table 2. Summary of flanking gene results.

	Post-mortem	*EN2* over-expression	*EN2* knock-down	*CUX1-NFIB* knock-down	*En2* knock-out
SHH	↑ [a]	↑	↓	↓	↓
CNPY1	↑ [b]	NS[d]	↓	↓	↓
INSIG1	↓ [c]	↑	NS	↓	NS
RBM33	NS	NS	↓	NS	ND[e]
HTR5A	NS	↑	↓	↓	ND

[a]increased in A-C/G-T individuals and affected individuals.
[b]increased in G-T/G-T individuals.
[c]decreased in affected individuals.
[d]NS-not significant.
[e]ND-not determined.

helps coordinate these developmental events [25,37,38]. Given the relevance to ASD etiology, mRNA levels were quantitated in micro-dissected mid-hindbrain junction from the *En2* knock-out and wild type littermates. Average *Shh* levels are significantly decreased in the knock-out (Fig 5a). We then examined the spatial expression pattern of *Shh* by ISH. *Shh* is expressed in a ventral domain in the embryonic mid-hindbrain. In the $En2^{ko/ko}$, the *Shh* expression domain is reduced (Fig 5c, d). To quantify this difference the entire mid-hindbrain was sectioned, all sections were then subjected to ISH and the average expression domain area was measured. A 24% decrease was observed which is consistent with the reduced mRNA levels (Fig 5a, b)

Transcript levels for some of the flanking genes are also increased or decreased in the above experiments but unlike *SHH* they are never affected in a consistent manner (Figure S4 in File S1). Thus only SHH is consistently positively correlated with EN2 - with over-expression leading to increased *SHH* levels while knock-down/knock-out results in decreased *SHH* levels. In sum all of the above experiments indicate that *SHH* and *EN2* are co-regulated, and suggest that increased levels of *EN2* in the post-mortem samples likely contribute to elevated levels of *SHH*.

Discussion

The present study demonstrates that *EN2* levels are elevated in affected A-C/G-T individuals, providing additional evidence that *EN2* is an ASD susceptibility gene. These data are consistent with our *in vitro* molecular and biochemical data indicating that the A-C haplotype functions as a transcriptional activator to increase reporter activity and endogenous *EN2* levels. Another recent post-mortem study also demonstrates increased *EN2* levels in cerebellar post-mortem samples but did not correlate expression with the ASD-associated haplotype [10]. Together, these results support the model that increased *EN2* levels contribute to ASD pathogenesis.

Our *EN2* post-mortem analysis demonstrates an interaction between affection status and *rs1861972-rs1861973* genotype. This result indicates that the *rs1861972-rs1861973* genotype functions differently depending upon the affection status. In the affected group, individuals with an A-C/G-T genotype express *EN2* at the highest levels. However, in the control group, G-T/G-T individuals display the highest *EN2* levels. These data suggest that other ASD genetic, epigenetic, environmental or treatment factors work in concert with the *rs1861972-rs1861973* haplotype to affect *EN2* levels. This finding is consistent with ASD being an epistatic, multi-factorial disorder. The identification of these other ASD factors will aid our understanding of how *rs1861972-rs1861973* function is regulated.

Interestingly, affected A-C/G-T individuals display higher *EN2* levels than the affected A-C/A-C group. Given the A-C haplotype functions as a transcriptional activator in cell culture analysis, the simplest model is A-C/A-C individuals should exhibit the highest levels of *EN2* levels. However previous in vitro molecular genetic analysis used standard over-expression and knock-down approaches that never examined the allelic dosage effect of *rs1861972-rs1861973* genotype. Possible explanations for why the A-C/A-C genotype did not result in higher EN2 levels include the following. One, autism-specific environmental factors diminish the effect of the A-C haplotype, reducing levels more in A-C/A-C than A-C/G-T or G-T/G-T individuals. For example, prescription drug use and associated comorbid disorders like epilepsy in the autism cohort could affect *EN2* levels through the A-C haplotype. Some information on medication, comorbidity, and severity of symptoms is available for a subset of affected individuals. Unfortunately the number of individuals with relevant information was not sufficient to warrant a formal statistical test. In addition other unrecorded variables specific to the A-C/A-C autism group likely exist, and these could impact *EN2* levels. Two, other ASD risk factors specifically interact with the A-C/G-T genotype to elevate *EN2* levels. Three, because ASD is a heterogeneous disorder, increased *EN2* levels might only be observed in a subset of affected A-C/A-C individuals, which might be detected if the number of samples was increased substantially. Four, it is possible that the A-C and G-T haplotypes function in trans to create a unique cis-regulatory element. Transvection is a phenomenon whereby cis-regulatory elements function in trans to control gene expression. Reports indicate that transvection regulates gene expression in both humans and Drosophila, suggesting this mechanism is possible [39,40]

Nevertheless, our post-mortem and molecular analysis is consistent with increased *EN2* levels contributing to ASD pathogenesis. Animal studies indicate that En2 regulates several important aspects of brain development relevant to ASD including connectivity, E/I balance, as well as serotonin and norepinephrine system development [15,16,24-26,41,42]. Over-expression and mis-expression studies in animal models have demonstrated that levels and proper spatial-temporal expression of *En2* is necessary for normal brain development [11,13–15,43–45]. Thus altered levels or mis-expression at a critical time points could affect any number of developmental processes relevant to ASD.

Levels for some of the flanking genes were also significantly increased or decreased in the post-mortem samples (Table 2). *SHH* levels were increased in affected individuals as well as individuals

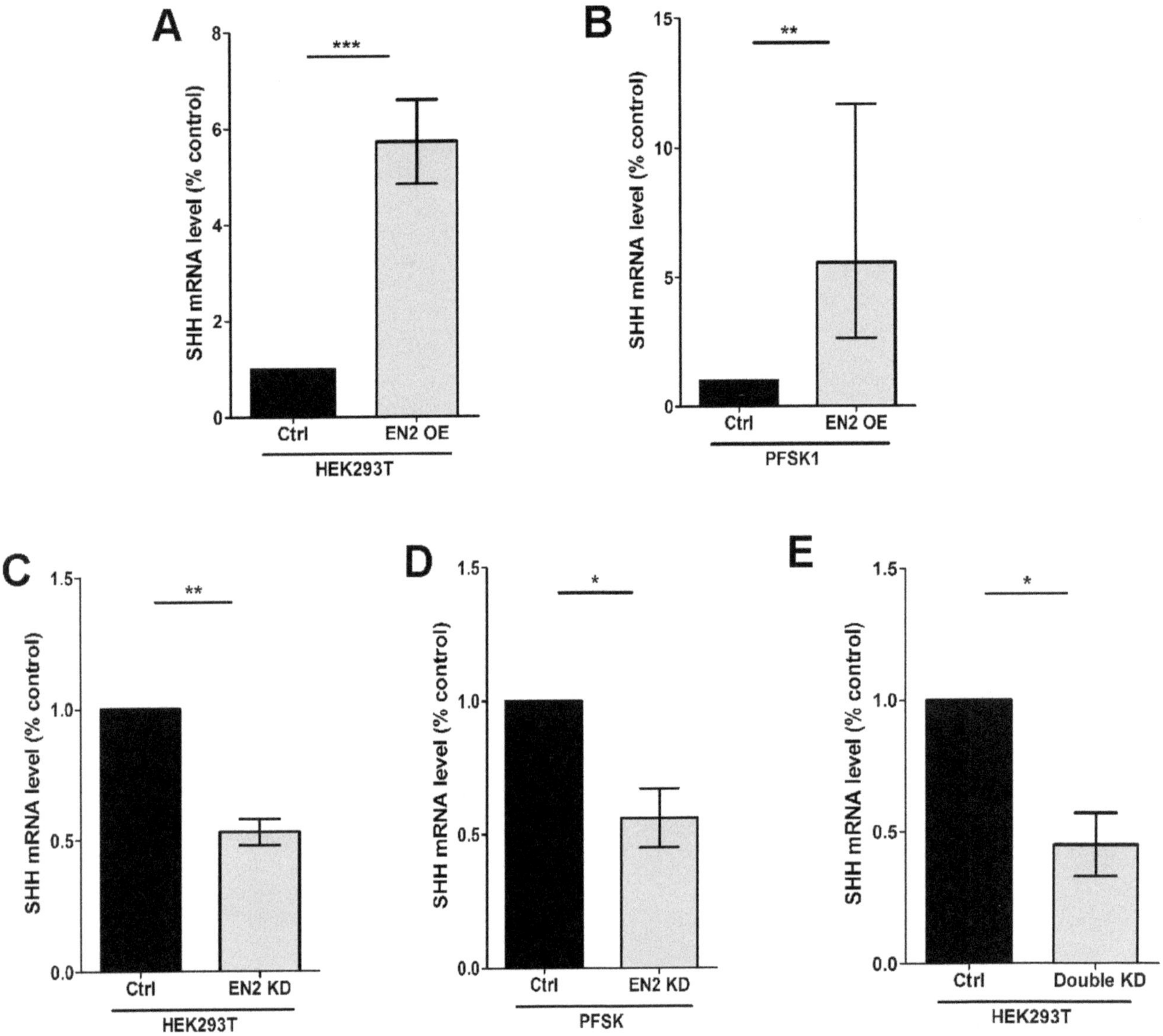

Figure 4. *SHH* expression is regulated by *EN2* levels. To investigate if *EN2* regulates flanking gene expression, over-expression and knock-down analyses were performed. (A, B) For over-expression analysis human *EN2* cDNA (EN2) or empty pCMV-Tag3B vectors (Ctrl) were transfected transiently into HEK293T (A) and PFSK1 (B) cells. SHH is expressed in both cell lines. mRNA levels were measured by Taqman qRT-PCR and normalized to GAPDH. Relative SHH mRNA levels are presented as fold difference of *EN2* over-expression versus control condition. qRTPCR was performed in triplicate and average ΔCt values were used for statistical analyses. N = 8–9, (C, D) *EN2* knock-down (KD) was achieved by transfecting shRNAmir constructs (Open Biosystems) into HEK293T cells (C) and PFSK1 (D) cells. A nonsilencing construct was used as a control (Ctrl). SHH mRNA levels were measured as described above. N = 3–6. (E) Both CUX1 and NFIB bind the *EN2* A-C haplotype and mediate its transcriptional activator function. To investigate the effect of CUX1 and NFIB on the flanking gene levels, stable double knock-downs (KD) were established in HEK293T cells and analyzed. A non-silencing control cell line (Ctrl) was also generated. mRNA levels for each gene were measured using Taqman qRT-PCR. N = 3. In sum *SHH* expression consistently mirrors *EN2* levels in all five experiments. Student T-test, two-tailed, paired, *P<.05, **P<.01, ***P<.001.

with an A-C/G-T genotype. *INSIG1* levels were decreased in affected individuals, while *CNPY1* was increased in G-T/G-T individuals (Table 2). None of these genes displayed an interaction between genotype and affection status, indicating that ASD only affects *rs1861972-rs1861973* regulation of *EN2*. Finally *RBM33* and *HTR5A* did not display any difference in expression.

Because *EN2*, *SHH*, *CNPY1* and *INSIG1* are co-expressed during development and regulate similar developmental processes, we investigated whether elevated levels of *EN2* may contribute to altered flanking gene expression. *SHH* levels were affected in all analyses. When *EN2* was over-expressed, *SHH* levels were also increased as observed in the post-mortem samples. When *EN2* levels were decreased by knock-down, the *CUX1-NFIB* double knock-down, or in the *En2* knock-out, *SHH* levels were also decreased. These results are consistent with *EN2* regulating *SHH* expression, which is supported by research in Drosophila [46-48]. Thus one likely down-stream effect of increased *EN2* levels is elevated SHH.

While EN2 regulation of *SHH* likely contributes to increased levels, other factors may also play a role. *SHH* is increased in all affected post-mortem samples regardless of genotype so other ASD risk factors also likely contribute to the increased expression. *SHH* levels are also increased in A-C/G-T individuals, suggesting that the *rs1861972-rs1861973* haplotype may regulate *SHH* at a

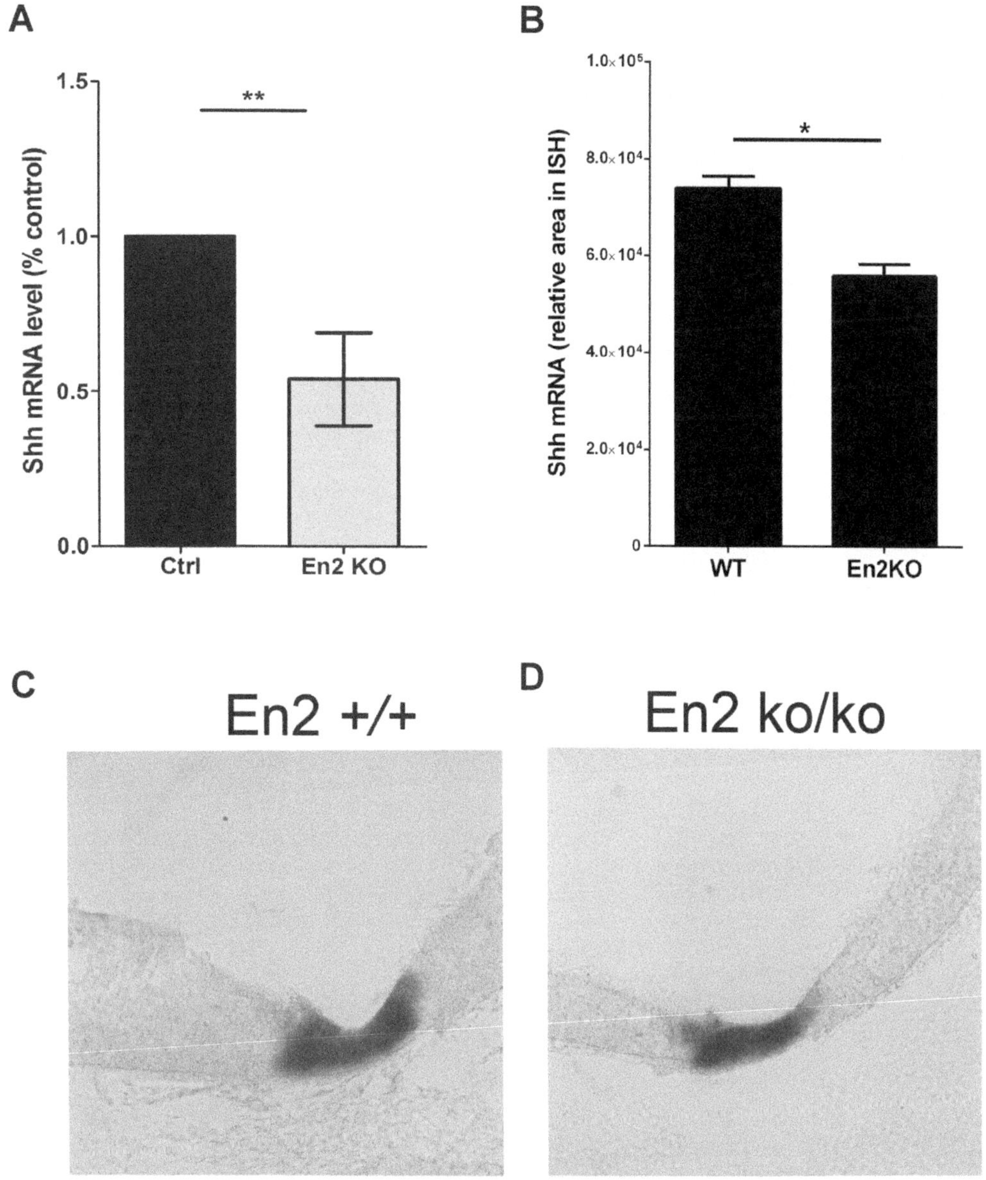

Figure 5. *Shh* levels are decreased in the ventral mid-hindbrain junction of *En2*$^{ko/ko}$. A) Ventral E10.5 mid-hind junction was dissected from *En2* knock-out (KO) embryos and wild-type (WT) littermates. *Shh* mRNA levels were measured by SYBR Green qRT-PCR and reduced expression is observed in the *En2*$^{ko/ko}$. N = 11 Student T-test, two-tailed, paired, **P<.01. B-D) *Shh* ISHs were performed at the same age and a reduced expression area was observed in the KO compared to WT. N = 5 Student T-test, two-tailed, paired, *P<.05.

distance. Consistent with this possibility the *CUX1-NFIB* double knock-down displays reduced *SHH* levels while the single CUX1 and NFIB knock-downs had no effect on *SHH* levels. It is well established that enhancers can function hundreds of kilobases away from transcriptional start sites. Interestingly, a classic example of long-range transcriptional regulation is *Shh* where spatially restricted expression in the developing limb, notochord, and floor plate is controlled by distant enhancers [49-51]. The cis-regulatory elements important for *Shh* cerebellar expression have not been identified.

Thus EN2 regulation, other ASD risk factors, and the *rs1861972-rs1861973* haplotype all likely contribute to increased *SHH* levels. Shh functions as a morphogen during development to coordinate numerous developmental processes including proliferation, neuronal specification, connectivity and synaptogenesis [52,53]. Shh also plays an essential role in the patterning of the mid-hindbrain to generate ventral dopaminergic, noradrenergic and serotonergic neurons [24,25,54,55]. These neurons then innervate the vast majority of the brain and control behaviors relevant to ASD such as attention, sleep-wake states and anxiety/mood. We observed diminished levels of Shh in the E10.5 *En2* knockout consistent with a possible effect on ventral neurotransmitter development. SHH is also potent mitogen [52]. While many studies point to synaptic defects in autism, macrocephaly and accelerated brain growth have also been consistently reported [56,57]. Elevated levels of SHH during brain development could contribute to this phenotype. Thus altered SHH levels may contribute to some of the neurodevelopmental phenotypes observed in individuals with ASD.

Finally, *CNPY1* and *INSIG1* levels are also affected in the post-mortem samples but unlike SHH these post-mortem effects do not seem to be due to increased *EN2* levels but instead other ASD factors likely play a more significant role.

In summary, our studies demonstrate that *EN2*, *SHH*, *CNPY1* and *INSIG1* levels are significantly altered in our post-mortem analysis. Increased *EN2* levels are consistent with our previous molecular genetic data for the ASD-associated A-C haplotype. The altered levels of *SHH* is likely to be due to a combination of other ASD-trans acting factors, long range cis-regulatory effects of the *rs1861972-rs1861973* haplotype, and regulation by EN2. The *CNPY1* and *INSIG1* effects are more likely due to other ASD risk factors. All four genes function in similar cell biological pathways relevant to ASD, and alterations in their levels could perturb CNS development and contribute to ASD pathogenesis.

Materials and Methods

All human post-mortem analysis and mouse studies were approved by the University of Medicine and Dentistry of New Jersey (UMDNJ) New Brunswick/Piscataway Institutional Review Board (IRB) and UMDNJ-Robert Wood Johnson Medical School (RWJMS) Institutional Animal Care and Use Committee (IACUC) (I12-013-3) committees. Written consent was obtained from both committees prior to initiating the analysis. All human post-mortem samples were obtained from NICHD Brain and Tissue Bank for Developmental Disorders and the Harvard Brain Tissue Resource Center. All samples are de-identified with no identifiable medical or personal information.

Post-mortem analysis

We obtained 90 frozen postmortem cerebellar tissue samples from 35 individuals with autism and 55 controls with no obvious diagnosable psychiatric disorder. Frozen cerebellar tissue was homogenized for isolation of RNA and DNA, and each post-mortem sample was genotyped for *rs1861972-rs1861973*. RNA integrity was assessed, cDNA was generated from 78 samples with RIN values greater than 3, and the QRTPCR was performed. See File S1 for details.

Post-mortem statistical analysis

Statistical analysis was performed in collaboration with biostatistician Yong Lin Ph.D. All results are adjusted for significant covariates. Only *EN2* levels displayed an interaction between genotype and affection status so comparisons were made considering both variables together. For all the other genes, no interaction was observed so comparisons were made for each variable (affection or genotype) separately. Since variations were not the same between the various genotype and affection groups, analysis of covariance with heterogeneous variance model was used to test if affection status or genotype is correlated with significant changes in mRNA levels. The response variable is the average ΔCt, which was generated by performing qRTPCR in triplicate for each transcript in every post-mortem sample. The full model for analysis of covariance includes 10 variables: affection, genotype, sex, and interaction between affection, genotype and sex (affection*genotype, affection*sex, genotype*sex, and affection*-genotype*sex), as well as age, post-mortem interval (PMI), and RIN. The Type 3 tests of fixed effects were performed, and insignificant covariates were removed one by one to obtain the final model, which includes only significant covariates. Pair-wise comparisons were conducted based on the final model so any difference in expression levels was adjusted for significant covariates. Since all analysis assumed normality, these assumptions were verified for the final model. Tests for normality of residuals were conducted, and QQ-plots as well as the residuals plots were generated for the final model. Based on these analyses, three potential outliers for *INSIG1* levels (AN16641 and AN00764 - affected G-T/G-T; UMB4899- affected A-C/G-T), one for *CNPY1* (AN16641- affected G-T/G-T), and one for *CUX1* (AN16641- affected G-T/G-T) were detected. For these three genes, sensitivity analysis was performed by removing outliers. Pair-wise comparisons were conducted based on this final model and any difference in expression levels was adjusted for significant covariates. Differences in gene expression levels were estimated for each comparison by calculating least squared mean of ΔΔCt values. Standard error was calculated for each least squared mean and significance was assessed using the Type 3 tests of fixed effects for *EN2* and all flanking genes. Tukey's adjustment was used for all pair-wise comparisons. Fold increase and decrease for each pair was calculated using the formula $2^{-\text{least squared mean}}$. A significance level of 5% was used for all the tests.

Over-expression, knock-down analysis and knockout analysis

Standard over-expression and knock-down analysis was performed. For the *En2* knock-out analysis, the $En2^{tm1Alj}$ knockout allele was maintained on a 12:12 light:dark cycle. Heterozygous matings were performed, impregnated females were identified and sacrificed. The mid-hindbrain junction was dissected underneath a Nikon stereo microscope in 1xPBS using forebrain-midbrain junction and rhombomere 4 as landmarks. The tissue was flash frozen, total RNA was isolated as described above and yolk sac DNA was used to determine genotype. For the over-expression, knock-down and knock-out analysis, flanking mRNA levels were measured by standard SYBR green QRTPCR. See File S1 for details.

Acknowledgments

We thank NICHD Brain and Tissue Bank for Developmental Disorders, the Harvard Brain Tissue Resource Center for the post-mortem samples, and all participating families for the post-mortem samples. We thank the Autism Tissue Program and especially Jane Pickett for all their help.

Author Contributions

Conceived and designed the experiments: JC PGM JHM. Performed the experiments: JC MRA MS. Analyzed the data: JC MRA MS YL PGM JHM. Contributed reagents/materials/analysis tools: LMB JHM. Wrote the paper: JC JHM.

References

1. Benayed R, Gharani N, Rossman I, Mancuso V, Lazar G, et al. (2005) Support for the homeobox transcription factor gene ENGRAILED 2 as an autism spectrum disorder susceptibility locus. Am J Hum Genet 77: 851–868.
2. Gharani N, Benayed R, Mancuso V, Brzustowicz LM, Millonig JH (2004) Association of the homeobox transcription factor, ENGRAILED 2, 3, with autism spectrum disorder. Molecular psychiatry 9: 474–484.

3. Yang P, Lung FW, Jong YJ, Hsieh HY, Liang CL, et al. (2008) Association of the homeobox transcription factor gene ENGRAILED 2 with autistic disorder in Chinese children. Neuropsychobiology 57: 3–8.
4. Yang P, Shu BC, Hallmayer JF, Lung FW (2010) Intronic single nucleotide polymorphisms of engrailed homeobox 2 modulate the disease vulnerability of autism in a han chinese population. Neuropsychobiology 62: 104–115.
5. Sen B, Singh AS, Sinha S, Chatterjee A, Ahmed S, et al. (2010) Family-based studies indicate association of Engrailed 2 gene with autism in an Indian population. Genes Brain Behav 9: 248–255.
6. Petit E, Herault J, Martineau J, Perrot A, Barthelemy C, et al. (1995) Association study with two markers of a human homeogene in infantile autism. Journal of medical genetics 32: 269–274.
7. Brune CW, Korvatska E, Allen-Brady K, Cook EH, Jr., Dawson G, et al. (2007) Heterogeneous association between engrailed-2 and autism in the CPEA network. American journal of medical genetics Part B, Neuropsychiatric genetics : the official publication of the International Society of Psychiatric Genetics.
8. Wang L, Jia M, Yue W, Tang F, Qu M, et al. (2008) Association of the ENGRAILED 2 (EN2) gene with autism in Chinese Han population. American journal of medical genetics Part B, Neuropsychiatric genetics : the official publication of the International Society of Psychiatric Genetics 147B: 434–438.
9. Choi J, Ababon MR, Matteson PG, Millonig JH (2012) Cut-like homeobox 1 and nuclear factor I/B mediate ENGRAILED2 autism spectrum disorder-associated haplotype function. Human molecular genetics 21: 1566–1580.
10. James SJ, Shpyleva S, Melnyk S, Pavliv O, Pogribny IP (2013) Complex epigenetic regulation of engrailed-2 (EN-2) homeobox gene in the autism cerebellum. Transl Psychiatry 3: e232.
11. Baader SL, Vogel MW, Sanlioglu S, Zhang X, Oberdick J (1999) Selective disruption of "late onset" sagittal banding patterns by ectopic expression of engrailed-2 in cerebellar Purkinje cells. J Neurosci 19: 5370–5379.
12. Herrup K, Kuemerle B (1997) The compartmentalization of the cerebellum. Annual review of neuroscience 20: 61–90.
13. Sillitoe RV, Gopal N, Joyner AL (2009) Embryonic origins of ZebrinII parasagittal stripes and establishment of topographic Purkinje cell projections. Neuroscience 162: 574–588.
14. Sillitoe RV, Stephen D, Lao Z, Joyner AL (2008) Engrailed homeobox genes determine the organization of Purkinje cell sagittal stripe gene expression in the adult cerebellum. J Neurosci 28: 12150–12162.
15. Sillitoe RV, Vogel MW, Joyner AL (2010) Engrailed homeobox genes regulate establishment of the cerebellar afferent circuit map. The Journal of neuroscience : the official journal of the Society for Neuroscience 30: 10015–10024.
16. Tripathi PP, Sgado P, Scali M, Viaggi C, Casarosa S, et al. (2009) Increased susceptibility to kainic acid-induced seizures in Engrailed-2 knockout mice. Neuroscience 159: 842–849.
17. Ritvo ER, Yuwiler A, Geller E, Ornitz EM, Saeger K, et al. (1970) Increased blood serotonin and platelets in early infantile autism. Archives of general psychiatry 23: 566-572.
18. Campbell M, Friedman E, Green WH, Collins PJ, Small AM, et al. (1975) Blood serotonin in schizophrenic children. A preliminary study. International pharmacopsychiatry 10: 213–221.
19. Cook EH, Jr., Rowlett R, Jaselskis C, Leventhal BL (1992) Fluoxetine treatment of children and adults with autistic disorder and mental retardation. J Am Acad Child Adolesc Psychiatry 31: 739–745.
20. McDougle CJ, Naylor ST, Cohen DJ, Aghajanian GK, Heninger GR, et al. (1996) Effects of tryptophan depletion in drug-free adults with autistic disorder. Archives of general psychiatry 53: 993–1000.
21. Wass S (2011) Distortions and disconnections: disrupted brain connectivity in autism. Brain and cognition 75: 18–28.
22. Minshew NJ, Keller TA (2010) The nature of brain dysfunction in autism: functional brain imaging studies. Current opinion in neurology 23: 124–130.
23. Rubenstein JL (2010) Three hypotheses for developmental defects that may underlie some forms of autism spectrum disorder. Current opinion in neurology 23: 118–123.
24. Alenina N, Bashammakh S, Bader M (2006) Specification and differentiation of serotonergic neurons. Stem cell reviews 2: 5-10.
25. Ye W, Shimamura K, Rubenstein JL, Hynes MA, Rosenthal A (1998) FGF and Shh signals control dopaminergic and serotonergic cell fate in the anterior neural plate. Cell 93: 755–766.
26. Simon HH, Scholz C, O'Leary DD (2005) Engrailed genes control developmental fate of serotonergic and noradrenergic neurons in mid- and hindbrain in a gene dose-dependent manner. Molecular and cellular neurosciences 28: 96–105.
27. Wechsler-Reya RJ, Scott MP (1999) Control of neuronal precursor proliferation in the cerebellum by Sonic Hedgehog. Neuron 22: 103–114.
28. Rossman ITaD-B, E (2008) ENGRAILED 2 and Cerebellar Development in the Pathogenesis of Autism Spectrum Disorders. Autism: Current Theories and Evidence Ed A W Zimmerman, Humana Press: 3–40.
29. Gong Y, Lee JN, Lee PC, Goldstein JL, Brown MS, et al. (2006) Sterol-regulated ubiquitination and degradation of Insig-1 creates a convergent mechanism for feedback control of cholesterol synthesis and uptake. Cell metabolism 3: 15–24.
30. Yang T, Espenshade PJ, Wright ME, Yabe D, Gong Y, et al. (2002) Crucial step in cholesterol homeostasis: sterols promote binding of SCAP to INSIG-1, a membrane protein that facilitates retention of SREBPs in ER. Cell 110: 489–500.
31. Porter FD (2008) Smith-Lemli-Opitz syndrome: pathogenesis, diagnosis and management. European journal of human genetics EJHG16: 535–541.
32. Hirate Y, Okamoto H (2006) Canopy1, a novel regulator of FGF signaling around the midbrain-hindbrain boundary in zebrafish. Current biology : CB 16: 421–427.
33. Matsui T, Thitamadee S, Murata T, Kakinuma H, Nabetani T, et al. (2011) Canopy1, a positive feedback regulator of FGF signaling, controls progenitor cell clustering during Kupffer's vesicle organogenesis. Proceedings of the National Academy of Sciences of the United States of America 108: 9881-9886.
34. Vaccarino FM, Grigorenko EL, Smith KM, Stevens HE (2009) Regulation of cerebral cortical size and neuron number by fibroblast growth factors: implications for autism. Journal of autism and developmental disorders 39: 511–520.
35. Lam KS, Aman MG, Arnold LE (2006) Neurochemical correlates of autistic disorder: a review of the literature. Res Dev Disabil 27: 254–289.
36. Bramham CR, Wells DG (2007) Dendritic mRNA: transport, translation and function. Nature reviews Neuroscience 8: 776–789.
37. Lam CS, Sleptsova-Friedrich I, Munro AD, Korzh V (2003) SHH and FGF8 play distinct roles during development of noradrenergic neurons in the locus coeruleus of the zebrafish. Mol Cell Neurosci 22: 501–515.
38. Hirate Y, Okamoto H (2006) Canopy1, a novel regulator of FGF signaling around the midbrain-hindbrain boundary in zebrafish. Curr Biol 16: 421–427.
39. Sandhu KS, Shi C, Sjolinder M, Zhao Z, Gondor A, et al. (2009) Nonallelic transvection of multiple imprinted loci is organized by the H19 imprinting control region during germline development. Genes & development 23: 2598–2603.
40. Liu H, Huang J, Wang J, Jiang S, Bailey AS, et al. (2008) Transvection mediated by the translocated cyclin D1 locus in mantle cell lymphoma. The Journal of experimental medicine 205: 1843–1858.
41. Brunet I, Weinl C, Piper M, Trembleau A, Volovitch M, et al. (2005) The transcription factor Engrailed-2 guides retinal axons. Nature 438: 94–98.
42. Wizenmann A, Brunet I, Lam JS, Sonnier L, Beurdeley M, et al. (2009) Extracellular Engrailed participates in the topographic guidance of retinal axons in vivo. Neuron 64: 355–366.
43. Millen KJ, Hui CC, Joyner AL (1995) A role for En-2 and other murine homologues of Drosophila segment polarity genes in regulating positional information in the developing cerebellum. Development 121: 3935–3945.
44. Millen KJ, Wurst W, Herrup K, Joyner AL (1994) Abnormal embryonic cerebellar development and patterning of postnatal foliation in two mouse Engrailed-2 mutants. Development 120: 695–706.
45. Baader SL, Sanlioglu S, Berrebi AS, Parker-Thornburg J, Oberdick J (1998) Ectopic overexpression of engrailed-2 in cerebellar Purkinje cells causes restricted cell loss and retarded external germinal layer development at lobule junctions. J Neurosci 18: 1763–1773.
46. Zecca M, Basler K, Struhl G (1995) Sequential organizing activities of engrailed, hedgehog and decapentaplegic in the Drosophila wing. Development 121: 2265–2278.
47. Guillen I, Mullor JL, Capdevila J, Sanchez-Herrero E, Morata G, et al. (1995) The function of engrailed and the specification of Drosophila wing pattern. Development 121: 3447–3456.
48. de Celis JF, Ruiz-Gomez M (1995) groucho and hedgehog regulate engrailed expression in the anterior compartment of the Drosophila wing. Development 121: 3467–3476.
49. Jeong Y, El-Jaick K, Roessler E, Muenke M, Epstein DJ (2006) A functional screen for sonic hedgehog regulatory elements across a 1 Mb interval identifies long-range ventral forebrain enhancers. Development 133: 761–772.
50. Jeong Y, Leskow FC, El-Jaick K, Roessler E, Muenke M, et al. (2008) Regulation of a remote Shh forebrain enhancer by the Six3 homeoprotein. Nature genetics 40: 1348–1353.
51. Lettice LA, Heaney SJ, Purdie LA, Li L, de Beer P, et al. (2003) A long-range Shh enhancer regulates expression in the developing limb and fin and is associated with preaxial polydactyly. Human molecular genetics 12: 1725–1735.
52. Traiffort E, Angot E, Ruat M (2010) Sonic Hedgehog signaling in the mammalian brain. J Neurochem 113: 576–590.
53. Harwell CC, Parker PR, Gee SM, Okada A, McConnell SK, et al. (2012) Sonic hedgehog expression in corticofugal projection neurons directs cortical microcircuit formation. Neuron 73: 1116–1126.
54. Cordes SP (2005) Molecular genetics of the early development of hindbrain serotonergic neurons. Clinical genetics 68: 487–494.
55. Lam CS, Sleptsova-Friedrich I, Munro AD, Korzh V (2003) SHH and FGF8 play distinct roles during development of noradrenergic neurons in the locus coeruleus of the zebrafish. Molecular and cellular neurosciences 22: 501–515.
56. DiCicco-Bloom E, Lord C, Zwaigenbaum L, Courchesne E, Dager SR, et al. (2006) The developmental neurobiology of autism spectrum disorder. J Neurosci 26: 6897–6906.
57. Redcay E, Courchesne E (2005) When is the brain enlarged in autism? A meta-analysis of all brain size reports. Biol Psychiatry 58: 1–9.

9

Prepulse Inhibition of the Acoustic Startle Reflex in High Functioning Autism

Sina Kohl[1]◔, Carolin Wolters[1]◔, Theo O. J. Gruendler[1,2,3], Kai Vogeley[1,4], Joachim Klosterkötter[1], Jens Kuhn[1]*

1 Department for Psychiatry and Psychotherapy, University Hospital of Cologne, Cologne, North Rhine-Westphalia, Germany, **2** Department of Economics, Otto-von-Guericke-University, Magdeburg, Saxony-Anhalt, Germany, **3** Center for Behavioral Brain Sciences, Magdeburg, Saxony-Anhalt, Germany, **4** Institute for Neuroscience and Medicine – Cognitive Neuroscience (INM3), Research Center Juelich, Juelich, North Rhine-Westphalia, Germany

Abstract

Background: High functioning autism is an autism spectrum disorder that is characterized by deficits in social interaction and communication as well as repetitive and restrictive behavior while intelligence and general cognitive functioning are preserved. According to the weak central coherence account, individuals with autism tend to process information detail-focused at the expense of global form. This processing bias might be reflected by deficits in sensorimotor gating, a mechanism that prevents overstimulation during the transformation of sensory input into motor action. Prepulse inhibition is an operational measure of sensorimotor gating, which indicates an extensive attenuation of the startle reflex that occurs when a startling pulse is preceded by a weaker stimulus, the prepulse.

Methods: In the present study, prepulse inhibition of acoustic startle was compared between 17 adults with high functioning autism and 17 sex-, age-, and intelligence-matched controls by means of electromyography.

Results: Results indicate that participants with high functioning autism exhibited significantly higher startle amplitudes than the control group. However, groups did not differ with regard to PPI or habituation of startle.

Discussion: These findings challenge the results of two previous studies that reported prepulse inhibition deficits in high-functioning autism and suggest that sensorimotor gating is only impaired in certain subgroups with autism spectrum disorder.

Editor: Harold A. Burgess, National Institutes of Health/NICHD, United States of America

Funding: The authors thank the Walter and Marga Boll Foundation, the German Research Foundation (KFO-219 grant), as well as the Center for Behavioral Brain Sciences for financial support. The funders had no role in study design, data collection and analysis, decision to publish, or preparation of the manuscript.

Competing Interests: The authors have declared that no competing interests exist.

* E-mail: jens.kuhn@uk-koeln.de

◔ These authors contributed equally to this work.

Introduction

In Leo Kanner's [1] original description of autism, he made the following observation:

> "Another intrusion comes from loud noises and moving objects, which are therefore reacted to with horror. Tricycles, swings, elevators, vacuum cleaners, running water, gas burners, mechanical toys, egg beaters, even the wind could on occasions bring about a major panic. (…) Yet it is not the noise or motion itself that is dreaded. The disturbance comes from the noise or motion that intrudes itself, or threatens to intrude itself, upon the child's aloneness." (p. 245)

In fact, about 90% of children with an autism spectrum disorder (ASD) exhibit sensory abnormalities [2,3,4]. Many of those show auditory hypersensitivity [5,6,7]. It was suggested that hypersensitivity is associated with an exceptional attention to detail in autism [5]. The weak central coherence theory of autism hypothesizes that the detail-focused processing style in children and adults with autism leads to a failure of central processing, which involves difficulties to extract global form or meaning [8]. Research regarding acoustic stimulation suggests that persons suffering from ASD are less susceptible to interference from melodic structure in music processing and to interference from visual to auditory perception (i.e. the *McGurk effect*). In addition, persons with autism show superior pitch and loudness processing and less distinctive auditory filtering [9,10]. Behavioral experiments showed that persons with ASD require a higher signal-to-noise ratio in comparison to control subjects to perceive noise or speech [11,12,13]. In addition, individuals with ASD have difficulties ignoring distracting sounds in peripheral spatial locations [14] and segregating incoming sounds [15].

Abnormal sensory processing may lead to sensorimotor integration deficits [16], which have been shown across different sensory modalities in ASD [17]. Sensorimotor gating is an adaptive mechanism that prevents overstimulation within the transformation of sensory input into motor action [18]. Abnormalities of motor behavior are highly prevalent in autism and have a great impact on everyday life abilities [19]. However, the etiology of these symptoms remains unclear [20].

In the present study, prepulse inhibition (PPI) of the acoustic startle reflex is used as a proxy of sensorimotor gating. PPI indicates an extensive attenuation of the startle reflex that occurs when a startle eliciting stimulus, the pulse, is preceded by a weaker stimulus, the prepulse, within a timeframe of 30–500 ms [21]. More than 90% of healthy subjects show a reduction of 40–80% of the startle reflex, if a pulse is preceded by a prepulse that does not elicit a startle response itself [22]. The protection of processing hypothesis proposes that the processing of sensory stimuli is protected against interference through other irrelevant or distracting stimuli by preattentive mechanisms [21].

The present study aimed at exploring sensorimotor gating in high functioning autism (HFA), a subgroup of ASD that is characterized by social and communication deficits as well as repetitive, restrictive and stereotyped behavior, interests, and activities with preservation of intelligence and general cognitive functioning [23].

We could identify five studies that focused on PPI deficits in ASD patients. McAlonan and colleagues [24] as well as Perry and colleagues [25] found attenuated PPI in adults with high functioning autism and Asperger syndrome. In contrast, three other groups did not find any significant differences in PPI in samples that included children [26] or children as well as adolescents [27,28]. Motivated by the inconsistent literature and with the idea that repetitive thoughts, behavior and activities might be a product of malfunctioning inhibition, it seemed important to us to conduct a study of high methodological quality in order to examine processing of auditory startle stimuli in a clearly defined subgroup of ASD patients. Derived from the above mentioned considerations we hypothesize that: participants with HFA will exhibit higher amplitudes of the startle reflex accompanied by reduced PPI in comparison to healthy controls.

Materials and Methods

The study was approved by the local ethics committee of the Medical Faculty of the University of Cologne, and conducted in accordance with the declaration of Helsinki. The ethics committee was also involved in compiling the patient information and consent form. All subjects were informed in speech and writing about the purpose and procedure of the study and had to give their written informed consent in order to participate. Also approved by the local ethics committee, a very experienced psychiatrist and expert in the field of autism spectrum disorders (KV) gave the diagnosis and assessed the capacity of each participant to give his/her consent. As further support of the evaluation and for diagnostic purpose an intelligence test has been conducted with each participant (German multiple choice test *Wortschatztest* (WST)) to confirm ability to give consent. We did not obtain any surrogate consents.

Materials

Autistic traits were estimated using the self-assessment questionnaire autism quotient (AQ) as screening instrument [29]. Empathy was measured by the self-report questionnaire empathy quotient (EQ) [30], and the tendency to systemize was acquired using the self-report questionnaire systemizing quotient (SQ) [31]. The Beck Depression Inventory (BDI) [32] was completed by all participants in order to measure depressive symptomatology. Intelligence was measured using the German multiple choice test *Wortschatztest (WST)* [33], which provides a short and valid estimation of general intelligence [34]. In addition, participants were asked to fill out a questionnaire, which included questions about any regular intake of medication, and the frequency and last point of time they consumed caffeine, alcohol, cannabis, and other drugs.

Subjects

23 subjects with HFA and 23 normal control (NC) subjects (both groups: 7 women, 16 men) were assessed. The experimental group was diagnosed and recruited in the Autism Outpatient Clinic of the Department of Psychiatry, University of Cologne. The diagnosis was made by two experienced clinicians in two independent interviews (one of them KV) according to the International Classification of mental disorders [23] and supplemented by comprehensive neuropsychological assessment. Only individuals with the diagnosis of HFA (F84.5) were included into the sample. Formally, criteria of the DSM-IV [35] for HFA were met as well.

Control subjects were matched to sex, age, and intelligence scores of the experimental group. In our screening procedure, none of the control subjects had a BDI score above the clinically critical value of 17 [36] or an AQ above the cutoff score of 32 suggested by Baron-Cohen, Wheelwright, Skinner, Martin, and Clubley [37]. None of the control subjects showed any signs or symptoms of any possible psychiatric comorbid disorder. According to self disclosure, none of the participants suffered from any kind of hearing impairment. All of the subjects had an intelligence quotient (IQ) above 70 (see table 1).

Three of the subjects with HFA and three of the NC subjects had to be excluded from the data analysis because they did not exhibit sufficient startle responses and were thus classified as non-responders. One participant with HFA had to be excluded from further data analysis because he fell asleep during the test sessions, and one data set of an HFA subject was not usable due to technical malfunction. Additionally, one of the subjects with HFA and three of the NC subjects were excluded because visual inspection of the data indicated startle responses to the prepulses and PPI was therefore not reliably calculable.

Thus, $n = 17$ subjects with HFA and $n = 17$ NC subjects (each with 5 women, 12 men) remained in the sample (Table 1–3). There were no significant group differences regarding age, intelligence, and years of education. However, the HFA group showed significantly higher BDI scores than the control group. In addition, participants with HFA showed significantly higher AQ and SQ scores, and significantly lower EQ scores than NC participants.

Procedure

The startle reflex was measured in a quiet laboratory by means of an EMG of the musculus orbicularis oculi (EMG SR-HLAB, San Diego Instruments, San Diego, CA). To this end, two miniature electrodes were placed below and next to the participant's right eye, and a ground electrode was placed behind the right ear. Participants were briefed to sit quietly in an armchair and to fix their gaze on a spot. The stimulus material was presented binaurally through headphones (TDH-39-P, Maico, Minneapolis, MN). During the course of the measurement, background white noise of 70 dB was presented. Acoustic stimuli consisted of bursts of broadband white noise. Startle eliciting stimuli were presented for 40 ms at intensities of 110 dB with uncontrolled instant rise time, while prepulses were presented for 20 ms at 80 dB. Each PPI session started with a 5 min acclimation

Table 1. Participants' characteristics.

Variable	HFA group		Control group		Statistical differences		
	M (SD)	Range	*M (SD)*	Range	*T*	*df*	*p*
Age	40.2 (9.93)	23–53	43.4 (10.55)	26–56	.090	32	.373
Education	18.2 (5.48)	10–30	20.4 (3.35)	15–27	1.38	32	.178
IQ	116.4 (16.14)	89–143	119.2 (7.0)	101–133	.66	22	.515
BDI	11 (9.76)	0–34	5.1 (4.98)	0–15	2.24	24	.035*
AQ	41.1 (3.64)	34–45	15.9 (7.05)	5–29	13.09	24	<.001*
EQ	16.9 (7.82)	6–30	42.4 (12.83)	21–65	3.77	23	<.001*
SQ	37.3 (15.42)	11–67	21.7 (7.24)	11–36	7.01	32	<.001*

HFA = High functioning autism; Education = Years of education; IQ = Intelligence Quotient; BDI = Beck Depression Inventory; AQ = Autism Quotient; EQ = Empathy Quotient; SQ = Systemizing Quotient; *significant at an alpha level of .05.

period of white noise. The first and the last block of the measurement comprised 5 pulse-alone trials. Intermittently, 10 pulse-alone trials, 10 prepulse-alone trials, and 30 prepulse-pulse trials were presented in a pseudorandom order. Prepulse-pulse stimulus onset asynchronies (SOAs) varied between 60, 120, and 240 ms. Intertrial intervals were 10, 15, 20, or 25 sec. Each trial was preceded by a baseline period of 60 ms, starting 80 ms before the stimulus onset.

Data analyses

EMG data were analyzed using a *Matlab* program (MathWorks, Inc., Natick, MA) that was developed in our clinic in order to visually inspect and calculate PPI data. Recorded EMG activity was high-pass filtered at 30 Hz and low-pass filtered at 300 Hz using a 4th order butterworth filter, and a 50 Hz notch filter with a width of 6 Hz was used to reduce power line interference (hier bitte den van Boxtel Artikel zitieren). The EMG signal was then rectified and smoothed using a 10 point moving average. By means of visual inspection, any trial featuring excessive noise in the EMG signal or a spontaneous blink in the period immediately preceding the stimulus onset or the minimal response onset were excluded from further analyses. Based on these criteria, 9.44% of trials had to be excluded from data analysis. In addition, the first two pulse-alone trials of each PPI measure were excluded from the analysis, as it was assumed that these trials evoke unrepresentatively high startle amplitudes [38].

Criteria for qualifying the EMG signal as an actual startle response were defined in accordance with guidelines for human startle eye blink EMG studies [38]. The latency window was set at 20 to 150 ms after pulse onset, and the minimum response amplitude was set at 2 *SD* above baseline. The response peak was identified by a computerized algorithm. If visual inspection indicated that response onset was outside the latency window or the criteria for minimal response size was not met, the trial was classified as a zero response trial. These trials were not considered in the calculation of the specific values. Participants were identified as non-responders and therefore excluded if they exhibited startle responses in less than half of the pulse-alone trials. Participants for whom visual inspection of the prepulse-alone trials revealed distinct reactions to the prepulses in half or more of the trials were excluded as well.

Statistical analyses

A commercial software package was used for statistical analysis of the data (SPSS for windows, version 21, IBM Corp., Armonk, NY).

Startle amplitudes. Mean startle amplitudes were calculated by averaging the response peaks of all included trials, and compared between groups using an unpaired Student's *t*-test. Differences in startle amplitudes within the different trial conditions were compared by means of a one-way repeated-measure ANOVA. In addition to startle amplitudes we calculated the response probability, the probability that a valid startle response follows the startle eliciting pulse. The response probability is given in percent.

PPI. Percentage PPI values were calculated according to the following formula: 100 – [(mean amplitude prepulse trials/mean amplitude pulse alone trials) x 100]. Besides comparing PPI between the HFA and NC group, PPI group differences were assessed using three different one-way repeated measures ANOVAs, including the between-subjects factor of group (1. male/female; 2. smoker/non-smoker; 3. HFA/NC), and within-subjects repeated measures of PPI across the different trial types. Mean startle amplitude across all pulse-alone trials was included as a

Table 2. Comorbid psychiatric disorders.

Number of participants (group)	Psychiatric disorder
1 (HFA)	Bipolar disorder
1 (HFA)	Depression
1 (HFA)	Dysthymia
1 (HFA)	Anxiety Disorder
2 (HFA)	ADHD
1 (HFA)	ADD

HFA = High functioning autism; ADHD = attention deficit/hyperactivity disorder; ADD = attention deficit disorder.

covariate. Furthermore, PPI differences across all three types of trials were calculated using Student's *t*-tests.

Correlations between PPI and autistic traits. To assess the relationship between PPI and autistic traits, the AQ, EQ, and SQ scores of the HFA subjects were correlated with percentage PPI of the three trial types using the Pearson's correlation coefficient.

Habituation. Primarily, group differences in habituation of the startle response across all pulse-alone trials were calculated. To this end, the altogether 20 pulse-alone trials were split into four blocks of five trials each. A one-way repeated measures ANOVA was conducted, including the between-subjects factor of diagnosis (HFA/NC) and the within-subjects factor of mean startle amplitude of the four pulse-alone blocks. Additionally, the overall habituation rate was examined by calculating the percent decrease from mean startle amplitude in the first five pulse-alone trials to mean amplitude in the last five trials and compared between groups by means of an unpaired Student's *t*-test.

Before conducting the ANOVAs, the assumption of sphericity was tested for the data, and degrees of freedom were corrected using Greenhouse-Geisser estimates of sphericity, if necessary. Effect sizes for ANOVAs were calculated using $\eta^2_{partial}$, effect sizes for post-hoc pairwise comparisons were calculated using Cohen's *d*.

Results

Startle amplitudes

Analysis of startle amplitudes for pulse-alone trials revealed significantly higher startle amplitudes ($M = 179.1$, $SD = 146.93$) for HFA patients than control subjects ($M = 96.6$, $SD = 62.93$), $T(32) = 2.13$, $p = .041$. The mean response probability for a significant startle amplitude in pulse alone trials for the HFA group ($M = 93.66$ $SD = 9.04$) was significantly higher compared to the control group ($M = 80.52$, $SD = 18.81$), $T(32) = 2.6$, $p = .014$.

PPI

Examining PPI differences between the HFA and NC group, Mauchly's test of sphericity was not significant, $\chi^2 = .17$, $df = 2$, $p = .435$. There was a significant main effect of trial type (60/120/240 ms SOA), $F(2) = 3.35$, $p = .041$, $\eta^2_{partial} = .098$. Post-hoc pairwise comparisons indicated that PPI was significantly lower in trials with an SOA of 240 ms than in those with an SOA of 60 ms, $p = .015$, $d = .61$, and 120 ms, $p = .001$, $d = .63$ (*p*-values were Bonferroni adjusted).

However, there was no significant effect of mean startle amplitude across pulse-alone trials, $F(1) = .30$, $p = .590$, and no significant interaction of startle amplitude and trial type, $F(2) = .12$, $p = .887$. Equally, there was no significant main effect of diagnosis on PPI, $F(1) = .02$, $p = .879$, and no significant interaction of diagnosis and trial type, $F(2) = .13$, $p = .877$. Figure 1 shows the PPI values of HFA and NC subjects across the three different types of trials. Likewise, there were no differences in overall PPI between participants with HFA ($M = 32.5$, $SD = 31.11$) and control participants (M = 36.8, SD = 22.11), T(32) = .46, p = .649.

The response probabilities for the prepulse trials did not differ significantly between the HFA Group ($M = 84.18$, $SD = 18.73$) and the controls ($M = 72.66$, $SD = 24.18$), $T(32) = 1.55$, $p = .13$.

Correlations between autistic traits and PPI

There were no significant correlations between AQ, EQ, and SQ scores and PPI in the different trial types among HFA participants (all $p > .1$).

Table 3. Medication.

Number of participants	Medication
5 (HFA), 1 (NC)	Antidepressant drug (2× Sertraline, 2× Mirtazepine,
	1× Citalopram, 1× Moclobemid)
2 (HFA), 1 (NC)	Beta blocker (1× Bisoprolol, 1× Metahexal,
	1× Mesoprolol)
1 (HFA), 1 (NC)	Irbesartan
1 (NC)	Ramiprile
1 (HFA)	Lamotrigine

HFA = High functioning autism; NC = normal controls.

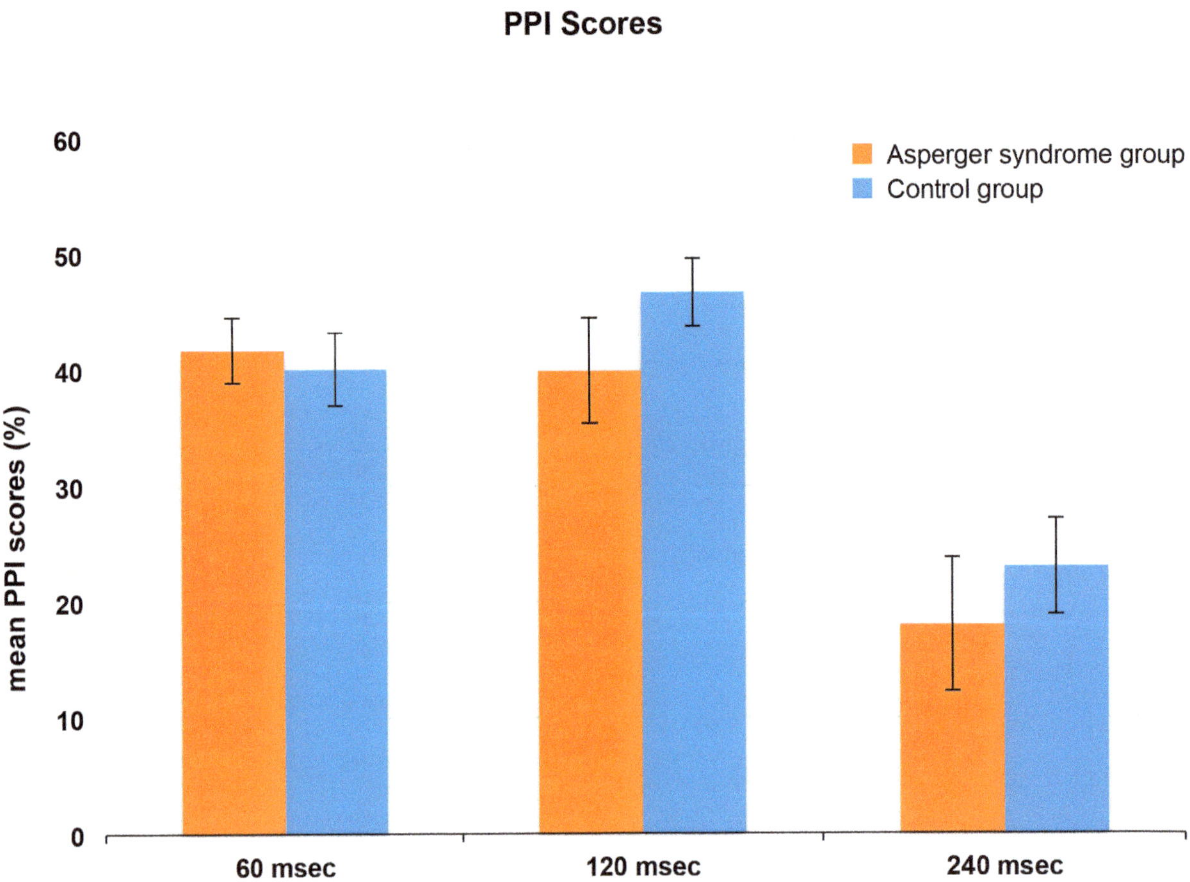

Figure 1. PPI scores. Mean PPI scores (± SEM) across the three trial conditions in subjects with high functioning autism (HFA) and normal control (NC) subjects.

Habituation

Mauchly's test indicated that the assumption of sphericity was not met for startle amplitude scores, $\chi^2 = 23.52$, $df = 5$, $p < .001$. Therefore, degrees of freedom were corrected using Greenhouse-Geisser estimates of sphericity. Results showed that the startle amplitude was significantly affected by block, $F(2) = 30.32$, $p < .001$, $\eta^2_{partial} = .486$, indicating habituation across the four blocks of pulse-alone trials. Pairwise comparisons determined that the mean startle amplitude decreased from the first block to the second, $p < .001$, $d = .47$, to the third, $p < .001$, $d = .67$, and to the fourth block, $p < .001$, $d = .75$. In addition, the startle amplitude significantly decreased from the second to the fourth block, $p < .001$, $d = .31$ (p-values were Bonferroni adjusted). Data analysis also revealed a significant main effect of diagnosis, $F(1) = 4.67$, $p = .038$, $\eta^2_{partial} = .127$, reflecting the differences in startle amplitude between HFA and NC participants. However, there was no significant block-by-group effect, $F(2) = .19$, $p = .834$. Visual inspection confirmed that the two groups had similar decreases in startle amplitude over the four blocks (see figure 2).

Analysis of overall percentage habituation from block 1 to block 4 did not show significant differences between HFA ($M = 48.0$, $SD = 26.31$) and NC participants ($M = 52.1$, $SD = 25.13$), $T(32) = .47$, $p = .641$.

Discussion

The present study assessed auditory sensorimotor gating by means of the acoustic startle reflex in subjects with HFA. Our results indicate significantly higher mean startle amplitudes in the HFA group and for the pulse alone condition significantly higher response probabilities compared to the control group. But groups did not differ significantly in terms of PPI, neither in the different SOA trial types, nor across all trials.

Startle amplitude

Increased startle amplitudes among HFA subjects may be caused by auditory hypersensitivity, which often occurs in autism [5]. Abnormalities in the processing of auditory information were also shown by neurophysiologic studies finding atypical neural activity in early auditory pathways in ASD [39]. Magnetoencephalography studies have linked auditory hypersensitivity to maturational abnormalities in the auditory cortex in autism, resulting in delayed responses of the auditory cortex to acoustic stimuli [40], and abnormalities in myelination processes, causing slower transmission rates in central auditory pathways [41,42]. In addition, reduced interneuron activity might lead to abnormal brain connectivity, which might in turn cause cortical hypersensitivity in the primary auditory cortex [43].

PPI

The other major hypothesis could not be proven by our results. Bearing in mind the weak central coherence theory of autism we hypothesized, subjects with HFA would show PPI deficits in comparison to the control group. But in accordance with three other studies [26,27,28] our results indicate that PPI does not

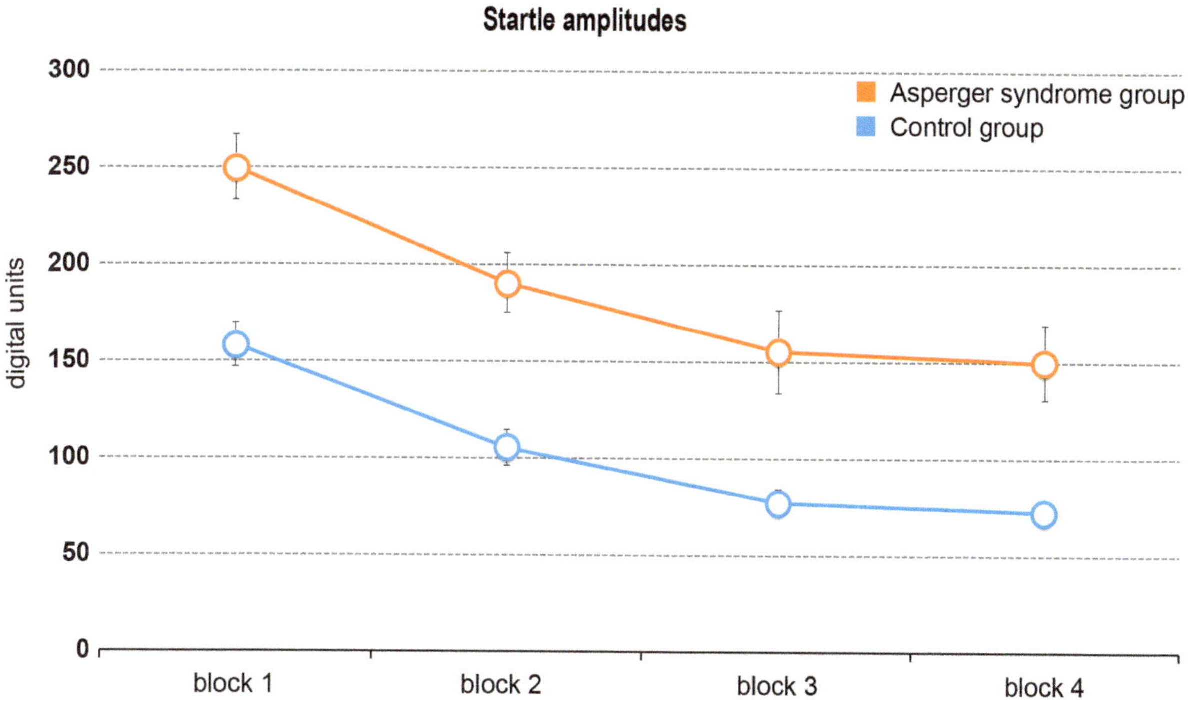

Figure 2. Startle amplitudes and habituation rates. Habituation rates across the four blocks of trials in the high functioning autism (HFA) and normal control (NC) group. Mean startle amplitudes (± SEM) of each five pulse-alone trials are shown. HFA participants showed significantly higher absolute startle amplitudes compared to NC participants, while habituation rates were similar.

differ between the HFA and the NC group. However, the aforementioned studies examined PPI in samples of children and young adults of different age on the autistic spectrum. As PPI is thought to mature with advancing age in childhood [44], PPI deficits might vary between children of different age groups, or may not be observable in children at all.

So far, only one study explicitly focused on adults with HFA [24]. The authors found significant PPI differences between subjects with HFA and the control group in only one condition (SOA 120 ms), while PPI in the HFA group was similar to or even higher than that of the control group in the other conditions (SOA 30 and 60 ms). In contrast, Perry et al. [25] found significantly reduced PPI in subjects with high-functioning autism in comparison to control subjects in the SOA 60 ms condition, but not in the SOA 30 and 120 ms conditions. However, these authors did not report the specific diagnoses of their participants. It must be emphasized that our cohort differs from the autism groups of previous studies in terms of age, sex, and IQ. These differences might have implications for our results. For example, our cohort has a higher mean IQ compared to previous studies, this might imply that our cohort is composed of pure HFA and not confounded by low intelligence or other cognitive dysfunctions.

Habituation

Even though individuals with HFA exhibited higher startle amplitudes than control subjects, habituation rates were similar in both groups. This finding is consistent with those of Ornitz et al. [27] and [24], who did not find any differences in habituation between subjects with ASD and control subjects. In contrast, Perry et al. [25] found that subjects with ASD show decelerated habituation, speculating that reduced habituation might lead to behavioral and cognitive deficits in autism. However, their sample comprised only male subjects with ASD, while the current study examined men and women with HFA. Then again, previous studies found reduced habituation to acoustic stimuli in children with autism [45] and at high risk for autism [46]. A cross-sectional questionnaire study found that less developmentally mature children with autism and other developmental disorders exhibited the highest rates of sensory processing difficulties [47]. Perhaps, habituation to sensory stimuli is associated with mental age, explaining normal habituation rates in normally intelligent adults with HFA.

Study limitations

Some factors might limit the degree to which the findings of the present study can be generalized. The determination of unimpaired hearing, potential psychiatric and neurological disorders as well as use of medication relied on self-report only. Therefore, information might be incomplete or unreliable. Seven HFA subjects reported an additional mental disorder. Studies consistently reported no alterations of PPI in depression and ADHD [48]. In bipolar disorder, PPI was found to be state dependent, while evidence regarding PPI deficits in anxiety disorders is still poor [48]. Although unlikely it can thus not completely be ruled out that comorbid disorders had an effect on sensorimotor gating. Drug intake of some participants in both groups might have influenced PPI, but here too an influence is more unlikely as animal and human studies showed that antidepressant drugs do not alter PPI [49]. However, evidence regarding the effects of other drugs, such as beta blockers, on PPI is still poor. In order to rule out such effects, subjects with comorbid psychiatric or neurological disorders and with drug intake should be excluded for less ambiguous results. Further, the mean PPI value of the healthy control group was relatively low compared to previous studies, which report PPI values between 40 to 80% in 90% of healthy adults [22]. Therefore there is a chance that comparison of control group and HFA group did not significantly differ due to relatively low PPI in controls.

Conclusions

While the results indicated no sensorimotor gating deficits, analysis of startle amplitudes revealed abnormalities in terms of exaggerated startle reaction in subjects with HFA. Individuals with HFA showed higher startle amplitudes than NC subjects, but exhibited similar rates of PPI and habituation of startle. These findings argue for functional pathophysiology on the level of the primary startle pathway, involving structures such as the caudal pontine reticular nucleus and ventrolateral tegmental nucleus in HFA. In contrast, the PPI circuit, including the pedunculopontine tegmental nucleus and inferior and superior colliculi, seems to be unimpaired.

Therefore, the extreme responses in individuals with autism to sensory stimulation that were already observed by Kanner in 1943 [1] are probably mainly due to a general hypersensitivity, but not difficulties in sensorimotor gating. Individuals with autism thus show unimpaired habituation of sensory stimuli and unimpaired transformation of these stimuli into motor action, while generally exhibiting more pronounced motor responses to sensory input in comparison to the healthy population.

The present study is the first to demonstrate normal PPI and habituation in a sample of adults with high-functioning autism. In consideration of previous studies, this finding suggests that sensorimotor gating deficits are not a distinctive feature of autism, but rather occur only in certain subgroups. For example, Yuhas et al. [28] found attenuated PPI in subjects with autism and Fragile-X-syndrome (FXS) in comparison to subjects with idiopathic autism and control subjects, indicating that FXS might be responsible for sensorimotor deficits in some individuals with autism. Therefore, future studies should focus on differential sample characteristics that might influence PPI, such as the occurrence of FXS. In order to minimize the possibility of type II errors, large sample sizes are needed. Future studies should particularly pay attention to careful sample selection and methodological aspects, as differences in methodology between the existing studies, such as reporting magnitude versus amplitude of the startle response, or different mean IQ or gender distributions, make a definite evaluation at this point in time impossible.

Moreover, it would be interesting to further explore the association between sensory processing and sensorimotor gating in autism. One possibility to explore sensory processing along with PPI is to measure gating of the auditory evoked potential by means of EEG [26]. Even though these authors did not find any significant differences between children and adolescents with and without autism, future research should examine possible associations between sensory gating and sensorimotor gating in higher-functioning adults.

Author Contributions

Conceived and designed the experiments: J. Kuhn SK CW. Performed the experiments: CW SK. Analyzed the data: TOJG CW SK J. Kuhn. Contributed reagents/materials/analysis tools: J. Kuhn J. Klosterkötter. Wrote the paper: SK CW TOJG KV J. Klosterkötter J. Kuhn. Diagnostics: KV.

References

1. Kanner L (1943) Autistic disturbances in affective contact. Nervous child 2: 217–250.
2. Kern JK, Trivedi MH, Garver CR, Grannemann BD, Andrews AA, et al. (2006) The pattern of sensory processing abnormalities in autism. Autism 10: 480–494.
3. Leekam SR, Neito C, Libby SJ, Wing L, Gould J (2001) Describing the sensory abnormalities of children and adults with autism. Journal of Autism Developmental Disorders 37: 894–910.
4. Tomchek SD, Dunn W (2007) Sensory processing in children with and without autism: a comparative study using the short sensory profile. Am J Occup Ther 61: 190–200.
5. Baron-Cohen S, Ashwin E, Ashwin C, Tavassoli T, Chakrabarti B (2009) Talent in autism: hyper-systemizing, hyper-attention to detail and sensory hypersensitivity. Philos Trans R Soc Lond B Biol Sci 364: 1377–1383.
6. Gomes E, Pedroso FS, Wagner MB (2008) Auditory hypersensitivity in the autistic spectrum disorder. Pro Fono 20: 279–284.
7. Hitoglou M, Ververi A, Antoniadis A, Zafeiriou DI (2010) Childhood autism and auditory system abnormalities. Pediatr Neurol 42: 309–314.
8. Frith U (1989) Autism: explaining the Enigma: Blackwell.
9. O'Connor K (2012) Auditory processing in autism spectrum disorder: a review. Neurosci Biobehav Rev 36: 836–854.
10. Ouimet T, Foster NE, Tryfon A, Hyde KL (2012) Auditory-musical processing in autism spectrum disorders: a review of behavioral and brain imaging studies. Ann N Y Acad Sci 1252: 325–331.
11. Alcantara JI, Weisblatt EJ, Moore BC, Bolton PF (2004) Speech-in-noise perception in high-functioning individuals with autism or Asperger's syndrome. J Child Psychol Psychiatry 45: 1107–1114.
12. DePape AM, Hall GB, Tillmann B, Trainor LJ (2012) Auditory processing in high-functioning adolescents with Autism Spectrum Disorder. PLoS One 7: e44084.
13. Groen WB, van Orsouw L, Huurne N, Swinkels S, van der Gaag RJ, et al. (2009) Intact spectral but abnormal temporal processing of auditory stimuli in autism. J Autism Dev Disord 39: 742–750.
14. Teder-Salejarvi WA, Pierce KL, Courchesne E, Hillyard SA (2005) Auditory spatial localization and attention deficits in autistic adults. Brain Res Cogn Brain Res 23: 221–234.
15. Lepisto T, Kuitunen A, Sussman E, Saalasti S, Jansson-Verkasalo E, et al. (2009) Auditory stream segregation in children with Asperger syndrome. Biol Psychol 82: 301–307.
16. Takarae Y, Luna B, Minshew NJ, Sweeney JA (2008) Patterns of visual sensory and sensorimotor abnormalities in autism vary in relation to history of early language delay. J Int Neuropsychol Soc 14: 980–989.
17. Fournier KA, Hass CJ, Naik SK, Lodha N, Cauraugh JH (2010) Motor coordination in autism spectrum disorders: a synthesis and meta-analysis. J Autism Dev Disord 40: 1227–1240.
18. Swerdlow NR, Braff DL, Geyer MA (2000) Animal models of deficient sensorimotor gating: what we know, what we think we know, and what we hope to know soon. Behav Pharmacol 11: 185–204.
19. Gowen E, Hamilton A (2013) Motor abilities in autism: a review using a computational context. J Autism Dev Disord 43: 323–344.
20. Miyahara M (2013) Meta review of systematic and meta analytic reviews on movement differences, effect of movement based interventions, and the underlying neural mechanisms in autism spectrum disorder. Front Integr Neurosci 7: 16.
21. Graham FK (1975) The More or Less Startling Effects of Weak Prestimulation. Psychophysiology 12: 238–248.
22. Filion DL, Dawson ME, Schell AM (1998) The psychological significance of human startle eyeblink modification: a review. Biol Psychol 47: 1–43.
23. Organization WH (1992) ICD-10 Classification of mental and behavioral disorders: Clinical descriptions and diagnostic guidelines. Geneva: World Helath Organization.
24. McAlonan GM, Daly E, Kumari V, Critchley HD, van Amelsvoort T, et al. (2002) Brain anatomy and sensorimotor gating in Asperger's syndrome. Brain 125: 1594–1606.
25. Perry W, Minassian A, Lopez B, Maron L, Lincoln A (2007) Sensorimotor gating deficits in adults with autism. Biol Psychiatry 61: 482–486.
26. Oranje B, Lahuis B, van Engeland H, Jan van der Gaag R, Kemner C (2013) Sensory and sensorimotor gating in children with multiple complex developmental disorders (MCDD) and autism. Psychiatry Res 206: 287–292.
27. Ornitz EM, Lane SJ, Sugiyama T, de Traversay J (1993) Startle modulation studies in autism. J Autism Dev Disord 23: 619–637.
28. Yuhas J, Cordeiro L, Tassone F, Ballinger E, Schneider A, et al. (2011) Brief report: Sensorimotor gating in idiopathic autism and autism associated with fragile X syndrome. J Autism Dev Disord 41: 248–253.
29. Baron-Cohen S, Hoekstra RA, Knickmeyer R, Wheelwright S (2006) The Autism-Spectrum Quotient (AQ)—adolescent version. J Autism Dev Disord 36: 343–350.
30. Baron-Cohen S, Wheelwright S (2004) The empathy quotient: an investigation of adults with Asperger syndrome or high functioning autism, and normal sex differences. J Autism Dev Disord 34: 163–175.
31. Baron-Cohen S, Richler J, Bisarya D, Gurunathan N, Wheelwright S (2003) The systemizing quotient: an investigation of adults with Asperger syndrome or high-functioning autism, and normal sex differences. Philos Trans R Soc Lond B Biol Sci 358: 361–374.

32. Hautzinger M, Bailer M, Worall H, Keller F (1995) Beck Depressions-Inventory (BDI). Bern: Huber.
33. Schmidt K-H, Metzler P (1992) Wortschatztest [Vocabulary test (WST)]. Weinheim: Beltz Test GmbH.
34. Lehrl S, Triebig G, Fischer B (1995) Multiple choice vocabulary test MWT as a valid and short test to estimate premorbid intelligence. Acta Neurol Scand 91: 335–345.
35. APA (2000) Diagnostic and Statistical Manual of Mental Disorders, foruth edition revised (DSM IV-TR). Washington, DC: American Psychiatric Association.
36. Beck AT, Ward C, Mendelson M (1961) Beck Depression Inventory (BDI). Archives of General Psychiatry 4: 561–571.
37. Baron-Cohen S, Wheelwright S, Skinner R, Martin J, Clubley E (2001) The autism-spectrum quotient (AQ): evidence from Asperger syndrome/high-functioning autism, males and females, scientists and mathematicians. J Autism Dev Disord 31: 5–17.
38. Blumenthal TD, Cuthbert BN, Filion DL, Hackley S, Lipp OV, et al. (2005) Committee report: Guidelines for human startle eyeblink electromyographic studies. Psychophysiology 42: 1–15.
39. Marco EJ, Hinkley LB, Hill SS, Nagarajan SS (2011) Sensory processing in autism: a review of neurophysiologic findings. Pediatr Res 69: 48R–54R.
40. Roberts TP, Khan SY, Rey M, Monroe JF, Cannon K, et al. (2010) MEG detection of delayed auditory evoked responses in autism spectrum disorders: towards an imaging biomarker for autism. Autism Res 3: 8–18.
41. Bruneau N, Roux S, Adrien JL, Barthelemy C (1999) Auditory associative cortex dysfunction in children with autism: evidence from late auditory evoked potentials (N1 wave-T complex). Clin Neurophysiol 110: 1927–1934.
42. Gage NM, Siegel B, Roberts TP (2003) Cortical auditory system maturational abnormalities in children with autism disorder: an MEG investigation. Brain Res Dev Brain Res 144: 201–209.
43. Matsuzaki J, Kagitani-Shimono K, Goto T, Sanefuji W, Yamamoto T, et al. (2012) Differential responses of primary auditory cortex in autistic spectrum disorder with auditory hypersensitivity. Neuroreport 23: 113–118.
44. Gebhardt J, Schulz-Juergensen S, Eggert P (2012) Maturation of prepulse inhibition (PPI) in childhood. Psychophysiology 49: 484–488.
45. Kemner C, Orange B, Verbaten MN, van Engeland H (2002) Normal P50 gating in children with autism. Journal of Clinical Psychiatry 63: 214–217.
46. Guiraud JA, Kushnerenko E, Tomalski P, Davies K, Ribeiro H, et al. (2011) Differential habituation to repeated sounds in infants at high risk for autism. Neuroreport 22: 845–849.
47. Baranek GT, David FJ, Poe MD, Stone WL, Watson LR (2006) Sensory Experiences Questionnaire: discriminating sensory features in young children with autism, developmental delays, and typical development. J Child Psychol Psychiatry 47: 591–601.
48. Kohl S, Heekeren K, Klosterkotter J, Kuhn J (2013) Prepulse inhibition in psychiatric disorders—apart from schizophrenia. J Psychiatr Res 47: 445–452.
49. Braff DL, Geyer MA, Swerdlow NR (2001) Human studies of prepulse inhibition of startle: normal subjects, patient groups, and pharmacological studies. Psychopharmacology (Berl) 156: 234–258.

10

Regional Gray Matter Volume Is Associated with Empathizing and Systemizing in Young Adults

Hikaru Takeuchi[1]*, Yasuyuki Taki[2], Yuko Sassa[2], Hiroshi Hashizume[2], Atsushi Sekiguchi[3], Ai Fukushima[3], Ryuta Kawashima[1,2,3]

1 Smart Ageing International Research Center, Institute of Development, Aging and Cancer, Tohoku University, Sendai, Japan, **2** Division of Developmental Cognitive Neuroscience, Institute of Development, Aging and Cancer, Tohoku University, Sendai, Japan, **3** Department of Functional Brain Imaging, Institute of Development, Aging and Cancer, Tohoku University, Sendai, Japan

Abstract

Empathizing is defined as the drive to identify the mental states of others for predicting their behavior and responding with an appropriate emotion. Systemizing is defined as the drive to analyze a system in terms of the rules that govern the system in order to predict its behavior. Using voxel-based morphometry and questionnaires in a large sample of normal, right-handed young adults, we investigated the regional gray matter volume (rGMV) correlates of empathizing and systemizing and additionally those of the D score, which is the difference between systemizing and empathizing, to reveal the comprehensive picture of those correlates. Negative rGMV correlates of empathizing and positive rGMV correlates of the D score (formed by the negative correlation between rGMV and empathizing), were found primarily in nodes in the default mode network, mirror neuron system, dorsal anterior cingulate cortex, and the lateral part of the prefrontal cortex together with other areas. Positive rGMV correlates of systemizing and of the D score (formed by the positive correlation between rGMV and systemizing) were found primarily in nodes in the external attention system, middle cingulate cortex, and other regions. Negative rGMV correlates of systemizing were found in an area close to the left posterior insula and putamen. These findings reconcile some previously inconsistent findings, provide other new findings and suggest that these areas contribute to empathizing–systemizing. Furthermore, the negative/positive rGMV correlates of empathizing and positive/negative rGMV correlates of systemizing overlapped substantially. This may be in line with the notion that empathizing and systemizing compete neurally in the brain.

Editor: Bogdan Draganski, Centre Hospitalier Universitaire Vaudois Lausanne - CHUV, UNIL, Switzerland

Funding: This study was supported by JST/RISTEX, JST/CREST (no particular numbers exist). The funders had no role in study design, data collection and analysis, decision to publish, or preparation of the manuscript.

Competing Interests: The authors have declared that no competing interests exist.

* E-mail: takehi@idac.tohoku.ac.jp

Introduction

Empathizing is defined as the drive to identify the mental states of others for predicting their behavior and responding with an appropriate emotion [1]. Systemizing is defined as the drive to analyze a system in terms of the rules that govern the system in order to predict its behavior [1]. Growing evidence shows that males exhibit greater systemizing than females, whereas females exhibit greater empathizing than males [2–4]. Moreover, the empathizing–systemizing theory posits that autism spectrum conditions (ASCs), such as Asperger's syndrome, represent an extreme disposition toward reduced empathizing and enhanced systemizing [1].

The systemizing quotient (SQ) and empathizing quotient (EQ) questionnaires [3,5], developed to evaluate individual differences of empathizing and systemizing, are self-report questionnaires. However, their validity in quantifying empathizing–systemizing has been established. Individuals with ASCs, males, and science students have higher SQ scores and lower EQ scores [2,4]. A higher EQ score is also associated with actors [6], larger individual social networks [7], and performance on a face perception task [8]. The Autism Spectrum Quotient (AQ), a measure of autistic traits, is well explained by a model including both EQ and SQ [9]. Furthermore, the D score, the difference between systemizing and empathizing, better describes ASCs and differentiates typical males from typical females than EQ and SQ alone [10]. However, the sum of the empathizing and systemizing scores does not differ between males and females [11]. On the basis of this evidence, it has been suggested that empathizing and systemizing compete neurally in the brain and that the D score provides information on the trade-off between the two [11]. However, other mechanisms may lead to the same sum of empathizing and systemizing between males and females. Moreover, little correlation exists between empathizing and systemizing [4,9]; therefore, this idea has been criticized and remains controversial [12].

The empathizing–systemizing theory posits that empathizing–systemizing can explain many behavioral and cognitive features of individuals with ASCs, such as inferior social, emotional, and empathetic skills [13,14]. These individuals have a reduced theory of mind (TOM) compared with those without [15]. TOM has been suggested as a key component of empathizing [16], and it is critical for detecting information related to the mental states, emotions, and intentions of others and for recognizing how the feelings of others may impact an individual [17]. Studies have shown that individuals with ASCs have enhanced abilities in math, physics, and engineering, all of which require a high level of systemizing [1], and enhanced spatial abilities that require systemizing in various ways, such as focusing on the details of an object and predicting how it can be transformed [1].

Two recently identified intrinsic brain networks, the default mode network (DMN) and the external attention system (EAS) [18,19], may be associated with empathizing–systemizing. DMN regions are active at rest, while they are usually suspended during externally directed, attention-demanding tasks. Regions of EAS, which is dedicated to external attention, respond to these tasks in the opposite manner [18–20]. Regions such as the medial prefrontal cortices (mPFCs), precuneus, and superior temporal sulcus (STS) belong to DMN, while regions such as the lateral PFC, inferior parietal lobe, dorsal anterior cingulate cortex (dACC), supplementary motor area, and temporoparietal cortex belong to EAS [18–21]. Furthermore, DMN regions are activated by various cognitions for which individuals with ASCs show inferiorities, including TOM, and the recognition of another's perspective [18,22]. However, empathy is a complex phenomenon and recruits a wide range of regions. Lesion and functional activation studies related to individual differences in empathy have consistently shown that mPFC, which is the key DMN node, plays a key role in individual differences in empathy [23–29]. On the other hand, EAS is divided into the dorsal attention network and the ventral attention network [30]. EAS works in opposition to DMN [21] but in association with other networks, such as the salience network [31]. Furthermore, EAS regions are activated by various cognitions, in which ASCs show superiority, or which are related to systemizing. These include spatial cognition [32], attention to detail [33,34], and modus tollens reasoning ("if p, then q") [33,34]. Furthermore, mathematicians have higher regional gray matter (rGM) density in EAS regions [35], and a functional imaging study has shown that individual systemizing is associated with functional activation of EAS regions [36]. However, the functions of the intrinsic network and of regions belonging to this network may differ; therefore, to the best of our knowledge, the idea that these functions are identical remains an assumption.

Much attention has been paid to empathizing–systemizing, and some studies have investigated the association between functional activity and empathizing–systemizing [36,37]. Lesion and GM structural studies of empathy have been conducted in patients with neurodegenerative diseases [23–25]. However, despite being strong, findings from the lesion studies may suffer from poor spatial resolution and an inability to investigate whole brain structures. Furthermore, structural correlates of certain cognitive functions may differ among patients with certain diseases and normal individuals [38] and among patients with different diseases [25]. The strength of structural imaging is that the results are not constrained by a specific functional task performed in a scanner. Thus, observing structural correlates of empathizing–systemizing in normal individuals can provide useful and distinctive information.

Anatomical correlates of empathy-related measures, systemizing, and the D score have previously been studied in normal populations [39–44]. **Table 1** summarizes the characteristics and results of these studies. However, several issues remain to be resolved. First, anatomical correlates of empathy reported in these studies have been inconsistent, which may be due to several factors including differences in methodology {subject characteristics, preprocessing, scale, and regions of interest (ROIs)} and relatively small sample sizes that result in insufficient statistical power. As noted earlier, empathizing is supposed to underlie a wide range of cognitions and many regions can contribute to empathizing, thus revealing all of these may require great statistical power. Second, in adults, the association between rGMV and systemizing (and also the D score) has only been investigated in males [40]. Thus, given that the empathizing–systemizing theory has tended to focus on sex-related differences, whether there are sex-related differences in rGMV correlates of systemizing remains to be determined. Furthermore, a very lenient cluster-determining threshold was used in the study by Lai et al. [40], and regardless of the cause, they identified rather large clusters. Because the cluster test cannot identify where exactly the significant effects of interest are in such large clusters [45], when the identified clusters are too large, it cannot localize the findings very well. Thus, more localized anatomical correlates of systemizing in normal adults remain undetermined.

Growing evidence suggests that ASCs exist on a continuum with normality [5] and that empathizing and systemizing are normally distributed in normal populations [1]. This suggests that studying correlates of empathizing and systemizing in normal populations is useful and has indeed been the case in psychological and neuroimaging studies. Several correlates of empathizing–systemizing have been investigated in typically developing young adults through these studies. Thus, investigating these correlates in typically developing young adults is important. The study aimed (a) to integrate previously reported inconsistent findings relating to rGMV correlates of empathy/empathizing using a large sample; (b) to identify localized anatomical correlates of systemizing; and (c) to identify sex-related differences in the rGMV correlates of empathizing and systemizing by investigating the correlates in a large sample of typically developing young adults. We additionally investigated those issues for the D score. We hypothesized that rGMV in regions associated with DMN and EAS would be associated with empathizing and systemizing, respectively. Specifically, we hypothesized that the key nodes of DMN and EAS, i.e., mPFC/precuneus/STS and the lateral PFC, would be associated with empathizing and systemizing, respectively. To address inconsistencies in the previous study findings, we recruited a large sample (567 subjects; 329 men and 238 women) of individuals of a specified age (20.8±1.9 years).

Materials and Methods

Ethics Statement

In accordance with the Declaration of Helsinki (1991), written informed consent was obtained from each subject. This study was approved by the Ethics Committee of Tohoku University.

Subjects

Five hundred and sixty-seven healthy, right-handed individuals {329 men and 238 women; mean age, 20.8 years (standard deviation, 1.9)} participated. All subjects were college, university, or postgraduate students, or had graduated within the previous year. For more details and related discussions of limitations regarding the study participants, see **Methods S1** and **Discussion S1**.

SQ–EQ Questionnaires

Japanese versions [4] of the SQ and EQ questionnaires [3,5] were administered. EQ and SQ scores were used as indices of empathizing and systemizing, respectively. These tests consist of 40 items for each quotient and 20 filler items that are not scored. The following are examples of items found on the SQ–EQ questionnaires:

"I can tune into how someone else feels rapidly and intuitively" (EQ)

"I am good at predicting how someone will feel" (EQ)

Table 1. Summary of previous gray matter structural studies of empathetic scales and systemizing and relevant measures in normal samples.

	Psychological measure	Subjects	GM measure	Areas
				Previous results related to empathy or sociality related to autistic traits
Banissy et al. [42]	EC (IRI) [127]*	118 healthy adults (66 females, mean age: 22.9 years, SD: 4.2 years)	rGMV	Negative correlation in the dACC, left insula, left IFG, and precuneus
Banissy et al. [42]	PT (IRI) [127]*	Same as the above	rGMV	Positive correlation in dACC
Cheng et al. [39]	ECS [128]	50 healthy adults (25 females, mean age: 27.1 years, range: 19–49 years)	rGMV	Positive correlation in the right IFG
Cheng et al. [39]	EETS [129]	Same at the above	rGMV	Positive correlation in the right IFG and right inferior parietal lobule
Cheng et al. [39]	EC (IRI)*	Same as the above	rGMV	Positive correlation in the right IFG, right inferior parietal lobule, and mPFC
Cheng et al. [39]	EQ	25 healthy males (mean age: 26.6 years, range: 19–49 years)	rGMV	Positive correlation in the right IFG and mPFC
Mutschler et al. [43]	E–S scale [130]	101 healthy females (mean age: 23.6 years, range: 13–35 years)	rGMD	Positive correlation in the left anterior insula
Sassa et al. [41]	EQ	290 healthy children (145 females, mean age: 10.6 years, range: 5.6–18.4 years)	rGMV	Positive correlation in the cluster that includes the left IFG, superior temporal gyrus, precentral gyrus, and middle to posterior insula.
Wallace et al. [44]	SRS [131]	323 typical (malinly) children (147 females, mean age: 10.6 years, SD: 3.7 years)	Cortical thickness	Negative correlation in the bilateral superior temporal gyrus, bilateral middle temporal gyrus, right angular gyrus, left superior parietal lobule, and precuneus
				Previous results related to systemizing (and D score)
Sassa et al. [41]	SQ	290 healthy children (145 females, mean age: 10.6 years, range: 5.6–18.4 years)	rGMV	Negative correlation in the cluster that includes the left posterior parietal cortex and precuneus.
Lai et al. [40]	SQ	88 normal males (mean age: 29 years, range: 18–45 years)	rGMV	Positive correlation in the cluster of the median GM structures (dorsal mPFC, ACC, middle cingulate cortices, and SMA) Negative correlation in the bilateral clusters that included the left hypothalamus, posterior insula, nucleus accumbens, caudate, putamen, and pallidum (only the left one included the insula**)
Lai et al. [40]	D score	Same as the above	rGMV	Positive correlation in the cluster of the median GM structures (dorsal medial prefrontal areas, anterior and middle cingulate cortices, and SMA) Negative correlation in the bilateral clusters that included the left hypothalamus, posterior insula, nucleus accumbens, caudate, putamen, and pallidum (only the left one included the insula**)

Previously reported rGM structural correlates of empathetic competence or relevant measures include the mPFC, dACC, IFG, insula, precuneus, inferior and superior parietal lobules, superior and middle temporal gyri, precentral gyrus, and angular gyrus. Those for systemizing include the median GM areas, subcortical areas, precuneus, and posterior parietal cortex.

*IRI has two other subscales, distress and fantasy. In accordance with Rankin et al.'s [25] contention that these two subscales do not measure empathetic competence well, they were not included in this table.

**The inclusion of the insula in the cluster was confirmed by the cordial offer of the mask for the clusters by the authors.

Abbreviations: dACC, dorsal anterior cingulate cortex; EC, empathetic concern from the Internal Reactivity Index; ECS, emotional contagion scale; EETS, emotional empathic tendency scale; EQ, empathizing quotient; GM, gray matter; IFG, inferior frontal gyrus; IRI, Internal Reactivity Index; mPFC, medial prefrontal cortex; PT, perspective taking from the Internal Reactivity Index; rGMD, regional gray matter density; rGMV, regional gray matter volume; SD, standard deviation; SMA, supplementary motor area; SQ, systemizing quotient; SRS, social responsiveness scale.

"I am fascinated by how machines work" (SQ)

"If I were buying a stereo, I would want to know about its precise technical features" (SQ)

The questionnaires comprise self-descriptive statements scored on a four-point scale ranging from Strongly Disagree to Strongly Agree. Half the items are worded to produce an "agree" response and the remaining to produce a "disagree" response. The items are randomized to avoid a response bias. Each strong systemizing/empathizing response is awarded 2 points, and each slight systemizing/empathizing response is awarded 1 point (i.e., each item is scored as 2, 1, or 0), resulting in a total score of 0–80 for each quotient.

These scales are known to be reliable. The internal consistency of EQ and SQ among normal subjects has a Cronbach's α coefficient of 0.86 and 0.88, respectively [4]. As noted earlier, the criterion-related validity of this questionnaire has been demonstrated, and individuals with ASCs have been shown to have higher SQ and lower EQ scores than those without [4]. Furthermore, males have higher SQ scores than females, while females have higher EQ scores than males [2]. For theoretical and practical issues relating to EQ and SQ, see **Discussion S1**.

The D score was calculated as described previously [11]. Raw SQ and EQ scores were standardized by subtracting the population mean from the score and then dividing the result by the maximum possible score: S = (raw SQ score − population mean of the raw SQ score)/80 and E = (raw EQ score − population mean of the raw EQ score)/80. For this computation, we used estimated population means (EQ: mean, 33.4; SQ: mean, 22.7) derived from a large sample (N = 1250) of Japanese university students in a previous study (which included an almost equal number of males and females) [4]. The discrepancy between systemizing and empathizing was then quantified as D = (S − E)/2. The greater the D score in a positive direction, the stronger one's systemizing relative to one's empathizing. D scores close to zero represent an equal drive to systemize and empathize. The D score is a measure widely used in research by leading experts in relevant areas [2,4,9,11,40,46]. The score is better at distinguishing ASCs from controls and differentiating typical males and females [2,4,9,11], predicting entry into physical sciences and humanities [2,46,47] and predicting programming aptitude [48] than EQ or SQ. However, because the D score has components of both S and E, examining correlates of the D score alone cannot reveal the whole picture. Thus, we also investigated the correlates of E and S scores. One of the problems with using the difference between two values is that when the difference is calculated, determining the source of variations of the value is not possible [49]. However, in the present study, the difference in SD of EQ and SQ scores was not substantial (EQ: SD, 9.63; SQ: SD, 8.44). Furthermore, z scores of the EQ and SQ scores can be used to calculate the D score [4], and this can control for differences in SD of the EQ and SQ scores. However, we used the present method to calculate the D score partly because it is more widely used [1,11,14,50,51] and partly because the distribution of the D score calculated using the z scores of EQ and SQ is very similar to that calculated using the present method and produced similar imaging findings [40].

Assessment of General Intelligence

General intelligence refers to the *g* factor [52], which contributes to success on diverse forms of cognitive tests, regardless of whether these are verbal or non-verbal. Raven's Advanced Progressive Matrix (RAPM) [53], which is the measure that is most correlated with *g* and is thus the best measure of general intelligence [53], was used to assess general intelligence. The test was used in the present study to adjust for the effect of individual psychometric measures of intelligence on brain structure. For more details on RAPM, see our previous studies [54,55].

Image Acquisition

MRI data acquisition was performed using a 3-T Philips Achieva scanner. High-resolution T1-weighted structural images (T1WIs: 240×240 matrix; TR, 6.5 ms; TE, 3 ms; FOV, 24 cm; slices, 162; slice thickness, 1.0 mm) were collected using a MPRAGE sequence.

Preprocessing of the Morphological Data

Preprocessing of the data from T1WIs was performed using VBM2 software [56], an extension of SPM2. Default parameter settings were used [56].

We used a scanner-specific customized GM anatomical template and prior probability maps from GM and white matter (WM) images constructed from T1WI taken using the same scanner as that used in our previous study [55], because T1WI obtained in the present study may have differed from the existing template and because each scanner introduces specific non-uniformities in image intensity and inhomogeneities in the B0 field. T1WIs of each subject were segmented into GM and WM partitions using the abovementioned customized GM and WM prior probability maps [55]. The resulting images included extracted GM and WM partitions in the native space. The GM partition was then normalized to the abovementioned customized GM probability map from the previous study [55]. The normalization parameters determined from this initial step were then applied to the native T1WI. These normalized T1-weighted structural images were then segmented into GM and WM partitions. Moreover, we performed a volume change correction (modulation) by modulating each voxel using the Jacobian determinants derived from spatial normalization, allowing for the determination of regional differences in the absolute amount of GM [57]. This resulted in rGMV-representing maps. Subsequently, all images were smoothed by convolving them with an isotropic Gaussian Kernel of 12-mm full width at half maximum. For the reasons for using VBM2, see our previous studies [58–61]; basically, VBM5/VBM8's preprocessing is not compatible with our T1-weighted structural images, and we cannot alter this.

Statistical Design

The morphological data were statistically analyzed using VBM5 software [56], an extension of SPM5. These analyses only included voxels with GM of >0.05 to avoid possible partial volume effects around the borders between GM and WM and between GM and cerebral spinal fluid. We tested for relationships between rGMV and the EQ/SQ scores and attempted to determine whether any such relationships differed between the sexes. We also investigated these relationships for D score.

Whole-brain multiple regression analysis was used to test for relationships between EQ/SQ scores and rGMV. This analysis included six covariates: sex, age, RAPM score, total brain volume, EQ score, and SQ score. For the reasons for choosing these models, see **Discussion S1**. Next, we tested whether the relationships between rGMV and the EQ/SQ score differed between the sexes (i.e., whether any interaction between sex and the EQ/SQ score affected rGMV). In the whole-brain analysis, we used a voxel-wise analysis of covariance (ANCOVA) with the sex-related difference as a grouping factor (using the full factorial option in SPM5). Age, RAPM score, total brain volume, EQ score, and SQ score were used as covariates. All of these covariates, except the total brain volume, were modeled in ANCOVAs so that the unique relationship between each covariate and rGMV could be detected for each sex (using the interactions option in SPM5). This allowed us to investigate the interaction effects of sex and each covariate. We used t-contrasts to assess the interaction effects between (a) sex and the EQ score (in the second ANCOVA) and (b) sex and the SQ score (in the second ANCOVA) on the basis of rGMV values.

We also performed another whole-brain multiple regression analysis and another whole-brain ANCOVA in which EQ and SQ scores were replaced with the D score.

Statistical Threshold

The significance level was generally set at $P<0.05$, corrected at the non-isotropic adjusted cluster level [62] with an underlying voxel level of $P<0.0025$. However, in the contrasts, where the cluster size test became theoretically inappropriate since the clusters formed were too big, a multiple comparison correction was performed using the false discovery rate (FDR) approach [63] as the second-best option. For details on the cluster size tests used and the selection of the present thresholding methods, see **Methods S1**. In these contrasts, we reported clusters that contained more than five voxels below the threshold of $P<0.05$, corrected for FDR.

Furthermore, the significance level was set at $P<0.05$ with the use of a small volume correction (SVC) for multiple comparisons (FDR) in ROIs for areas with a strong *a priori* hypothesis but without significant results in the whole-brain analyses. These areas included mPFC/precuneus/STS for the analyses of empathizing and the D score and the right lateral PFC for the analysis of systemizing and the D score. As described earlier, these regions are key nodes of DMN and EAS and the core of our hypotheses. Furthermore, the right dorsolateral PFC (DLPFC) and right ventrolateral PFC are consistently correlated with systemizing in different types of brain activities of interest [36]. The mask image comprised a sphere (12 mm radius; smoothing size) around peak voxels in mPFC.

The peak voxels in mPFC ($x, y, z = -1, 47, -4$) and precuneus ($x, y, z = -5, -49, 40$) were selected from a previous representative study of DMN [21]. The peak voxels in the bilateral STS ($x, y, z = \pm55, -55, 11$) were selected from a previous study of autism spectrum traits (ASQ) in the normal population that focused on this region [64]. The peak voxels in the right DLPFC ($x, y, z = 38, 39, 33$) and the ventrolateral PFC ($x, y, z = 50, 23, -1$) were selected from the results of a previous functional imaging study on systemizing [36]. The peak voxels of these regions were selected on the basis of the representativeness of the previous study [21] or because of similar themes.

Results

Behavioral Data

Table 2 shows the average score, standard deviation, age range, EQ/SQ/D score, RAPM score for each sex, and the statistical values for the comparison between males and females (two-tailed *t*-tests). **Table 3** presents simple correlation coefficients among the EQ/SQ/D and RAPM scores in all subjects, male subjects, and female subjects.

Correlation between rGMV and EQ/SQ Scores Across Sexes

Multiple regression analysis, including age, sex, general intelligence, total brain volume, and SQ score, showed that the EQ score was significantly and negatively correlated with GMV in a large anatomical cluster that included regions of the bilateral mPFCs, bilateral superior frontal gyrus, middle frontal gyrus, left inferior frontal gyrus (IFG) and regions of the precuneus, right orbital frontal gyrus, right superior parietal lobule, medial frontal gyrus, and anterior cingulate gyrus (Figs. 1b, 2b, 3b). SVC using FDR were applied in ROIs for areas with a strong *a priori* hypothesis but without significant results in the whole-brain analyses. These areas included mPFC/precuneus/STS for the analyses of empathizing and the D score and the right lateral PFC for the analysis of systemizing and the D score. As described in Introduction, these regions are key nodes of DMN and EAS and the core of our hypotheses. For more details of the procedures and reasons, please refer to the subsection 2.4 of the Methods. But there were no other significant results in this contrast. Among these areas, as seen the subsection below, the rGMV in the right orbital frontal gyrus was not significantly positively correlated with the D score. As described below, rGMV in a region in the left IFG showed a significant negative correlation with the D score probably mainly as a result of a trend-level negative correlation with the EQ score ($x, y, z = -52, 22, 28, t = 3.23, P = 0.053$, corrected for FDR).

Multiple regression analysis, including age, sex, general intelligence, total brain volume, and EQ score, showed that the SQ score was significantly negatively correlated with rGMV in an anatomical cluster that included the left posterior insula and the left putamen at the whole-brain level. No other significant results were observed at the whole brain level, although a trend-level negative correlation was observed between rGMV and the SQ score in an anatomical cluster that included areas in the right posterior insula and right putamen ($x, y, z = 31, -16, 6, t = 3.94, P = 0.326$, corrected at the non-stationary cluster level). SVCs were used for regions with an *a priori* hypothesis, and significant positive correlations were found in the right middle frontal gyrus (Figs. 1c, 2c, 3c).

Tables 4, 5, and **6** show all of the significant results.

Correlation between rGMV and D Scores Across Sexes

Multiple regression analysis, including age, sex, general intelligence, and total brain volume, showed that the D score was significantly and positively correlated with rGMV in a large

Table 2. Demographic variables for males and females and statistical results of the comparisons between males and females (two-tailed *t*-tests).

	Males			Females			*P* value	*t* value
Measure	**Mean**	**Standard deviation**	**Range**	**Mean**	**Standard deviation**	**Range**		
Age	20.89	1.94	18–27	20.78	1.82	18–27	0.544	0.61
RAPM	28.72	3.72	15–36	28.08	3.71	18–36	0.045	2.01
EQ score	29.69	9.63	9–66	35.11	9.40	14–63	$5.36*10^{-11}$	−6.70
SQ score	27.76	8.44	9–56	21.62	7.11	8–45	$1.82*10^{-19}$	9.37
D score	0.0548	0.0736	−0.152 to 0.298	−0.0174	0.0715	−0.221–0.192	$2.41*10^{-28}$	11.73

RAPM, EQ, SQ, and D scores showed sex-related differences.
Abbreviations: RAPM, Raven's Advanced Progressive Matrix; EQ, empathizing quotient; SQ, systemizing quotient.

Table 3. Simple correlation coefficients between psychological variables (and *P* values) in all subjects (MF), male subjects (M), and female subjects (F).

	EQ score	SQ score	D score	RAPM score
EQ score	–	–		–
SQ score	MF: 0.012 (0.780)	–	–	–
	M: 0.157 (0.004**)			
	F: 0.060 (0.353)			
D score	MF: 0.757 (2.36*10^{-106}***)	MF: 0.645 (5.71*10^{-68}***)	–	–
	M: 0.707 (6.95*10^{-51}***)	M: 0.589 (4.52*10^{-32}***)		
	F: 0.784 (7.97*10^{-51}***)	F: 0.571 (4.48*10^{-22}***)		
RAPM score	MF: −0.095(0.023*)	MF: 0.128 (0.002**)	MF: 0.156 (1.90*10^{-4}***)	–
	M: −0.010(0.854)	M: 0.118 (0.032*)	M: 0.093 (0.092)	
	F: −0.168(0.009**)	F: 0.083 (0.200)	F: 0.190 (0.003**)	

*$P<0.05$,
**$P<0.01$,
***$P<0.001$.
Abbreviations: RAPM, Raven's Advanced Progressive Matrix; EQ, empathizing quotient; SQ, systemizing quotient.

anatomical cluster that included regions of the bilateral mPFCs, bilateral superior frontal gyrus, middle frontal gyrus, left IFG and regions of the precuneus, middle cingulate gyrus, anterior cingulate gyrus, right superior parietal lobule, and right extranuclear area close to the caudate, thalamus, and right temporal pole (Figs. 1a, 2a, 3a). **Table 7** shows all of these results. No significant negative correlation was observed between rGMV and the D score in the whole-brain analysis.

SVC detected significant negative correlations in the right STS in areas with a strong *a priori* hypothesis that lacked significance in the whole-brain analysis (**Table 8**). A trend-level negative correlation was also found between rGMV and the D score in an anatomical cluster that included the left posterior insula and left putamen ($x, y, z = -28, -11, 5$, $t = 3.85$, $P = 0.061$, corrected at the non-stationary cluster level), and significant correlations were observed between rGMV and the SQ score, as described below.

Because the D score is the difference between S and E, rGMV correlates of the D score are likely to be also correlated with one or both SQ and EQ scores. To reveal how the relationship between rGMV and the EQ and/or SQ score contributed to the significant relationship between the D score and rGMV, we performed the following procedures: (1) We created mask images for each significant cluster of the relationship between the D score and rGMV (described in **Table 8**). (2) We applied these mask images to the whole-brain multiple regression analysis of EQ/SQ (the same multiple regression analysis model described above). (3) We investigated whether EQ and/or SQ scores showed significant relationships with rGMV using SVC and FDR in the areas of the mask images where significant clusters showing a correlation between rGMV and the D score were found. The largest of these clusters was a cluster in the anterior part of the brain (the uppermost cluster in **Table 7**) that did not appear to be a homogeneous area. Therefore, we subdivided this cluster into seven major areas (areas that belonged to the right/left middle/superior frontal gyrus, anterior cingulate gyrus, medial frontal gyrus, and left IFG) before the analyses. To determine the anatomical areas used in these analyses, we used the WFU PickAtlas Tool (http://www.fmri.wfubmc.edu/cms/software#PickAtlas) [65,66] with the Talairach Daemon [67] option. This method was also used to divide the large cluster in the analyses described in subsection 3.4.

The significant positive correlation between rGMV in the right extra-nuclear area close to the caudate and the D score was formed by the correlation between rGMV in this area and the SQ score. A significant negative correlation between rGMV in the right STS and the D score and significant positive correlations between rGMV in the anterior cingulate gyrus and right middle frontal gyrus in the largest anterior cluster, in the precuneus and middle cingulate gyrus, in one of the two clusters in the left IFG, and in the right temporal pole and the D score were formed by both of positive correlations between rGMV and the SQ score and negative correlations between rGMV and the EQ score The significant correlations between rGMV and the D score in all of the other areas were formed by negative correlations between rGMV and the EQ score.

Interaction Effects between Sex and EQ/SQ/D Score on rGMV in both Sexes

ANCOVAs using data from both sexes detected no interaction effects between (a) the EQ score and sex on rGMV; (b) between the SQ score and sex on rGMV; and (c) between the D score and sex on rGMV.

Discussion

This study investigated rGMV correlates of empathizing and systemizing and their sex-related differences in a large sample of typically developing young adults. We aimed to clarify the following unresolved issues: (a) integration of previously reported inconsistent findings of rGMV correlates of empathy/empathizing using a large sample; (b) identification of localized anatomical correlates of systemizing; and (c) identification of sex-related differences in rGMV correlates of empathizing and systemizing. We also investigated these issues for D scores.

Summary

In agreement with our hypothesis, rGMVs in regions in the DMN were correlated with empathizing, while those in EAS regions were correlated with systemizing. Further, consistent with

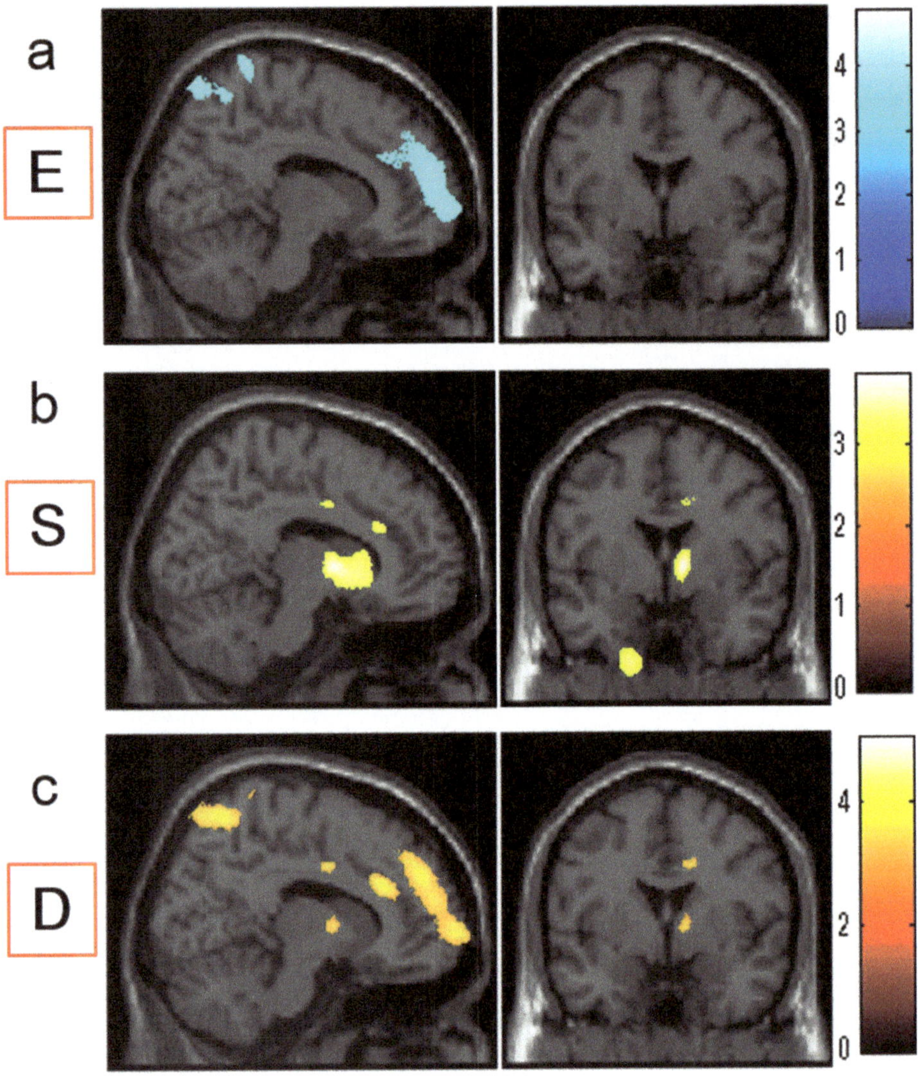

Figure 1. Regions with correlations between empathizing, systemizing, D score, and rGMV in or close to the lateral parts of the brain. (a) Regions with negative correlations between rGMV and empathizing. Results are shown with $P<0.0025$, uncorrected. Regions with correlations are shown in clusters, which were mainly located in a wide range of frontal and parietal areas. (b) Regions with positive correlations between rGMV and systemizing. Results are shown with $P<0.0025$, uncorrected. Regions with correlations are shown in the right middle frontal gyrus and other regions. (c) Regions with positive correlations between rGMV and the D score. Results are shown with $P<0.0025$, uncorrected. Regions with correlations are shown in clusters, which were mainly located in a wide range of frontal and parietal areas and in other regions.

the previously suggested link between the mirror neuron system (MNS) and empathy, rGMVs in part of MNS were correlated with empathizing. In agreement with a previous study, systemizing was negatively correlated with rGMV in a region around the left posterior insula and left putamen and positively correlated with rGMV in the middle cingulate gyrus. The D score was correlated with rGMV in most of these areas. In addition to our other significant results, these findings reconciled with the findings of previous analyses of rGMV correlates of empathizing/empathy in typically developing young adults and localized rGMV correlates of empathizing, systemizing, and the D score. The significant results that agreed with our hypothesis showed that empathizing was generally negatively correlated with rGMV in these DMN areas, whereas systemizing was positively correlated with rGMV in these EAS areas. Several regions exhibiting a significant correlation between rGMV and the D score, a positive correlation between rGMV and systemizing and a negative correlation between rGMV and empathizing were observed simultaneously (in the same regions), suggesting an overlap between these two despite the low correlation between empathizing and systemizing. This overlap suggests the involvement of developmental or cognitive mechanisms, as discussed later, and this might be in line with the suggestion that empathizing and systemizing compete neurally in the brain [11]. Finally, rGMV correlates of empathizing included areas close to the midline and also extended well into the lateral parts of the brain, thus covering DLPFCs. We therefore integrated most previously reported inconsistent findings of the rGMV correlates of empathy/empathizing. We identified several localized anatomical correlates of empathizing, systemizing, and the D score in EAS, DMN, and MNS areas. We did not find sex-related differences in rGMV correlates of empathizing, systemizing, or the D score.

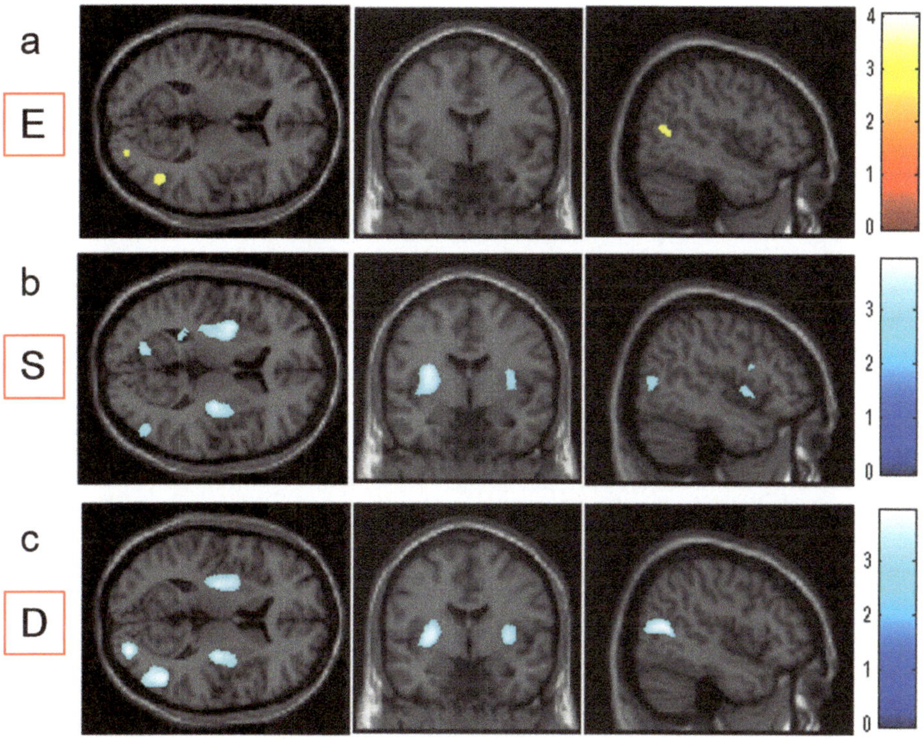

Figure 2. Regions with correlations between empathizing, systemizing, D score, and rGMV. (a), (b), (c) Regions with correlations are overlaid on a single subject T1 image of SPM5 in sagittal (left panels; x = 12) and coronal (right panels; y = 0) views. Results are shown with $P<0.0025$, uncorrected. (a) Regions with negative correlations between rGMV and empathizing. Regions with correlations are shown in clusters, which were mainly located in the medial prefrontal, anterior cingulate, and medial parietal areas. (b) Regions with positive correlations between rGMV and systemizing. Regions with correlations are shown in areas of dACC, middle cingulate cortex, and areas around the caudate and extranuclear regions. (c) Regions with positive correlations between rGMV and the D score. Regions with correlations are shown in the medial prefrontal areas, anterior cingulate cortex, middle cingulate cortex, medial parietal regions, and the extranuclear area close to the caudate.

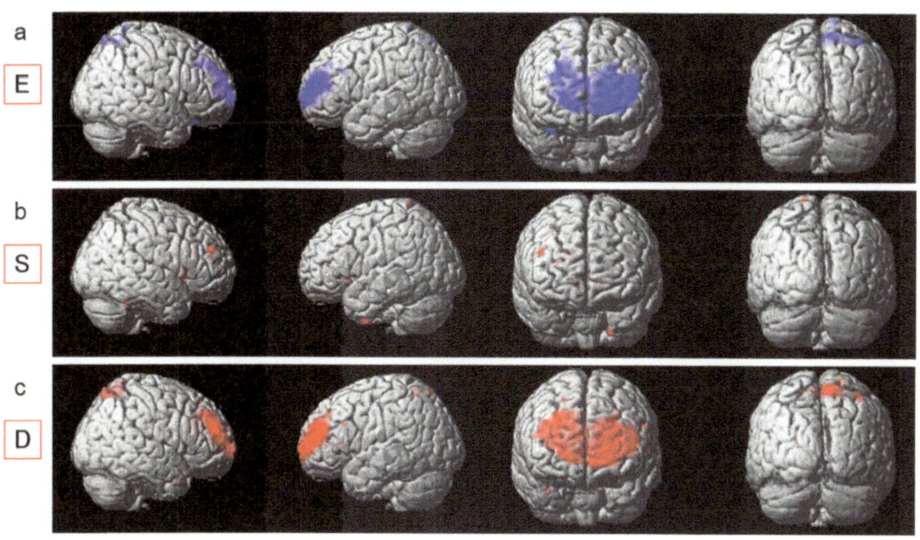

Figure 3. Regions with correlations between empathizing, systemizing, D score, and rGMV. (a), (b), (c) Regions with correlations are overlaid on a single subject T1 image of SPM5 in the axial (left panels; z = 47), coronal (middle panels; y = −63), and sagittal (right panels; x = 11) views. Results are shown with $P<0.0025$, uncorrected. (a) Regions with positive correlations between rGMV and empathizing. Regions with correlations are shown in the right STS. (b) Regions with negative correlations between rGMV and systemizing. Regions with correlations are shown in the right STS, a cluster that included the left posterior insula and left putamen, and other regions. (c) Regions with negative correlations between rGMV and the D score. Regions with correlations are shown in the right STS, a cluster that included the left posterior insula and left putamen, and other regions.

Table 4. Brain regions with significant negative correlations between regional gray matter volume (rGMV) and empathizing {Whole-brain analysis (voxel-level FDR correction, >5 voxels)}.

Area		x	y	z	t score	Corrected P value (FDR)	Cluster size (mm³)
Superior frontal gyrus (B)/Medial frontal Gyrus/middle frontal gyrus (B)/Inferior frontal gyrus (L)/Anterior cingulate gyrus		−21	53	20	4.86	0.011	24611
-Anterior cingulate gyrus							54
-Medial frontal gyrus							4613
-Inferior frontal gyrus	L						45
-Middle frontal gyrus	L						5324
-Superior frontal gyrus	L						7426
-Middle frontal gyrus	R						571
-Superior frontal gyrus	R						2362
Precuneus		3	−57	61	4.13	0.014	551
Orbital frontal gyrus	R	34	28	−26	3.81	0.023	342
Superior parietal lobule	R	10	−76	67	3.58	0.033	106
Precuneus		12	−46	76	3.51	0.037	28
Superior parietal lobule	R	38	−72	59	3.50	0.038	49
Superior medial frontal gyrus		4	32	40	3.48	0.038	19
Anterior cingulate gyrus		−7	35	16	3.44	0.041	45

Empathizing was negatively correlated with rGMV of various areas in the prefrontal cortex, anterior cingulate gyrus, right superior parietal lobule, and precuneus.
Abbreviations: B, bilateral; EQ, empathizing quotient; FDR, false discovery rate; L, left; R, right; SQ, systemizing quotient; SVC, small volume correction.

Comparison of Our Results Regarding Empathizing with Our Hypothesis and with Previous Study Results and Functions of Identified Areas

Areas showing significant correlations between (a) rGMV and empathizing or (b) significant correlations between rGMV and the D score (formed by a correlation between rGMV and empathizing) were largely consistent with previous reports and our hypothesis and the previously suggestion that that MNS plays a key role in empathy. These areas involve parts of DMN (mPFC, orbital frontal gyrus, precuneus, right STS, and right temporal pole), MNS (left IFG and right posterior parietal lobule), and the anterior cingulate gyrus. The mPFC, orbital frontal gyrus, precuneus, STS, and right temporal pole are robust DMN regions [21,68] and are key nodes in areas related to social cognition [69]. The mPFC and contingent regions are involved in assessing the psychological attributes of a person, regardless of whether this is self [22,70] or non-self [22]. Several studies have shown that the precuneus is involved in perspective taking [71], which plays a key role in empathy [3]. STS plays a key role in the perception of social signals [72], and the regional GM structure of the right STS is positively correlated with the skill of processing social cues [73] and with interpersonal emotional intelligence [74]. The main function of the right temporal pole is to link high-level sensory representations with emotional responses and social memory [75]. The right temporal pole is involved in empathy- and TOM-related tasks [76] and in other tasks that require the consideration of another individual's thoughts and emotions, possibly via the utilization of this basic function [75]. These regions may facilitate empathizing through these functions. An area in mPFC was identified as an anatomical correlate of empathizing by Cheng et al. [39], and lesion studies have consistently detected an association between this area and empathy, as described earlier. An area in the left frontal gyrus and precuneus was identified as an rGMV correlate of a subfactor in another questionnaire related to empathy [77]. In the present study, rGMV in the precuneus was negatively correlated with an empathic concern subfactor, i.e., the tendency to experience feelings of sympathy and compassion for unfortunate individuals. The rGMV and WM structure of the right STS are negatively correlated with ASQ, which evaluates social and communication skills, and may well be related to

Table 5. Brain regions with significant positive correlations between regional gray matter volume (rGMV) and systemizing.

Area		x	y	z	t score	Corrected P value (FDR)
ROI analysis (SVC)						
Middle frontal gyrus	R	48	48	30	3.46	0.029

Systemizing was positively correlated with rGMV of the right middle frontal gyrus.
Abbreviations: FDR, false discovery rate; R, right; ROI, region of interest; SVC, small volume correction.

Table 6. Brain regions with significant negative correlations between regional gray matter volume (rGMV) and systemizing {Whole-brain analysis (non-stationary cluster size)}.

Area		x	y	z	t score	Corrected P value
Insula/putamen	L	−31	−3	15	3.71	0.026

Systemizing was negatively correlated with rGMV of an anatomical cluster including the left insula and left putamen.
Abbreviations: L, left.

Table 7. Brain regions with significant positive correlations between regional gray matter volume (rGMV) and the D score { Whole-brain analysis (voxel-level FDR correction, >5 voxels)}.

Area		x	y	z	*t* score	Corrected *P* value	Cluster size (mm^3)	Regions with a negative correlation with EQ	Regions with a positive correlation with SQ
Superior frontal gyrus (B)/Medial frontal Gyrus/middle frontal gyrus (B)/ Inferior frontal gyrus (L)/Anterior cingulate gyrus		−12	61	6	5.02	0.009	38316		
–Anterior cingulate gyrus							952	99.5	96.3
–Medial frontal gyrus							6696	100	0
–Inferior frontal gyrus	L						144	99.3	0
–Middle frontal gyrus	L						6304	100	0
–Superior frontal gyrus	L						9520	100	0
–Middle frontal gyrus	R						3648	99.8	76.0
–Superior frontal gyrus	R						6688	100	0
Precuneus		3	−56	63	3.97	0.015	3383	100%	76.1%
Middle cingulate gyrus	R	15	−2	36	3.66	0.024	133	99.2%	99.2%
Anterior cingulate gyrus		−3	34	19	3.62	0.026	863	99.9%	0%
Superior parietal lobule	R	38	−75	58	3.58	0.027	247	99.6%	0%
Inferior frontal gyrus	L	−62	24	6	3.32	0.039	6	100%	83.3%
Superior medial frontal gyrus		6	35	41	3.31	0.039	32	100%	0%
Inferior frontal gyrus	L	−57	22	29	3.21	0.045	7	100%	0%
Extra-nuclear		12	0	4	3.19	0.046	12	0%	100%
Temporal pole	R	37	8	−28	3.17	0.048	6	83.3%	83.3%

The D score was positively correlated with rGMV of various areas in the prefrontal cortex, anterior cingulate gyrus, right superior parietal lobule, precuneus, right extra-nuclear area, and right temporal pole.
Abbreviations: B, bilateral; EQ, empathizing quotient; FDR, false discovery rate; L, left: R, right; SQ, systemizing quotient.

Table 8. Brain regions with significant negative correlations between regional gray matter volume (rGMV) and the D score.

Area		x	y	z	*t* score	Corrected *P* value (FDR)	Cluster size (mm^3)	Regions with a positive correlation with EQ	Regions with a negative correlation with SQ
ROI analysis (SVC)									
Superior temporal sulcus	R	47	−63	11	3.85	0.012	1303	74.4	96.5

The D score was negatively correlated with rGMV of the right superior temporal sulcus.
Abbreviations: EQ, empathizing quotient; FDR, false discovery rate; R, right; ROI, region of interest; SQ: systemizing quotient; SVC: small volume correction.

empathizing and other symptoms of ASCs [44,64]. The right temporal pole has not been correlated with empathy scales in normal samples, but atrophy of this region has been associated with a lack of empathy in clinical patients [25]. The left IFG and right superior parietal lobule are parts of MNS [78]. The more anterior regions of the posterior parietal lobule are often considered as MNS, but the superior parietal lobule area is also included in MNS and responds to the action of a movement [78]. The involvement of these areas in empathizing is consistent with the widely held view that MNS facilitates understanding of the intentions of others and plays important roles in empathy and empathic dysfunction in ASCs [79,80]. The correlation between rGMV in the left IFG/right posterior parietal cortex and empathizing agrees with a previously reported correlation between rGMV in IFG and empathic concern [77]; a correlation between rGMV in IFG and empathizing in children [41]; a correlation between rGMV in the right parietal lobule, including the superior posterior lobule, and empathy scales [39]; and clinical studies that have linked empathic dysfunction with lesions in IFG [24]. Previous studies of rGMV and empathy, such as the study of Banissy et al. (2012), detected an association between high rGMV and dACC. dACC is believed to play a central role in empathy because it is consistently active when perceiving the pain of others and is related to the unpleasantness of pain [81,82]. The brain structure in this area may relate to empathizing via this function, although there are other possibilities. This area has a wide range of functions, although its underlying function is considered to be negative surprise [83]. Higher rGMV in this area is associated with several conditions related to negative emotions such as anxiety and fear in normal samples [84–86]. Low rGMV in this area was also associated with a higher quality of life (QOL) in our previous study [61]. Furthermore, it is well known that positive emotions are strongly associated with empathy [87]. This association was confirmed in our study where there was a robust correlation between QOL [88] and empathizing ($r = 0.299$, $P = 5.51*10^{-12}$, simple regression analysis; both datasets were obtained from 509 subjects). Low rGMV in this area may result in fewer negative emotions, which may lead to greater empathizing. However, we could not find rGMV correlates of empathizing in the insula despite three previous GM studies [41–43] and our own previous WM study having identified anatomical correlates in this area [89]. For a related discussion on possible reasons for these discrepancies, see the two paragraphs below.

Comparison of Our Results Regarding Systemizing with Our Hypothesis and Previous Study Results and Functions of Identified Areas

Areas with significant correlations between (a) rGMV and systemizing and (b) rGMV and the D score (formed by the correlation between rGMV and systemizing) observed in the present study that were consistent with our hypothesis and with those of other studies included areas in EAS, such as the right middle frontal gyrus, dorsal part of the anterior cingulate gyrus, and middle cingulate gyrus, and an anatomical cluster that included part of the basal ganglia (putamen) and the posterior insula. rGMV in an anatomical cluster that included the dorsal part of the anterior to the middle cingulate cortex was positively correlated with systemizing and the D score, while rGMV in a cluster around the architecture of the basal ganglia was negatively correlated with systemizing and the D score in a previous study of empathizing and systemizing [40]. We here utilized different statistical methods and successfully identified more localized rGMV correlates of systemizing/D score. Unlike a previous study [40], a dissociation was observed in the correlation with systemizing/D score between the putamen (negative correlation) and a region around the caudate (positive correlation). This could have been due to a difference such as the use of a more conservative voxel-level threshold. The right middle frontal gyrus and dACC are robust parts of EAS [21]. This part of the middle frontal gyrus is DLPFC, which is involved in the manipulation or mental operation of objects retained in the mind of an individual [90]. dACC is involved in the prediction, monitoring, and detection of errors, possibly via the aforementioned main function of this region, i.e., negative surprise [83]. The middle cingulate gyrus has an important role in tracking higher-order probabilistic statistics related to the environment [91]. The caudate is not part of the resting-state functional connectivity network involved with DLFPC [21], although this area is usually coactive with DLPFC during a wide range of tasks [92]. The area is considered to be deeply involved in learning, memory, and feedback processing [93]. These functions may allow these regions to support the analysis of a system in terms of the rules that govern the system in order to predict its behavior. Conversely, the posterior insula and putamen are involved with distressing emotions such as hatred [94], romantic love [95], disgust [96], and anger [97,98], which drive an individual to think and behave according to these emotions [94,99]. The negative correlation between rGMV and systemizing in this area may reflect less distressing emotions in subjects with higher systemizing, which may make it easier to observe objects without these distressing emotions and to analyze the system logically rather than emotionally. In agreement with this notion, systemizing has been reported to be consistently negatively correlated with neuroticism [100], which is the tendency to experience distressing feelings [101].

Discrepancies between the Present Results and Our Hypothesis/Expectations and Previous Study Results

Some discrepancies were observed between the present results and our hypothesis/expectations and previous study results. These are classified as follows: (a) differences in the positivity or negativity of correlations between studies; (b) differences in the positivity or negativity of correlations between regions; (c) differences in the positivity or negativity of correlations between the different types of cognitive functions; (d) overlap between rGMV correlates of systemizing and empathizing.

Differences in the positivity or negativity of correlations between different studies may have arisen because lower rGMV reflects advanced cortical development and better functioning in some regions in typically developing young adults, but neuronal degeneration or advanced aging in older adults and clinical samples, immature development in small children, and worse functioning in these populations. Significant negative correlations between empathizing and rGMV were found in the mPFC, precuneus, right temporal pole, left IFG, and right superior parietal lobule. As discussed earlier, we interpreted lower rGMV as indicative of higher functioning in these regions. The negative correlations between rGMV and empathy measures in the left IFG and precuneus and their interpretations are consistent with those observed in a previous study of young adults [77]. Indeed, the association between better social or self-related cognitive functioning and lower rGMV in regions around areas close to mPFC has been well demonstrated in young adults [74,102]. In other cases, cortical thinning was associated with greater or increased cognitive functioning [103]. In clinical and older samples, however, positive correlations were found between empathy measures and rGMV in the mPFC, IFG, posterior parietal lobule, and right temporal pole [25]. As discussed previously, the cortices exhibit developmental thinning after adolescence [104]. Thinned cortices are thought to represent advanced development in young adult samples with better functioning [74,77,102] but may represent the loss of synapses and neurons and degeneration in older or clinical samples [105,106]. In small children who have not reached the age of cortical thinning, lower rGMV may reflect delayed development. These differences in physiological mechanisms underlying individual differences in GMV in different populations may explain the aforementioned differences in the positivity or negativity of correlations between different studies. However, as discussed previously [60,74], regions around STS and the posterior insula do not show developmental cortical thinning [104], and in these regions, the link between greater cortical thinning and advanced development was not supported. Thus, the present results together with those of previous studies of young adults and children support the interpretations for these areas [41,44,60,73]. The lack of the rGMV correlates of empathizing in the anterior insula in the present study differs from previous studies [41–43,89] that have reported such an association and may also be related to this point since these areas show a peak rGMV at around the age of the present study sample [107]. It is also possible that the difference may be explained by statistical fluctuations or the fact that these areas show rGMV reduction not only during development but also in a wide range of psychiatric diseases [108].

As for the difference in the positivity or negativity of the correlation according to the cognitive function type, contrary to the notion above, positive correlations were observed between rGMV and systemizing in areas that exhibited developmental cortical thinning after adolescence, such as the middle frontal gyrus [104]. In cognitively intact younger adults, thicker cortices are associated with facilitated cognitive functioning linked to externally directed attention-demanding tasks. The opposite may be true for social and emotional cognitive functions. Contrary to this hypothesis, however, a negative correlation was observed between cognitive functions and cortical thickness, and studies of intelligence often show that thicker cortices are associated with higher intelligence [109]. On the basis of these studies, greater GMV and thicker cortices are hypothesized to link to more efficient cognitive functioning [110]. In agreement with this hypothesis, our previous study of young adults showed that higher creativity, greater ability to resolve cognitive interferences, and a greater working memory span, which are considered to be externally directed attention-demanding tasks, were associated with more rGM in the lateral PFC [55,111] (the GM link to the working memory span is from unpublished data). Based on these findings, we suggest that in cognitively intact younger adults (a) cognitive functions such as social and emotional abilities and empathizing are preferentially associated with lower rGMV in relevant brain regions and are possibly increased by synaptic pruning; (b) cognitive functions such as those measured by externally directed attention-demanding tasks (i.e., tasks measured by psychometric intelligence tests) and systemizing are associated with higher rGMV. Alternatively, cognitive functions with more complex and refined information processing may be facilitated by synaptic pruning and thinned cortices [112], while cognitive functions that require a larger capacity, strength, or faster speed may be facilitated by more neurons or synapses and thicker cortices. However, this is simply pure speculation based on imaging study results and more data are required to test this hypothesis. The causes of the positive correlations between rGMV and systemizing (and other related cognitive functions) and negative correlations between rGMV and empathizing (and social and emotional cognitive functions) may be related to autistic traits and a lack of synaptic pruning. Interestingly, autistic subjects, who have a low ability for empathizing and other related cognitive functions but a high ability for systemizing and its related cognitive functions, also have cortices with higher rGMVs in some of the lateral and medial prefrontal and parietal areas [113]. Cortices with higher rGMVs detected in autistic subjects are believed to be related to a lack of synaptic pruning in the brain [114]. Individual differences in empathizing and systemizing and in traits associated with the autistic spectrum are observed even among normal samples [115]. These individual trait differences may be partly due to a lack of synaptic pruning in the brain. This hypothesis may be consistent with the hypothesis that autism and Asperger's syndrome lie on a continuum where Asperger's syndrome is a "bridge" between autism and normality [116]. Interestingly, the aforementioned cognitive functions positively correlated with rGMV in young adults (i.e., working memory span, resolution of cognitive interference, and creativity measured by divergent thinking) were not necessarily compromised in higher functioning autistic subjects [117–119], although this point may be disputed, while the self-, social-, and emotion-related cognitive functions negatively correlated with rGMV [74] were robustly impaired in individuals with ASCs [120]. However, whether the same neurophysiological mechanisms underlie individual differences in normal and clinical samples is not guaranteed and may be case-specific. Furthermore, some meta-analyses have shown decreased rGMV in some areas in ASCs (especially in the medial temporal structures, which were not included in the present study) and increases in rGMV [113,121–123] and interaction effects between age and ASCs on brain structures [121,123,124]. There are discrepancies and congruencies among these meta-analytic studies, and the abovementioned discussions have to be viewed cautiously.

Finally, we suggest a few possible explanations for the overlap of negative/positive rGMV correlates of empathizing and positive/negative rGMV correlates of systemizing. Significant correlations of empathizing and systemizing in areas with an *a priori* hypothesis or areas that had been previously identified as significant were described above. However, there were also overlaps of negative/positive rGMV correlates of empathizing and positive/negative rGMV correlates of systemizing in many areas, particularly the rGMV correlates of empathizing that extended far into the lateral PFCs. This pattern was very consistent with the results of our previous study of empathizing/systemizing and WM volume [89]. The overlaps described above cannot be explained by a negative correlation between SQ and EQ because no such relationship was observed in this study. This contrasts with the results of a previous study where regions belonging to DMN and those belonging to EAS were clearly segregated by functional activity and functional connectivity analyses [21]. However, associations of the GM structures of DMN (especially mPFC) and those of EAS with psychometric intelligence tests (during which only EAS regions are activated [125]) are actually common in structural studies [110]. One possible explanation for this phenomenon from recent findings is related to the development of the brain structure, namely that rGMV in one area has a very strong correlation with rGMV in the contralateral area and contingent areas regardless of the networks to which these contingent areas belong [126]. Given this strong correlation and rGMV co-development in contingent regions, when rGMV in mPFC is correlated with empathizing, it is not surprising that rGMV in DLPFC has a similar correlation with empathizing. Another possibility suggested is that empathizing and systemizing compete neurally in the brain and that the D score provides information on the trade-off between the two [11]. This type of relationship may result from cognitive mechanisms such as higher systemizing that cannot coexist with higher empathizing in some senses [14] or physiological mechanisms such as advanced synaptic pruning that may underlie higher empathizing and lower systemizing, as suggested above. Other possibilities include higher smoothing values, insufficient normalizing, and fundamental individual differences in the precise anatomical locations of certain functions.

Clinical Implications

As discussed above, the present findings were, in part, congruent with the previous findings of a meta-analytic study of the brain structures of autistic subjects, although there were some apparent discrepancies in the medial temporal structures, as discussed. Thus, the present findings may be, at least in part, in line with the notion that ASCs exist on a continuum with normality [5] and may imply the ASC cognitive patterns that can be explained largely by higher systemizing and lower empathizing [9]. The brain structures of autistic subjects may thus be partly explained by anatomical correlates of systemizing and empathizing. However, as discussed, the remaining incongruencies among the structural studies of empathizing and systemizing in normal subjects, discrepancies among the meta-analytic studies of autistic subjects, may be due to differences in subjects' characteristics, such as age, which can affect the pattern of anatomical correlates of cognition. Thus, these findings should be considered cautiously until well-controlled direct comparisons of brain structures and of empathizing and systemizing are performed in large samples of normal and autistic subjects.

Supporting Information

Methods S1 Supplemental methods. Supplemental descriptions of details of methods.

Discussion S1 Supplemental discussion. Supplemental discussion regarding limitations of the study.

Acknowledgments

We thank Y. Yamada for operating the MRI scanner; M. Asano, H. Ambo, and J. Tayama for helping to find the testers for the psychological tests; the participants of the study for their contribution; the testers for their work; and all our other colleagues at IDAC, Tohoku University for their support. We would also like to thank A. Wakabayashi for providing the questionnaire. The authors would also like to thank Enago (www.enago.jp) for the English language review.

Author Contributions

Conceived and designed the experiments: HT YT RK. Performed the experiments: HT YT YS HH AS AF. Analyzed the data: HT. Wrote the paper: HT.

References

1. Baron-Cohen S, Knickmeyer RC, Belmonte MK (2005) Sex differences in the brain: implications for explaining autism. Science 310: 819–823.
2. Wakabayashi A, Baron-Cohen S, Wheelwright S, Goldenfeld N, Delaney J, et al. (2006) Development of short forms of the Empathy Quotient (EQ-Short) and the Systemizing Quotient (SQ-Short). Personality and individual differences 41: 929–940.
3. Baron-Cohen S, Wheelwright S (2004) The empathy quotient: an investigation of adults with Asperger syndrome or high functioning autism, and normal sex differences. Journal of Autism and Developmental Disorders 34: 163–175.
4. Wakabayashi A, Baron-Cohen S, Uchiyama T, Yoshida Y, Kuroda M, et al. (2007) Empathizing and systemizing in adults with and without autism

spectrum conditions: cross-cultural stability. Journal of Autism and Developmental Disorders 37: 1823–1832.
5. Baron-Cohen S, Richler J, Bisarya D, Gurunathan N, Wheelwright S (2003) The systemizing quotient: an investigation of adults with Asperger syndrome or high-functioning autism, and normal sex differences. Philosophical Transactions of the Royal Society of London Series B: Biological Sciences 358: 361–374.
6. Nettle D (2006) Psychological profiles of professional actors. Personality and individual differences 40: 375–383.
7. Stileman E (2007) Construction of the Social Network Score (SNS) Questionnaire for undergraduate students, and an examination of the pre-requisites for large social networks in humans? Undergraduate thesis. Edinburgh: University of Edinburgh.
8. Penton-Voak IS, Allen T, Morrison ER, Gralewski L, Campbell N (2007) Performance on a face perception task is associated with empathy quotient scores, but not systemizing scores or participant sex. Personality and individual differences 43: 2229–2236.
9. Wheelwright S, Baron-Cohen S, Goldenfeld N, Delaney J, Fine D, et al. (2006) Predicting autism spectrum quotient (AQ) from the systemizing quotient-revised (SQ-R) and empathy quotient (EQ). Brain Research 1079: 47–56.
10. Baron-Cohen S (2004) The essential difference: Male and female brains and the truth about autism New York: Basic Books.
11. Goldenfeld N, Baron-Cohen S, Wheelwright S (2005) Empathizing and systemizing in males, females and autism. Clinical Neuropsychiatry 2: 338–345.
12. Andrew J, Cooke M, Muncer S (2008) The relationship between empathy and Machiavellianism: An alternative to empathizing–systemizing theory. Personality and Individual Differences 44: 1203–1211.
13. Hall JA (1978) Gender effects in decoding nonverbal cues. Psychological bulletin 85: 845–857.
14. Baron-Cohen S (2003) The essential difference: The truth about the male and female brain. New York: Perseus Books Group.
15. Baron-Cohen S (2002) The extreme male brain theory of autism. Trends in Cognitive Sciences 6: 248–254.
16. Krill AL, Platek SM, Wathne K (2008) Feelings of control during social exclusion are partly accounted for by empathizing personality. Personality and individual differences 45: 684–688.
17. Bachevalier J, Loveland KA (2006) The orbitofrontal-amygdala circuit and self-regulation of social-emotional behavior in autism. Neuroscience & Biobehavioral Reviews 30: 97–117.
18. Buckner RL, Andrews-Hanna JR, Schacter DL (2008) The Brain's Default Network. Annals of the New York Academy of Sciences 1124: 1–38.
19. Corbetta M, Shulman GL (2002) Control of goal-directed and stimulus-driven attention in the brain. Nature Reviews Neuroscience 3: 201–215.
20. Laird AR, McMillan KM, Lancaster JL, Kochunov P, Turkeltaub PE, et al. (2005) A comparison of label-based review and ALE meta-analysis in the Stroop task. Human Brain Mapping 25: 6–21.
21. Fox MD, Snyder AZ, Vincent JL, Corbetta M, Van Essen DC, et al. (2005) The human brain is intrinsically organized into dynamic, anticorrelated functional networks. Proceedings of the National Academy of Sciences 102: 9673–9678.
22. Amodio DM, Frith CD (2006) Meeting of minds: the medial frontal cortex and social cognition. Nature Reviews Neuroscience 7: 268–277
23. Shamay-Tsoory SG, Tomer R, Berger BD, Aharon-Peretz J (2003) Characterization of empathy deficits following prefrontal brain damage: the role of the right ventromedial prefrontal cortex. Journal of Cognitive Neuroscience 15: 324–337.
24. Shamay-Tsoory SG, Aharon-Peretz J, Perry D (2009) Two systems for empathy: a double dissociation between emotional and cognitive empathy in inferior frontal gyrus versus ventromedial prefrontal lesions. Brain 132: 617–627.
25. Rankin KP, Gorno-Tempini ML, Allison SC, Stanley CM, Glenn S, et al. (2006) Structural anatomy of empathy in neurodegenerative disease. Brain 129: 2945–2956.
26. Masten CL, Eisenberger NI, Pfeifer JH, Dapretto M (2010) Witnessing peer rejection during early adolescence: Neural correlates of empathy for experiences of social exclusion. Social Neuroscience 5: 496–507.
27. Wagner DD, Kelley WM, Heatherton TF (2011) Individual differences in the spontaneous recruitment of brain regions supporting mental state understanding when viewing natural social scenes. Cerebral Cortex 21: 2788–2796.
28. Rameson LT, Morelli SA, Lieberman MD (2011) The Neural Correlates of Empathy: Experience, Automaticity, and Prosocial Behavior. Journal of Cognitive Neuroscience. 1–11.
29. Zaki J, Weber J, Bolger N, Ochsner K (2009) The neural bases of empathic accuracy. Proceedings of the National Academy of Sciences 106: 11382–11387.
30. Fox MD, Corbetta M, Snyder AZ, Vincent JL, Raichle ME (2006) Spontaneous neuronal activity distinguishes human dorsal and ventral attention systems. Proceedings of the National Academy of Sciences 103: 10046–10051.
31. Zhou Y, Wang K, Liu Y, Song M, Song SW, et al. (2010) Spontaneous brain activity observed with functional magnetic resonance imaging as a potential biomarker in neuropsychiatric disorders. Cognitive Neurodynamics 4: 275–294.
32. Cohen MS, Kosslyn SM, Breiter HC, DiGirolamo GJ, Thompson WL, et al. (1996) Changes in cortical activity during mental rotation A mapping study using functional MRI. Brain 119: 89.
33. Baron-Cohen S, Ashwin E, Ashwin C, Tavassoli T, Chakrabarti B (2009) Talent in autism: hyper-systemizing, hyper-attention to detail and sensory hypersensitivity. Philosophical Transactions of the Royal Society B: Biological Sciences 364: 1377–1383.
34. Kroger JK, Sabb FW, Fales CL, Bookheimer SY, Cohen MS, et al. (2002) Recruitment of anterior dorsolateral prefrontal cortex in human reasoning: a parametric study of relational complexity. Cerebral Cortex 12: 477–485.
35. Aydin K, Ucar A, Oguz KK, Okur OO, Agayev A, et al. (2007) Increased gray matter density in the parietal cortex of mathematicians: a voxel-based morphometry study. American Journal of Neuroradiology 28: 1859.
36. Billington J, Baron-Cohen S, Bor D (2008) Systemizing influences attentional processes during the Navon task: An fMRI study. Neuropsychologia 46: 511–520.
37. Chakrabarti B, Bullmore E, Baron-Cohen S (2006) Empathizing with basic emotions: Common and discrete neural substrates. Social Neuroscience 1: 364–384.
38. Antonova E, Kumari V, Morris R, Halari R, Anilkumar A, et al. (2005) The relationship of structural alterations to cognitive deficits in schizophrenia: a voxel-based morphometry study. Biological psychiatry 58: 457–467.
39. Cheng Y, Chou KH, Decety J, Chen IY, Hung D, et al. (2009) Sex differences in the neuroanatomy of human mirror-neuron system: a voxel-based morphometric investigation. Neuroscience 158: 713–720.
40. Lai MC, Lombardo MV, Chakrabarti B, Ecker C, Sadek SA, et al. (2012) Individual differences in brain structure underpin empathizing–systemizing cognitive styles in male adults. Neuroimage 61: 1347–1354.
41. Sassa Y, Taki Y, Takeuchi H, Hashizume H, Asano M, et al. (2012) The correlation between brain gray matter volume and empathizing and systemizing quotients in healthy children. Neuroimage 60: 2035–2041.
42. Banissy MJ, Kanai R, Walsh V, Rees G (2012) Inter-individual differences in empathy are reflected in human brain structure. Neuroimage 62: 2034–2039.
43. Mutschler I, Reinbold C, Wankerl J, Seifritz E, Ball T (2013) Structural basis of empathy and the domain general region in the anterior insular cortex. Frontiers in Human Neuroscience 7: article 177.
44. Wallace GL, Shaw P, Lee NR, Clasen LS, Raznahan A, et al. (2012) Distinct Cortical Correlates of Autistic versus Antisocial Traits in a Longitudinal Sample of Typically Developing Youth. The Journal of neuroscience 32: 4856–4860.
45. Friston KJ, Holmes A, Poline JB, Price CJ, Frith CD (1996) Detecting activations in PET and fMRI: levels of inference and power. NeuroImage 4: 223–235.
46. Billington J, Baron-Cohen S, Wheelwright S (2007) Cognitive style predicts entry into physical sciences and humanities: Questionnaire and performance tests of empathy and systemizing. Learning and Individual Differences 17: 260–268.
47. Focquaert F, Steven MS, Wolford GL, Colden A, Gazzaniga MS (2007) Empathizing and systemizing cognitive traits in the sciences and humanities. Personality and Individual Differences 43: 619–625.
48. Wray S (2007) SQ minus EQ can predict programming aptitude. Proceedings of the PPIG 19th Annual Workshop, Finland.
49. DeGutis J, Mercado RJ, Wilmer J, Rosenblatt A (2013) Individual Differences in Holistic Processing Predict the Own-Race Advantage in Recognition Memory. PLoS One 8: e58253.
50. Auyeung B, Baron-Cohen S, Ashwin E, Knickmeyer R, Taylor K, et al. (2009) Fetal testosterone and autistic traits. British Journal of Psychology 100: 1–22.
51. Wakabayashi A, Baron-Cohen S, Wheelwright S (2006) Individual and gender differences in Empathizing and Systemizing: measurement of individual differences by the Empathy Quotient (EQ) and the Systemizing Quotient (SQ). Shinrigaku Kenkyu 77: 271–277.
52. Spearman C (1904) General intelligence, objectively determined and measured. American Journal of Psychology 15: 201–293.
53. Raven J (1998) Manual for Raven's progressive matrices and vocabulary scales. Oxford: Oxford Psychologists Press.
54. Takeuchi H, Taki Y, Sassa Y, Hashizume H, Sekiguchi A, et al. (2010) White matter structures associated with creativity: Evidence from diffusion tensor imaging. Neuroimage 51: 11–18.
55. Takeuchi H, Taki Y, Sassa Y, Hashizume H, Sekiguchi A, et al. (2010) Regional gray matter volume of dopaminergic system associate with creativity: Evidence from voxel-based morphometry Neuroimage 51: 578–585.
56. Gaser C (2007) VBM Toolbox for SPM2, VBM Toolbox for SPM5. http://dbmneurouni-jenade/vbm/(Accessed 2008 March 1).
57. Ashburner J, Friston KJ (2000) Voxel-based morphometry-the methods. Neuroimage 11: 805–821.
58. Takeuchi H, Taki Y, Nouchi R, Hashizume H, Sekiguchi A, et al. (2013) Anatomical correlates of self-handicapping tendency. Cortex 49: 1148–1154.
59. Takeuchi H, Taki Y, Nouchi R, Hashizume H, Sassa Y, et al. (2012) Associations among imaging measures (2): The association between gray matter concentration and task-induced activation changes. Human Brain Mapping Article first published online.
60. Takeuchi H, Taki Y, Nouchi R, Sekiguchi A, Kotozaki Y, et al. (2012) Regional gray matter density is associated with achievement motivation:

evidence from voxel-based morphometry. Brain Structure & Function Epub ahead of print.

61. Takeuchi H, Taki Y, Nouchi R, Hashizume H, Sassa Y, et al. (2013) Anatomical correlates of quality of life: Evidence from voxel-based morphometry. Human Brain Mapping Epub ahead of publication.
62. Hayasaka S, Phan KL, Liberzon I, Worsley KJ, Nichols TE (2004) Nonstationary cluster-size inference with random field and permutation methods. Neuroimage 22: 676–687.
63. Genovese CR, Lazar NA, Nichols T (2002) Thresholding of statistical maps in functional neuroimaging using the false discovery rate. Neuroimage 15: 870–878.
64. von dem Hagen EAH, Nummenmaa L, Yu R, Engell AD, Ewbank MP, et al. (2011) Autism spectrum traits in the typical population predict structure and function in the posterior superior temporal sulcus. Cerebral Cortex 21: 493–500.
65. Maldjian JA, Laurienti PJ, Burdette JH (2004) Precentral gyrus discrepancy in electronic versions of the Talairach atlas. Neuroimage 21: 450–455.
66. Maldjian JA, Laurienti PJ, Kraft RA, Burdette JH (2003) An automated method for neuroanatomic and cytoarchitectonic atlas-based interrogation of fMRI data sets. Neuroimage 19: 1233–1239.
67. Lancaster JL, Woldorff MG, Parsons LM, Liotti M, Freitas CS, et al. (2000) Automated Talairach atlas labels for functional brain mapping. Human Brain Mapping 10: 120–131.
68. Buckner RL, Andrews-Hanna JR, Schacter DL (2008) The brain's default network. Annals of the New York Academy of Sciences 1124: 1–38.
69. Pelphrey KA, Carter EJ (2008) Brain Mechanisms for Social Perception. Annals of the New York Academy of Sciences 1145: 283–299.
70. Christoff K, Gabrieli JDE (2000) The frontopolar cortex and human cognition: Evidence for a rostrocaudal hierarchical organization within the human prefrontal cortex. Psychobiology 28: 168–186.
71. Cavanna AE, Trimble MR (2006) The precuneus: a review of its functional anatomy and behavioural correlates. Brain 129: 564–583.
72. Milligan K, Astington JW, Dack LA (2007) Language and Theory of Mind: Meta-Analysis of the Relation Between Language Ability and False-belief Understanding. Child Development 78: 622–646.
73. Kanai R, Bahrami B, Duchaine B, Janik A, Banissy MJ, et al. (2012) Brain Structure Links Loneliness to Social Perception. Current Biology 22: 1975–1979.
74. Takeuchi H, Taki Y, Sassa Y, Hashizume H, Sekiguchi A, et al. (2011) Regional gray matter density associated with emotional intelligence: Evidence from voxel-based morphometry. Human Brain Mapping 32: 1497–1510.
75. Olson IR, Rao H, Moore KS, Wang J, Detre JA, et al. (2006) Using perfusion fMRI to measure continuous changes in neural activity with learning. Brain and cognition 60: 262–271.
76. Völlm BA, Taylor ANW, Richardson P, Corcoran R, Stirling J, et al. (2006) Neuronal correlates of theory of mind and empathy: a functional magnetic resonance imaging study in a nonverbal task. Neuroimage 29: 90–98.
77. Banissy MJ, Kanai R, Walsh V, Rees G (2012) Inter-individual differences in empathy are reflected in human brain structure. Neuroimage.
78. Cattaneo L, Rizzolatti G (2009) The mirror neuron system. Archives of Neurology 66: 557–560.
79. Rizzolatti G, Craighero L (2005) Mirror neuron: a neurological approach to empathy. Neurobiology of human values: 107–123.
80. Iacoboni M, Dapretto M (2006) The mirror neuron system and the consequences of its dysfunction. Nature Reviews Neuroscience 7: 942–951.
81. Singer T, Frith C (2005) The painful side of empathy. Nature Neuroscience 8: 845–846.
82. Fan Y, Duncan NW, de Greck M, Northoff G (2011) Is there a core neural network in empathy? An fMRI based quantitative meta-analysis. Neuroscience & Biobehavioral Reviews 35: 903–911.
83. Egner T (2011) Surprise! A unifying model of dorsal anterior cingulate function? Nature Neuroscience 14: 1219–1220.
84. Fornito A, Yung AR, Wood SJ, Phillips LJ, Nelson B, et al. (2008) Anatomic abnormalities of the anterior cingulate cortex before psychosis onset: an MRI study of ultra-high-risk individuals. Biological Psychiatry 64: 758–765.
85. Carlson JM, Beacher F, Reinke KS, Habib R, Harmon-Jones E, et al. (2011) Nonconscious attention bias to threat is correlated with anterior cingulate cortex gray matter volume: A voxel-based morphometry result and replication. Neuroimage 59: 1713–1718.
86. Pujol J, López A, Deus J, Cardoner NI, Vallejo J, et al. (2002) Anatomical variability of the anterior cingulate gyrus and basic dimensions of human personality. Neuroimage 15: 847–855.
87. Strayer J, Roberts W (2004) Empathy and Observed Anger and Aggression in Five-Year-Olds. Social Development 13: 1–13.
88. Tazaki M, Nakane M (2007) Revised manual of WHO QOL 26. Tokyo: Kaneko-syobou.
89. Takeuchi H, Taki Y, Thyreau B, Sassa Y, Hashizume H, et al. (2013) White matter structures associated with empathizing and systemizing in young adults. Neuroimage 77: 222–236.
90. Owen AM (2000) The role of the lateral frontal cortex in mnemonic processing: the contribution of functional neuroimaging. Experimental brain research 133: 33–43.
91. Behrens TEJ, Woolrich MW, Walton ME, Rushworth MFS (2007) Learning the value of information in an uncertain world. Nature Neuroscience 10: 1214–1221.
92. Postuma RB, Dagher A (2006) Basal ganglia functional connectivity based on a meta-analysis of 126 positron emission tomography and functional magnetic resonance imaging publications. Cerebral Cortex 16: 1508–1521.
93. Packard MG, Knowlton BJ (2002) Learning and memory functions of the basal ganglia. Annual Review of Neuroscience 25: 563–593.
94. Zeki S, Romaya JP (2008) Neural correlates of hate. PLoS One 3: e3556.
95. Bartels A, Zeki S (2004) The neural correlates of maternal and romantic love. Neuroimage 21: 1155–1166.
96. Phillips ML, Young A, Senior C, Brammer M, Andrew C, et al. (1997) A specific neural substrate for perceiving facial expressions of disgust. Nature 389: 495–498.
97. Paulus MP, Simmons AN, Fitzpatrick SN, Potterat EG, Van Orden KF, et al. (2010) Differential brain activation to angry faces by elite warfighters: neural processing evidence for enhanced threat detection. PloS one 5: e10096.
98. Schultheiss OC, Wirth MM, Waugh CE, Stanton SJ, Meier EA, et al. (2008) Exploring the motivational brain: Effects of implicit power motivation on brain activation in response to facial expressions of emotion. Social Cognitive and Affective Neuroscience 3: 333–343.
99. Haruno M, Kawato M (2006) Different neural correlates of reward expectation and reward expectation error in the putamen and caudate nucleus during stimulus-action-reward association learning. Journal of Neurophysiology 95: 948–959.
100. Nettle D (2007) Empathizing and systemizing: What are they, and what do they contribute to our understanding of psychological sex differences? British Journal of Psychology 98: 237–255.
101. Costa PT, McCrae RR (1992) Professional manual: revised NEO personality inventory (NEO-PI-R) and NEO five-factor inventory (NEO-FFI). Odessa, FL: Psychological Assessment Resources.
102. Takeuchi H, Taki Y, Sassa Y, Hashizume H, Sekiguchi A, et al. (2013) Brain structures associated with executive functions during everyday events in a non-clinical sample. Brain Structure and Function 218: 1017–1032.
103. Kanai R, Rees G (2011) The structural basis of inter-individual differences in human behaviour and cognition. Nature Reviews Neuroscience 12: 231–242.
104. Sowell ER, Peterson BS, Thompson PM, Welcome SE, Henkenius AL, et al. (2003) Mapping cortical change across the human life span. Nature Neuroscience 6: 309–315.
105. Taki Y, Goto R, Evans A, Zijdenbos A, Neelin P, et al. (2004) Voxel-based morphometry of human brain with age and cerebrovascular risk factors. Neurobiology of Aging 25: 455–463.
106. Baron J, Chetelat G, Desgranges B, Perchey G, Landeau B, et al. (2001) In vivo mapping of gray matter loss with voxel-based morphometry in mild Alzheimer's disease. Neuroimage 14: 298–309.
107. Shaw P, Kabani NJ, Lerch JP, Eckstrand K, Lenroot R, et al. (2008) Neurodevelopmental trajectories of the human cerebral cortex. The Journal of Neuroscience 28: 3586–3594.
108. Nagai M, Kishi K, Kato S (2007) Insular cortex and neuropsychiatric disorders: A review of recent literature. European Psychiatry 22: 387–394.
109. Haier RJ, Jung RE, Yeo RA, Head K, Alkire MT (2004) Structural brain variation and general intelligence. Neuroimage 23: 425–433.
110. Jung RE, Haier RJ (2007) The parieto-frontal integration theory (P-FIT) of intelligence: Converging neuroimaging evidence. Behavioral and Brain Sciences 30: 135–154.
111. Takeuchi H, Taki Y, Sassa Y, Hashizume H, Sekiguchi A, et al. (2012) Regional gray and white matter volume associated with Stroop interference: Evidence from voxel-based morphometry. Neuroimage 59: 2899–2907.
112. Chechik G, Meilijson I, Ruppin E (1999) Neuronal regulation: A mechanism for synaptic pruning during brain maturation. Neural Computation 11: 2061–2080.
113. Yu KK, Cheung C, Chua SE, McAlonan GM (2011) Can Asperger syndrome be distinguished from autism? An anatomic likelihood meta-analysis of MRI studies. Journal of psychiatry & neuroscience: JPN 36: 412–421.
114. Hill EL, Frith U (2003) Understanding autism: insights from mind and brain. Philosophical Transactions B 358: 281–289.
115. Baron-Cohen S, Wheelwright S, Skinner R, Martin J, Clubley E (2001) The autism-spectrum quotient (AQ): evidence from Asperger syndrome/high-functioning autism, males and females, scientists and mathematicians. Journal of Autism and Developmental Disorders 31: 5–17.
116. Baron-Cohen S (1995) Mindblindness: As essay on autism and theory of mind. Boston, MA: Wiley Online Library.
117. Liu MJ, Shih WL, Ma LY (2011) Are children with Asperger syndrome creative in divergent thinking and feeling? A brief report. Research in Autism Spectrum Disorders 5: 294–298.
118. Ambery FZ, Russell AJ, Perry K, Morris R, Murphy DGM (2006) Neuropsychological functioning in adults with Asperger syndrome. Autism 10: 551–564.
119. Sinzig J, Morsch D, Bruning N, Schmidt MH, Lehmkuhl G (2008) Inhibition, flexibility, working memory and planning in autism spectrum disorders with and without comorbid ADHD-symptoms. Child and adolescent psychiatry and mental health 2: 4.
120. Montgomery JM, McCrimmon AW, Schwean VL, Saklofske DH (2010) Emotional intelligence in Asperger syndrome: Implications of dissonance

between intellect and affect. Education and Training in Autism and Developmental Disabilities 45: 566–582.
121. Duerden EG, Mak-Fan KM, Taylor MJ, Roberts SW (2012) Regional differences in grey and white matter in children and adults with autism spectrum disorders: an activation likelihood estimate (ALE) meta-analysis. Autism Research 5: 49–66.
122. Via E, Radua J, Cardoner N, Happé F, Mataix-Cols D (2011) Meta-analysis of gray matter abnormalities in autism spectrum disorder: should Asperger disorder be subsumed under a broader umbrella of autistic spectrum disorder? Archives of General Psychiatry 68: 409–418.
123. Nickl-Jockschat T, Habel U, Maria Michel T, Manning J, Laird AR, et al. (2012) Brain structure anomalies in autism spectrum disorder–a meta-analysis of VBM studies using anatomic likelihood estimation. Human Brain Mapping 33: 1470–1489.
124. Redcay E, Courchesne E (2005) When is the brain enlarged in autism? A meta-analysis of all brain size reports. Biological Psychiatry 58: 1–9.
125. Duncan J, Seitz RJ, Kolodny J, Bor D, Herzog H, et al. (2000) A Neural Basis for General Intelligence. Science 289: 457–460.
126. Zielinski BA, Gennatas ED, Zhou J, Seeley WW (2010) Network-level structural covariance in the developing brain. Proceedings of the National Academy of Sciences 107: 18191–18196.
127. Davis MH (1980) A multidimensional approach to individual differences in empathy. JSAS Catalog of Selected Documents in Psychology 10: 989–1015.
128. Doherty RW (1997) The emotional contagion scale: A measure of individual differences. Journal of nonverbal Behavior 21: 131–154.
129. Mehrabian A, Epstein N (1972) A measure of emotional empathy. Journal of Personality 40: 525–543.
130. Leibetseder M, Laireiter A-R, Riepler A, Köller T (2001) E-Skala: Fragebogen zur Erfassung von Empathie–Beschreibung und psychometrische Eigenschaften. Zeitschrift für Differentielle und diagnostische Psychologie 22: 70–85.
131. Constantino JN, Przybeck T, Friesen D, Todd RD (2000) Reciprocal social behavior in children with and without pervasive developmental disorders. Journal of Developmental & Behavioral Pediatrics 21: 2–11.

11

Facial Trustworthiness Judgments in Children with ASD Are Modulated by Happy and Angry Emotional Cues

Frances Caulfield, Louise Ewing*, Nichola Burton, Eleni Avard, Gillian Rhodes

Australian Research Council Centre of Excellence in Cognition and its Disorders, School of Psychology, University of Western Australia, Perth, Western Australia, Australia

Abstract

Appearance-based trustworthiness inferences may reflect the misinterpretation of emotional expression cues. Children and adults typically perceive faces that look happy to be relatively trustworthy and those that look angry to be relatively untrustworthy. Given reports of atypical expression perception in children with Autism Spectrum Disorder (ASD), the current study aimed to determine whether the modulation of trustworthiness judgments by emotional expression cues in children with ASD is also atypical. Cognitively-able children with and without ASD, aged 6–12 years, rated the trustworthiness of faces showing happy, angry and neutral expressions. Trust judgments in children with ASD were significantly modulated by overt happy and angry expressions, like those of typically-developing children. Furthermore, subtle emotion cues in neutral faces also influenced trust ratings of the children in both groups. These findings support a powerful influence of emotion cues on perceived trustworthiness, which even extends to children with social cognitive impairments.

Editor: Valerie W. Hu, The George Washington University, United States of America

Funding: This research was supported by the Australian Research Council Centre of Excellence in Cognition and its Disorders (CE110001021), an ARC Professional Fellowship to Rhodes (DP0877379) and an ARC Discovery Outstanding Researcher Award to Rhodes (DP130102300). The funders had no role in study design, data collection and analysis, decision to publish, or preparation of the manuscript.

Competing Interests: The authors have declared that no competing interests exist.

* E-mail: louise.ewing@uwa.edu.au

Introduction

The face plays an important role in social cognition, with people routinely inferring personality traits from an individual's appearance [1]. Evaluations of an individual's trustworthiness are one of the many important appearance-based trait inferences made on a daily basis [2]. Although not necessarily accurate, adults make reliable, automatic trustworthiness attributions after very brief exposure to faces and these judgments can have a substantial impact on social interactions, influencing how people behave towards others [3–6].

There has recently been increasing interest in trait inferences in Autism Spectrum Disorder (ASD), which is characterised by social cognitive impairments [7]. Individuals with ASD often have difficulties understanding the mental state of others and reading social information from faces [8–10], which may be critical for these appearance-based trait inferences. Trustworthiness judgments are of particular interest in this group because imaging studies have revealed that the amygdala, which is involved in trust perception [11–13], may be atypical in individuals with ASD [8,14–16].

Current findings regarding facial trustworthiness judgments in ASD are mixed. Some studies report no significant differences in trustworthiness judgments between typical adults and adults with ASD [17–19]. Other studies report that individuals with ASD significantly overrate the trustworthiness of negatively valenced faces [11,20,21]. Critically however, in these latter studies the responses of adults with ASD are highly variable and overlap considerably with the responses of the typical adults [11] and in one study the group differences did not survive correction for multiple comparisons [20]. Taken together, these findings provide limited support for differences in facial trust perception between adults with and without ASD. Still, there may be other atypicalities in responses to trustworthy and untrustworthy faces in individuals with ASD. For example, there have been some reports of atypical neural [18] and autonomic [17] responses in adults with ASD during trust evaluation tasks.

A critical feature of trust perception that is yet to be investigated in individuals with ASD is the role of emotional expression cues. Researchers propose that facial expressions of emotion may convey not only an individual's current affective state, but also more stable trait impressions, such as trustworthiness, consistent with that emotion [22–24]. In particular, happy and angry expressions have been associated with perceived trustworthiness, with happy expressions found to increase the appearance of trustworthiness and angry expressions found to diminish it [25–30]. When these expressions are overtly expressed the process is known as temporal extension [24]. When these expressions are very subtle, such as those perceptible in neutral faces, the phenomenon is known as emotion overgeneralization [31]. There is also evidence that this association between perceived trustworthiness and facial cues to emotion is bidirectional. For example, computer-modelling studies have shown that manipulating the trustworthiness of faces influences their perceived emotional expressions [26]. These findings suggest a strong association between emotional expressions and perceived facial trustworthiness.

The same may not be the case however for individuals with ASD, who often demonstrate difficulties extracting emotional information from faces. Indeed the Diagnostic and Statistical Manual of Mental Disorders-IV (DSM-IV) criteria for ASD include items related to deficits in identifying and processing emotion, such as the use of facial expressions, lack of emotional sharing and impaired responses to others emotions [7]. The extent of emotion processing deficits in ASD remains a topic of much debate [32,33–35], but the conclusions of a recent meta-analysis of 48 studies support a general impairment in emotion recognition in individuals with ASD [32]. Given the association between perceived emotion and trustworthiness, it seems plausible that difficulties reading emotional information from faces could disrupt the typical modulation of trust inferences by expression cues.

The current study aimed to directly examine the influence of emotional expressions on trust judgments in children with ASD. Children with and without ASD, aged 6 to 12 years, made trustworthiness ratings of neutral faces and faces displaying happy and angry expressions. We created two intensity levels of overtly expressed happiness and anger (25% and 50%) and looked for evidence of temporal extension. We also looked for evidence of overgeneralization of emotion cues present in neutral expression faces. Temporal extension and emotion overgeneralization have both been shown to occur in trust judgments of typical adults [26–30], older adults [25] and typically-developing children [36]. Here, we were interested to see whether these effects also extend to children with ASD. Specifically, we were interested in whether cues to anger diminish the appearance of trustworthiness for children with ASD and whether cues to happiness increase it.

We also measured expression recognition ability to assess whether any differences in the modulatory effects of emotion are related to differences in expression sensitivity between our two participant groups. Evidence of impaired expression processing *and* reduced modulation of trust judgments by expression in children with ASD could signal that expression recognition is critical for trustworthiness attribution. In contrast, evidence of intact expression processing without modulation of trust judgments could suggest that children with ASD have atypical sensitivity to the social affordances of expression cues.

Method

Ethics Statement

This study was approved by the Human Research Ethics Committee at the University of Western Australia and all parents provided written consent prior to their child's participation in the project. All children also gave verbal and written consent before taking part. The individual displayed in figure 1 of this manuscript has given written informed consent (as outlined in PLOS consent form) to publish a recognizable image.

Participants

Fifteen cognitively-able boys with ASD aged 6 years 9 months to 12 years 8 months (M = 9:3, SD = 1:10) were recruited from the West Australian Register for Autism Spectrum Disorders, local schools and community groups. They had all received an independent diagnosis of an ASD by a multidisciplinary team following DSM-IV criteria [37]. Parents completed the Social Communication Questionnaire (SCQ) [38], a retrospective questionnaire measure of their children's autism symptomatology. All children scored at or above the cut-off for clinically significant levels of autistic symptomatology (score of 12) [39]. Children also completed Module 3 of the Autism Diagnostic Observation Schedule-2 (ADOS-2) [40], with six participants scoring below the cut-off (score of 7) on this semi-structured standardized assessment of current autism symptomatology. Note - When the data were reanalysed including only those children with ASD who scored above the ADOS-2 cut-off for *current* ASD symptoms the pattern of results remained unchanged (see Appendix S1).

In addition, 15 typically-developing children (8 male) aged between 6 years 3 months and 11 years 6 months (M = 8:10, SD = 1:9) were recruited from local schools and community groups. These children were well matched to the children with ASD on chronological age, non-verbal IQ and full-scale IQ, and did not differ significantly in terms of verbal IQ (see Table 1). Six additional children were excluded prior to matching due to inattention (ASD = 1, Typical = 1) or difficulties understanding the concept of trustworthiness (ASD = 2, Typical = 2) during testing. No typically-developing child displayed clinically significant levels of ASD symptomatology, as indicated by scores on the SCQ. Face recognition was significantly impaired in the children with ASD relative to this typical group (see Table 1), as indexed by scores on the Cambridge Face Memory Test – for Children (CFMT-C) [41].

An additional 16 adults (18–54 years, M = 29.1, SD = 10.9; 4 male) were recruited to rate the neutral face stimuli from the trust rating task on their resemblance to happy and angry expressions.

Procedure

The trust rating task and expression recognition task were run on a 15-inch MacBook Pro laptop computer and were part of a larger battery of unrelated tasks conducted with participants over two or three 90–120 minute activity sessions in the family home, school or at the University of Western Australia. The experimenter sat alongside the child throughout all tasks to monitor engagement and provide verbal encouragement.

Trust ratings. Participants rated the trustworthiness of faces displaying happy, angry and neutral expressions. Children were told that an Alien named Zeb needed help to complete a mission to learn more about human trustworthiness. They were given a brief description of trustworthiness that focused on three key elements of trust: honesty, reliability and emotional trust [42,43]. They then answered three questions to confirm they understood our operationalization of trustworthiness: Sarah watched her little

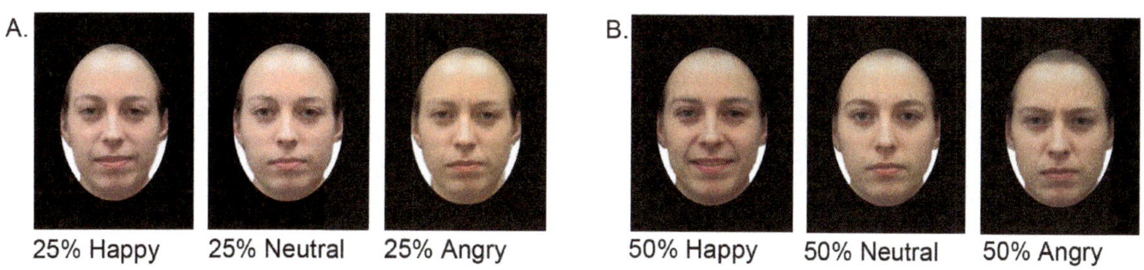

Figure 1. An example of expression stimuli used in the trust rating task. A happy, neutral and angry expression at 25% intensity (A) and 50% intensity (B). The identity displayed here did not appear in the stimulus set.

Table 1. Descriptive statistics for age, cognitive ability and autism symptomatology measures.

Measure	Group					
	ASD (n = 15)		Typical (n = 15)			
	M (SD)	Range	*M (SD)*	Range		Cohen's *d*
Age (months)	110.9 (21.6)	81–152	106.0 (20.9)	75–138	$t(28) = -.63$, $p = .54$	0.24
Nonverbal IQ[a]	107.8 (17.6)	84–134	105.3 (13.4)	81–129	$t(28) = -.43$, $p = .67$	0.16
Verbal IQ[a]	96.5 (11.1)	81–118	102.1 (7.3)	87–114	$t(24.22) = 1.64$, $p = .12$[e]	0.67
Full Scale IQ[a]	101.6 (12.7)	87–125	104.0 (6.5)	88–112	$t(20.89) = .65$, $p = .52$[e]	0.28
SCQ[b]	25.5 (6.8)	12–34	1.7 (2.4)	0–8	$t(17.41) = -12.84$, $p < .001$[e]	6.16
ADOS-2[b,c]	7.9 (5.3)	0–21				
CFMT-C[d]	69.3 (9.1)	52–82	77.1 (12.1)	57–97	$t(28) = 1.99$, $p = .03$[f]	0.75

[a]Nonverbal and verbal IQ were measured with the WASI [65]: Matrix Reasoning and Block Design (nonverbal IQ) and Similarities and Vocabulary (verbal IQ). Full-scale IQ (FSIQ) was derived by standardizing the sum of both verbal and performance ability scores against age-based norms.
[b]Higher scores on both the SCQ [38] and ADOS-2 [40] indicate a greater degree of autism symptomatology.
[c]ADOS-2 score reported = Communication+Social Interaction algorithm total (cut-off = 7).
[d]Accuracy (total percentage correct) on the Cambridge Face Memory Test - for Children [41].
[e]Equal variances not assumed.
[f]One-tailed independent samples t-test.

brother like she promised. Would you trust Sarah?; Jake copied the test answers from the person sitting next to him. Would you trust Jake?; Mia hasn't told anyone that her best friend is afraid of the dark. Would you trust Mia? If participants responded incorrectly to any item, we repeated our description of trust and repeated all three questions (one child with ASD required repetition). Any participant who still could not respond correctly to all questions was excluded (see above).

The stimuli were images of faces displaying happy, angry and neutral expressions (Figure 1). They were generated from 20 neutral Caucasian faces (10 male) [44], with mid-range trustworthiness ratings (adults used a scale ranging from 1 "not at all trustworthy" to 9 "extremely trustworthy"; $M = 5.0$, $SD = 0.4$) [45]. Each identity was morphed, using Fantamorph v5.3.1 (http://www.fantamorph.com), with three composite faces displaying happy, angry and neutral expressions respectively (each an average of 50 identities) [46]. We morphed the original (neutral expression) images towards a neutral composite, for the neutral face condition, to ensure that all stimuli were morphs. Standard morphing procedures were used to create morphs at 25% and 50% by blending the original faces with the composites in different proportions, e.g. a 25% angry morph was a 75/25 blend of an original face and the angry composite. There were 120 stimuli in total: 3 expressions (happy, angry, neutral)×2 intensities (25%, 50%)×20 identities.

On each trial, a face was presented on screen for 1500 ms for participants to rate with the number keys using a 7-point scale consisting of numbered cups (1 = not very trustworthy to 7 = very trustworthy) [47]. Faces subtended an average visual angle of $8.4° \times 6.3°$ at an approximate viewing distance of 50 cm. Each trial was initiated with a space-bar press. The 120 faces were presented in randomized order in 6 blocks of 20 trials. Between each block participants were given a break in which they were told 'fun facts' about Zeb the alien. Participants began with 10 practice trials: 4 trials using well-known cartoon faces (2 trustworthy, 2 male) and 6 trials using real faces (3 expressions×2 intensities). Stimuli used for practice trials were not used in the main task.

The neutral expressions were also rated on their resemblance to happy and angry facial expressions by a group of typical adults. Ratings of emotional expressions (happy, angry) were obtained using a 7-point scale (1 = not at all happy/angry to 7 = very happy/angry). Participants were informed that all faces would be emotionally neutral but could nevertheless show subtle variations in emotional information. They were encouraged to use the whole range of the scale.

Expression recognition. The expression recognition task was adapted from Gao and Maurer [48,49]. Children were told that they would be shown the faces of people who were watching different movies that made them feel different things. They were told to select the expression, from five cartoon emoticon-style faces, which best matched what the person was feeling. The experimenter emphasized that there could be different intensity expressions.

The stimuli were photographs of four models (two male) from the NimStim Face Stimulus Set [50] each posing happy, angry, sad, fearful and neutral expressions. Eight levels of intensity (0, 10, 20, 30, 40, 60, 80, 100) were created for each of the four expressions by morphing between neutral (0%) expressions and 100% intensity levels in varying degrees [48]. This resulted in 128 stimuli: (4 expressions×7 intensity levels×4 models)+(4 neutral expressions×4 models).

Each trial began with a face presented on screen for 1000 ms followed by a response screen that prompted the participant to indicate the expression that corresponded to what the person was feeling. Children pointed to the appropriate icon and the experimenter pressed the corresponding key to reduce the cognitive demands of the task. There were 128 trials in total presented in randomized order. To ensure task duration was age-appropriate the task was split into two sessions. Two different models (one male) were presented in each session (64 trials in total), with order of model presentation counterbalanced between participants.

Results

Two extreme scores defined by SPSS (one ASD 50% angry difference score and one ASD happy expression recognition threshold) were replaced with the next lowest score. Following replacement of these scores all distributions of trust and expression judgments for each group were normal and therefore appropriate for parametric analysis [51].

Trustworthiness from Expressive Faces (Temporal Extension)

We were interested in the extent to which overt happy and angry expressions modulated trust judgments in children with ASD, relative to typically-developing children. Given the absence of any specific predictions about the relative magnitude of effects for the two expressions, we did not equate the intensity of the happy and angry expressions and we consider them separately in our analysis. In each case we used a 2×2 mixed ANOVA to investigate the effects of group (ASD, typical) and intensity (25%, 50%) on the influence of expression on trust ratings, indexed as the difference between trust ratings of expressive faces and neutral faces (see below). Descriptive statistics for each group's trustworthiness ratings of the angry, neutral and happy expression faces are shown in Table 2.

Angry faces. The dependent variable was the mean difference between trustworthiness ratings of the angry and neutral faces (neutral minus angry). One sample t-tests revealed that this value was significantly greater than zero for the typically-developing children for the 25% and 50% angry faces, all *t*s >2.21, *p*s <.05, Cohen's *d*s >1.18, which confirms that angry expressions had the predicted negative effect on perceived trustworthiness. The children with ASD also showed a significant difference from zero for the 50% angry expressions, $t(14) = 3.15$, $p = .007$ and Cohen's $d = 1.68$, and a marginal difference from zero for the 25% expressions, $t(14) = 2.02$, $p = .063$ and Cohen's $d = 1.08$ (Figure 2).

Our ANOVA revealed a significant main effect of intensity on the influence of anger, $F(1, 28) = 7.58$, $p = .01$, *partial* $\eta^2 = .21$. Angry expressions influenced trustworthiness more at 50% ($M = 0.7$, $SD = 0.8$) than at 25% ($M = 0.3$, $SD = 0.5$). There was no main effect of group, $F(1, 28) = 0.40$, $p = .53$, *partial* $\eta^2 = .01$, and no interaction of group and intensity, $F(1, 28) = 0.31$, $p = .58$, *partial* $\eta^2 = .01$ (Figure 2).

Happy faces. The dependent variable was the mean difference between trustworthiness ratings assigned to the happy and neutral faces (happy minus neutral). One sample t-tests indicated that this value was significantly greater than zero for children with ASD and typically-developing children at both intensities, all *t*s >2.30, *p*s <.05, Cohen's *d*s >1.23 (Figure 3). Thus cues to happiness had a positive effect on perceived facial trustworthiness in children with and without ASD.

Our ANOVA revealed a significant main effect of intensity on the influence of happiness, $F(1, 28) = 12.35$, $p = .002$, *partial* $\eta^2 = .31$. Happy expressions influenced trustworthiness judgments more at 50% ($M = 1.6$, $SD = 1.9$) than at 25% ($M = 1.0$, $SD = 1.3$). As with the angry cues, there was no significant difference between the groups, $F(1, 28) = 0.006$, $p = .94$, *partial* $\eta^2 < .001$, and no interaction between group and intensity, $F(1, 28) = 0.03$, $p = .86$, *partial* $\eta^2 = .001$, indicating that the influence of happy cues on trustworthiness judgments did not differ for the children with ASD and typically-developing children (Figure 3).

We also investigated whether the influence of emotion expressions on trust judgments was associated with ASD symptomatology, as indexed by SCQ scores, in our sample of children. This analysis revealed no significant correlations between the modulatory power of 25% happy expressions, 50% happy expressions, or 50% angry expressions and SCQ scores (see Table 3). However, there was a significant positive correlation between symptom severity and the modulatory power of the 25% angry expressions. This correlation suggests that greater symptom severity was associated with greater influence of the 25% angry expressions on trust judgments.

Trustworthiness from Neutral Faces (Emotion Overgeneralization)

To assess whether there was also an association between perceived trustworthiness and more subtle emotional expressions for children with ASD we looked at the relationship between the children's trustworthiness ratings and adults' ratings of the subtle emotion cues present in the neutral expression face stimuli. The internal consistency of the adult expression ratings was high (Cronbach's alpha = .86 and.93 for angry and happy expressions respectively) but the internal consistency of the trust ratings was low and did not support averaging across participants (Cronbach's alpha = −.30 and −.44 for the ASD and typical group respectively). We therefore computed separate correlation coefficients for the association between trust ratings and mean expression ratings (happy, angry) of each identity for each participant. Fisher's r to z transformation was applied to these correlation coefficients prior to analysis [52].

One-tailed, one sample t-tests indicated that the mean correlation between trust and anger ratings was significantly different from zero (i.e., negative) for children with ASD ($M = -.10$, $SD = .20$), as well as the typically-developing children ($M = -.14$, $SD = .21$), both *t*s>−1.80, *p*s <.05, Cohen's *d*s >0.97. The mean correlation between trust and happiness ratings was significantly greater than zero for the typically-developing children ($M = .14$, $SD = .21$), $t(14) = 2.56$, $p = .02$, Cohen's $d = 1.37$, and showed a similar trend for the children with ASD ($M = .09$, $SD = .24$), but this value did not reach significance, $t(14) = 1.40$, $p = .09$, Cohen's $d = 0.75$. These results suggest subtle emotion cues in neutral faces influence trust ratings of children with ASD as well as typically-developing children.

A 2×2 mixed ANOVA on the trust correlations, with group (ASD, typical) as a between-participants factor and expression (angry, happy) as a within-participants factor revealed no main effect of group, $F(1, 28) = 0.06$, $p = .81$, *partial* $\eta^2 = .002$, and no interaction between group and expression, $F(1, 28) = 0.43$, $p = .52$, *partial* $\eta^2 = .015$. These results indicate that the children with ASD

Table 2. Descriptive statistics for trustworthiness ratings of the 25% and 50% angry, neutral and happy faces for each group.

	25%			50%		
	Angry	Neutral	Happy	Angry	Neutral	Happy
	M (SD)	M (SD)	M (SD)	M (SD)	M (SD)	M (SD)
ASD	3.4 (1.3)	3.7 (1.2)	4.7 (1.0)	3.1 (1.4)	3.7 (1.4)	5.4 (1.3)
Typical	3.6 (0.9)	3.9 (0.8)	4.9 (0.8)	3.1 (1.3)	4.0 (0.9)	5.5 (1.0)

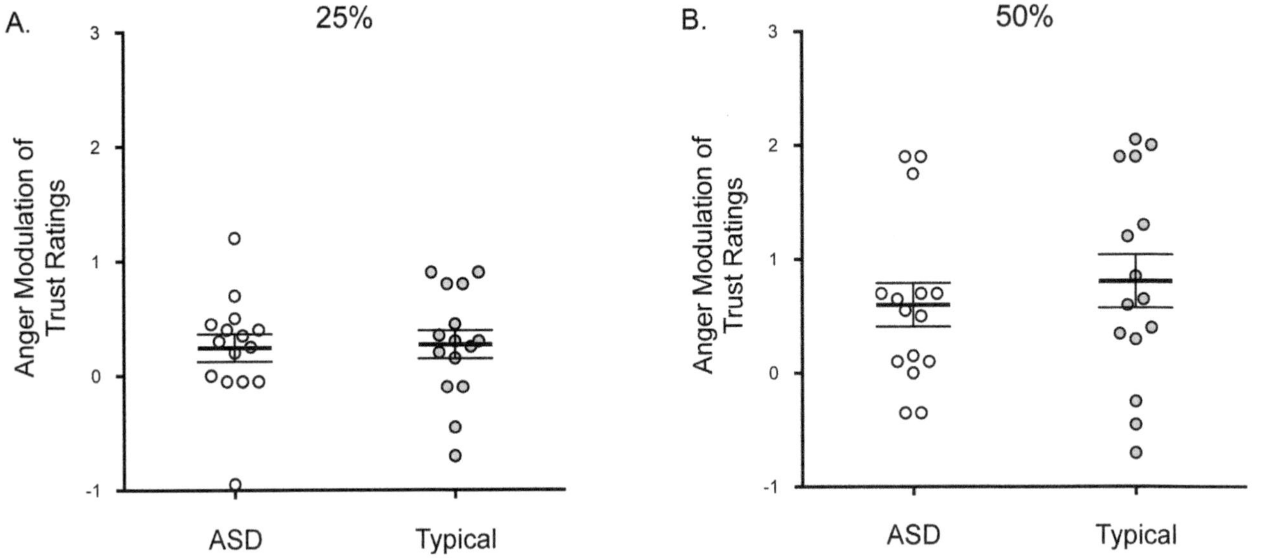

Figure 2. Anger modulation of trust ratings. Mean difference (SEM) in trustworthiness ratings for angry and neutral expressions at 25% (A) and 50% (B) intensity for each group. Larger values indicate greater modulation of angry expressions on trust judgments and zero indicates no modulation. Individual participants are shown.

did not differ from typical children with regard to the influence of subtle emotion cues from neutral faces on trust judgments. There was a main effect of expression, $F(1, 28) = 9.34$, $p = .005$, *partial* $\eta^2 = .25$, which reflected the difference between the negative association between trust and anger ratings ($M = -.12$, $SD = .20$) and the positive association between trust and happiness ratings ($M = .11$, $SD = .22$).

Expression Recognition

We calculated children's thresholds for correctly identifying happy and angry expressions on our recognition task [48,49]. For each participant we fitted a cumulative Gaussian function to the responses for each intensity level for each expression in Graphpad Prism 5. The threshold level represents the intensity level at which the face was correctly identified as happy or angry (50% of the time). The data for two participants (one typical and one ASD) were removed due to poor fits ($R^2 < .5$).

We used a 2×2 mixed ANOVA to examine the effects of expression (happy, angry) and group (ASD, typical) on this measure of expression sensitivity. There was a significant main effect of expression, $F(1, 26) = 5.78$, $p = .024$, *partial* $\eta^2 = .18$, with children more sensitive to the happy expressions ($M = 0.3$, $SD = 0.1$) than the angry expressions ($M = 0.4$, $SD = 0.1$). There

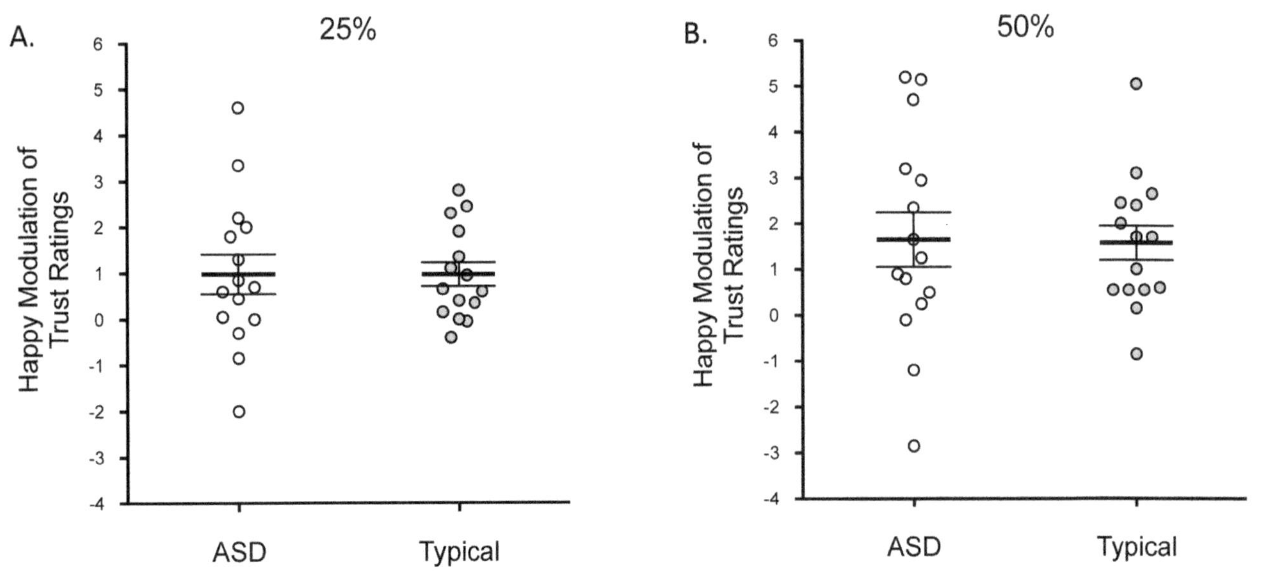

Figure 3. Happy modulation of trust ratings. Mean difference (SEM) in trustworthiness ratings for happy and neutral expressions at 25% (A) and 50% (B) intensity for each group. Larger values indicate greater influence of happy expressions on trust judgments and zero indicates no modulation. Individual participants are shown.

Table 3. Correlations between the influence of happy and angry expressions on trustworthiness judgments and autism symptom scores in the children with ASD.

Intensity	Expression	SCQ scores ($n = 15$)	
		p	*r*
25%	Angry	.63	.01
	Happy	−.14	.62
50%	Angry	.08	.77
	Happy	.05	.86

was no main effect of group, $F(1, 26) = 0.29$, $p = .59$, *partial* $\eta^2 = .01$, and no interaction between group and expression, $F(1, 26) = 2.19$, $p = .15$, *partial* $\eta^2 = .08$. This indicates that the children with ASD did not differ from the typical group with respect to their sensitivity to happy and angry expressions (Figure 4).

Discussion

We found that facial trustworthiness judgments in children with ASD were significantly modulated by happy and angry emotional expressions, like typically-developing children. These results suggest that facial expressions of emotion not only communicate emotional states but also contribute to impressions of trustworthiness for cognitively-able children with ASD.

Our findings extend previous trust perception research in ASD, which has solely focused on adults' trust attributions [11,17–21]. Here, we show that children with ASD, who may be less likely than adults to have developed compensatory mechanisms to overcome social cognitive difficulties, draw upon emotion cues when making inferences of trustworthiness from faces. Specifically, overt angry expressions diminished the appearance of trustworthiness and overt happy expressions increased the appearance of trustworthiness in faces for them. Although the effects of the 25% angry expressions did not reach significance, there was a large effect size and no group differences relative to the typical children, which suggests that the non-significant result reflected our small sample size rather than reduced modulatory power for subtle angry cues. These results suggest that trait attributions in children with ASD may reflect the temporal extension of transient facial cues as signals of more enduring characteristics.

We also provide evidence that this relationship between emotion perception and trustworthiness judgments extends to even very subtle emotion cues present in neutral faces. Our results revealed that the children with ASD did not differ from typical children with regard to the influence of subtle emotion cues from neutral faces on trust judgments. There was a negative association between trust and anger ratings and a positive association between trust and happiness ratings for both groups of children. Although the correlation between trust and happiness ratings did not reach significance for the children with ASD, there was again a moderate effect size, suggesting that this non-significant result reflects low statistical power. These results indicate that children with ASD may also be sensitive to the effects of emotion overgeneralization and provide further support for an association between emotional expressions and trust attributions in children with ASD.

Our findings are consistent with previous adult studies reporting no significant differences in trustworthiness judgments between typical adults and adults with ASD [17–19]. However, there are

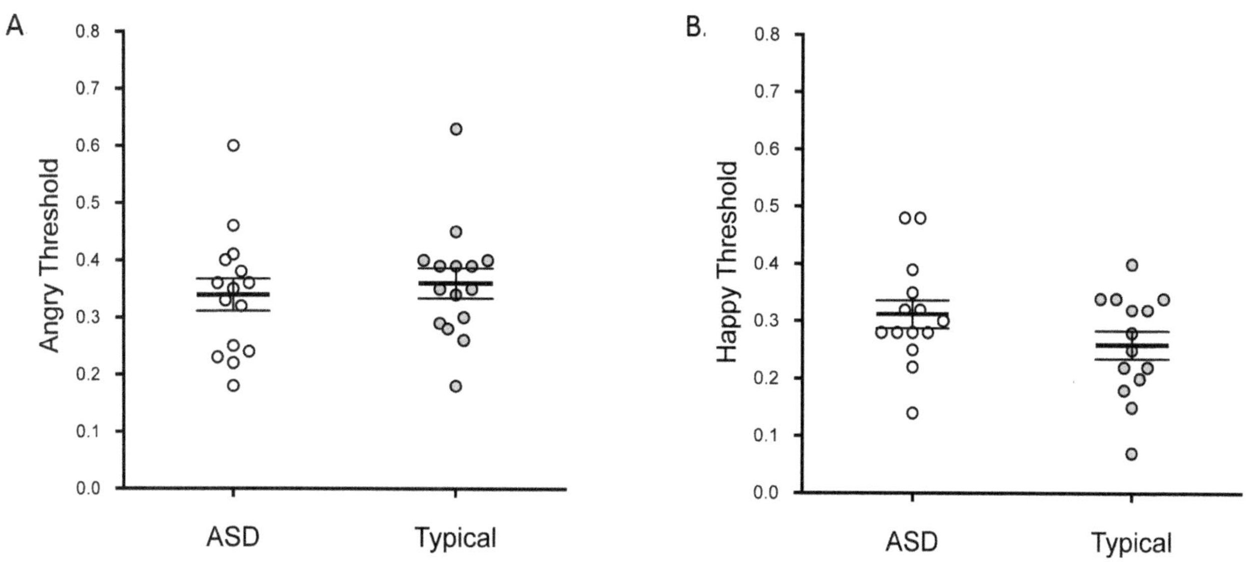

Figure 4. Expression recognition ability. Mean thresholds (SEM) for recognition of the angry (A) and happy (B) expressions for each group. Lower thresholds indicate greater sensitivity to the expression. Individual participants are shown.

also studies that *have* reported atypicalities in response to trustworthy and untrustworthy faces in adults with ASD [11,20,21]. It is likely that considerable variation in participant demographics, matching strategies and task format across studies contributes to the heterogeneity of results. Moreover, differences in expression recognition ability between participant groups may also, in part, account for inconsistencies. This latter explanation seems plausible given that two of the previous studies reporting differences in trustworthiness judgments between typical adults and adults with ASD also report emotion processing impairments in the ASD group [20,21].

Perhaps critically, the children with ASD in the current study did not exhibit expression processing impairments. Previous studies have reported expression recognition difficulties in similar samples [53,54,55]. However, this group of children with ASD demonstrated an intact sensitivity to happy and angry expressions on our measure of expression recognition, which was designed to be sensitive to detect subtle processing atypicalities. Our study is not the first to find intact expression processing in individuals with ASD [56,57–60]. Indeed, despite considerable research attention the literature remains divided as to whether or not individuals with ASD show reliable emotion processing impairments [32–35]. Based on our findings, we can conclude that when expression processing is intact in children with ASD, emotional expressions influence impressions of trustworthiness from faces.

Clearly, however, an important extension of the current study will be to investigate trust perception in children with ASD who *do* show significant emotion processing impairments. Such research would allow us to determine whether the modulatory power of emotion cues on trust judgments can be dissociated from expression recognition ability. It seems likely that impairments reading expression information would limit the influence of these cues on trustworthiness judgments. However, it is also possible that the modulation of trait judgments by emotion cues may be independent of explicit expression recognition ability, particularly given the automatic nature of these appearance-based trait inferences [4,61].

Interpretation of the current results must take into consideration the characteristics of our cognitively-able ASD sample. Though low levels of *current* autism symptoms in a subset of our sample, as indexed by scores on the ADOS-2 [40], could limit the generalizability of our findings, we highlight that all participants had received an ASD diagnosis from a multidisciplinary team and were scored above the criterion for ASD on a well-validated retrospective symptom measure (SCQ) [38]. In addition, our sample demonstrated other perceptual atypicalities in face perception, e.g. significant impairments in face recognition, relative to typical children, as indexed by scores on the CFMT-C. Moreover, when we reanalyzed our data including only those children with ASD who met the more conservative current symptom criterion (score of 7 or above on the ADOS-2), the modulatory effects of the happy and angry expressions remained in the predicted direction, with moderate-large effect sizes across all conditions.

Interestingly, results of our correlational analysis between symptom severity and the influence of emotion expressions on trust judgments suggested that children with more severe ASD symptomatology may *overuse* certain expression cues. Our results revealed a positive correlation between symptom severity and the modulatory power of 25% angry expressions on trust judgments. That is, more severe ASD symptoms were associated with greater influence of the 25% angry expressions when judging trustworthiness. This overuse of the angry expression cues may constitute evidence of atypical trust perception. It would be interesting to see whether the same profile of trust perception is observed in a larger sample of children with more severe ASD symptomatology.

The current study adds to a growing body of evidence detailing intact aspects of social cognition in individuals with ASD. Other studies have revealed that adults with ASD spontaneously infer traits, such as whether a person is clever, honest and friendly, from descriptions of behaviour [62] and children with ASD have been shown to use social stereotypes to predict behaviour [63,64]. Together these findings suggest that, despite significant impairments in interpersonal understanding, social knowledge is not universally disrupted in individuals with ASD. Our findings suggest that trust perception may be another spared social capacity in ASD. Continued research into other social judgments and trait attributions will help further our understanding of the complex profile of social cognitive ability and impairment in individuals with ASD.

In conclusion, we have shown that impressions of trustworthiness from facial appearances in cognitively-able children with ASD are significantly modulated by emotional expressions. Angry expressions diminished the appearance of trustworthiness and happy expressions increased the appearance of trustworthiness for the children with ASD, just like for the typically-developing children. The associations between perceived emotion and trustworthiness also extended to subtle expression cues present in neutral faces. These findings indicate that cognitively-able children with ASD draw upon emotion cues when judging facial trustworthiness, which suggests that similar mechanisms may drive trustworthiness inferences in typical children and children with ASD.

Supporting Information

Appendix S1 This supporting information describes the results for each task when the data were reanalysed with only those children with ASD who scored above the ADOS-2 cut-off for *current* ASD symptoms ($n = 9$).

Acknowledgments

We thank Xiaoqing Gao and Daphne Maurer for providing us with their expression recognition task and Andy Skinner and Christopher Benton for providing us with their composite expression stimuli. We also thank Ainsley Read, Samantha Bank and Libby Taylor for assistance with testing and all of the children, families, community groups and schools who kindly volunteered their time to participate.

Author Contributions

Conceived and designed the experiments: FC LE GR. Performed the experiments: FC LE NB EA. Analyzed the data: FC LE GR. Wrote the paper: FC LE GR.

References

1. Hassin R, Trope Y (2000) Facing faces: Studies on the cognitive aspects of physiognomy. Journal of Personality and Social Psychology 78: 837–852.
2. Cosmides L, Tooby J (1992) Cognitive adaptations for social exchange. In: Barkow J, Cosmides L, Tooby J, editors. The adapted mind: Evolutionary psychology and the generation of culture. New York: Oxford University Press. 163–228.
3. Rule NO, Krendl AC, Ivcevic Z, Ambady N (2013) Accuracy and consensus in judgments of trustworthiness from faces: Behavioral and neural correlates. Journal of Personality and Social Psychology 104: 409–426.
4. Willis J, Todorov A (2006) First impressions: Making up your mind after 100 ms exposure to a face. Psychological Science 17: 592–598.

5. Todorov A, Pakrashi M, Oosterhof NN (2009) Evaluating faces on trustworthiness after minimal time exposure. Social Cognition 27: 813–833.
6. Chang LJ, Doll BB, van't Wout M, Frank MJ, Sanfey AG (2010) Seeing is believing: Trustworthiness as a dynamic belief. Cognitive Psychology 61: 87–105.
7. American Psychiatric Association (2013) Diagnostic and Statistical Manual of Mental Disorders. Arlington, VA: American Psychiatric Publishing.
8. Baron-Cohen S, Ring HA, Bullmore ET, Wheelwright S, Ashwin C, et al. (2000) The amygdala theory of autism. Neuroscience & Biobehavioral Reviews 24: 355–364.
9. Webb SJ, Faja S, Dawson G (2011) Face Processing in Autism. In: Calder AJ, Rhodes G, Johnson MH, Haxby JV, editors. The Oxford Handbook of Face Perception. Oxford: Oxford University Press. 839–856.
10. Frith U (2008) Autism: A very short introduction. New York: Oxford University Press.
11. Adolphs R, Sears L, Piven J (2001) Abnormal processing of social information from faces in autism. Journal of Cognitive Neuroscience 13: 232–240.
12. Adolphs R, Tranel D, Damasio AR (1998) The human amygdala in social judgment. Nature: 470–473.
13. Winston JS, Strange BA, O'Doherty J, Dolan RJ (2002) Automatic and intentional brain responses during evaluation of trustworthiness of faces. Nature Neuroscience 5: 277–283.
14. Ashwin C, Baron-Cohen S, Wheelwright S, O'Riordan M, Bullmore ET (2007) Differential activation of the amygdala and the 'social brain' during fearful face-processing in Asperger Syndrome. Neuropsychologia 45: 2–14.
15. Critchley HD, Daly EM, Bullmore ET, Williams SCR, Van Amelsvoort T, et al. (2000) The functional neuroanatomy of social behaviour. Brain 123: 2203–2212.
16. Di Martino A, Ross K, Uddin LQ, Sklar AB, Castellanos FX, et al. (2009) Functional brain correlates of social and nonsocial processes in autism spectrum disorders: an activation likelihood estimation meta-analysis. Biological Psychiatry 65: 63–74.
17. Mathersul D, McDonald S, Rushby JA (2013) Psychophysiological correlates of social judgement in high-functioning adults with autism spectrum disorder. International Journal of Psychophysiology 87: 88–94.
18. Pinkham AE, Hopfinger JB, Pelphrey KA, Piven J, Penn DL (2008) Neural bases for impaired social cognition in schizophrenia and autism spectrum disorders. Schizophrenia Research 99: 164–175.
19. White S, Hill E, Winston J, Frith U (2006) An islet of social ability in Asperger Syndrome: judging social attributes from faces. Brain and Cognition 61: 69–77.
20. Couture S, Penn D, Losh M, Adolphs R, Hurley R, et al. (2010) Comparison of social cognitive functioning in schizophrenia and high functioning autism: more convergence than divergence. Psychological Medicine 40: 569–579.
21. Losh M, Adolphs R, Poe MD, Couture S, Penn D, et al. (2009) Neuropsychological profile of autism and the broad autism phenotype. Archives of General Psychiatry 66: 518–526.
22. McArthur LZ, Baron RM (1983) Toward an ecological theory of social perception. Psychological Review 90: 215–238.
23. Zebrowitz LA, Collins MA (1997) Accurate social perception at zero acquaintance: The affordances of a Gibsonian approach. Personality and Social Psychology Review 1: 204–223.
24. Secord P (1958) Facial features and inference processes in interpersonal perception. In: Tagiuri R, Luigi P, editors. Person Perception and Interpersonal Behavior. Standford: Standford University Press. 300 315.
25. Franklin R, Zebrowitz LA (2013) Older Adults' Trait Impressions of Faces Are Sensitive to Subtle Resemblance to Emotions. Journal of Nonverbal Behavior 37: 139–151.
26. Oosterhof NN, Todorov A (2008) The functional basis of face evaluation. Proceedings of the National Academy of Sciences 105: 11087–11092.
27. Oosterhof NN, Todorov A (2009) Shared perceptual basis of emotional expressions and trustworthiness impressions from faces. Emotion 9: 128–133.
28. Said CP, Sebe N, Todorov A (2009) Structural resemblance to emotional expressions predicts evaluation of emotionally neutral faces. Emotion 9: 260–264.
29. Sutherland CA, Oldmeadow JA, Santos IM, Towler J, Michael Burt D, et al. (2013) Social inferences from faces: Ambient images generate a three-dimensional model. Cognition 127: 105–118.
30. Zebrowitz LA, Kikuchi M, Fellous J-M (2007) Are effects of emotion expression on trait impressions mediated by babyfaceness? Evidence from connectionist modeling. Personality and Social Psychology Bulletin 33: 648–662.
31. Zebrowitz LA, Montepare JM (2008) Social psychological face perception: Why appearance matters. Social and Personality Psychology Compass 2: 1497–1517.
32. Uljarevic M, Hamilton A (2013) Recognition of emotions in autism: a formal meta analysis. Journal of Autism and Developmental Disorders 43: 1–10.
33. Harms MB, Martin A, Wallace GL (2010) Facial emotion recognition in autism spectrum disorders: A review of behavioral and neuroimaging studies. Neuropsychology Review 20: 290–322.
34. Nuske HJ, Vivanti G, Dissanayake C (2013) Are emotion impairments unique to, universal, or specific in autism spectrum disorder? A comprehensive review. Cognition & Emotion 27: 1042–1061.
35. Gaigg SB (2012) The interplay between emotion and cognition in Autism Spectrum Disorder: implications for developmental theory. Frontiers in Integrative Neuroscience 6.
36. Caulfield F, Ewing L, Rhodes G (2014) Judging Trustworthiness from Faces: Emotion Cues Modulate Trustworthiness Judgments in Children as well as Adults. Manuscript submitted for publication.
37. American Psychiatric Association (2000) Diagnostic and Statistical Manual of Mental Disorders. Washington, DC: American Psychiatric Association.
38. Rutter M, Bailey A, Lord C, Berument S (2003) Social Communication Questionnaire. Los Angeles, CA: Western Psychological Services.
39. Corsello C, Hus V, Pickles A, Risi S, Cook EH, et al. (2007) Between a ROC and a hard place: decision making and making decisions about using the SCQ. Journal of Child Psychology and Psychiatry 48: 932–940.
40. Lord C, Rutter M, DiLavore P, Risi S, Gotham K, et al. (2012) Autism Diagnostic Observation Schedule, Second Edition (ADOS-2) Manual (Part I): Modules 1–4. Torrance, CA: Western Psychological Services.
41. Pellicano E, Pimperton H, Duchaine B (2014) The Cambridge Face Memory Test for Children. Manuscript submitted for publication.
42. Rotenberg KJ (1994) Loneliness and interpersonal trust. Journal of Social and Clinical Psychology 13: 152–173.
43. Rotenberg KJ, Fox C, Green S, Ruderman L, Slater K, et al. (2005) Construction and validation of a children's interpersonal trust belief scale. British Journal of Developmental Psychology 23: 271–293.
44. Rhodes G, Simmons LW, Peters M (2005) Attractiveness and sexual behavior: Does attractiveness enhance mating success? Evolution and Human Behavior 26: 186–201.
45. Haynes S (2011) Judgments of trustworthiness from faces: Do children and adults judge alike?: The University of Western Australia.
46. Skinner A, Benton C (2010) Anti-expression aftereffects reveal prototype-referenced coding of facial expressions. Psychological Science 21: 1248–1253.
47. Cooper PA, Geldart S, Mondloch CJ, Maurer D (2006) Developmental changes in perceptions of attractiveness: A role of experience? Developmental Science 9: 530–543.
48. Gao X, Maurer D (2009) Influence of intensity on children's sensitivity to happy, sad, and fearful facial expressions. Journal of Experimental Child Psychology 102: 503–521.
49. Gao X, Maurer D (2010) A happy story: Developmental changes in children's sensitivity to facial expressions of varying intensities. Journal of Experimental Child Psychology 107: 67–86.
50. Kim YS, Leventhal BL, Koh Y-J, Fombonne E, Laska E, et al. (2011) Prevalence of autism spectrum disorders in a total population sample. American Journal of Psychiatry 168: 904–912.
51. Field A (2009) Discovering Statistics Using SPSS. London: Sage Publications.
52. Silver NC, Dunlap WP (1987) Averaging correlation coefficients: Should Fisher's z transformation be used? Journal of Applied Psychology 72: 146–148.
53. Davies S, Bishop D, Manstead ASR, Tantam D (1994) Face perception in children with autism and Asperger's syndrome. Journal of Child Psychology and Psychiatry 35: 1033–1057.
54. Hobson RP (1986) The autistic child's appraisal of expressions of emotion. Journal of Child Psychology and Psychiatry 27: 321–342.
55. Celani G, Battacchi MW, Arcidiacono L (1999) The understanding of the emotional meaning of facial expressions in people with autism. Journal of Autism and Developmental Disorders 29: 57–66.
56. Castelli F (2005) Understanding emotions from standardized facial expressions in autism and normal development. Autism 9: 428–449.
57. Piggot J, Kwon H, Mobbs D, Blasey C, Lotspeich L, et al. (2004) Emotional attribution in high-functioning individuals with autistic spectrum disorder: a functional imaging study. Journal of the American Academy of Child & Adolescent Psychiatry 43: 473–480.
58. Lacroix A, Guidetti M, Roge B, Reilly J (2009) Recognition of emotional and nonemotional facial expressions: A comparison between Williams syndrome and autism. Research in Developmental Disabilities 30: 976–985.
59. Jones CR, Pickles A, Falcaro M, Marsden AJ, Happe F, et al. (2011) A multimodal approach to emotion recognition ability in autism spectrum disorders. Journal of Child Psychology and Psychiatry 52: 275–285.
60. Evers K, Kerkhof I, Steyaert J, Noens I, Wagemans J (2014) No differences in emotion recognition strategies in children with autism spectrum disorder: Evidence from hybrid faces. Autism Research and Treatment 2014: 1–8.
61. Rule NO, Ambady N (2008) The face of success. Psychological Science 19: 109–111.
62. Ramachandran R, Mitchell P, Ropar D (2009) Do individuals with autism spectrum disorders infer traits from behavior? Journal of Child Psychology and Psychiatry 50: 871–878.
63. Hirschfeld L, Bartmess E, White S, Frith U (2007) Can autistic children predict behavior by social stereotypes? Current Biology 17: R451–R452.
64. Hamilton AFC, Krendl AC (2007) Social cognition: Overturning stereotypes of and with autism. Current Biology 17: R641–R642.
65. Wechsler D (1999) Wechsler Abbreviated Scale of Intelligence. San Antonio, TX: The Psychological Corporation.

12

Massively Parallel Sequencing of Patients with Intellectual Disability, Congenital Anomalies and/or Autism Spectrum Disorders with a Targeted Gene Panel

Maggie Brett[1], John McPherson[2], Zhi Jiang Zang[3], Angeline Lai[4], Ee-Shien Tan[4], Ivy Ng[4], Lai-Choo Ong[5], Breana Cham[4], Patrick Tan[2,3], Steve Rozen[2], Ene-Choo Tan[1]*

1 KK Research Centre, KK Women's & Children's Hospital, Singapore, Singapore, **2** Duke-NUS Graduate Medical School, Singapore, Singapore, **3** National Cancer Centre, Singapore, Singapore, **4** Genetic Services, KK Women's & Children's Hospital, Singapore, Singapore, **5** Universiti Malaya Medical Centre, Petaling Jaya, Malaysia

Abstract

Developmental delay and/or intellectual disability (DD/ID) affects 1–3% of all children. At least half of these are thought to have a genetic etiology. Recent studies have shown that massively parallel sequencing (MPS) using a targeted gene panel is particularly suited for diagnostic testing for genetically heterogeneous conditions. We report on our experiences with using massively parallel sequencing of a targeted gene panel of 355 genes for investigating the genetic etiology of eight patients with a wide range of phenotypes including DD/ID, congenital anomalies and/or autism spectrum disorder. Targeted sequence enrichment was performed using the Agilent SureSelect Target Enrichment Kit and sequenced on the Illumina HiSeq2000 using paired-end reads. For all eight patients, 81–84% of the targeted regions achieved read depths of at least 20×, with average read depths overlapping targets ranging from 322× to 798×. Causative variants were successfully identified in two of the eight patients: a nonsense mutation in the *ATRX* gene and a canonical splice site mutation in the *L1CAM* gene. In a third patient, a canonical splice site variant in the *USP9X* gene could likely explain all or some of her clinical phenotypes. These results confirm the value of targeted MPS for investigating DD/ID in children for diagnostic purposes. However, targeted gene MPS was less likely to provide a genetic diagnosis for children whose phenotype includes autism.

Editor: Hao Sun, The Chinese University of Hong Kong, Hong Kong

Funding: This study is funded by Grant number BMRC 06/1/50/19/485 from the Agency for Science and Technology and Research; and NMRC/PPG/KKH12010-Theme3 from the National Medical Research Council, Ministry of Health, Republic of Singapore. The funders had no role in study design, data collection and analysis, decision to publish, or preparation of the manuscript.

Competing Interests: The authors have declared that no competing interests exist.

* E-mail: tanec@bigfoot.com

Introduction

Developmental delay and/or intellectual disability (DD/ID) affects 1–3% of all children and at least half of these are thought to have a genetic etiology. The genetic causes include microscopically visible chromosomal imbalances, copy number variants as well as point mutations. However, the genetic etiology remains unknown for at least 50% of all cases of DD/ID [1]. Diagnosis of DD/ID is challenging due to the broad spectrum of phenotypic presentations, as patients with DD/ID often have congenital anomalies and/or autism spectrum disorders. With the advent of massively parallel sequencing (MPS) or next generation sequencing (NGS), there has been expectation of an increased detection of the genetic causes of DD/ID. In particular, exome sequencing has been identified as an effective tool for discovery of new disease genes. However, many technical challenges remain including the uneven depth of coverage across the exome, gaps in coverage and mapping problems. In addition, there is the challenge of interpreting the clinical significance of the thousands of variants generated by exome sequencing.

An alternative approach is to perform MPS with a targeted gene panel. Studies using panels of targeted genes have been reported for various disease entities like cardiomyopathies [2], hearing loss [3], epilepsy [4] and retinal disorders [5]. These studies have shown that targeted MPS is particularly suited for clinical diagnostic testing for genetically heterogeneous conditions where there are a large number of known candidate genes.

We describe our experiences with using massively parallel sequencing of a targeted gene panel of 355 genes for investigating the genetic etiology of eight patients with a range of phenotypes including DD/ID, congenital anomalies and autism spectrum disorder.

Materials and Methods

Ethics Statement

This study is approved by the Institutional Review Board of KK Women's and Children's Hospital and SingHealth Centralised Institutional Review Board A. The patients were recruited with written informed parental consent by the Genetics Service, KK Women's & Children's Hospital, Singapore.

Patient phenotypes

Eight patients with phenotypes ranging from developmental delay, multiple congenital anomalies and/or autism spectrum disorders were selected for the targeted sequencing (Table 1). Prior

Table 1. Phenotypes and genetic testing of the eight patients.

Patient	Age	Gender	Phenotypes	Previous genetic testing
Patient 1	11	Male	DD/ID, hydrocephalus, adducted thumbs, agenesis of corpus callosum, spasticity, optic atrophy, CTEV, no speech	Karyotype, aCGH
Patient 2	4	Male	DD, microcephaly, dysmorphism (hypertelorism, low set ears, posteriorly rotated, microstomia with tented upper lip, high forehead with cowlick), hypotonia, short fingers, bilateral CTEV, bifid scrotum, undescended testes, speech delay, family history of neurodevelopmental disorders and early deaths	aCGH
Patient 3	4	Female	Dandy-Walker malformation, bilateral post-axial polydactyly, ventricular septal defect; anal stenosis, hearing loss, omphalocoele minor, hypoplastic nipple, sacral dimple, low set ears, deep set eyes, significant tendency to keloid formation	Karyotype, fluorescent in-situ hybridization for 6p deletion, aCGH
Patient 4	11	Female	DD, autism spectrum disorder diagnosed at age 3½.	Karyotype, Angelman Syndrome, aCGH
Patient 5	5	Male	DD, no speech, no eye contact	Karyotype, FragX, aCGH
Patient 6	5	Male	Speech delay, autism spectrum disorder, sister with DD and Turner's syndrome	Karyotype, FragX, aCGH
Patient 7	11	Male	Normal IQ, mild autism, does not interact with peers, hyperactive	Karyotype, aCGH
Patient 8	7	Female	DD, intellectual disability? autism spectrum disorder, speech delay, moderate IQ, hypertelorism, depressed nasal bridge, prominent jaw, brother with ADHD	Karyotype, FragX, aCGH,

DD = developmental delay; ID = intellectual disability; CTEV = congenital talipes equinovarus; ADHD = attention deficit hyperactivity disorder; aCGH = array comparative genomic hybridization; FragX = Fragile X

genetic tests were normal and array comparative genomic hybridization did not detect any copy number changes associated with known microdeletion and microduplication syndromes.

DNA extraction

Genomic DNA was isolated from peripheral blood using the Gentra Puregene blood kit (Qiagen Inc.,USA) according to the manufacturer's instructions.

Targeted gene panel and MPS

A total of 355 genes were targeted for capture and deep sequencing. They include candidate genes associated with DD/ID, microdeletion/microduplication syndromes, congenital anomalies, and autism spectrum disorders (Table S1). Using the eArray system (Agilent Technologies Inc. USA), the capture was designed to include exons with at least 30 bp of the flanking intronic sequence. In addition, 5 kb of the flanking sequence in the 5′UTR and 3′UTR regions were added to the targeted regions. A total of 4150 regions from the 355 genes were targeted for a final capture size of 4.79 Mb.

Targeted sequence enrichment was performed using the Agilent SureSelect Target Enrichment Kit (Agilent Technologies Inc. USA). Genomic DNA was sheared using a Covaris S1 Ultra-sonicator (Covaris, MA). Adaptor-ligated libraries were constructed using Paired-End Genomic DNA kits (Illumina, CA). The multiplexed samples were sequenced on the Illumina Hiseq platform using 76-bp paired-end reads.

Variant analysis and prioritization

Sequencing data were aligned to hg19 using the Burrows-Wheeler Aligner (BWA) software. PCR duplicates were removed with the 'samtools' software, and variants called using the Genome Analysis Toolkit (GATK, version 1.0) software from the Broad Institute.

Variants were annotated based on CCDS, Refseq and Ensembl gene transcripts. Identified variants that are listed in the NCBI dbSNP (version 132) were filtered out, along with variants that had poor depth or low average base quality scores. Prioritization of variants was carried out by the following criteria: selection of candidate genes based on patient's phenotype, severity of the predicted impact on gene function, conservation of amino acid affected, and frequency of the variant in the literature and databases including the Human Gene Mutation Database (HGMD http://www.biobase-international.com/), Leiden Open Variation Databases (LOVD http://www.lovd.nl/3.0/home), Exome Variant Server (EVS, http://evs.gs.washington.edu/EVS/) and 1000 genomes database (http://browser.http://browser.1000genomes.org/index.html). PolyPhen-2 (http://genetics.bwh.harvard.edu/pph2/) and SIFT (http://sift.bii.a-star.edu.sg/) were used to predict the pathogenicity of non-synonymous variants. The candidate variants were confirmed by Sanger sequencing and familial segregation testing was performed whenever possible. The workflow is summarized in Figure 1.

Genotype data has been deposited at the European Genome-phenome Archive (EGA, http://www.ebi.ac.uk/ega/), which is hosted by the EBI, under accession number EGAS00001000683.

Sanger Dideoxy Terminator Sequencing

Selected variants were confirmed by Sanger dideoxy terminator sequencing. Primers were designed with Primer3 software. PCR was carried out with HotStarTaq PCR kit (Qiagen Inc.,USA) and GC-Rich PCR kit (Roche Diagnostics GmbH, Mannheim, Germany) was used for GC rich regions. Sequencing products were resolved on an ABI3730 capillary sequencing instrument (Applied Biosystems) and chromatograms were analysed with Mutation Surveyor version 3.3 (SoftGenetics, LLC, State College, PA, USA).

RNA extraction and cDNA sequencing

RNA was extracted from freshly collected whole blood using the NucleoSpin RNA blood kit (Machery-Nagel GmbH, Germany) and cDNA was synthesized using the Qiagen OneStep RT-PCR kit (Qiagen Inc., USA). PCR primers were designed within exons and PCR was performed using cDNA as template. PCR products were visualised on gels and sequenced as described above.

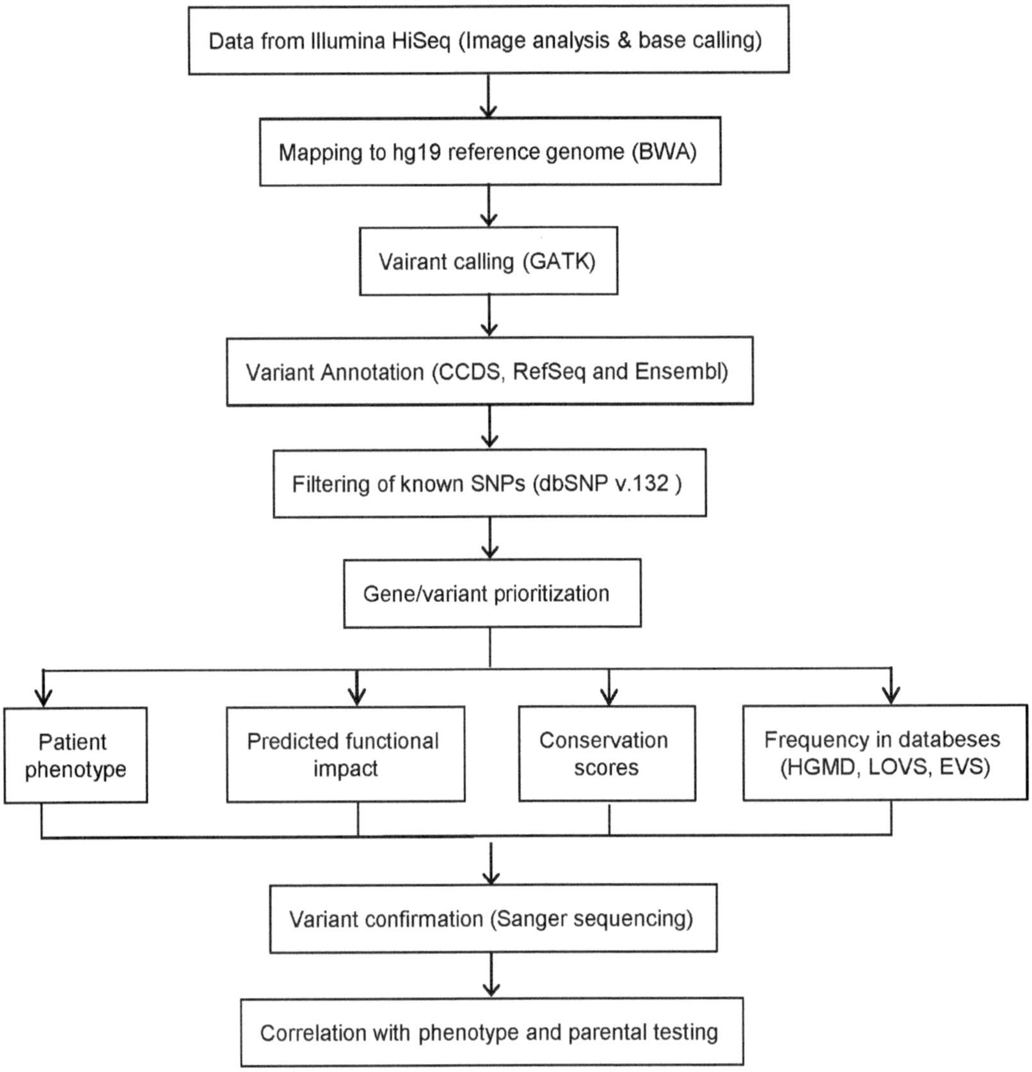

Figure 1. Variant analysis and prioritization workflow. Summary of our variant evaluation process for identifying candidate mutations

Results

Data output and quality

For all eight patients, 81–84% of the targeted regions achieved read depths of at least 20×, with average read depths overlapping targets ranging from 322× to 798× (Table 2). There were a few genes with very poor coverage. In particular, coverage of *IKBKG*, *CFC1* and *GTF21* was generally poor. In addition, read depths were <10× for a few exons in genes like *ARX*, *SHANK3*, *MECP2*, *SALL1*, *TBX1*, *PGA5*, *NF1*, *CHRNA7*, *NIPA1*, *DMD*. These were usually either in exon 1 or within GC rich regions.

Variant detection and prioritization

After filtering out the common variants present in dbSNP and variants with MAF >1% in EVS and the 1000 Genome browser, 1505 single nucleotide variants (SNVs) were identified in the eight patients, with a range of 131 to 236 SNVs per patient. A small number of variants were selected for validation by Sanger sequencing based on the prioritization criteria shown in Figure 1.

Patient 1

A total of 172 SNVs were detected in Patient 1 who is male with a 46,XY karyotype. Of the SNVs affecting exons, the top candidate mutation was a putative splice site mutation in the *L1CAM* gene, c.3458-1G>A, located at chrX: 153129005 (hg19) which was sequenced at 88× (Figure 2A). This variant was confirmed by Sanger sequencing (Figure 2B) and parental testing confirmed that the hemizygous mutation was inherited from his healthy mother. The variant affects the invariant AG acceptor splice site of intron 25 and is predicted to affect the splicing of exon 26. cDNA sequencing confirmed that splicing is affected at exon 26 and that the variant results in a deletion of 5 bp (r.3458_3462delTGAAG) from exon 26,which causes a frame shift and a premature stop leading to a predicted truncated protein of 1153 amino acids (Figure 2C).

Patient 2

Patient 2 is male with a 46,XY karyotype. Among the 129 SNVs detected in this patient, the top candidate was a c.7156C>T

Table 2. Summary of MPS data for the eight patients.

Sample	Read Pairs (M)	% Aligned to Reference	Reads overlapping target (%)	Ave Target Depth	Target ≥20× (%)	Total SNV	Variants in dbSNP	Novel variants
Patient 1	32.30	82.6	53.4	487	82	15482	14368	172
Patient 2	20.53	87.6	55.4	322	81	9699	9183	129
Patient 3	51.92	80.5	54.4	798	83	23885	21794	236
Patient 4	48.25	81.7	52.8	719	84	23716	21946	228
Patient 5	18.93	88.1	56.5	304	81	9204	8603	158
Patient 6	30.44	86.0	55.7	478	83	13726	12803	179
Patient 7	48.76	81.0	51.4	707	83	26268	23517	272
Patient 8	24.33	86.1	57.1	392	82	10598	9955	131

(p.R2386X) mutation in the *ATRX* gene, located at chr X: 76776310 (Figure 3A). The mutation was validated by Sanger sequencing (Figure 3B), and extended family testing showed that the mutation was present in the unaffected mother and in an affected brother (Figure 3C), but was absent in the father and unaffected sister.

Patient 3

A total of 236 SNVs were detected in Patient 3, who is female with a 46,XX karyotype. The top candidate SNVs included potential splice site SNVs in *USP9X* and *FGFR2*, and non-synonymous variants in *RELN*, *DMD*, *MAP7D2* and *ZNF41*. Indels in exonic regions of *SHROOM4*, *ZIC2* and *MED12* were also investigated. All the SNVs and indels were confirmed by Sanger sequencing and parental testing showed that all the variants were inherited except for the *USP9X* splice site variant. The *de novo* c.1986-1G>T variant in *USP9X* (chrX: 41025124) is the likely causative mutation (Figure 4A & 4B). This variant is novel and is predicted to affect the acceptor splice site of intron 15 of the *USP9X* gene. cDNA sequencing with primers in exon 13 and exon 17 showed the normal transcript together with the low-level presence of an altered transcript. The altered transcript showed a deletion of 13 bases (r.1986_1998delATTTTTATTGAAG) which is predicted to result in an altered protein and a premature stop codon p.F663Mfs*18 (Figure 4C & 4E). A second, independent pair of primers in exons 13 and 16 also showed the presence of this low-level altered transcript. Sequencing of the RT-PCR product from a control RNA only showed the presence of the normal transcript with no altered transcript seen (Figure 4D)

Patients 4–8

The top candidate variants of patients 4–8 are listed in Table 3. All these variants have been confirmed by Sanger sequencing and their inheritance was tested if parental samples were available. In addition to the variants detected by MPS, previous array CGH using Affymetrix SNP6 for Patient 5 showed a 134 kb deletion at 9p21.1 extending from 28,609,725–28,743,782 (hg19) involving the *LINGO2* gene (data not shown). This copy number change was initially thought to have no clinical significance.

Discussion

The average read depths achieved for the targeted regions were very high (>322×) and read depths of >20× were achieved for 81–84% of the targets. There was some variation in coverage, with overall poor coverage for just three genes and poor coverage in a few exons for another 10 genes.

Targeted MPS detected the causative mutations in *L1CAM* in Patient 1 and *ATRX* in Patient 2, which were consistent with their respective phenotypes. In Patient 1 the c.3458-1G>A mutation in the *L1CAM* gene affected the splicing process and cDNA sequencing confirmed the presence of a truncated transcript. Mutations in the *L1CAM* gene are associated with L1 syndrome, an X-linked recessive disorder. The major features of L1 syndrome include congenital hydrocephalus, adducted thumbs, spastic paraplegia, agenesis of the corpus callosum and cognitive impairment [6]. These features were all present in Patient 1. The c.3458-1G>A mutation in Patient 1 is novel but a splice site mutation at the same position (c.3458-1G>C) has been reported in a male with L1 syndrome [7].

In Patient 2, a p.R2386X mutation in the *ATRX* gene segregated with the clinical phenotypes in the family. Mutations in *ATRX* cause X-linked alpha thalassaemia mental retardation (ATR-X syndrome) in males, which is associated with profound

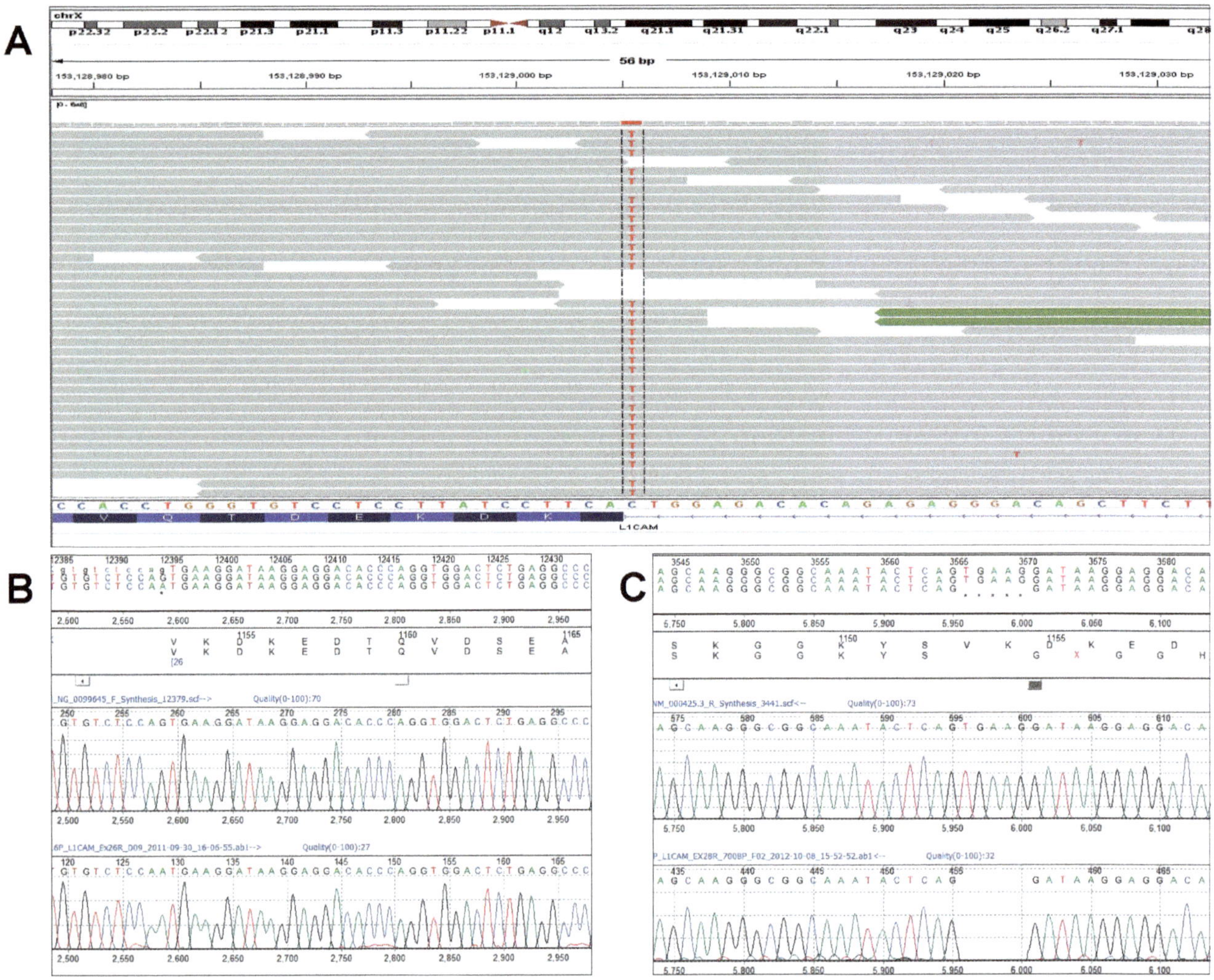

Figure 2. *L1CAM* splice site mutation in Patient 1. (A) IGV snapshot of c.3458-1G>A variant in the *L1CAM* gene (Chr X:153129005, hg19). (B) Sanger sequencing confirmation of c.3458-1G>A variant (NM_000425.3) (C) Partial cDNA sequence showing the mutant allele with the 5 bp deletion.

developmental delay, facial dysmorphism, genital abnormalities and alpha thalassemia [8]. The features in Patient 2 were largely consistent with ATR-X syndrome. The p.R2386X mutation occurs in exon 34 of the ATRX protein. This mutation has been reported in three separate instances in the literature and all cases have involved severe mental retardation and genital abnormalities [9]. Independent testing of this family by conventional ATRX molecular testing corroborated our MPS result [10].

Patient 3 has multiple congenital anomalies. A *de novo* c.1986G>T mutation in the *USP9X* gene is likely to be causative for all or some of her clinical phenotypes. We showed the presence of a truncated cDNA sequence which is predicted to result in a truncated protein. It is possible that the truncated protein might have a dominant negative effect or impaired protein function. USP9X is a member of the USP family of deubiquinating enzymes (DUBs) which process ubiquitin precursors and ubiquinated proteins. It has an important regulatory role in protein turnover and is an essential component of the TGFβ/BMP signalling cascade through its control of SMAD4 monoubiquitination [11]. The drosophila homolog (FAF) is essential for normal eye development and embryonic viability and the mouse homolog (FAM) has been shown to play essential roles in embryonic development [12–14]. There has been one published report of a truncating mutation in *USP9X* which segregated with disease in an X-linked mental retardation family [15]. Identification of more patients with mutations in the *USP9X* gene will be needed to confirm the association with ID and congenital anomalies.

Patients 4, 5, 6, 7, 8 have phenotypes that included autism spectrum disorders. Autism spectrum disorders are complex disorders. Despite the compelling argument for a genetic basis for autism, it is estimated that a specific genetic cause has been established for only 15% of cases [16]. Recent large exome studies in trios have implicated a number of genes, but did not identify any gene as a major cause of autism [17–19]. The exome studies all showed the extreme heterogeneous nature of autism and also indicated that many of the genes implicated were interconnected by shared pathways. The exome trio studies also showed the importance of *de novo* point mutations in autism.

Single variants in a number of genes were detected but variants in *AHI1* and *MAP7D3* were seen in Patient 5 and Patient 7. *AHI1*

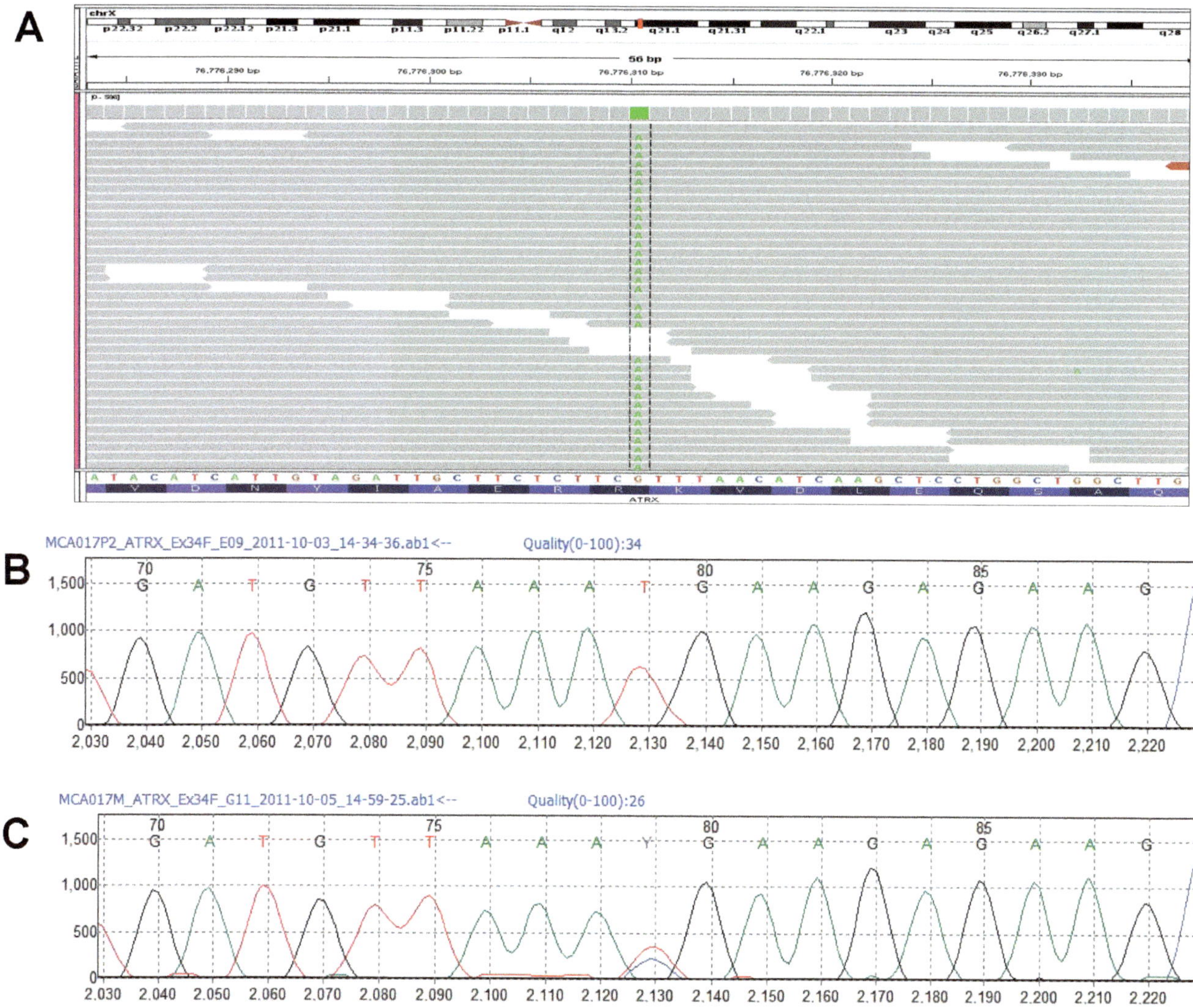

Figure 3. *ATRX* p.R2386X mutation in Patient 2. (A) IGV snapshot of c.7156C>T variant in *ATRX* (Chr X:76776310, hg19). (B) Sanger sequencing confirmation of c.7156C>T (p.R2386X, NM_00489.3) in Patient 2. (C) Sanger sequencing showing heterozygous c.7156C>T variant in the mother.

is highly expressed in fetal brain and also in the cerebellum and cerebral cortex of the adult brain, and mutations in *AHI1* cause Joubert Syndrome [20]. Genetic association has also been reported between *AHI1* and autism [21]. The *AHI1* variant E1086G is a pathogenic mutation in a case of Joubert syndrome [22]. The E1086G and D1179Y variants have been reported in the EVS database with a frequency of 0.008% and 0.033% respectively. *MAP7D3* has not been associated with autism spectrum disorders. There was one report of a truncating variant in *MAP7D3* in an X-linked mental retardation family that did not segregate with disease. The T335M variant has been reported in the EVS database with a frequency of 0.019% (2 of 10444 alleles).

Novel variants in *CREBBP*, *TSC1* and *FMR1* were detected in Patient 4. These genes have been associated with syndromic autism and were probably unlikely to be causative of her phenotypes as they were inherited from her healthy parents. Similarly there were interesting candidate variants in Patient 6 in *NIPA1* gene which has been associated with autism. Again these variants were inherited and thus less likely to be causative of his autism spectrum disorder.

In Patient 7, variants were found in *SYNGAP1* and *SEMA5A* which have been linked to autism [23]. This patient also had a V528M variant in *FLNA* that has been reported in a case of bilateral periventricular nodular heterotopia [24] and also as a functional polymorphism [25]. Novel variants in *FOXP1*, *ATRX*, *AUTS2*, *CSMD1* were detected in Patient 8. All these genes have been associated with autism and other neurodevelopmental disorders. However, all these variants are inherited from her healthy parents and thus their role in her phenotype remains uncertain. In particular mutations and deletions in *FOXP1* have been shown to cause autism, mental retardation and speech and language deficits [26,27]. The A100G variant in *FOXP1* has been predicted to be damaging by PolyPhen 2 and SIFT. The novel V260I variant in *AUTS2* is also of interest. This variant is present only in AUTS2 isoform 3, the shortest isoform comprised of 266 amino acids. The *AUTS2* gene was first identified as a candidate gene for autism when it was shown to be disrupted by a

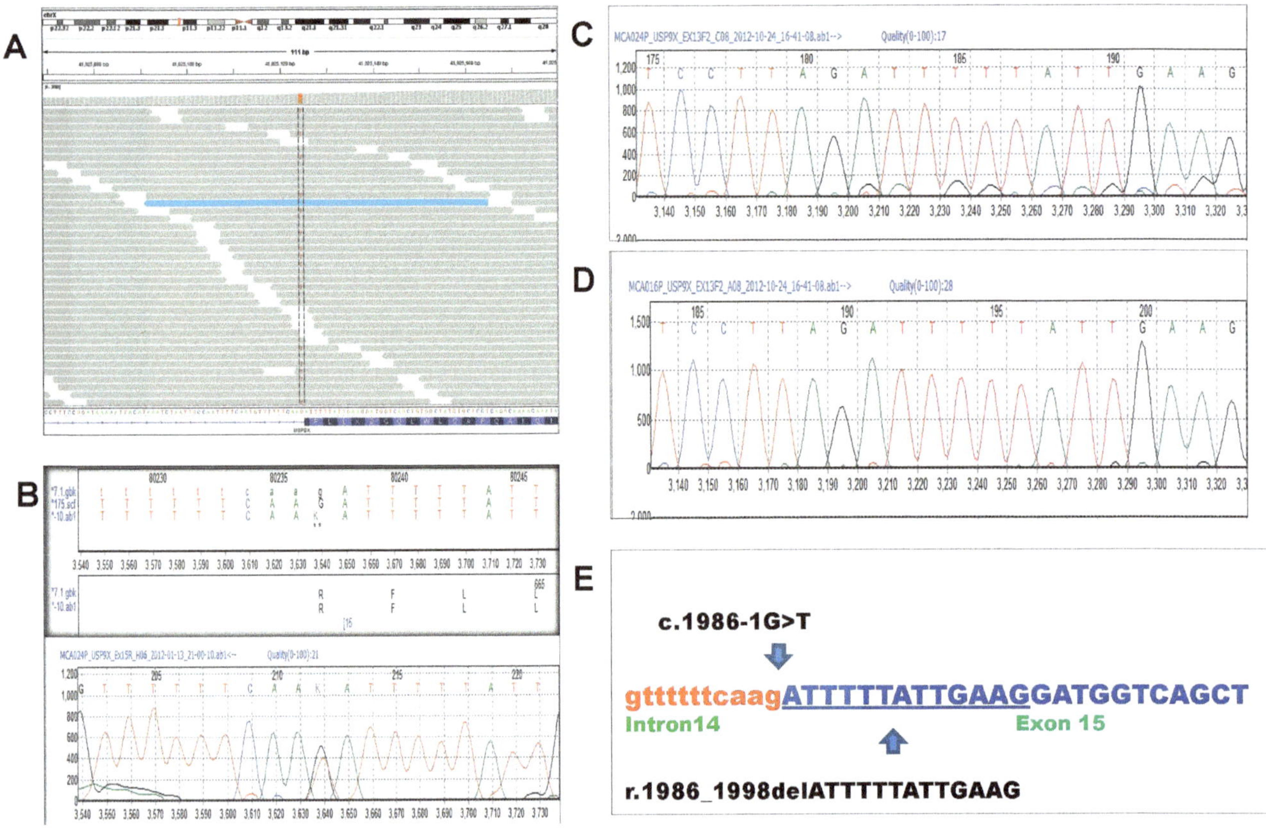

Figure 4. ***USP9X*** **splice site mutation in Patient 3.** (A) IGV snapshot of c.1986-1G>T variant in *USP9X* (Chr X:41025124, hg19). (B) Sanger sequencing confirmation of c.1986-1G>T variant (NM_001039590.2) in Patient 3. (C) Partial cDNA sequence showing expression of both the wild type and low level mutant allele with the 13 bp deletion. (D) Partial cDNA sequence of control patient. (E) Partial genomic DNA sequence of exon 15 (uppercase, blue) and intron 14 (lowercase, red) of *USP9X* gene showing the c.1986-1G>T variant (arrow) and the 13 bp deletion (r.1986_1998delATTTTTATTGAAG) which is underlined.

translocation breakpoint in a pair of autistic twins [28]. Mutations in the *AUTS2* gene have also been identified in patients with mental retardation [29].

Patient 5 also had a 134 kb deletion at 9p21.1 affecting the 5′UTR and first two exons of the *LINGO2* gene. This deletion was not present in his mother and the father's DNA was not available for testing. Deletions affecting the *LINGO2* gene have been reported in a cohort of Utah autism patients [30]. There is a possibility that the 9p21.1 deletion could act in conjunction with other SNVs in Patient 5 to influence his phenotype. Recent publications have highlighted the potential effects of polygenic mutational events, variable expressivity, variable penetrance, and CNV burden on complex disorders like autism [31–34]. All these factors complicate the diagnosis of the causes of autism spectrum disorders. The unavailability of some parental samples and the lack of complete phenotyping of parents in our study also limit the ability to predict the causality of some of the variants detected.

Despite the progress in genetic testing, 50–60% of the causes of DD/ID remain unknown. This is unfortunate as a clinical diagnosis of DD/ID provides crucial information for diagnostics and helps in understanding the mechanisms of the disease including the options for management and treatment. In addition, it puts an end to the testing odyssey and gives families closure and may also be important for future reproductive decisions.

This pilot study has confirmed the value of targeted MPS for investigating DD/ID and multiple congenital anomalies in children for diagnostic purposes. Causative mutations were found in two of the eight patients tested and a likely causal mutation was found in another patient. For the other five patients, no conclusions can be made about the variants as no compelling *de novo* variants were found. Thus, targeted gene MPS was less likely to provide a genetic diagnosis for children whose phenotype includes autism.

The advantages of targeted gene sequencing as opposed to whole exome sequencing is the increase in numbers of patients who could be sequenced and hence an increase in the number of patients who might receive a diagnosis. With targeted gene sequencing a greater depth of coverage could be achieved at a lower cost. The increased depth will facilitate the detection of indels that might be missed by exome sequencing. Targeted sequencing also obviates the problem of incidental results. Clinical interpretation of novel variants remains challenging but should gradually become easier with the continued development of variant databases of healthy controls as well as locus-specific disease databases.

Table 3. Assessed candidate variants found in patients 4–8.

Patient	Gene	Coordinates (hg19)	Nucleotide change	Amino acid change	Prediction		Inheritance
					PolyPhen-2	SIFT	
4	*CREBBP*	Chr16:3820816	G>A	p.P879S	Benign	Tolerated	Maternal
	CTNNA3	Chr10:67829183	T>C	p.K681R	Benign	Tolerated	Paternal
	TSC1	Chr9:135804244	T>C	p.N6D	Benign	Tolerated	Maternal
	FMR1	ChrX:147019073	A>G	p.E360G	Benign	Tolerated	Maternal
	GPR50	ChrX:150348482	C>T	p.R143C	Probably damaging	Deleterious	Maternal
5	*ANKRD11*	Chr16:89346082	C>T	p.P2290S	Benign	Tolerated	Maternal
	CACNA1C	Chr12:2800220	A>G	p.N2091S	Benign	Tolerated	Not maternal[a]
	AHI1	Chr6:135611614	C>A	p.D1179Y	Benign	Deleterious	Not maternal[a]
	MAP7D3	ChrX:135314112	G>A	p.T335M	Benign	Tolerated	Maternal
6	*NIPA1*	Chr15:23049158	G>A	p.P221S	Possibly damaging	Tolerated	Maternal
	NIPA1	Chr15:23049147	C>G	p.Q224H	Benign	Tolerated	Maternal
	CTNND2	Chr5:11411650	T>G	p.E146A	Possibly damaging	Tolerated	Paternal
7	*SYNGAP1*	Chr6:33411463	C>G	p.A1045G	Benign	Tolerated	Not tested
	SEMA5A	Chr5:9318508	C>A	p.Q82H	Benign	Deleterious	Not tested
	AHI1	Chr6:135644371	T>C	p.E1086G	Probably damaging	Deleterious	Not tested
	MAP7D3	ChrX:135310836	C>T	p.R611H	Probably damaging	Tolerated	Not tested
	FLNA	ChrX:153593613	C>T	p.V528M	Probably damaging	Deleterious	Not tested
8	*FOXP1*	Chr3:71102908	G>C	p.A100G	Probably damaging	Deleterious	Maternal
	AUTS2	Chr7:69755471	G>A	p.V260I	Unknown	Tolerated	Maternal
	ATRX	ChrX:76938923	G>C	p.P609A	Benign	Tolerated	Maternal
	CNTN3	Chr3:74420458	T>A	p.I183L	Benign	Tolerated	Maternal
	CSMD1	Chr8:2800085	C>T	p.G1374S	Unknown	Deleterious	Paternal
	DMD	ChrX:32364161	G>C	p.Q1829E	Benign	Tolerated	Maternal

[a]Father's DNA not available.

Supporting Information

Table S1 List of 355 genes in the targeted sequencing panel.

Author Contributions

Conceived and designed the experiments: MB PT ECT. Performed the experiments: ZJZ PT. Analyzed the data: MB JM SR. Contributed reagents/materials/analysis tools: AL EST IN LCO BC. Wrote the paper: MB SR ECT.

References

1. Chelly J, Khelfaoui M, Francis F, Cherif B, Bienvenu T (2006) Genetics and pathophysiology of mental retardation. Eur J Hum Genet 14: 701–713.
2. Meder B, Haas J, Keller A, Heid C, Just S, et al. (2011) Targeted next-generation sequencing for the molecular genetic diagnostics of cardiomyopathies. Circ Cardiovasc Genet 4: 110–122.
3. Brownstein Z, Friedman LM, Shahin H, Oron-Karni V, Kol N, et al. (2011) Targeted genomic capture and massively parallel sequencing to identify genes for hereditary hearing loss in Middle Eastern families. Genome Biol 12: R89.
4. Lemke JR, Riesch E, Scheurenbrand T, Schubach M, Wilhelm C, et al. (2012) Targeted next generation sequencing as a diagnostic tool in epileptic disorders. Epilepsia 53: 1387–1398.
5. Neveling K, Collin RW, Gilissen C, van Huet RA, Visser L, et al. (2012) Next-generation genetic testing for retinitis pigmentosa. Hum Mutat 33: 963–972.
6. Finckh U, Schroder J, Ressler B, Veske A, Gal A (2000) Spectrum and detection rate of L1CAM mutations in isolated and familial cases with clinically suspected L1-disease. Am J Med Genet 92: 40–46.
7. Rehnberg M, Jonasson J, Gunnarsson C (2011) Novel L1CAM splice site mutation in a young male with L1 syndrome. Am J Med Genet A 155A: 439–441.
8. Gibbons R (2006) Alpha thalassaemia-mental retardation, X linked. Orphanet J Rare Dis 1: 15.
9. Gibbons RJ, Wada T, Fisher CA, Malik N, Mitson MJ, et al. (2008) Mutations in the chromatin-associated protein ATRX. Hum Mutat 29: 796–802.
10. Latiff ZA OS, Lau D, Wong SW, Ong LC, Aziz DA, et al. (2013) Alpha-thalassemia mental retardation syndrome: A case report of two affected siblings. Journal of Pediatric Neurology 11: 67–70.
11. Dupont S, Mamidi A, Cordenonsi M, Montagner M, Zacchigna L, et al. (2009) FAM/USP9x, a deubiquitinating enzyme essential for TGFbeta signaling, controls Smad4 monoubiquitination. Cell 136: 123–135.
12. Jolly LA, Taylor V, Wood SA (2009) USP9X enhances the polarity and self-renewal of embryonic stem cell-derived neural progenitors. Mol Biol Cell 20: 2015–2029.
13. Jones MH, Furlong RA, Burkin H, Chalmers IJ, Brown GM, et al. (1996) The Drosophila developmental gene fat facets has a human homologue in Xp11.4 which escapes X-inactivation and has related sequences on Yq11.2. Hum Mol Genet 5: 1695–1701.
14. Pantaleon M, Kanai-Azuma M, Mattick JS, Kaibuchi K, Kaye PL, et al. (2001) FAM deubiquitylating enzyme is essential for preimplantation mouse embryo development. Mech Dev 109: 151–160.
15. Tarpey PS, Smith R, Pleasance E, Whibley A, Edkins S, et al. (2009) A systematic, large-scale resequencing screen of X-chromosome coding exons in mental retardation. Nat Genet 41: 535–543.
16. Carter MT, Scherer SW (2013) Autism spectrum disorder in the genetics clinic: a review. Clin Genet 83: 399–407.
17. Neale BM, Kou Y, Liu L, Ma'ayan A, Samocha KE, et al. (2012) Patterns and rates of exonic de novo mutations in autism spectrum disorders. Nature 485: 242–245.
18. O'Roak BJ, Vives L, Fu W, Egertson JD, Stanaway IB, et al. (2012) Multiplex targeted sequencing identifies recurrently mutated genes in autism spectrum disorders. Science 338: 1619–1622.
19. Sanders SJ, Murtha MT, Gupta AR, Murdoch JD, Raubeson MJ, et al. (2012) De novo mutations revealed by whole-exome sequencing are strongly associated with autism. Nature 485: 237–241.
20. Ferland RJ, Eyaid W, Collura RV, Tully LD, Hill RS, et al. (2004) Abnormal cerebellar development and axonal decussation due to mutations in AHI1 in Joubert syndrome. Nat Genet 36: 1008–1013.
21. Alvarez Retuerto AI, Cantor RM, Gleeson JG, Ustaszewska A, Schackwitz WS, et al. (2008) Association of common variants in the Joubert syndrome gene (AHI1) with autism. Hum Mol Genet 17: 3887–3896.
22. Kroes HY, van Zon PH, Fransen van de Putte D, Nelen MR, Nievelstein RJ, et al. (2008) DNA analysis of AHI1, NPHP1 and CYCLIN D1 in Joubert syndrome patients from the Netherlands. Eur J Med Genet 51: 24–34.
23. Betancur C (2011) Etiological heterogeneity in autism spectrum disorders: more than 100 genetic and genomic disorders and still counting. Brain Res 1380: 42–77.
24. Kakita A, Hayashi S, Moro F, Guerrini R, Ozawa T, et al. (2002) Bilateral periventricular nodular heterotopia due to filamin 1 gene mutation: widespread glomeruloid microvascular anomaly and dysplastic cytoarchitecture in the cerebral cortex. Acta Neuropathol 104: 649–657.
25. Kunishima S, Ito-Yamamura Y, Hayakawa A, Yamamoto T, Saito H (2010) FLNA p.V528M substitution is neither associated with bilateral periventricular nodular heterotopia nor with macrothrombocytopenia. J Hum Genet 55: 844–846.
26. Hamdan FF, Daoud H, Rochefort D, Piton A, Gauthier J, et al. (2010) De novo mutations in FOXP1 in cases with intellectual disability, autism, and language impairment. Am J Hum Genet 87: 671–678.
27. Horn D, Kapeller J, Rivera-Brugues N, Moog U, Lorenz-Depiereux B, et al. (2010) Identification of FOXP1 deletions in three unrelated patients with mental retardation and significant speech and language deficits. Hum Mutat 31: E1851–1860.
28. Sultana R, Yu CE, Yu J, Munson J, Chen D, et al. (2002) Identification of a novel gene on chromosome 7q11.2 interrupted by a translocation breakpoint in a pair of autistic twins. Genomics 80: 129–134.
29. Kalscheuer VM, FitzPatrick D, Tommerup N, Bugge M, Niebuhr E, et al. (2007) Mutations in autism susceptibility candidate 2 (AUTS2) in patients with mental retardation. Hum Genet 121: 501–509.
30. Matsunami N, Hadley D, Hensel CH, Christensen GB, Kim C, et al. (2013) Identification of rare recurrent copy number variants in high-risk autism families and their prevalence in a large ASD population. PLoS One 8: e52239.
31. Coe BP, Girirajan S, Eichler EE (2012) The genetic variability and commonality of neurodevelopmental disease. Am J Med Genet C Semin Med Genet 160C: 118–129.
32. Devlin B, Scherer SW (2012) Genetic architecture in autism spectrum disorder. Curr Opin Genet Dev 22: 229–237.
33. Girirajan S, Rosenfeld JA, Cooper GM, Antonacci F, Siswara P, et al. (2010) A recurrent 16p12.1 microdeletion supports a two-hit model for severe developmental delay. Nat Genet 42: 203–209.
34. Leblond CS, Heinrich J, Delorme R, Proepper C, Betancur C, et al. (2012) Genetic and functional analyses of SHANK2 mutations suggest a multiple hit model of autism spectrum disorders. PLoS Genet 8: e1002521.

13

Automatic Conversational Scene Analysis in Children with Asperger Syndrome/High-Functioning Autism and Typically Developing Peers

Alessandro Tavano[1,2], Anna Pesarin[3], Vittorio Murino[4], Marco Cristani[3,4]*

1 Institute of Psychology, University of Leipzig, Leipzig, Germany, **2** Scientific Institute "E.Medea", San Vito al Tagliamento (Pordenone), Italy, **3** Department of Computer Science, University of Verona, Verona, Italy, **4** Italian Institute of Technology (IIT), Genova, Italy

Abstract

Individuals with Asperger syndrome/High Functioning Autism fail to spontaneously attribute mental states to the self and others, a life-long phenotypic characteristic known as mindblindness. We hypothesized that mindblindness would affect the dynamics of conversational interaction. Using generative models, in particular Gaussian mixture models and observed influence models, conversations were coded as interacting Markov processes, operating on novel speech/silence patterns, termed Steady Conversational Periods (SCPs). SCPs assume that whenever an agent's process changes state (e.g., from silence to speech), it causes a general transition of the entire conversational process, forcing inter-actant synchronization. SCPs fed into observed influence models, which captured the conversational dynamics of children and adolescents with Asperger syndrome/High Functioning Autism, and age-matched typically developing participants. Analyzing the parameters of the models by means of discriminative classifiers, the dialogs of patients were successfully distinguished from those of control participants. We conclude that meaning-free speech/silence sequences, reflecting inter-actant synchronization, at least partially encode typical and atypical conversational dynamics. This suggests a direct influence of theory of mind abilities onto basic speech initiative behavior.

Editor: Michel Botbol, University of Western Brittany, France

Funding: The study was funded by the Italian Ministry of Health (www.salute.gov.it) as part of a two-year project on "Neurorehabilitation of prosodic and pragmatic skills in individuals with High-functioning Autism, Specific Language Impairment and Williams syndrome", Principal Investigator Alessandro Tavano, RC-2007/8, 3:06, "E. Medea" Research Institute. Alessandro Tavano was also supported at the University of Leipzig by a DFG (German Research Foundation) Reinhart-Koselleck Project grant, awarded to Professor E. Schröger. Psychologist Elisa Cravello was employed within the project for data analysis purposes and participated to the present study acting as the adult conversational partner. The funders had no role in study design, data collection and analysis, decision to publish, or preparation of the manuscript.

Competing Interests: The authors have declared that no competing interests exist.

* E-mail: marco.cristani@univr.it

Introduction

Human beings are more aptly defined as conversational mammals, rather than simply as articulate mammals [1]. We effortlessly engage in verbal exchanges, seeking for informative as well as emotionally rewarding experiences. It has been recently acknowledged that the biological universality of such talent stands in sheer contrast with the complex set of abilities it requires, such as the tightly timed coordination of speech, facial gestures, respiratory kinematics, bodily posture, visual and auditory attention [2–4]. How are these different levels of behavior and sensory experience successfully integrated? Some philosophers suggest that individuals might use normative frames of reference to reach a sufficient degree of mutual knowledge, and therefore infer (predict) each other's next conversational move [5]. However, while verbal interaction certainly involves normative elements, they hardly help capturing its causal dynamics. A cognitive account has been proposed that sets dialog exchanges as the primary site of language experience [6–8]. A central tenet of this account is that successful dialogs depend on the fast interactive alignment of procedural and representational contents between interlocutors (see [6], p. 170). Notably, this would be achieved via "resource-free" processes such as priming. For example, as the conversation progresses each interactant will tend to use a common set of words, sentences, communicative styles, thereby establishing mutual resonance relationships at different levels of complexity [9].

Indeed, such perspective matches the intuition that when a conversation is successful we end up speaking "the same language" as our interlocutor. However, everyday conversations also implicate spontaneous adaptation to new, unpredicted discourse paths. For example, changes in one's own or other's beliefs or desires determine the introduction of a new topic or, at times, highlight the chance for a metaphoric or ironic statement [2,10,11]. We continuously make room for other minds [12] using our ability to "mentalize", that is, to promptly and spontaneously attribute mental states such as beliefs and desires to the self and others [13].

Mentalizing is a core social skill operative since infancy in neurotypical development [14,15]. Explicit reflection upon one's own and others' true or false beliefs emerges between the ages of 4 and 6 years, when children begin to distinguish between belief-based and reality-based thoughts [16]. Importantly enough, 5- and 6-year-old children become also faster in responding correctly than incorrectly to false-belief tasks, suggesting that

Table 1. Average percentage of silence and speech samples in the conversations of the two classes of participants.

Class	speech	silence
Asperger/HFA	0.4292	0.5708
Controls	0.4447	0.5553

decision-making skills develop along with mentalizing abilities [17]. From age 8–10 years onwards, children can master higher-order mentalizing activities, and conversation becomes a central focus of emotional and cognitive development [18].

However, in some cases the ability to mentalize is severely impaired. Individuals with Asperger Syndrome or High Functioning Autism (hereafter, HFA) are phenotypically characterized by a marked impairment in spontaneous mentalizing, while intelligence and formal language skills are preserved [19,20]. Individuals with Asperger Syndrome/HFA can learn to handle conversational interaction as a task [21,22]. However, explicit strategies are unlikely to compensate for the absence of spontaneous adaptation to dynamic changes. Consequently, social relation problems commonly surface in adolescents and young adult individuals with Asperger syndrome/HFA [23]. So far, the impact of mindblindness on the dynamics that characterize conversational behavior has not been investigated.

In this work, we captured conversational blueprints by resorting to human computational modeling. We designed a meaning-free, low-level acoustic serial generative framework, composed by a Gaussian mixture model (GMM) [24], followed by an observed influence model (OIM) at the top level [25]. OIMs are built upon Markov models, which offer a stochastic interpretation of time series, and thus are apt for the analysis and recognition of event sequences in speech recognition and natural language processing [26]. Interaction effects within each conversation were modeled assuming that the two speech streams were cooperative, binary (silence vs. speech) stochastic processes. Further, we posited that whenever a process changes its state, it injects a corresponding auto-transition state in the other process, forcing synchronization and creating novel low-level auditory segments termed Steady Conversational Periods (SCPs) [27]. SCPs permit the calculation of transition probabilities both intra- and inter-processes, thereby picturing the fast mutual effects of dialogic exchanges. The resulting influence matrix shows how much the state one participant is in at time t_1 influences the state the other participant will be in at time t_2 (inter-chain influence), as well as the how each participant proactively influences his/her own transition from state to state (intra-chain influence) [27,28]. Using this approach, we aimed at verifying if the dynamics of flat (non arguing) dialogs depend on theory of mind abilities.

Materials and Methods

Participants

Data collection was run at the Scientific Institute "E.Medea" in S. Vito al Tagliamento (Pordenone, Italy). A young female psychologist acted as moderator in binary conversations with selected participants. The moderator was not aware of the study aims, clinical characteristics of the participant population, or individual clinical status (patient vs. control). She was introduced to all participants as a researcher who was interested in hearing their opinion on a set of topics.

Nine children and adolescents with a diagnosis of Asperger syndrome/HFA (8 males, 1 female, age range 7–14 years, mean = 11) following the DSM IV (1994) criteria and the support of either the Childhood Autism Rating Scale (CARS, [29]) or the Autism Diagnostic Observation Schedule (ADOS, [30]) participated in the study. Nine gender- and age-matched typically developing peers were selected. All participants (N = 18) were made familiar with the moderator (acquaintance phase, about 10 minutes, not recorded). All individuals with Asperger syndrome/HFA had a clinical history of extensive rehabilitative training programs focused on limiting repetitive behaviors and enhancing social relationships in one-to-one and group interactions (range of program duration: 2–5 years). At the time of the experiment they were all still receiving rehabilitative training.

Ethics statement. Our research adheres to the basic ethical considerations for the protection of human participants in research according to the Declaration of Helsinki, and has been approved by the Ethics Committee of the Scientific Institute "E.Medea" (Bosisio Parini, Lecco, IT). The parents of potential participants first received a letter describing the study. Then a short phone colloquium cleared any remaining doubts. Both parents signed a written informed consent and at least one of them (or a caring relative, e.g. grandfather) accompanied the participant to take part in the experimental session. Children and adolescents were explicitly asked whether they would agree to talk with the moderator and exchange views on a set of familiar topics, which would later be analyzed by researchers. All participants gave their verbal consent.

Data collection. Participants entered an anecohic soundproof room which contained two boots separated by a transparent glass pane. They sat on one side of the glass pane and were always in full visual contact with the moderator, who sat on the other side. Participants were offered puppets and toys to play out during the acquaintance phase. All participants as well as the moderator wore headphones and spoke to a calibrated recording microphone in order to output two synchronized but separate (unmixed) audio sources [27]. The headphones and microphone were explored as a playful practice. We adhered to a type of participatory research in which participants with and without disabilities are encouraged to actively contribute their views and find their own solution to establishing a pleasant interactive setting [31]. Children and adolescents were gradually involved in a dyadic conversation lasting about 10 minutes (experimental recording). It has been shown that topic change constitutes the second major type of variation in children's language samples [32]. To control for this issue, the moderator introduced five topics in a flexible sequence (school activities, hobbies, friends, food, family), prompting an active conversational exchange. The moderator was instructed to follow the participants' reasoning path and react appropriately, avoiding a rigid question-answer scheme. A total of 18 semi-structured conversational samples were collected. A speech/silence thresholding was performed on the raw signals, obtaining a signal D, formed by two binary arrays $D^{(1)}$ and $D^{(2)}$, each one of length T, and each related to a particular interactant (participant/moderator). The percentage of speech and silence samples for the two classes are reported in Table 1, highlighting a similar profile.

Neuropsychological profile. After the recording session, all participants received a neuropsychological screening targeting: a) linguistically mediated short-term/working memory and narrative memory; b) executive skills; 3) verbal prosodic abilities. The tests were: forward and backward digit span [33]; narrative memory, Tower of London and visual face recognition [34]; rhythm perception task (targeting the ability to reproduce rhythmical beat sequences [35]); verbal fluency [36]; comprehension and repetition

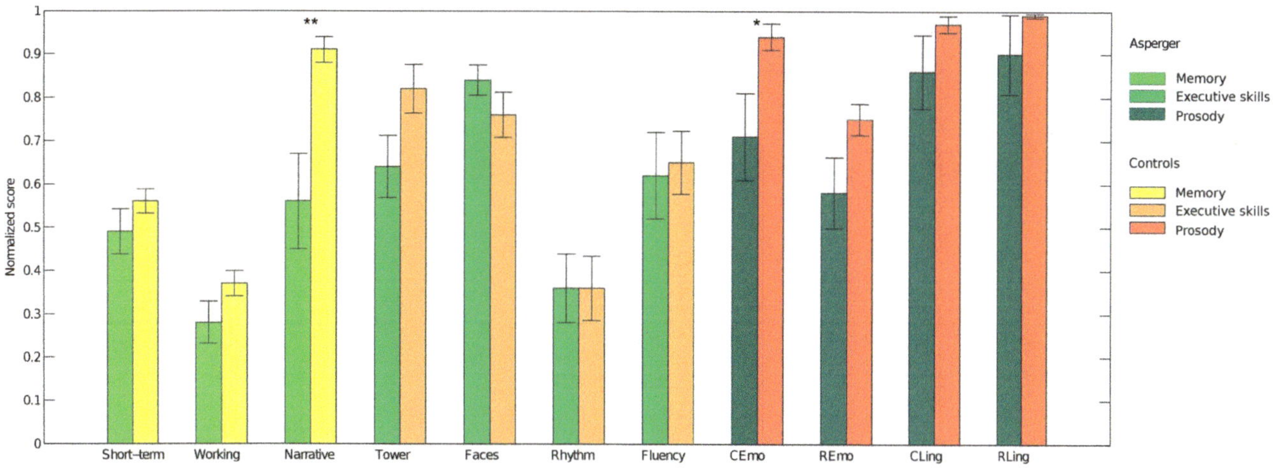

Figure 1. Neuropsychological profile. Legend: C/REmo = Emotional prosody comprehension/repetition; C/RLing = Linguistic prosody comprehension/repetition. Significance flags: ** $=p<0.01$; * $= p<0.05$.

of emotional (happy, sad, angry) and linguistic (affirmative, interrogative, imperative) prosodic contours [37]. Accuracy/performance data were normalized to max = 1 before entering statistical analyses (for the verbal fluency test, a global mean value was obtained by collapsing the number of uttered words across target letters F, A, S). Two-tailed t-tests were used to verify the presence of significant differences between the groups ($p<0.05$). Fig. 1 displays the neuropsychological profile of Asperger syndrome/HFA and neurotypical control participants.

A significant difference was found for the narrative memory test ($t(16) = -3{,}057$, $p=0.008$), suggesting poor verbal long-term memory storage in the Asperger/HFA group. As expected, participants with Asperger syndrome/HFA showed difficulties in emotional prosody comprehension ($t(16) = -2{,}199$, $p=0.043$), and a tendency to significance was evident for emotional prosody repetition ($t = -1{,}852$, $p=0.083$), and the Tower of London score ($t = -1{,}909$, $p=0.074$), with participants with Asperger syndrome/HFA showing emotional repetition/planning difficulties. No significant differences were found in short-term/working memory, face recognition, linguistic prosody, rhythm perception and verbal fluency skills (all ps ≥ 0.15).

The observed influence model

The observed influence model (OIM) is a simplified version of the influence model [25]; while OIM relies on interacting Markov chains, the influence model focuses on hidden Markov chains. We define the state variable of a Markov chain as $S_t \in \{1,\ldots,N\}$, and $P(S_t|S_{t-1})$ as the transition probability of a first-order Markov chain. OIM factorizes the multi-process conditional relations among C Markov chains by means of a weighted linear combination of pairwise *inter-chain* and *intra-chain* transition probabilities. Considering first-order Markov chains with N states, the (full) factorization of the multi-chain transition probability is:

$$P({}^{c}S_t|\ S_{t-1},\ldots,\ {}^{C}S_{t-1}) = \sum_{d=1}^{C} {}^{(c,d)}\theta P({}^{c}S_t\ |{}^{d}S_{t-1}) \qquad (1)$$

with $c,d\in\{1,\ldots,C\}$, ${}^{(c,d)}\theta\geq 0$, $\sum_{d=1}^{C} {}^{(c,d)}\theta=1$. The value $P({}^{c}S_t|{}^{d}S_{t-1})$ represents the probability of going from state S_{t-1} of the chain d to state S_t of the chain c. The weight ${}^{(c,d)}\theta$ represents the influence that chain d exerts on chain c. A sketch of the model is depicted in Fig. 2 a.

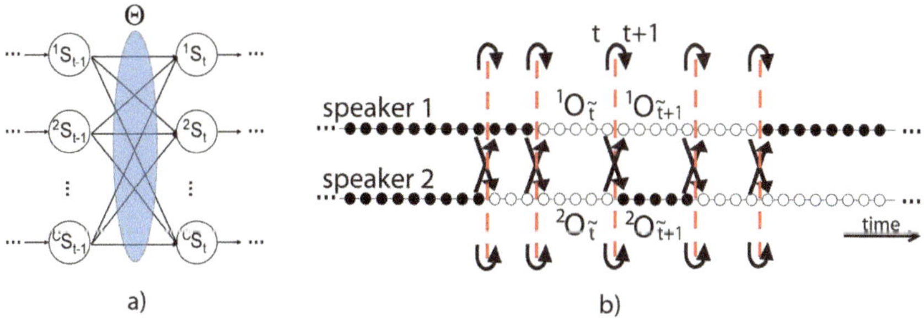

Figure 2. The generative framework. The Figure represents two main aspects: a) State factorization exploited in an observed influence model. The area named Θ indicates the influence factors that apply to the state transitions, depicted as directed arrows. b) Synchronization through Steady Conversational Periods. There are two audio processes, *speaker*1 and *speaker*2, sampled at a given frequency, where audio samples are shown as *speech* (black dots) and *silence* (white dots) values. Continuous periods of speech or silence are not synchronized, so it is not possible to evaluate a first-order statistical transition probability among the periods. Global transitions (dashed red lines) define the SCPs, thus allowing the calculation of first-order transition probabilities (black arrows).

Table 2. Cluster boundaries (in seconds) for the SCP durations, for the speech and silence SCP typology.

SCP type	short	medium	long
silence	[0,53]	[53,165]	[165,440]
speech	[0,12]	[12,86]	[86,480]

A first-order influence model is thus defined as $\lambda=\left\{\left\{{}^{(c,d)}A\right\}_{c,d\in\{1,\dots,C\}},\Theta,\left\{{}^{c}\pi\right\}_{c\in\{1,\dots,C\}}\right\}$, where ${}^{(c,d)}A$ is the *intra* -chain transition matrix when $c=d$, and represents the dynamics of a single process *per se*. When $c\neq d$, we consider the *inter* -chain matrices, modeling how much a state of a chain conditions the next state of the other chain. The $C\times C$ matrix Θ contains the influence weights, and $\{{}^{c}\pi\}$ contains the (independent) initial probability distributions for all processes, *i.e.*, ${}^{c}\pi=\{{}^{c}\pi_i\}_{i\in\{1,\dots,N\}}$, where ${}^{c}\pi_i=P({}^{c}S_1=i)$.

The OIM transition factorization has space complexity $O(C^2N^2+C^2)$, where C^2N^2 is due to the transition tables parameters, and C^2 to the influence coefficients. OIM learning of the $\{\theta\}$ coefficients is performed by standard constrained gradient descent [24,38], while the $\{{}^{(c,d)}A\}$, $\{{}^{c}\pi\}$ parameters are estimated by simple state counting.

The SCP model. Let us suppose to have a dialog with T instants. Within the recording setting described above, a dialogue can be represented as an OIM, but the lack of effective synchronization between the start/end instants of the speech/silence periods leads to problems in evaluating inter-chain conditional dependencies.

Thus, we proposed to use a novel feature based on the core assumption that turn-taking dynamics are interactionally controlled [39], called Steady Conversational Period (SCP). SCPs are built on the duration of continuous slots of silence or speech [27]. The SCP extraction procedure assumes that whenever a process (i.e, silence or speech) changes its state, it causes a *global* transition that affects also the opposite process, inserting a novel auto-transition state (see the red dashed lines in Fig. 2 b). The fragmentation caused by global transitions synchronizes the processes, creating $\tilde{T}<T$ different SCPs ${}^{c}O_{\tilde{t}}$, where the apex $c\in1,2$ indexes the speaker and $\tilde{t}=1,\dots,\tilde{T}$ enumerates the different SCPs. The introduction of SCPs in the model makes it feasible to evaluate first-order intra- and inter-chain conditional probabilities (black solid line in Fig. 2 b).

In order to take into account the different durations of each silence and speech segment, all SCPs related to speech and silence were labelled as $\langle$*short, medium, long*$\rangle$, after a Gaussian clustering over a training dataset, performed with the Expectation Maximization algorithm [40].

More formally, given the clustering, each SCP ${}^{c}O_{\tilde{t}}$ takes one label among 1,...,6, where 1,2,3 address short, medium and long continuous periods of speech, respectively, and the same applies with 4,5,6 for the silence periods. The number of states was decided as to maximize classification accuracies (see Table 2). It is worth noticing that the obtained performances were similar if 4 states were chosen (short and long periods), while suboptimal results were obtained with only 2 states, and more than 6. This quantization gives rise to *quantized* SCPs sequences ${}^{1}\mathbf{Q},\dots,{}^{C}\mathbf{Q}$; pooled together, these sequences form a dialog $\mathbf{D}$.

Table 3. Ordered features: each feature is ordered based on its frequency in the pool of features selected by the 3 feature selection strategies.

Feature	Frequency	Parameter
17	0.83	$P({}^{1}S_t=5\vert{}^{1}S_{t-1}=3)$
80	0.46	$P({}^{1}S_t=2\vert{}^{2}S_{t-1}=2)$
82	0.36	$P({}^{1}S_t=4\vert{}^{2}S_{t-1}=2)$
89	0.32	$P({}^{1}S_t=5\vert{}^{2}S_{t-1}=3)$
15	0.3	$P({}^{1}S_t=3\vert{}^{1}S_{t-1}=3)$
107	0.3	$P({}^{1}S_t=5\vert{}^{2}S_{t-1}=6)$
53	0.24	$P({}^{2}S_t=5\vert{}^{1}S_{t-1}=3)$
38	0.21	$P({}^{2}S_t=2\vert{}^{1}S_{t-1}=1)$
14	0.15	$P({}^{1}S_t=2\vert{}^{1}S_{t-1}=3)$
55	0.14	$P({}^{2}S_t=1\vert{}^{1}S_{t-1}=4)$

On the right, the corresponding parameter for each feature. For the sake of clarity, only 10 features are reported.

After that, an observed influence model $\lambda=\left\{\left\{{}^{(c,d)}A\right\}_{c,d\in\{1,\dots,C\}},\Theta,\left\{{}^{c}\pi\right\}_{c\in\{1,\dots,C\}}\right\}$; was fitted to a dialog $\mathbf{D}$.

The intra-chain parameters of the model intuitively indicate the conversational trend of each participant considered separately. The inter-chain transition parameters encode first-order state dependencies among processes, and influence factors mirror the influence that a process exerts on the other, independently on the state assumed by the single processes.

A classification involving the OIM has to be carried out considering carefully the order with which the observation sequences are organized. For example, within a dyad, in which the second process/speaker exerts a strong influence on the first one, a model is learnt where the weight ${}^{(1,2)}\theta$ is high. In order to recognize such situation in a classification scenario, the relative ordering of the sequences has to be preserved, *i.e.*, the second sequence has to be the one related to the process that influences the opposite one. If this cannot be ensured, a reasonable strategy for extracting the "correct" classification score would be the following: the dialogs $\{\mathbf{D}={}^{1}\mathbf{Q},\dots,{}^{C}\mathbf{Q}\}$ are presented to the model in all their possible orderings (having diads, only two), indexed by o, collecting all corresponding likelihood scores $\{P(\mathbf{D}_o|\lambda)\}$. The correct likelihood score would thus be the highest one.

The generative score space. In order to increase the classification accuracy of the generative framework, and, at the same time, get an insight on how the model works in encoding the dialogs, we built a generative score space $\mathcal{I}$. Following [41], a generative score space can be built by considering each dialog $\mathbf{D}$ as completely represented by a generative model λ with its parameters, which was trained on the dialog. Formally, the observed dialog $\mathbf{D}$ is mapped through φ into a fixed-length score vector $\varphi^{f}_{F}(\mathbf{D})\in\mathcal{I}$,

$$\varphi^{f}_{F}(\mathbf{D})=\varphi_{F}f\left(\hat{P}(\mathbf{D}|\lambda)\right), \tag{2}$$

where $\hat{P}(\mathbf{D}|\lambda)$ is the set of distributions that define a generative model, f is a function of these distributions and F is some operator applied afterwards. For instance, in case of the Fisher score [42], f is the log likelihood, and the operator F produces the first-order

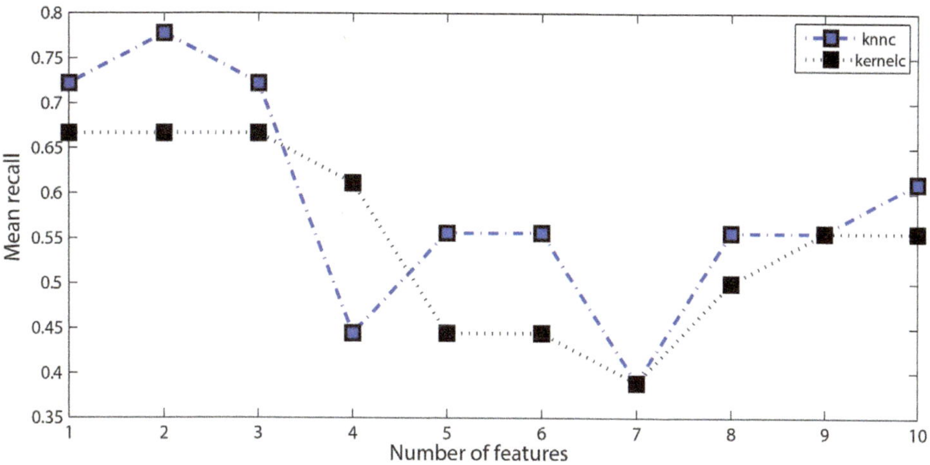

Figure 3. Feature analysis. Classification accuracies (measured in term of mean recall of the two classes) depending on the number of features employed, where the features are considered in order of importance (see Table 3).

derivatives with respect to the parameters. Another example is the TOP kernel [43] for which the function f is the posterior log-odds and F is still the gradient operator.

In these cases, the generative score-space approaches help to distill the relationship between a model parameter contained in λ and a particular data sample modeled by that parameter. After the mapping, a score-space metric must be defined in order to calculate the distances in that space.

In our case, f was the parameter extractor function (*i.e.*, the function that estimates the parameters of a statistical distribution), F the identity operator, and as a metric we selected the Euclidean one. In synthesis, f extracted the transition parameters (by simple counting) and the influence coefficients (by gradient descent).

Given a set of M classes of dialogs, each formed by W sequences, the space $\mathcal{I}$, could be seen as formed by a set of multidimensional class-labeled samples; actually, on each sequence, a model is trained, that provides a set of features/parameters. Therefore, standard tools of data analysis can be applied. We wanted to highlight the discriminative power of the features in a classification context, and therefore we applied a feature selection (or ranking) strategy, and, subsequently, we applied different discriminative classifiers on the feature subset. The feature selection/ranking strategies together with the discriminative classifiers employed will be detailed in the next section. Discriminative classifiers were preferred, because they directly focus on estimating class posterior probabilities instead of modeling class distributions. Such classifiers should also be less affected by the dimensionality problem.

Encapsulating OIMs in the SCP-based generative framework is straightforward. The embedding in $\mathcal{I}$ produces an ensemble of features $\varphi^f_F(\mathbf{D}) = \left\{ \left\{ ^{(c,d)}A \right\}_{c,d\in\{1,\ldots,C\}}, \Theta, \left\{ ^{c}\pi \right\}_{c\in\{1,\ldots,C\}} \right\}$, for each dialog: considering that the space complexity of the whole model is C^2N^2 (the transition matrices) $+C^2$ (the influence coefficients) $+NC$ (the initial distributions), and fixing $N=6$ (corresponding to 3 states for the speech duration and 3 for the silence duration) and $C=2$ (two speakers), we obtained 160 values. This parameter setting was used in all the reported experiments.

The rationale underlying the choice of this score space is that by employing parameters as features, and analysing the features with feature selection strategies, we can understand which portions of a model are more effective in capturing the unique characteristics of the classes. For example, capturing the fact that a particular state transition is strongly discriminant for a certain class implies that such transition is peculiar for that model. This property cannot be mimicked by Fisher score based approaches, where the basic tool is the differentiation with respect to particular quantities (i.e., the log-likelihood in the Fisher score), which can suffer of the so-called "wrap around" problem, where very different data points may map to the same derivative (see [44] for an example).

Table 4. Leave-One-Out classification performances, considering only the best features 17 and 80.

Classifier	Asperger		Controls	
	Precision	Recall	Precision	Recall
knnc	0.69	1	1	0.56
kernelc	0.64	0.78	0.71	0.56

Results

As mentioned, for each of the $W=18$ participants we learned an individual dialog model, giving rise to 160 parameter values (having $N=6$, $C=2$) per participant; in the following we will use the term "feature" as a synonym of parameter.

The point was to understand how well the two classes of participants could be separated, i.e., how different the parameters of the two classes were. To this aim, we adopted a classification framework, in which one of the participants (the *test* participant) has to be classified in one of the two classes, considering the similarity between his/her model parameters (i.e., features) and the ones of the remaining participants (the *training* participants).

We applied the classification procedure considering iteratively each of the W participants as the test element, keeping the remaining ones as training. This strategy is termed *cross-validation* since it validates the classification performance shuffling the elements that are used to represent (or train) a class and the ones employed as test. This particular cross-validation strategy is dubbed *leave-one-out* (LOO) since, in turns, a single element is assumed as test element. Its use is particularly suited for limited samples.

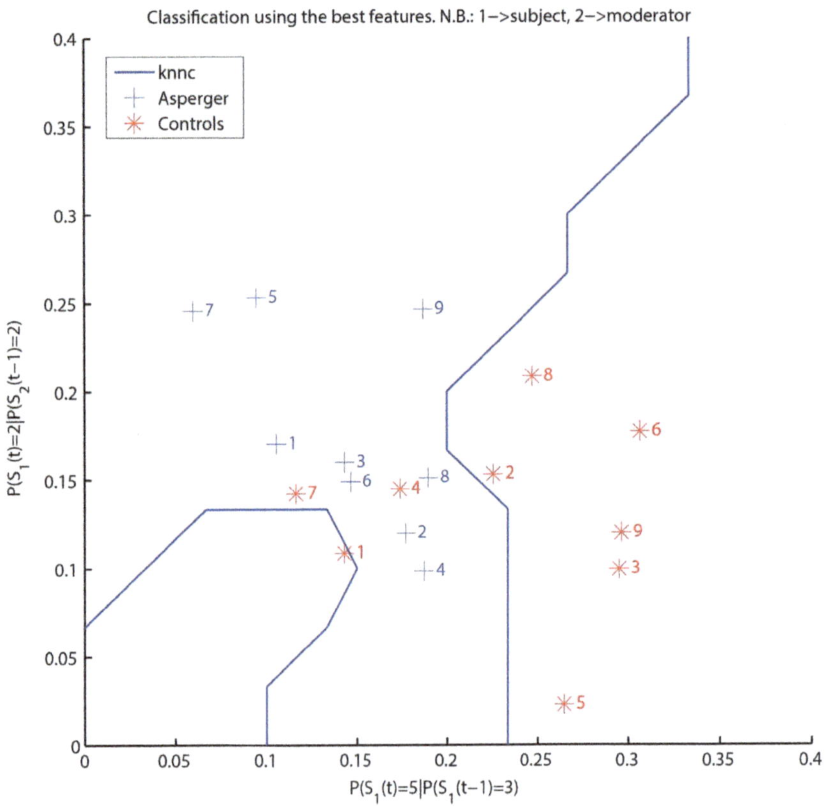
Classification using the best features. N.B.: 1->subject, 2->moderator
knnc
Asperger
Controls
P(S1(t)=2|P(S2(t-1)=2)
P(S1(t)=5|P(S1(t-1)=3)

a)

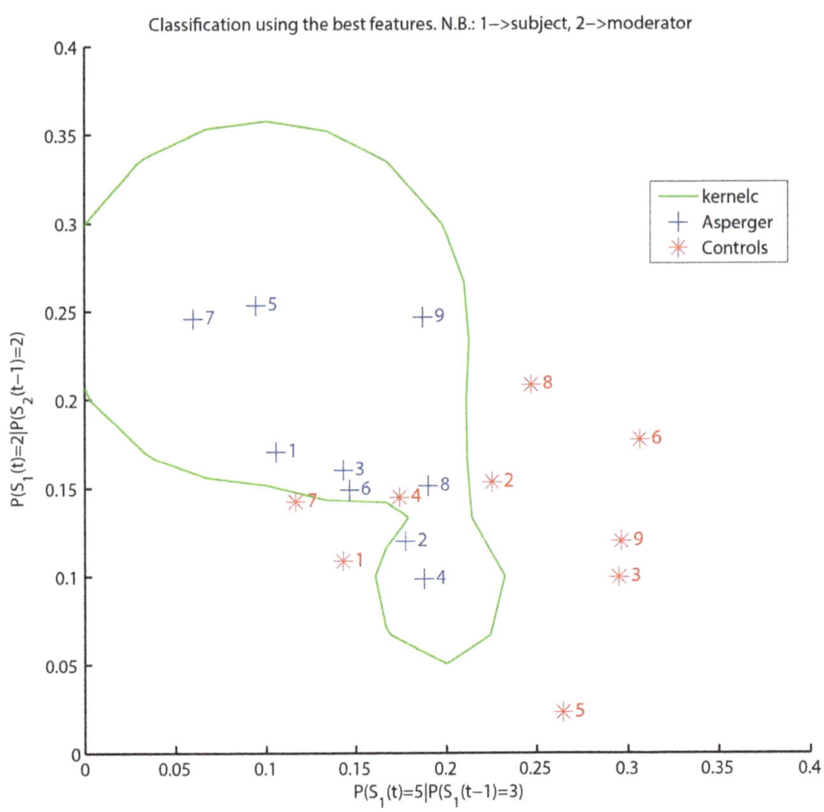
Classification using the best features. N.B.: 1->subject, 2->moderator
kernelc
Asperger
Controls
P(S1(t)=2|P(S2(t-1)=2)
P(S1(t)=5|P(S1(t-1)=3)

b)

Figure 4. The generative score space. Separation boundaries in the generative score space with a) the K-nearest neighbor classifier and b) the Support Vector Machine classifier (the kernelc implementation of Prtools), both performed on the best features found by feature selection.

Due to the high number of parameters, and for the purpose of understanding intuitively in which sense the two classes differ, we used a feature selection strategy. This allowed us to find out which one of the 160 parameters was most important for class separation; in other words, we highlighted the parameters that are most discriminant.

Feature selection is an open research field of pattern recognition, and many policies have been designed so far. One of the most widely employed is based on the concept of stability [45]. In simple terms, at each iteration of the LOO strategy a pool of features is selected as the most informative (*i.e.*, giving rise to a high classification performance) employing a particular feature selection approach, namely, the forward feature selection strategy [24]; if this set is consistent across different iterations of the cross-validation strategy, then it is considered to be stable, i.e. invariant to the nature of the training and the testing set.

We employed a slightly different approach, as more apt to deal with different feature selection policies. By fixing H feature selection policies, and for each policy a cross-validation LOO strategy, we evaluated how many times a feature is selected as discriminant for that particular policy, considering at the end all the different policies for choosing the final subset. As a classifier for the feature selection step we used the K-nearest neighbor classifier (K = 3) [24].

In our case, we employed $H = 3$ different policies of feature selection, that is, forward feature selection [46], branch and bound [47], and min-redundancy max-relevance [48]. Each policy may provide a subset of ν best features. In our case, we defined $\nu = 10$.

At each iteration of the cross-validation of a single policy, an instance of ν features is produced. With 18 participants, this corresponds to 18 instances. Considering the three policies of feature selection, 64 instances were obtained. After that, each of the 160 features was evaluated, counting how many times it appeared in an instance, thus assigning a frequency score to each feature. The scored features were then ordered (see Table 3, where 10 features are reported); together with the number of the features, we report their functional significance, i.e., the parameters they represent. These features can be thought of as independent on the particular strategy of feature selection. Manifestly, only transition parameters are present, while influence coefficients and initial probabilities are not present.

At this point we evaluated which subset ensured maximal classification accuracy. We thus considered one feature at a time, starting from the most frequent one, feeding two different classifiers and evaluating the LOO classification accuracy. As classifiers, we considered the K-nearest neighbor classifier (K = 3) and the linear Support Vector Machine, both implemented using the MATLAB Prtools [49]. The classification performances are reported in Fig. 3, in relation to the number of features employed.

The curves indicate that the first 2 features are the most important for the classification. They represent the probability of the moderator to speak for a long time after a medium silence interval (feature 17), and the probability of the moderator to speak for a medium interval after the participant (Asperger/HFA or control) has spoken for a medium-length segment (feature 80). Keeping these two features, the LOO classification performances are detailed in Table 4.

In addition, we report the values of the two features for all the participants in a 2D space (see Fig. 4), showing also the classification boundaries identified by the two different classifiers: boundaries are obtained by opportunely sampling the feature space, assigning a label to each point, and defining a boundary where the classification labels change from one class to the other. Employing the K-nearest neighbor classifier (knnc) and the linear support vector machine (kernelc) we obtained the separation accuracies, in terms of precision and recall, reported in Table 5. These values reflect the degree of certainty (max = 1) with which the two classes can be separated based on the selected features.

To increase the reliability of our findings, we replicated the classification procedure in a subsample of our data. Participants with Asperger syndrome/HFA number 5 and number 7 had the lowest scores across groups on the narrative memory test (0.03 and 0.06, respectively) and emotional prosody comprehension (0.33, 0.08). To investigate if automatic classification was influenced by neuropsychological differences in single participants, we first we re-run the statistical comparisons on the mentioned tests without Asperger syndrome/HFA participants 5 and 7, and the corresponding age-matched control individuals. We still found a significant difference for the narrative memory test ($t(12) = -2.541$, $p = 0.026$), but no difference in emotional prosody comprehension ($t(12) = -1.448$, $p = 0.173$). We then highlighted the position occupied by each participant in the classifier space, according to each feature. At visual inspection, Fig. 4 suggest that participants 5 and 7 with Asperger syndrome/HFA cluster with patients 1 and 9, and control participants 9, 8, 6, and 3 form a separate cluster of their own. This observation deems unlikely that specific problems with emotional prosody recognition or complex language memory tasks in participants 5 and 7 with Asperger syndrome/HFA would drive the classification effects. To verify this point, we excluded participants 5 and 7 from both groups and re-run the classification procedure using the K-nearest neighbor classifier; surprisingly, the classification performances were almost the same than considering the whole sample population, that is: Asperger, Precision = 0.7, Recall = 1; Controls, Precision = 1.0, Recall = 0.57. For a comparison, see the LOO classification results of Table 4.

Table 5. Separation performances, considering only the best features 17 and 80.

Classifier	Asperger		Controls	
	Precision	Recall	Precision	Recall
knnc	0.81	1	1	0.78
kernelc	0.9	1	1	0.89

Discussion

We used pattern recognition as a lens into meaning-free conversational blueprints [50]. We were able to model the mutual effects of dialogic exchanges by forcing synchronization of silence/speech sequences (Steady Conversational Periods, SCPs). By analyzing both intra- and inter-processes (speech/silence) transition probabilities, the conversations of individuals with Asperger syndrome/HFA were reliably and automatically distinguished from those of gender- and age-matched peers. The synchronization assumption was sufficient to tear apart the clinical from the non-clinical group without relying on any higher-order feature (e.g., meaning, word frequency, syntactic complexity).

Previous work showed the effectiveness of such a novel approach on groups with either extremely different speech rates (e.g., children vs. adults) or speech modes (e.g., flat conversations vs. lively discussions) [27,28]. We now classified two samples with a similar speech rate, similar age and a compatible higher-order cognitive profile, but crucially different in the spontaneous attribution of mental states to the self and others [18–20,23]. It follows that theory of mind skills exert a sizable influence onto basic speech initiative behavior.

This result is in line with theories that try to capture the biological bases of human conversational talent as stemming from the coordination of speech, gestures, kinematics and sensory attention [2]. We suggest that across-level interactant synchronization might be a key concept in investigating conversational speech dynamics [50], thereby extending the entrainment approach beyond purely linguistic representations [6].

The creation of the SCPs as a relevant index is motivated by several reasons, not restricted to a mere algebraic point of view or to the assumption of synchronicity. At a basic level, they partially reflect the respiratory kinematics which co-determine the dynamics of self-initiated speech [51,52]. Such kinematics provide the basis for the coordination of prosodic and syntactic planning [53]. SCPs might thus reflect a significant subset of the variance characterizing the real-time interplay of physiological, neuropsychological and intentional factors which determine the dynamics of speech alternation in a dialog, including turn-taking strategies usually negotiated via audiovisual intentional cues [54,55].

The crucial point of our work was to obtain a successful classification. However, the extracted features also provide some insights into the underlying processes (see Fig. 4). For example, the moderator displayed a tendency to self-influence the change between silence and speech while conversing with control participants, suggesting a more directive role. Instead, consistent instances of speech activity on the part of individuals with Asperger syndrome/HFA determined segments of silence on the part of the moderator, suggesting that what the children said, or the way they said it, interrupted the flow of the verbal exchange. The fact that in our analysis we abstracted away from meaning must not be taken to imply that meaning has no influence, but simply that SCPs highlight the reverberations of meaningful or less meaningful verbal exchanges on lower functional levels. It is likely that with larger group samples the interactions can be more finely pictured by more significant features.

We did not test theory of mind skills directly because all patients had already been exposed to similar tests many times during clinical assessment and rehabilitative training. We could document the correlated difficulty in emotional recognition using a novel test setting ([37], see Fig. 1). We also found a significant difference in narrative memory between Asperger/HFA and neurotypically developing participants. Recalling complex verbal material relies on inferential bridges that the listener must make to obtain a coherent picture of the different characters. As the spontaneous attribution of mental states is a key stage in this process, individuals with Asperger syndrome/HFA are likely to fail in tasks requiring the retrieval of a coherent story [56]. Finally, a recent work suggests that Asperger syndrome/HFA individuals may use inner speech for short-term/working memory tasks, as control peers do, but not for planning [57], a fact that could explain the planning difficulties in our group of patients.

Human beings might use forms of entrainment via resource-free processes such as priming to share information among each other and within themselves across functional levels. Conversational entrainment need not be representational in format, but can determine the game of parts of influencing each other's next move [50]. This perspective is not in contradiction with the idea that we can predict or infer the interlocutor's possible next move based on general cooperation assumptions [5]. Simply, rational inference now becomes a local-value strategy, capturing the mechanics of some single frames within the dynamic, effortless and kaleidoscopic flow of conversational speech, which we just began to tackle. For example, much research is needed on how the brain effectively manages the inherent complexity that our analysis highlighted [58]. From a neurocognitive viewpoint, the concept of mutual knowledge implies that information from multiple sources must be at the same time flexibly integrated within an individual's perceptual focus [59,60], as well as shared with the interlocutor. Future research will tell us how much the brain synchronizes to the pleasure of a chat.

Acknowledgments

The authors wish to thank Psychologist Elisa Cravello for acting as moderator conversational partner. We also thank Clinical Psychologist Elisabetta Pigat of the "E.Medea" Research Institute for her help with patient selection. Finally, we thank each and every participant, and their families, for providing us with the exceptional opportunity to learn from and with them.

Author Contributions

Conceived and designed the experiments: AT AP VM MC. Performed the experiments: AT AP MC. Analyzed the data: AT AP VM MC. Contributed reagents/materials/analysis tools: AT AP MC. Wrote the paper: AT AP VM MC.

References

1. Aitchison J (2008) The articulate mammal: An introduction to psycholinguistics. London: Routledge.
2. Scott S, McGettigan C, Eisner F (2009) A little more conversation, a little less action. Candidate roles for the motor cortex in speech perception. Nat Rev Neurosci 10: 295–302.
3. Iacoboni M, Molnar-Szakacs I, Gallese V, Buccino G, Mazziotta J, et al. (2005) Grasping the intentions of others with one's own mirror neuron system. PLoS Biol 3: e79.
4. Vuilleumier P, Armony J, Driver J, Dolan R (2003) Distinct spatial frequency sensitivity for procesing faces and emotional expressions. Nat Neurosci 6: 624–631.
5. Grice H (1989) Studies in the Way of Words. Cambridge (Mass.): Harvard University Press.
6. Pickering M, Garrod S (2004) Toward a mechanistic psychology of language. Behav Brain Sci 27: 169–226.
7. Schiller N, de Ruiter J (2004) Some notes on priming, aligning and self-monitoring. Behav Brain Sci 27: 208–209.
8. Goldinger S, Azuma T (2004) Resonance within and between linguistic beings. Behav Brain Sci 27: 199–200.
9. Brennan S, Clark H (1996) Conceptual pacts and lexical choice in conversation. J Exp Psychol Learn 22: 1482–1493.
10. Rapp A, Mutschler D, Erb M (2012) Where in the brain is nonliteral language? A coordinate-based meta-analysis of functional magnetic resonance imaging studies. Neuroimage 63: 600–610.
11. Uchiyama H, Saito D, Tanabe H, Harada T, Seki A, et al. (2012) Distinction between the literal and intended meanings of sentences: A functional magnetic resonance imaging study of metaphor and sarcasm. Cortex 48: 563–583.
12. Austin J (1946) Other minds. Proceedings of the Aristotelian Society 20: 148–187.
13. Miller G (2005) Reecting on another's mind. Science 308: 945–947.
14. Onishi K, Baillargeon R (2005) Do 15-month-old infants understand false beliefs? Science 308: 255–258.
15. Kovacs A, Teglas E, Endress A (2010) The social sense: Susceptibility to others' beliefs in human infants and adults. Science 330: 1830–1834.

16. Frith U, Frith C (2003) Development and neurophysiology of mentalizing. Philos Trans R Soc Lond B 358: 459–473.
17. Talwar V, Gordon H, Lee K (2007) Lying in the elementary school years. Verbal deception and its relation to second-order belief understanding. Dev Psychol 43: 804–810.
18. Frith C, Singer T (2008) The role of social cognition in decision making. Philos Trans R Soc Lond B 363: 3875–3886.
19. Frith U (2003) Autism: Explaining the Enigma. Oxford: Blackwell.
20. Senju A, Southgate V, White S, Frith U (2009) Mindblind eyes: An absence of spontaneous theory of mind in Asperger syndrome. Science 325: 883–885.
21. Solomon M, Goodlin-Jones B, Anders T (2004) A social adjustment enhancement intervention for high functioning autism, Asperger's syndrome, and pervasive developmental disorder. J Autism Dev Disord 34: 649–668.
22. Adams C, Green J, Gilchrist A, Cox A (2002) Conversational behaviour of children with Asperger syndrome and conduct disorder. J Child Psychol Psychiatry 43: 679–690.
23. Lai M, Lombardo M, Pasco G, Ruigrok A, Sadek S, et al. (2011) A behavioral comparison of male and female adults with high functioning autism spectrum conditions. PloS ONE 6: e20835.
24. Duda R, Hart P, Stork D (2001) Pattern Classification. John Wiley and Sons.
25. Asavathiratham C (2000) A Tractable Representation for the Dynamics of Networked Markov Chain. Ph.D. thesis, Dept. of ECS, MIT.
26. Manning C, Schütze H (1999) Foundations of Statistical Natural Language Processing. Cambridge (MA): The MIT Press.
27. Cristani M, Pesarin A, Drioli C, Tavano A, Perina A, et al. (2011) Generative modeling and classification of dialogs by a low-level turn-taking feature. Pattern Recognition 44: 1785–1800.
28. Pesarin A, Cristani M, Murino V, Drioli C, Perina A, et al. (2008) A statistical signature for automatic dialogue classification. In: Proceedings of International Conference on Pattern Recognition (ICPR 2008). 1–4.
29. Schopler E, Reichler R, DeVellis R, Daly K (1980) Toward objective classification of childhood autism: Childhood autism rating scale (cars). J Autism Devel Dis 10: 91103.
30. Lord C, Rutter M, Di Lavore P, Risi S (2005) Autism diagnostic observation schedule. Florence, Italy: Giunti OS. (Adapted by R Tancredi and M. Saccani and A.M. Persico and B. Parrini and R. Igliozzi and R. Faggioli).
31. Lewis A, Porter J (2004) Interviewing children and young people with learning disabilities: Guidelines for researchers and multi-professional practice. Br J Learn Disabil 32: 191–197.
32. Heilmann J, DeBrock L, Riley-Tillman TC (2013) Stability of measures from children's interviews: The effects of time, sample length, and topic. Am J Speech Lang Pathol 22: 463–475.
33. Wechsler D (1986) Wechsler Intelligence Scale for Children – Scala di intelligenza Wechsler per bambini. Florence, Italy: Organizzazioni Speciali.
34. Korkman M, Kirk U, Kempi S (2011) NEPSY-II. A developmental neuropsychological assessment. Florence, Italy: Giunti OS. (Adapted by C Urgesi and F. Campanella and F Fabbro).
35. Stambak M (1980) Tre prove di ritmo. Florence, Italy: Organizzazioni Speciali.
36. Novelli G, Papagno C, Capitani E, Laiacona N, Vallar G, et al. (1986) Tre test clinici di ricerca e produzione lessicale. Taratura su soggetti normali. Archivio di Psicologia Neurologia e Psichiatria 47: 477–506.
37. Tavano A, Côté H, Ferré P, Ska B, Joanette Y (2013) MEC – Protocollo Montréal per la valutazione delle abilità comunicative. Milan, Italy: Springer Verlag.
38. Basu S, Choudhury T, Clarkson B, Pentland A (2001) Learning human interaction with the inuence model. Technical Report 539, MIT MediaLab.
39. Sacks H, Schegloff EA, Jefferson G (1974) A simplest systematics for the organization of turn-taking for conversation. Language 50: 696–735.
40. Bilmes J (1997) A gentle tutorial on the EM algorithm and its application to parameter estimation for Gaussian mixture and hidden Markov models. Technical Report ICSI-TR-97-021, ICSI.
41. Smith N, Gales M (2001) Speech recognition using SVMs. In: NIPS. 1197–1204.
42. Jaakkola T, Haussler D (1999) Exploiting generative models in discriminative classifiers. In: Proceedings of the 1998 conference on Advances in neural information processing systems II. Cambridge, MA, USA: MIT Press, 487–493.
43. Tsuda K, Kawanabe M, Rätsch G, Sonnenburg S, Müller K (2002) A new discriminative kernel from probabilistic models. Neural Comput 14: 2397–2414.
44. Perina A, Cristani M, Castellani U, Murino V, Jojic N (2009) Free energy score space. In: Bengio Y, Schuurmans D, Lafferty J, Williams CKI, Culotta A, editors, Advances in Neural Information Processing Systems 22. 1428–1436.
45. Kuncheva L (2007) A stability index for feature selection. In: IASTED International Multi-Conference Artificial Intelligence and Applications. 390–395.
46. Pudil P, Novovičová J, Kittler J (1994) Floating search methods in feature selection. Pattern recognition letters 15: 1119–1125.
47. Narendra PM, Fukunaga K (1977) A branch and bound algorithm for feature subset selection. IEEE Transactions on Computers 100: 917–922.
48. Peng H, Fulmi L, Ding C (2005) Feature selection based on mutual information criteria of maxdependency, max-relevance, and min-redundancy. Pattern Analysis and Machine Intelligence, IEEE Transactions on 27: 1226–1238.
49. Duin R, Juszczak P, Paclk P, Pekalska E, DeRidder D, et al. (2004). Prtools version 4.1: A matlab toolbox for pattern recognition. Internet. Http://www.prtools.org.
50. Wilson M, Wilson TP (2005) An oscillator model of the timing of turn-taking. Psychonomic Bulletting and Review 12: 957–968.
51. RM Warner, Waggener T, Kronauer R (1983) Synchronized cycles in ventilation and vocal activity during spontaneous conversational speech. J Appl Physiol 54: 1324–1334.
52. McFarland D (2001) Respiratory markers of conversational interaction. J Speech Lang Hearing Res 44: 128–143.
53. Hird K, Kirsner K (2002) The relationship between prosody and discourse in spontaneous discourse. Brain and Language 80: 536–555.
54. Fisher III J, Darrell T (2004) Speaker association with signal-level audiovisual fusion. IEEE Trans on Multimedia 6: 406–413.
55. Richardson D, Dale R, Kirkham N (2007) The art of conversation is coordination. Psychological Science 18: 407–413.
56. Mason R, Williams D, Kana R, Minshew N, Just M (2008) Theory of mind disruption and recruitment of the right hemisphere during narrative comprehension in autism. Neuropsychologia 46: 269–280.
57. Williams D, Bowler D, Jarrold C (2012) Inner speech is used to mediate short-term memory, but not planning, among intellectually high-functioning adults with autism spectrum disorder. Dev Psychopathol 24: 225–239.
58. Miller V, Jansen B (2008) Oscillatory neural network for pattern recognition: Trajectory based classification and supervised learning. Biol Cybern 99: 459–471.
59. Zion-Golumbic E, Schroeder C (2012) Attention modulates "speech-tracking" at a cocktail party. Trends Cogn Sci 16: 363–364.
60. Zion-Golumbic E, Ding N, Bickel S, Lakatos P, Schevon C, et al. (2013) Mechanisms underlying selective neuronal tracking of attended speech at a cocktail party. Neuron 77: 980–991.

14

Aspergers – Different, Not Less: Occupational Strengths and Job Interests of Individuals with Asperger's Syndrome

Timo Lorenz*, Kathrin Heinitz

Department of Psychology, Freie Universität Berlin, Berlin, Germany

Abstract

Rooted in the neurodiversity approach, this study provides an overview of the strengths and interests of individuals with Asperger's Syndrome. We interviewed136 individuals with Asperger's Syndrome and 155 neurotypical individuals via an online survey with regards to (a) demography, (b) occupational strengths, (c) general self-efficacy, (d) occupational self-efficacy, and (e) the job interest profile according to Holland. The vocational and educational fields of the individuals with Asperger's in the sample are more diverse than and surpass those classical fields stated in research and biographical literature. The comparison of both groups in cross-tables showed that the indicated strengths differ in several areas ($\Phi_{Cramer} = .02–.47$), which means that a specific strength profile can be derived, and this profile goes beyond the clinical view of the diagnostic criteria. Individuals with Asperger's indicate lower self-efficacy, both general and occupational. Furthermore, a high concentration of individuals with Asperger's can be found in the areas I (Investigative) and C (Conventional) of Holland's RIASEC model.

Editor: Gabriel S. Dichter, UNC Chapel Hill, United States of America

Funding: The authors have no support or funding to report.

Competing Interests: The authors have declared that no competing interests exist.

* Email: timo.lorenz@fu-berlin.de

Introduction

The diagnostic concept of Asperger's Syndrome, which is part of the autistic spectrum, was introduced in the diagnostic manuals of both the APA and the WHO in the 1990s [1]. Since the introduction of this diagnosis and due to the improvement in diagnostics, many children have been diagnosed with Asperger's, which with the release of the DSM-V [2] has now become part of the autism spectrum disorder. Many of these children have by now completed school or university [3]. The school system is struggling to meet the needs of this group of people, and individuals with Asperger's still encounter obstacles upon entering careers. Individual biographies, interviews and media reports show that individuals with Asperger's work in professional fields such as research, IT, electrical engineering or mechanics [4,5,6]. To this day, however, no general survey exists to show which professional areas are frequented by employed individuals with Asperger's.

Several pragmatic approaches have been established to streamline the process of entering professional life for individuals with Asperger's, among them guidebooks [7] and organizations (e.g. "specialisterne" in Denmark, "Passwerk" in Belgium or "auticon" in Germany). These organizations function as intermediaries between individuals with Asperger's and businesses, yet the approaches still lack evidence-based tools to optimize the person-job-fit of individuals with Asperger's. Person-job-fit however affects job performance, turnover intentions, engagement and financial outcomes [8,9]. It minimizes a person's boredom and anxiety while maximizing effort and enjoyment [8] and has a strong correlation with job satisfaction [10].

Progress in this field would be beneficial on two fronts: it would help individuals with Asperger's enter employment in jobs that fit their qualifications, all the while helping to meet the market's demand for qualified personnel.

The purpose of this study is to provide a primary overview of the professions, strengths and job interest profiles of individuals with Asperger's. This in turn will help lay the foundation for the development of approaches towards improving the occupational situation of individuals with Asperger's.

Neurodiversity and strengths

Our approach is based on the theory of neurodiversity, a concept with footholds in neuroscience, evolutionary psychology and other fields, which considers autism a regular variant of the human brain [11]. This neuronal variance, which is regarded as natural, causes difficulties for individuals with Asperger's in areas such as empathy and social skills [12].

Regarding individuals with Asperger's as solely impaired or deficient would discount their strengths and capabilities [3,13]. Their skills of concentration during long-lasting routine work, identification of logical rules and patterns, processing visual information, and the ability to remember facts, surpass neurotypical individuals [14–20] (a designation for persons with no divergent neurological development, in this case with no form of autism; [21]). These strengths can be an advantage in certain professions and thereby offer good prospects to integrate individuals with Asperger's into the professional world according to their abilities, creating a better person-job-fit. This is based on the strength philosophy, which assumes that persons can achieve more when they build on their strengths rather than try to balance their weaknesses [22].

Hence one aim of this study is to provide a summary of the task-relevant strengths (e.g. attention to detail, fine motor skills, logical reasoning, concentrativeness or visual skills) that individuals with Asperger's recognize in themselves, and to compare these with the descriptions of neurotypical individuals.

Self-efficacy

Self-efficacy is another important intrapersonal factor that has an impact on several work-related outcomes. Among these are job performance [23], job satisfaction, intention to quit the profession [24] or career choice and development [25] and its predictive value for well-being and dealing with life's challenges [26–28]. Self-efficacy is defined as "belief in one's capabilities to mobilize the motivation, cognitive resources, and courses of action needed to meet given situational demands" [29]. Persons with high self-efficacy confront difficult situations with the certainty that they will remain in control [30]. Self-efficacy consists of two different facets, a generalized trait-like self-efficacy and a task-specific self-efficacy [31].

To our knowledge, no studies regarding individuals with Asperger's and self-efficacy have been conducted so far. Self-efficacy could be an explanation for a possible capacity-to-function-gap, i.e. that the available strengths (the capacity to function) of individuals with Asperger's are not made use of in (occupational) situations, leading to problems in the job or even to unemployment.

The social categorization of Asperger's Syndrome as a "disorder" or "disability" [13], and a high unemployment rate among this subgroup [32] has psychosocial effects such as low self-esteem, stress, social isolation [33,34] and low self-efficacy.

This study will examine if individuals with Asperger's have lower general self-efficacy and a lower task-specific, in this case occupational, self-efficacy than neurotypical individuals. This yields two hypotheses:

1) *Individuals with Asperger's have a lower general self-efficacy than neurotypical individuals.*
2) *Individuals with Asperger's have a lower occupational self efficacy than neurotypical individuals.*

Job interest types

A work situation that matches the person's job interest type fulfills their psychological needs, leading to higher intrinsic motivation, attention, and job satisfaction [35]. Aside from their strengths, the professional interests of individuals with Asperger's will also be assessed in this study, since this will allow for an optimal identification and adaptation of the fit for specific professions.

The analysis of job interests will be based on Holland's RIASEC model [35] as a theoretical foundation. This model consists of six categories or interest types (Realistic, Investigative, Artistic, Social, Enterprising and Conventional) These classify persons according to their main interests (accordingly: manual, investigative, artistic, social, enterprising or organizing) and list specific prototypic professions for the respective types. Tests based on Holland's model generate a three-digit code out of the three interest types with the highest values.

The above-mentioned biographies, interviews and media coverage of individuals with Asperger's in professional fields such as research, IT and engineering lead to this study's hypothesis 3 for the model of job interest types:

3) *Individuals with Asperger's have a higher amount of interest type codes of one of the possible combinations in the categories R. I and C.*

Method

Participants and Procedure

This study has a total of 306 participants. Fifteen people were excluded from the data set (one due to implausible response behavior with no variance in answers, three on account of young age, two due to missing information regarding their Asperger's diagnosis, nine due to an AQ-10 score of <6 despite their declaration of an Asperger's diagnosis). The AQ-10 was employed to re-affirm the already existing diagnosis. It was by no means used as a diagnostic tool, which is why we did not exclude any neurotypical individuals. In total 291 persons were included in the analysis. Of these, 136 were individuals with Asperger's (86 women, 46 men, 4 other), between ages 18–65 ($M_{age} = 35.54$ years, $SD = 10.59$) and 155 were neurotypical individuals (91 women, 62 men, 2 other) between 18–60 years of age ($M_{age} = 33.5$ years, $SD = 9.05$). Participants were recruited by approaching group administrators on Facebook with the request to publish the link to the survey as well as by publishing the link in specialized internet forums. Individuals with Asperger's have time and again stated that they find online communication to be more comfortable than face-to-face communication [36]. Hence, this way of data acquisition was chosen in order to guarantee barrier-free access to the survey. The survey was administered in German. Participation was strictly voluntary, no compensation was supplied.

Materials

Demographics. Participants were interviewed with regards to their country of residence, age, gender ("male", "female", and "other" – in order to accommodate individuals who do not identify with the gender binary), vocational training, college education, and current employment. The open input for current employment was encoded for analysis according to the Klassifikation der Berufe (Classification of occupations) 2010 [37], and the open input for college education was encoded according to the OECD [38].

Strengths. Participants were asked to pick one to five outstanding strengths from a list of 26 strengths (attention to detail, focus, team work, multitasking, numbers, repetitive tasks, creative solutions, systemizing, empathy, emotional control, physical work, fine motor skills stamina, consistency, flexibility, logical reasoning, concentrativeness, visual skills, auditory skills, apprehension, retentiveness, social skills, proactiveness, verbal skills). An open input-field allowed the participants to add their own concepts of strengths. Merely 136 of the 291 participants abided by the instruction to indicate one to five strengths. No difference between individuals with Asperger's and neurotypical individuals could be found in the compliance of this instruction, X^2 (1, $N = 155$) = 3.48, $p = .06$. Individuals with Asperger's ($M = 6.65$, $SD = 3.70$) named more strengths than neurotypical individuals ($M = 5.69$, $SD = 2.74$).

Asperger's diagnosis. Participants were asked whether they had received an official Asperger's Syndrome diagnosis. In addition, they completed the Autism Spectrum Quotient Test with 10 items (AQ-10) [39] with a 4-point scale, ranging from 1 = "*definitely agree*" to 4 = "*definitely disagree*" (e.g. "I find it difficult to work out people's intentions"). The test has an adult sensitivity of .88 and a specificity of .91, the cut-off was placed at 6 [39]. Cronbach's α of the AQ-10 was .89.

General self-efficacy. General self-efficacy was evaluated using the General Self-Efficacy scale (GSE) [40]. Participants responded to 10 items with a 4-point scale ranging from 1 = "*definitely agree*" to 4 = "*definitely disagree*" (e.g. "It is easy for me to stick to my aims and accomplish my goals."). Cronbach's α was .90. We ran our analysis referring to the mean score of the GSE.

Occupational self-efficacy. Occupational self-efficacy was evaluated with the occupational self-efficacy scale [41]. Participants responded to 8 items with a 4-point scale ranging from 1 = "*definitely agree*" to 4 = "*definitely disagree*" (e.g. "I feel that I meet most occupational demands.") Cronbach's α of this scale was .91. We ran our analysis referring to the mean score of the occupational self-efficacy scale.

Job interest type. Participants completed the revised German version of the General Interest Structure Test (AIST-R) [42]. Participants responded to 60 items with a 5-point scale ranging from 1 = "*I am not interested at all; I do not enjoy this at all*" to 5 = "*I am highly interested; I very much enjoy this*" (e.g. "Reading academic articles" or "Working with metal/wood, building something out of metal/wood"). The responses result in a three-digit code, which consists of a subsequent ranking of the six categories, from highest to lowest score. The three highest scores in this ranking then make up the code. Cronbach's α was .88. We ran our analysis referring to the standard scores of the AIST-R.

Data analysis

The data was checked for the appropriate prerequisites to conduct our data analysis doing t-tests and X^2-tests. Due to forced choice in the standardized questionnaires there was no missing data.

Results

Demographics

The largest part of the persons in the sample originated from Germany 93%), followed by Switzerland (2%) and Austria (1%). Altogether, 3% came from non-German speaking countries and 1% of the participants did not answer the question about their current country of residence.

Of the individuals with Asperger's, 55.9% stated to have absolved occupational training, as did 39.4% of neurotypical individuals. University degrees were held by 36.8% of individuals with Asperger's and 71% of neurotypical individuals. Table 1 relates the courses of study stated in the survey to the total amount of students in Berlin, Germany, in the winter semester of 2012/13 [43]. In comparison to the students in Berlin the number of individuals with Asperger's in this sample that state to be enrolled in social sciences (psychology, economics and business, educational sciences, sociology, law, political science, social and economic geography, media and communications) and natural sciences (mathematics, computer and information sciences, physical sciences, chemical sciences, earth and related environmental sciences and biological sciences) is disproportionately high. The number of neurotypical individuals in the social sciences is disproportionately high as well, whereas the number in natural sciences is disproportionately low. The corresponding numbers can be seen in table 1.

44.9% of individuals with Asperger's stated to be currently employed. This number is lower than the information regarding employment given by the neurotypical individuals in this sample (71.6%), X^2 $(1, N = 291) = 21.46$, $p < .001$, $\Phi_{Cramer} = .27$. Table 2 gives an overview of the open input about the current field of work. The majority of both groups can be found in the categories

Table 1. The courses of study of the individuals in the sample vs. the total amount of students in Berlin, Germany in the winter semester of 2012/13.

	Humanities	Social Sciences	Agricultural Sciences	Medical and Health Sciences	Engineering and Technology	Natural Sciences	other
Students Berlin	24.61%	27.17%	2.49%	6.29%	21.84%	16.64%	0.98%
Aspergers	18.8%	39.6%	4.20%	6.30%	2.10%	29.2%	0.00%
NT	22.3%	57.6%	3.00%	2.00%	11.1%	4.00%	0.00%

Note: Aspergers = individuals with Asperger's in the sample, NT = neurotypical individuals in the sample.

Table 2. Current employment of individuals with Asperger's vs neurotypical individuals.

		Classification according to KldB 2010 Code									total
		Agriculture, forestry, animal husbandry, and horticulture	Production of raw materials	Construction, architecture, surveying, and building technology	Natural sciences, geography and computer science	Transportation, logistics, protection and security	Commercial services, retail, sales and distribution, hotels and tourism	Business organization, accounting, law and administration	Health care, social affairs, and education	Humanities, social sciences, and economic sciences, media, art, culture and design	
Aspergers	qty	0	6	0	6	1	2	12	21	4	52
	%	.0%	11.5%	.0%	11.5%	1.9%	3.8%	23.1%	40.4%	7.7%	100.0%
NT	qty	1	3	3	5	2	10	19	42	16	101
	%	1.0%	3.0%	3.0%	5.0%	2.0%	9.9%	18.8%	41.6%	15.8%	100.0%
total	qty	1	9	3	11	3	12	31	63	20	153
	%	.7%	5.9%	2.0%	7.2%	2.0%	7.8%	20.3%	41.2%	13.1%	100.0%

Note: KldB = Klassifikation der Berufe (classification of occupations), Aspergers = individuals with Asperger's, NT = neurotypical individuals, qty = quantity.

"health care, social affairs, and education" and "business organization, accounting, law and administration". The comparison shows that more individuals with Asperger's work in the categories "production of raw materials" and "natural sciences, geography and computer science".

AQ-10

In this sample the mean of the autism quotient scores for individuals with Asperger's is 8.86 (SD = 1.13), for neurotypical individuals it is 3.55 (SD = 2.90).

Strengths

Cross-tables were generated to compare the distribution of the individual strengths in both groups. For an overview of the percent frequency of strengths for both groups and the results of the X^2 (1, N = 291) tests, see table 3. The level of significance was Bonferroni-Holm corrected. 16 of 26 strengths were reported differently comparing the two groups. The three strongest effect sizes could be found with empathy (Φ_{Cramer} = .47), attention to detail (Φ_{Cramer} = .39) and social skills (Φ_{Cramer} = .39). No relation of strengths with respect to the individuals with Asperger's AQ-10 score or gender could be determined.

Self-efficacy

Individuals with Asperger's reported a lower general self-efficacy (M = 21.44, SD = 5.32) than neurotypical individuals (M = 28.39, SD = 5.59), $t(289) = -10.81$, $p<.001$, r = .54. Furthermore, individuals with Asperger's also reported a lower occupational self-efficacy (M = 16.91, SD = 5.75) than neurotypical individuals (M = 22.72, SD = 5.20), $t(289) = -9.05$, $p<.001$, r = .47. These results are in favor of hypothesis 1 and 2.

The correlations between the statement of being currently employed and both self-efficacy scores were analyzed in an explorative data analysis. This showed the correlation with general self-efficacy to be statistically non-significant (r = .03, p = .70), and the correlation to occupational self-efficacy to be statistically significant (r = .26, $p<.001$) for individuals with Asperger's. Both self-efficacies, general self-efficacy (r = .20, p = .011) and occupational self-efficacy (r = .25, p = .002), show statistically significant relations with employment status for neurotypical individuals.

Furthermore, we tested whether or not a connection between the stated strengths of individuals with Asperger's and their self-efficacy scores exists. For the general self-efficacy 'score, visual skills (r = .27, p = 001) and proactiveness (r = .30, $p<.001$) proved to be statistically significant. For occupational self-efficacy, a statistically significant correlation with proactiveness (r = .30, $p<.001$) was found.

Job interest type

Table 4 provides an overview of the group statistics results for the individual job interest types. Individuals with Asperger's score especially high in the interest types I (Investigative) and C (Conventional) and low in S (Social) and E (Enterprising) In order to test hypothesis 3 a cross-table was generated (see table 5). Individuals with Asperger's have a job interest code consisting of the types R (Realistic), I (Investigative) and C (Conventional) more often than neurotypical individuals, X^2 (1, N = 291) = 25.93, $p<.001$, Φ_{Cramer} = .30. Due to this data, results are in favor of hypothesis 3.

Due to the data and the high scores in the job interest types I and C of individuals with Asperger's, an explorative data analysis was conducted to determine the results of reducing the job interest code to these two interest types. A cross-table was generated and table 5 provides an overview of the percent distribution within the groups; the effect size in this analysis compared to the RIC-code analysis increases from a moderate to a relatively strong association [43], $\Phi_{Cramer}=.49$, X^2 (1, $N=291$) = 70.64, $p<.001$.

Discussion

Results of this study show that the indicated occupational and educational fields of the individuals with Asperger's that participated in this study (Table 2) are more diverse than the hitherto existing literature [4,5,6] will have us believe, exceeding the fields of natural science, engineering, and IT. It becomes clear that future research and projects on the occupational integration of individuals with Asperger's generally can and should include more occupational areas than natural science, engineering and IT in order to better meet the needs of a diverse group of people, i.e. librarianship and fields of social science. When it comes to strengths, the data suggests that the strengths areas that were rarely indicated by individuals with Asperger's, i.e. empathy and flexibility, directly reflect the clusters of diagnostic criteria for Asperger's syndrome as provided by the DSM-IV [45] or, respectively, of autism spectrum disorder as provided by the DSM-V [2]. These criteria can result in a cluster of possible problems in everyday life [1]. The frequently indicated strengths, i.e. attention to detail or focus, form a cluster of their own, comprised of areas that, when combined, result in a very distinct strength profile. These strengths provide a perspective - beyond the clinical view - on areas in which individuals with Asperger's can draw on their strengths in order to fully tap into their potential within specific jobs.

Individual, tailored coaching could help to further a goal-oriented integration of individuals with Asperger's into the working world, drawing on available strengths while acknowledging problematic areas such as team work or social skills in face-to-face communication [46,47]. Areas that require these exact strength profiles can be pinpointed within most occupational fields. Here, individuals with Asperger's could not just be integrated but might also be able to specifically show achievements superior to other candidates. Individual results on job-interests can further be used to determine corresponding occupational areas. Müller et al. [48] have shown that a high person-job-fit positively influences how individuals with Asperger's experience occupational life.

The data of this study shows that individuals with Asperger's have a lower general and occupational self-efficacy with a relation between employment and occupational self-efficacy. These results

Table 3. Frequency of indicated strengths of individuals with Asperger's vs. neurotypical individuals.

	%	%			
strength	**Aspergers**	**NT**	X^2	p	Φ_{Cramer}
Attention to detail	73	34	43.26	.000*	.39
Logical reasoning	60	35	18.86	.000*	.26
Reliability	49	44	0.63	.426	.05
Focus	48	17	30.91	.000*	.33
Systemizing	47	29	10.05	.002*	.19
Consistency	40	19	14.61	.000*	.22
Visual skills	36	18	12.02	.001*	.20
Creative solutions	35	26	2.65	.104	.10
Retentiveness	35	14	16.61	.000*	.24
Repetitive tasks	32	10	23.04	.000*	.28
Numbers	29	08	20.32	.000*	.26
Organizing ability	24	29	1.13	.288	.06
Apprehension	24	21	0.35	.553	.04
Verbal skills	24	41	9.45	.002*	.18
Auditory skills	23	05	21.32	.000*	.27
Stamina	22	20	0.19	.667	.03
Proactiveness	17	19	0.16	.690	.02
Fine motor skills	11	06	1.93	.164	.08
Concentrativeness	10	05	2.10	.148	.09
Emotional control	09	15	2.96	.085	.10
Physical work	09	08	0.02	.895	.00
Flexibility	04	26	24.91	.000*	.29
Social skills	04	35	43.52	.000*	.39
Multitasking	01	17	22.14	.000*	.28
Empathy	01	41	65.50	.000*	.47
Team work	00	25	39.52	.000*	.37

* = statistically significant after Bonferroni-Holm correction.
Note: Aspergers = individuals with Asperger's, NT = neurotypical individuals.

suggest that individuals with Asperger's could benefit from training programs that specifically target an increase in occupational self-efficacy. Generally, our findings concur with previous literature regarding individualized off-and on-the-job coaching for individuals with Asperger's that includes both the general aims of targeting job tasks, acclimation to the job site, and social integration [49,50,51,52]. Additionally, a specific focus on occupational self-efficacy would bring further benefits.

Future directions

Future research should attempt to replicate the data in the same context, as well as in other ethnic backgrounds, and with groups outside of the World Wide Web, in order to test and possibly increase the conclusions' generalizability.

Longitudinal studies and qualitative data can help to find the causes of the low self-efficacy scores, specifically of occupational self-efficacy. Furthermore, they could help to identify barriers in specific transition phases, i.e. the transition from school to vocational training or higher education, as well as entering and sustaining employment. The combination of these measures could help to develop programs for the transition to employment that would help to integrate individuals with Asperger's into the working world, and to accept them as full-fledged members of society.

Limitations

Results of this study should be interpreted with the following limitations in mind. Firstly, participants were all recruited online. It is possible that findings may not generalize to people who are not using the internet or are not using social networks. The fact that more women participated in this study than would be expected when it comes to ASD could be explained by (a hypothetical) greater use of social media in women. More concerns about generalizability are warranted because this study used a nonprobability sample. Furthermore, participants were all of German-speaking descent, and were therefore relatively ethnically homogeneous. It is possible that individuals from other ethnic backgrounds would have reported different strengths or job interests. The participants were not diagnosed by means of a singular diagnostic method. Instead, they were asked to provide information about their Asperger's diagnosis. Due to the strong variation within the diagnostic process, we had to rely upon the participants' self-reported data of an existing diagnosis. Future research should include individuals with a confirmed diagnosis, possibly diagnosed by the same institution or at least using the same diagnostic process. This procedure would forgo self-reported data. Furthermore, it would provide insight into the differences within the spectrum by allowing for the comparison of individual scores.

The sample of neurotypical individuals shows a slight deviation from the results of the AIST-R reference sample. The aberration for the interest type "Realistic" with a lower mean score could serve to explain the significant results in comparison with the surveyed individuals with Asperger's, because the mean score of individuals with Asperger's in the sample is equal to the mean score of the reference sample.

Ethics statement

This study does not involve any conflict of ethics, since no clinical intervention was performed. Neither were blood or tissue samples taken for study purposes.

Participants were informed before participating that their responses would be treated confidentially and anonymously throughout and that all data would be analyzed in a generalized

Table 4. Results t-tests job interest type scores – individuals with Asperger's vs. neurotypical individuals.

Interest	*M*	*SD*	*M*	*SD*	*M*	*df*	*t*	*p*
type	Aspergers	Aspergers	*NT*	NT	difference			
R	100.69	9.16	97.23	8.66	3.46	289	3.23	.001*
I	110.83	8.76	102.66	8.19	8.17	289	8.21	.000*
A	102.12	9.51	105.00	10.35	−2.88	289	−2.46	.014
S	90.56	12.94	102.11	12.83	−12.29	289	−8.12	.000*
E	87.76	10.22	102.86	11.45	−13.45	289	−10.51	.000*
C	110.32	10.32	102.88	9.80	7.44	289	6.30	.000*

* = statistically significant after Bonferroni correction.

Note: Aspergers = individuals with Asperger's, NT = neurotypical individuals, RIASEC refers to Holland's job interest types (R = Realistic, I = Investigative, A = Artistic, S = Social, E = Enterprising and C = Conventional) measured with the AIST-R.

Table 5. Comparison of RIC- and IC-Code – individuals with Asperger's vs. neurotypical individuals.

RIC-Code				**total**
		no	**yes**	
Aspergers	quantity	91	45	136
	%	66.9%	33.1%	100.0%
NT	quantity	141	14	155
	%	91.0%	9.0%	100.0%
total	quantity	232	59	291
	%	79.7%	20.3%	100.0%
IC-Code				**total**
		no	**yes**	
Aspergers	quantity	32	104	136
	%	23.5%	76.5%	100.0%
NT	quantity	113	42	155
	%	72.9%	27.1%	100.0%
total	quantity	145	146	291
	%	49.8%	50.2%	100.0%

Note: Aspergers = individuals with Asperger's, NT = neurotypical individuals, RIC and IC refers to Holland's job interest types (R = Realistic, I = Investigative and C = Conventional) measured with the AIST-R.

manner so that no conclusions could be drawn about individual persons.

Hence, we were not required to obtain approval from the ethics committee.

Furthermore, a consent form is not applicable, since an online survey was conducted. There was no contact between researchers and participants. The subjects participated voluntarily and were informed about the study's objectives and at all times giving their consent by filling out the online survey.

Author Contributions

Conceived and designed the experiments: TL KH. Performed the experiments: TL KH. Analyzed the data: TL KH. Contributed reagents/materials/analysis tools: TL KH. Wrote the paper: TL KH.

References

1. Attwood T (2006) The complete guide to Asperger's syndrome. Philadelphia: Jessica Kingsley Publishers.
2. American Psychiatric (2013) Diagnostic and statistical manual of mental disorders (5th edition). Arlington, VA: American Psychiatric Publishing.
3. Griffin E, Pollak D (2009) Student experiences of neurodiversity in higher education: Insights from the BRAINHE Project. Dyslexia 15: 23–41.
4. Grandin T (2006) Thinking in pictures: And other reports from my life with autism. New York: Vintage.
5. Robison JE (2008) Look me in the eye: My life with Asperger's. New York: Random House.
6. Alexander C (2013) IT-Consultants mit Autismus gesucht. Der SPIEGEL. Available: http://www.spiegel.de/karriere/berufsleben/berliner-firma-stellt-autisten-als-it-spezialisten-ein-a-885080.html. Accessed 2013 Oct 8.
7. Simone R, Grandin T (2010) Asperger's on the job: Must-have advice for people with Asperger's or High Functioning Autism, and their employers, educators, and advocates. Arlington: Future Horizons Inc.
8. Harter JK, Blacksmith N (2010) Employee engagement and the psychology of joining, staying in and leaving organizations. In: P Linley, S Harrington and N Garcea, editors. Oxford handbook of positive psychology and work. New York: Oxford Press. pp. 121–130.
9. Schmidt FL, Hunter JE (1998) The validity and utility of selection methods in personnel psychology: Practical and theoretical implications of 85 years of research findings. Psych. Bull 124: 262.
10. Kristof-Brown AL, Zimmerman RD, Johnson EC (2005) Consequences of indiviudals' fit at work: A meta-analysis of person-job, person-organization, person-group, and person-supervisor fit. Pers Psychol 58: 281–342.
11. Jaarsma P, Welin S (2012) Autism as a natural human variation: Reflections on the claims of the neurodiversity movement. Health Care Anal 20: 20–30.
12. Kapp SK, Gillespie-Lynch K, Sherman LE, Hutman T (2012) Deficit, difference, or both? Autism and neurodiversity. Dev Psychol 49: 59–71.
13. Armstrong T (2010) Neurodiversity: Discovering the extraordinary gifts of autism, ADHD, dyslexia, and other brain differences. Cambridge: Da Capo.
14. Chown N, Beavan N (2011) Intellectually capable but socially excluded? A review of the literature and research on students with autism in further education. Journal of Further and Higher Education: 1–17.
15. Grandin T (2009) How does visual thinking work in the mind of a person with autism? A personal account. Philos Trans R Soc Lond B Biol Sci 364: 1437–1442.
16. Asperger H (1944) Die "Autistischen Psychopathen" im Kindesalter. Eur Arch Psychiatry Clin Neurosci 117: 76–136.
17. Happé F, Vital P (2009) What aspects of autism predispose to talent? Philos Trans R Soc Lond B Biol Sci 364: 1369–1375.
18. James I (2010) Autism and mathematical talent. Mathematical Intell 32: 56–58.
19. Kunda M, Goel AK (2008) How thinking in pictures can explain many characteristic behaviors of autism. 7th IEEE International Conference on Development and Learning. Monterey, CA IEEE. pp. 304–309.
20. Mottron L, Dawson M, Soulières I, Hubert B, Burack J (2006) Enhanced perceptual functioning in autism: An update, and eight principles of autistic perception. J Autism Dev Disord 36: 27–43.
21. Attwood T (1998) Asperger's syndrome: A guide for parents and professionals. London: Jessica Kingsley Publishers.
22. Clifton DO, Harter JK (2003) Investing in strengths. In: K. S Cameron, J. E Dutton and R. E Quinn, editors. Positive organizational scholarship: Foundations of a new discipline. San Francisco: Berrett-Koehler. pp. 111–121.
23. Stajkovic AD, Luthans F (1998) Self-efficacy and work-related performance: A meta-analysis. Psych Bull 124: 240.
24. Saks AM (1995) Longitudinal field investigation of the moderating and mediating effects of self-efficacy on the relationship between training and newcomer adjustment. J Appl Psychol 80: 211.
25. Bandura A (1994) Self-efficacy. In: V. S Ramachandran, editor. Encyclopedia of human behavior. New York: Academic Press. pp. 71–81.
26. Jerusalem M (1990) Persönliche Ressourcen, Vulnerabilität und Stresserleben. Göttingen: Hogrefe.
27. Schwarzer R (1992) Self-efficacy: Thought control of action. Washington, DC: Hemisphere.
28. Schwarzer R (1994) Optimistische Kompetenzerwartung: Zur Erfassung einer personellen Bewältigungsressource. Diagnostica 40: 92–116.
29. Wood R, Bandura A (1989) Impact of conceptions of ability on self-regulatory mechanisms and complex decision making. Pers Soc Psychol Bull 56: 407.

30. Bandura A (1977) Self-efficacy: toward a unifying theory of behavioral change. Psych Rev 84: 191.
31. Bandura A (1997) Self-efficacy: The exercise of control. New York: Freeman.
32. Howlin P (2013) Social disadvantage and exclusion: adults with autism lag far behind in employment prospects. J Am Acad Child Adolesc Psychiatry 52: 897–899.
33. Hofvander B, Delorme R, Chaste P, Nydén A, Wentz E, et al. (2009) Psychiatric and psychosocial problems in adults with normal-intelligence autism spectrum disorders. BMC psychiatry 9: 35.
34. Taylor JL, Hodapp RM (2012) Doing nothing: Adults with disabilities with no daily activities and their siblings. Am J Intellect Dev Disabil 117: 67–79.
35. Holland JL (1997) Making vocational choices: A theory of vocational personalities and work environments. Odessa: Psychological Assessment Resources.
36. Benford P, Standen P (2009) The internet: a comfortable communication medium for people with Asperger syndrome (AS) and high functioning autism (HFA)? J Assist Technol 3: 44–53.
37. Bundesagentur für Arbeit (2011) Klassifikation der Berufe 2010. In: Bundesagentur für Arbeit, editor. Nürnberg: Bundesagentur für Arbeit.
38. Organisation for Economic Co-operation and Development (2007) Revised Fields of Science and Technology. In: Organisation for Economic Co-operation and Development, editor. Paris: Organisation for Economic Co-operation and Development.
39. Allison C, Auyeung B, Baron-Cohen S (2011) Toward brief "red flags" for autism screening: The short Autism Spectrum Quotient and the short quantitative checklist in 1,000 cases and 3,000 controls. J Am Acad Child Adolesc Psychiatry 51: 202–212.e207.
40. Schwarzer R, Jerusalem M (1995) Generalized Self-Efficacy scale. In: J Weinman, S Wright and M Johnston, editors. Measures in health psychology: A user's portfolio causal and control beliefs. Windsor, England: NFER-NELSON. pp. 35–37.
41. Schyns B, von Collani G (2012) Berufliche Selbswirksamkeitserwartung. In: A Glöckner-Rist, editor. Zusammenstellung sozialwissenschaftlicher Items und Skalen ZIS Version 1500. Bonn: GESIS.
42. Bergmann C, Eder F (2005) Allgemeiner Interessen-Struktur-Test (AIST-R) mit Umwelt-Struktur-Test (UST-R)-Revision. Göttingen: Beltz Test.
43. Amt für Statistik Berlin-Brandenburg (2013) B III 1 – j/2012 - Studierende an Hochschulen in Berlin Wintersemester 2012/2013. In: Amt für Statistik Berlin-Brandenburg, editor. Potsdam: Amt für Statistik Berlin-Brandenburg.
44. Rea LM, Parker RA (1992) Designing and conducting survey research. San Francisco: Jossey-Boss.
45. American Psychiatric Association (2000) Diagnostic and statistical manual of mental disorders (4th edition, text revised). Washington, DC: American Psychiatric Association.
46. Hendricks D (2010) Employment and adults with autism spectrum disorders: Challenges and strategies for success. J Vocat Rehabil 32: 125–134.
47. Hurlbutt K, Chalmers L (2004) Employment and adults with Asperger syndrome. Focus Autism Other Dev Disabl 19: 215–222.
48. Müller E, Schuler A, Burton BA, Yates GB (2003) Meeting the vocational support needs of individuals with Asperger Syndrome and other autism spectrum disabilities. J Vocat Rehabil 18: 163–175.
49. Griffith GM, Totsika V, Nash S, Hastings RP (2012) 'I just don't fit anywhere': support experiences and future support needs of individuals with Asperger syndrome in middle adulthood. Autism 16: 532–546.
50. Hillier A, Campbell H, Mastriani K, Izzo MV, Kool-Tucker AK, et al. (2007) Two-year evaluation of a vocational support program for adults on the autism spectrum. Career Dev Transit Except Individ 30: 35–47.
51. Howlin P, Alcock J, Burkin C (2005) An 8 year follow-up of a specialist supported employment service for high-ability adults with autism or Asperger syndrome. Autism 9: 533–549.
52. Mesibov GB, Shea V (2010) The TEACCH program in the era of evidence-based practice. J Autism Dev Disord 40: 570–579.

Heterogeneous Pattern of Selective Pressure for PRRT2 in Human Populations, but No Association with Autism Spectrum Disorders

**Guillaume Huguet[1,2,3], Caroline Nava[4,5,6,7], Nathalie Lemière[1,2,3], Etienne Patin[8], Guillaume Laval[8], Elodie Ey[1,2,3], Alexis Brice[4,5,6,9], Marion Leboyer[10,11], Pierre Szepetowski[12,13,14], Christopher Gillberg[15,16,17], Christel Depienne[4,5,6,9], Richard Delorme[1,2,11,18], Thomas Bourgeron[1,2,3,11]*

1 Human Genetics and Cognitive Functions, Institut Pasteur, Paris, France, **2** CNRS URA 2182 'Genes, synapses and cognition', Institut Pasteur, Paris, France, **3** University Denis Diderot Paris 7, Paris, France, **4** INSERM, U975—CRICM, Institut du cerveau et de la moelle épinière (ICM), Hôpital Pitié-Salpêtrière, Paris, France, **5** CNRS 7225—CRICM, Hôpital Pitié-Salpêtrière, Paris, France, **6** Université Pierre et Marie Curie-Paris-6 (UPMC), UMR_S 975, Paris, France, **7** Département de Génétique et de Cytogénétique, Unité fonctionnelle de génétique clinique, AP-HP, Hôpital Pitié-Salpêtrière, Paris, France, **8** Unit of Human Evolutionary Genetics, Institut Pasteur, Paris, France, **9** Département de Génétique et de Cytogénétique, Unité fonctionnelle de neurogénétique moléculaire et cellulaire, AP-HP, Hôpital Pitié-Salpêtrière, Paris, France, **10** INSERM, U955, Psychiatry Genetic team, Creteil, France, **11** Fondation FondaMental, Créteil, France, **12** INSERM, UMR_S901, Marseille, France, **13** Aix-Marseille University, Marseille, France, **14** Mediterranean Institute of Neurobiology (INMED), Marseille, France, **15** Gillberg Neuropsychiatry Centre, University of Gothenburg, Göteborg, Sweden, **16** Institute of Neuroscience and Physiology, Department of Pharmacology, Gothenburg University, Gothenburg, Sweden, **17** Institute of Child Health, University College London, London, United Kingdom, **18** Assistance Publique-Hôpitaux de Paris, Robert Debré Hospital, Department of Child and Adolescent Psychiatry, Paris, France

Abstract

Inherited and *de novo* genomic imbalances at chromosome 16p11.2 are associated with autism spectrum disorders (ASD), but the causative genes remain unknown. Among the genes located in this region, *PRRT2* codes for a member of the synaptic SNARE complex that allows the release of synaptic vesicles. *PRRT2* is a candidate gene for ASD since homozygote mutations are associated with intellectual disability and heterozygote mutations cause benign infantile seizures, paroxysmal dyskinesia, or hemiplegic migraine. Here, we explored the contribution of *PRRT2* mutations in ASD by screening its coding part in a large sample of 1578 individuals including 431 individuals with ASD, 186 controls and 961 individuals from the human genome Diversity Panel. We detected 24 nonsynonymous variants, 1 frameshift (A217PfsX8) and 1 in-frame deletion of 6 bp (p.A361_P362del). The frameshift mutation was observed in a control with no history of neurological or psychiatric disorders. The p.A361_P362del was observed in two individuals with autism from sub-Saharan African origin. Overall, the frequency of *PRRT2* deleterious variants was not different between individuals with ASD and controls. Remarkably, *PRRT2* displays a highly significant excess of nonsynonymous (pN) *vs* synonymous (pS) mutations in Asia (pN/pS = 4.85) and Europe (pN/pS = 1.62) compared with Africa (pN/pS = 0.26; Asia *vs* Africa: P = 0.000087; Europe *vs* Africa P = 0.00035; Europe *vs* Asia P = P = 0.084). We also showed that whole genome amplification performed through rolling cycle amplification could artificially introduce the A217PfsX8 mutation indicating that this technology should not be performed prior to *PRRT2* mutation screening. In summary, our results do not support a role for *PRRT2* coding sequence variants in ASD, but provide an ascertainment of its genetic variability in worldwide populations that should help researchers and clinicians to better investigate the role of *PRRT2* in human diseases.

Editor: Mathias Toft, Oslo University Hospital, Norway

Funding: This work was funded by the Institut Pasteur, CNRS, INSERM, AP-HP, University Paris Diderot, the Bettencourt-Schueller foundation, the Orange foundation, the FondaMental foundation, the Conny-Maeva foundation, the Cognacq-Jay foundation, the ANR (SynDivAutism), Neuron-ERANET (EUHF-AUTISM). The funders had no role in study design, data collection and analysis, decision to publish, or preparation of the manuscript.

Competing Interests: The authors have declared that no competing interests exist.

* E-mail: thomasb@pasteur.fr

Introduction

Autism Spectrum Disorders (ASD) are characterized by impairments in reciprocal social communication, and repetitive, stereotyped and ritualistic behaviors [1]. ASD include autism, Asperger syndrome and pervasive developmental disorder not otherwise specified (PDD-NOS). The prevalence of ASD overall is about 1/100, but closer to 1/300 for autism with intellectual disability (ID) [2]. The susceptibility genes to ASD remain largely unknown, but mutations affecting genes such as *NLGN3/4X*, *SHANK2/3*, *NRXN1* and *CNTNAP2* were shown to alter synaptic function and increase the risk for ASD [3]. Several large-scale studies have reported an enrichment of copy number variants (CNVs) in individuals with ASD [4,5], suggesting that gene dosage plays a key role in the susceptibility to ASD [6]. Among the recurrent genomic alterations associated with ASD, *de novo* or inherited submicroscopic microdeletion/duplication at 16p11.2 have been associated with a variety of developmental/neuropsychiatric disorders including ASD, intellectual disability (ID), schizophrenia, or bipolar disorders, but also with body mass index [7–14]. A meta-analysis of 6 studies including more than 2000 individuals and 30000 controls provided strong support for the role of recurrent 16p11.2 genomic imbalances as risk factors for ASD (duplication OR:20.7 and $P = 1.9 \times 10^{-7}$; deletion OR:38.7 and 2.3×10^{-13}) [13]. The deleted/duplicated region at 16p11.2 spans 500–600 kb and is flanked by large and highly similar 147 kb low copy repeats with >99% homology, predisposing to unequal crossing-over during meiosis [10–14]. Among the 27 genes located within the interval, Kumar *et al.* (2009) screened for rare variations in 8 candidate genes selected for their function and expression in the brain (*ALDOA, DOC2A, HIRIP3, MAPK3, MAZ, PPP4C, SEZ6L2* and *TAOK2*). None of them showed a significant association with ASD at the exception of *SEZ6L2* for which a suggestive association was detected [15], but not confirmed [16]. Smaller deletions at 16p11.2 were identified in individuals with ASD narrowing the critical region and including the *PRRT2* gene [8,9]. *PRRT2* codes for a membrane protein that interacts with SNAP25, a protein from the synaptic vesicles release machinery (the SNARE complex). *PRRT2* is a compelling candidate gene for ASD and other psychaitric diseases since a homozygote frameshift mutation (A217PfsX8) was shown to segregate with non-syndromic ID in one consanguineous family with 9 affected individuals [17]. Furthermore numerous heterozygote frameshift, nonsense and missense *PRRT2* mutations (including the recurrent frameshift A217PfsX8) were identified in individuals and families with benign infantile seizures (BIS), paroxysmal kinesigenic dyskinesia (PKD), hemiplegic migraine (HM), or episodic ataxia, variably associated (*e.g.* the ICCA syndrome that associates BIS with PKD) [18–21]. Following these results, we compared the frequency of deleterious mutations in 431 individuals with ASD and 186 controls. In addition, we ascertained the genetic variability of *PRRT2* in a sample of 961 individuals from worldwide populations.

Materials and Methods

Individuals and control samples

Mutation screening of *PRRT2* was performed in individuals with ASD recruited by the PARIS (Paris Autism Research International Sibpair) study at specialized clinical neuropsychiatric centers disposed in France and Sweden (Table S1). Diagnosis was based on comprehensive clinical evaluation by experienced clinicians using DSM IV-TR criteria; most individuals were assessed with the Autism Diagnostic Interview-Revised (ADI-R) and some of them also with the Autism Diagnostic Observation Scale (ADOS). In Sweden, in some cases, the Diagnostic Interview for Social and Communication Disorders (DISCO-10) was used instead of the ADI-R. Cases were included only after a thorough clinical evaluation, including psychiatric and neuropsychological examination, standard karyotyping, and fragile-X testing, as well as brain imaging and EEG whenever possible. For comparison between cases and controls, only individuals from European descent were considered (Table S2). The Human Genome Diversity Panel (HGDP) is a collection of 961 individuals from worldwide populations [22]. This study was approved by the local Institutional Review Board (IRB). The local IRB are the Comités de Protection des Personnes Île-de-France VI Sis Hôpital Pitié-Salpêtrière 75013 PARIS for France and the Sahlgrenska Academy Ethics committee, University of Gothenburg for Sweden. For all probands written inform consent was signed by the individuals or parents or the legal representative.

Mutation screening of PRRT2

We obtained DNA of 431 unrelated individuals with ASD, 180 controls and 961 individuals without known clinical status from the Human Genome Diversity Panel (HGDP) from blood leukocytes or B-lymphoblastoid cell lines, and was extracted with phenol-chloroform (Table S1, S2). All coding exons of *PRRT2* were screened by direct sequencing of the PCR products (Table S3). The 3 coding exons of PRRT2 (NP_660282.2) and one supplementary exon present in the splicing isoforms (Q7Z6L0-1, Q7Z6L0-2, Q7Z6L0-3) were sequenced. For the amplicon of exon 2, that contains the frameshift mutation A217PfsX8, we screened an additional sample of 295 individuals with ASD and 92 controls. For all exons, the amplification of 20 ng of DNA template was performed using a standard PCR protocol with the FastStart Taq polymerase (Roche): 95°C for 15 min, followed by 35 cycles of 95°C for 30 s, 55 to 64°C (depending on the Tm) for 30 s, 72°C for 30 s to 1 min (depending on the product size), with a final cycle at 72°C for 10 min. Direct sequencing of the PCR products was performed using the BigDye Terminator Cycle V3.1 Sequencing Kit, and an ABI PRISM genetic analyzer (Applied Biosystems). For all nonsynonymous variations, the genotype was confirmed by sequencing an independent PCR product. Because of the low quantity of DNA for 3 individuals with ASD, we used whole genome amplification (WGA), using two commercially available Multiple Displacement Amplification kits. For the GenomiPhi DNA Amplification Kit (Amersham Pharmacia, Uppsala, Sweden), 25 ng of genomic DNA (in 2.5 µl) were mixed with 22.5 µl of

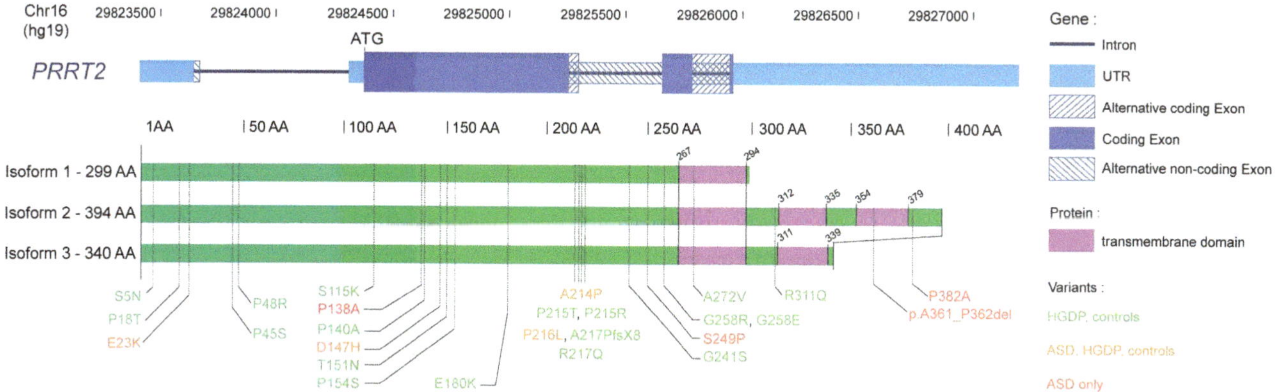

Figure 1. *PRRT2* coding variants identified in this study. Schematic diagram of the *PRRT2* gene and of the three PRRT2 protein isoforms. Mutation identified in this study are indicated in green (controls and HGDP), orange (controls, HGDP, and patients) and red (patients only).

GenomiPhi sample buffer. For the Repli-G Whole Genome Amplification kit (Qiagen Sciences Inc. Germantown, MD), 25 ng of genomic material were diluted in TE to a final volume of 2.5 µl. For comparison with the exome variant server, we verified that the coverage of the *PRRT2* exons was satisfactory (92% of the coding region had a coverage >20; Figure S1).

Statistical analyses and software

The significance of differences in *PRRT2* variants in individuals and controls was determined by a two-sided Fisher's exact test on a two-by-two contingency table. PolyPhen-2 (http://psort.hgc.jp) and PSORT (http://genetics.bwh.harvard.edu/pph2) were used to predict the functional impact of amino acid substitutions and trans-membrane segments, respectively. To estimate the selective pressure on PRRT2 in different populations (pN/pS), the number of synonymous SNPs or nonsynonymous SNPs was divided by the total number of synonymous or nonsynonymous positions in PRRT2. The number of synonymous and nonsynonymous sites of PRRT2 were calculated by DnaSP v5 [23].

Results

We sequenced all coding exons of *PRRT2* in a large cohort of 1578 individuals including 431 individuals with ASD, 186 controls and 961 individuals from the HGDP [22]. None of the patients tested were deleted or duplicated for the 16p11.2 locus. Overall, we identified 24 nonsynonymous variants, 1 frameshift A217PfsX8 and 1 in-frame deletion of 6 bp (Del 361A-362P) (Table 1, Figure 1, Table S4 and S5). Among those, 18 were not reported before (S5N, P18T, P48R, S115K, P140A, T151N, P154S, E180K, A214P, P215T, G241S, S249P, G258E, G258R, A272V, R311Q, p.A361_P362del), 1 (A217PfsX8) was repeatedly found in individuals with BIS, PDK and/or HM as well as in unaffected carriers, and 7 (E23K, P45S, P138A, D147H, P215R, P216L, R217Q) were previously observed in the general population (listed in Exome Variant Server, dbSNP or in the 1000 genomes project, Table S6). After stratification for European ancestry, we did not observe significant enrichment of coding sequence variants in the patient sample compared with controls (Table 1). This absence of enrichment was also observed when only variants predicted as deleterious were taken into account.

In the patient sample, we were able to ascertain the inheritance of the variants for 10 families and found that all mutations were inherited. Interestingly, the majority of the mutations were inherited from the mother (9/10; P = 0.012). In two individuals with ASD from sub-Saharan African origin, a 6 bp in-frame deletion (p.A361_P362del) was identified. The variant was transmitted by unaffected mothers and never observed in any individuals from our study and from other *PRRT2* mutation screening or in the 1000 genomes (>2000 controls). The genomes of these two individuals were investigated using the Illumina 1M Duo SNP array. Using Identity by state (IBS) analysis, we showed that these two individuals were not relatives (Table S7), but were clustered with individuals from South Africa and Kenya (Fig. S2). This *PRRT2* deletion of 2 conserved amino acids occurs in a predicted transmembrane domain of a specific isoform of *PRRT2* (Figure 1). *In silico* prediction using the PSORT software suggests however that the deletion does not disrupt the transmembrane domain of this isoform.

In the control sample, we identified one individual carrying the frameshift mutation A217PfsX8 already described as causing autosomal dominant ICCA, BIS, PKD, HM or epilepsy) [18–21]. This control individual had no history of psychiatric and neurological disorders. To further explore the prevalence of

Table 1. *PRRT2* coding variants identified in individuals with ASD and controls.

Variants	dbSNP/EVS/1KG	Inheritance	Ethnicity	Polyphen2	ASD (All; European ancestry)	Controls from European ancestry	Odds ratio [.95 CI][c]	P value[c]
E23K[a]	1KG_16_29824442	ND	2 Europe	Benign	2/431; 2/261	0/186		
P138A[a]	rs79182085	ND	1 Asia	Benign	1/431; 0/261	0/186		
D147H[a]	rs79568162	Maternal	1 Asia	Benign	1/431; 0/261	0/186		
A214P[a]	-	4 Maternal	1 Asia, 1 Europe, 2 Africa	Damaging	4/726; 1/474	0/272		
P216L[a]	rs76335820	2 Maternal, 1 Paternal, 5 ND	6 Europe, 1 mixed, 1 ND	Damaging	8/726; 6/474	8/272		
A217PfsX8	-	ND	1 Europe	Damaging	0/726; 0/474	1/272		
S249P	-	ND	1 mixed	Damaging	1/726; 0/474	0/272		
p.A361_P362del	-	2 Maternal	2 Sub Saharan Africa	Damaging[b]	2/431; 0/261	0/186		
P382A	-	Maternal	1 mixed	Damaging	1/431; 0/261	0/186		
All variants					17/431; 6/261	6/186	0.71 [0.23–2.24]	0.77
All damaging					13/431; 3/261	6/186	0.36 [0.09–1.44]	0.17

[a]Variants observed in the human genome diversity panel.
[b]The p.A361_P362del was considered as probably damaging since it affects conserved amino acids of PRRT2.
[c]Odds ratio, confidence intervals (CI) and P values were calculated only for populations from European ancestry using a 2-tailed Fisher exact test.

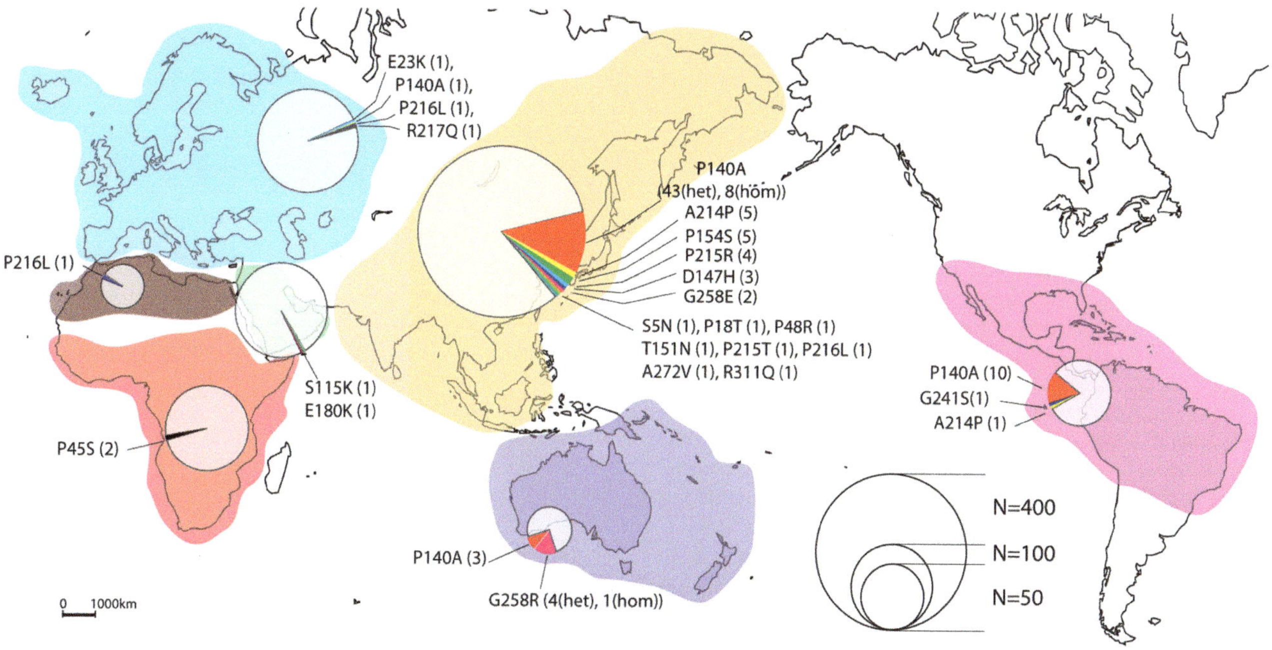

Figure 2. *PRRT2* variants identified in individuals from worldwide populations. A total of 961 individuals from the human genome diversity panel (HGDP) were sequenced for all *PRRT2* exons. The diameter of each circle is proportional to the number of individuals who were sequenced for *PRRT2*.

A217PfsX8, we screened an additional sample of 295 individuals with ASD and 92 controls. Overall, A217PfsX8 was observed only in the control described above and not detected in any of the other 277 controls, 726 individuals with ASD and in any of the 961 individuals from the HGDP.

We used a panel of DNA from individuals originated from worldwide populations (Figure 2, Table S4 and S5). We could identify 21 nonsynonymous *PRRT2* variants and trace the possible origin of them. For example, the predicted damaging P140A is a relatively frequent polymorphism present in Asia (7%), Oceania (5%), in Native American (7%), but more rare in Europe (allele frequency <1%). The A214P variant was observed in Asian (allele frequency <1%) and Native American populations. The P216L was observed in North Africa (allele frequency 1,7%), Europe (<1%) and Asia (<1%). Interestingly, we observed a higher ratio of nonsynonymous *vs* synonymous variants in Asia compared with Africa. In Asia, we found only 1 synonymous variant (E127E) carried by a single individual (allelic frequency of synonymous variants: 1/878 = 0.12%) and 15 nonsynonymous variants (S5N, P18T, P48R, P140A, D147H, T151N, P154S, A214P, P215T, P215R, P216L, G258E, A272V, R311Q) carried by 78 individuals (allelic frequency of nonsynonymous variants: 86/878 = 9,8%). In contrast, in Africa, we found 3 synonymous variants (P215P, L251L, C276C) carried by 7 individuals (allelic frequency of synonymous variants: 8/216 = 3.7%) and only 1 nonsynonymous variant (P45S) carried by 2 individuals (allelic frequency of nonsynonymous variants: 2/216 = 0.92%).

To evaluate selective constraints on PRRT2 in the different populations, we estimated pN/pS the ratio of nonsynonymous (pN) to synonymous polymorphism (pS) in each population sample (Table 2). Usually, most nonsynonymous changes would be expected to be eliminated by purifying selection, but under certain conditions positive Darwinian selection may lead to their retention [24]. Investigating the number of synonymous and non-synonymous substitutions therefore provides information about the degree of selection operating on a gene. A pN/pS ratio greater

Table 2. Synonymous and nonsynonymous variations of *PRRT2* in worldwide populations.

Ethnic	Nonsynonymous variants	Synonymous variants	pN (nonsynonymous variants/ nonsynonymous sites)[a]	pS (synonymous variants/ synonymous sites)[a]	pN/pS
EVS Europe (N = 4300)	14	3	0.021	0.013	1.62
EVS African-American (N = 2012)	6	8	0.009	0.035	0.26
HGDP Asia (N = 439)	14	1	0.021	0.004	4.85
HGDP Africa (N = 108)	1	2	0.001	0.009	0.17
HGDP Europe (N = 159)	4	0	0.006	0.000	>1.5[b]

[a]Number of nonsynonymous and synonymous sites for PRRT2 are 668.5 and 231.5, respectively.
[b]For the calculation of the pN/pS for Europe, the value of pS was set to 0.004 (the minimum of 1 synonymous variant observed in 159 individuals).

than one implies positive Darwinian selection; less than one implies purifying (stabilizing) selection; and a ratio of one indicates neutral (i.e. no) selection [25]. The calculation of the pN/pS ratio in the different populations revealed sign of positive Darwinian selective pressure on PRRT2 in Asia (pN/pS = 4.85) compared to Africa (pN/pS = 0.17; Fischer exact test P = 0.000087). For Europe (pN/pS>1.5), there was a trend for higher nonsynonymous mutations compared to Africa (Fischer exact test P = 0.057). We therefore tested if this difference was also observed between American European and American African populations available in the Exome Variant Server database (Table 2). Using this large dataset of 4300 individuals from European ancestry and 2012 individuals from African ancestry, we could confirm that there was a significant increase of nonsynonymous variants in Europe (pN/pS = 1.62) compared to Africa (pN/pS = 0.26) (Fischer exact test P = 0.00035). Finally, we observed a trend for higher frequency of nonsynonymous variants in Asia compared to Europe (Fischer exact test P = 0.084). As expected, there was no difference between populations from the HGDP and those from EVS (Africa HGDP *vs* Africa EVS P = 0.67; Europe HGDP *vs* Europe EVS P = 1). In order to test whether this difference in selective pressure was specific to *PRRT2*, we used the data from EVS and extended our pN/pS calculation to all genes included in the 16p11.2 deletion (Figure 3; Table S8). We observed that the majority of the genes had a very similar pN/pS in Europe and Africa. Only C16orf92 showed a higher pN/pS in Africa compared to Europe. In contrast, ASPHD1, YPEL3, MAPK3 and PRRT2 showed a higher pN/pS in Europe compared to Africa. However, *PRRT2* was the only gene with a pN/pS significantly different in Europe and Africa after correction for multiple testing.

During the screening of the recurrent frameshift mutation 'A217PfsX8', we used whole genome amplified DNA for three individuals with ASD. Strikingly, we observed the A217PfsX8 mutation in these three samples for which the DNA was amplified using rolling circle amplification protocol (Genomiph from GEHealthcare) (Figure 4). We obtained the native DNA from these three individuals and found that they were actually not carrying the A217PfsX8 mutation. We then re-amplified the native DNA from these three individuals using another RCA protocol (REPLI-g Mini method from QIAGEN). After direct sequencing of the PCR products, the A217PfsX8 frameshift mutation was again present. Based on these results, we strongly advise that *PRRT2* mutation screening should not be performed on DNA previously amplified through RCA.

Discussion

Both deletions and duplications at 16p11.2 increase the risk for ASD, but the genes and the mechanisms involved remain largely unknown. Whereas several other strong candidate genes including the *KCTD13* gene are located within the deletion and can be considered possible driver(s) as well [26], *PRRT2* was indeed a very compelling candidate. Homozygous PRRT2 mutations were associated with clinical features also observed in a subset of individuals with ASD such as intellectual disability and epilepsy. *PRRT2* encodes a putative membrane protein, localized at the synaptic membrane and interacting with SNAP25, a member of the SNARE protein complex involved in the release of synaptic vesicles. Our study was designed to identify new coding variants of *PRRT2* in a relatively large sample of individuals with ASD and to ascertain the genetic variability of the gene in worldwide populations.

We could not find any deleterious *PRRT2* mutation enrichment in individuals with ASD compared with controls. None of the patients tested were deleted or duplicated for the 16p11.2 locus. In addition, we did not find causative *PRRT2* mutations previously associated with neurological diseases such as PDK, ICCA, epilepsy or migraine in our cohort of patients. We observed a significant enrichment of maternally transmitted mutations in the individuals with ASD (9/10 transmitted by the mother). However, this apparent disequilibrium might have occurred by chance since to our knowledge, no transmission disequilibrium was reported for

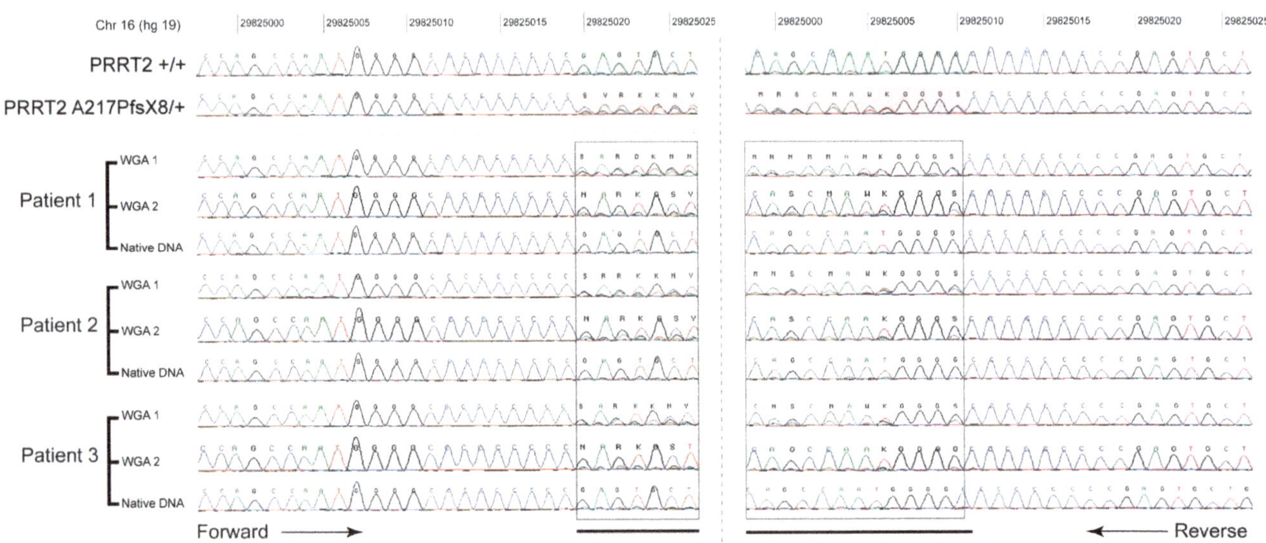

Figure 3. Genetic variability in Europe and Africa for all genes located within the 16p11.2 deletion. A. Nonsynonymous mutations per nonsynonymous sites (pN) and synonymous mutations per synonymous sites (pS) were estimated using the data from 4300 individuals from European ancestry and 2012 individuals from African ancestry available at the Exome Variant Server (http://evs.gs.washington.edu/EVS/). The horizontal lanes correspond to the means of pN and pS for the 27 genes. Difference of pN/pS between Europe and Africa were calculated using a 2-tailed Fisher exact test and the $-\text{Log}_{10}$ P value is indicated. B. Plot of the $-\text{Log}_{10}$ P values obtained for the difference between the pN/pS ratio in Africa and in Europe in relation the ratio (Europe pN/pS)/(Africa pN/pS).

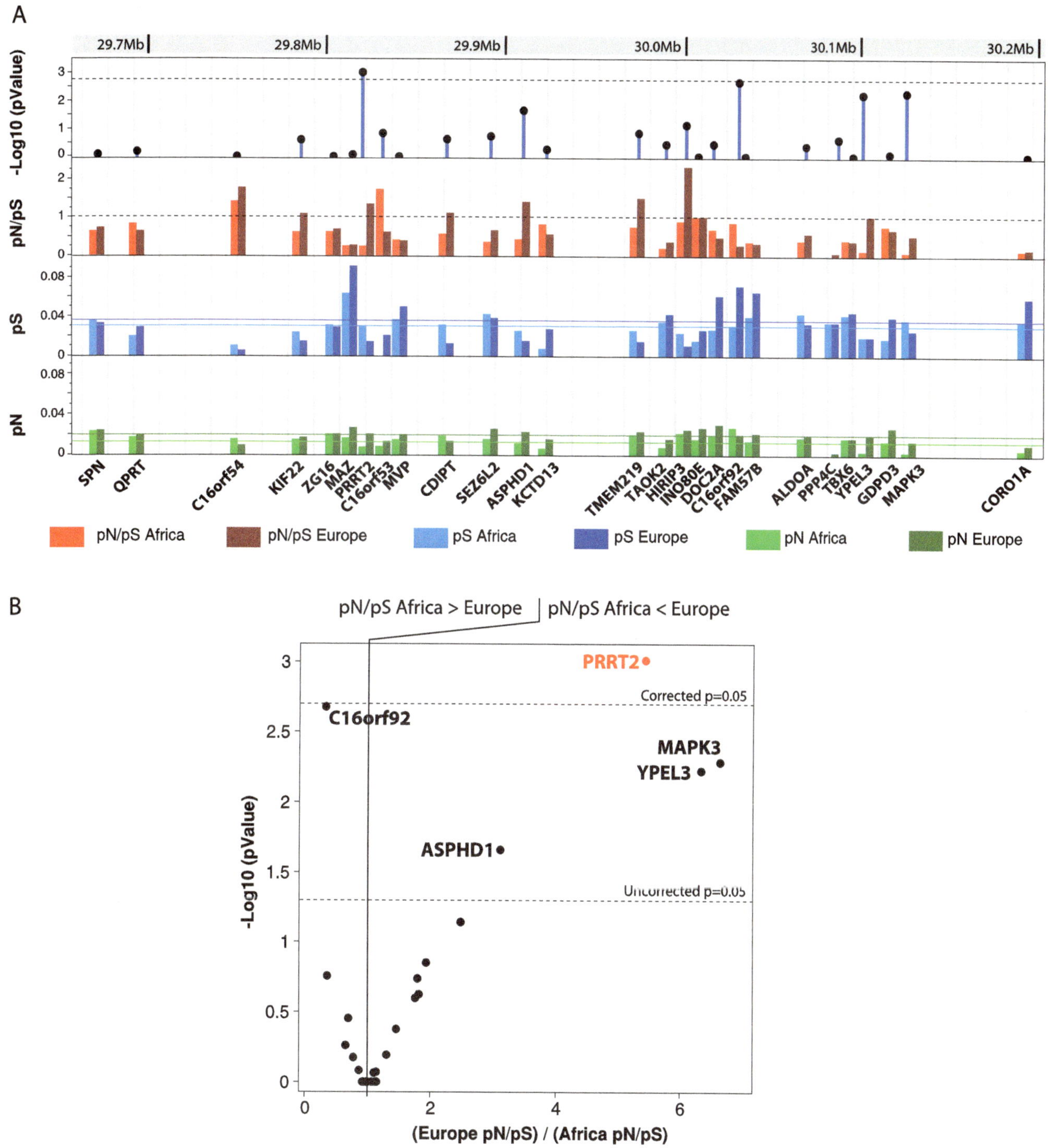

Figure 4. Chromatograms of the *PRRT2* A217PfsX8 mutation before and after whole genome amplification. The chromatograms of *PRRT2* sequence before (Native DNA) and after whole genome amplification of the DNA from three independent patients using two different protocols GenomiPhi DNA Amplification Kit (WGA-1) or Repli-G Whole Genome Amplification kit (WGA-2). The mutation was not present in the native DNA, but was detected after whole genome amplification.

PRRT2 mutations in other neurological diseases. Taken together, these results indicate that mutations in *PRRT2* are not a frequent cause of autism. Our study cannot however exclude that, in individuals with 16p11.2 deletions, haploinsufficiency of *PRRT2* could increase the risk of ASD.

Secondly, we detected the presence of the deleterious truncating mutation A217PfsX8 in a control (of note the DNA of this individual was not whole genome amplified). This man had no psychiatric diseases and, to his knowledge, no history of any psychiatric disorders in his first and second degree relatives (parents and grand parents). This individual had no diagnostic for migraine and epilepsy, but was unavailable for further clinical explorations in order to detect mild signs of neurological problems. Similar incomplete penetrance of the A217PfsX8 mutation was observed in carriers from families with ICCA syndrome [21]. Based on the literature, the penetrance of the A217PfsX8 mutation was estimated to 94% [27]. It remains unknown if additional genetic variants could act as suppressors in the unaffected individuals carrying the A217PfsX8 mutation.

Thirdly, we ascertained the genetic variability of *PRRT2* in worldwide populations. We identified 21 novel nonsynonymous variants including 17 never reported before and 4 already listed in the nucleotide variant database (Table S6). Despite the relatively large number of chromosomes tested and the population diversity, we did not observe any truncating mutations. Most of the nonsynonymous variants are restricted to one population (D147H, P154S, E180K, P215R, G241S, G258E and G258R) or to closely related populations (A214P and P216L). One variant P140A was frequently observed in different populations with a shared genetic origin (Asia, Native American and Oceania). Overall, the low rate (<1%) of nonsynonymous mutation indicates that *PRRT2* is under strong selective pressure. Nevertheless, our results also revealed a heterogenous pattern of selective pressure acting on *PRRT2* in human populations. The low pN/pS ratio in Africa indicates *PRRT2* is under the usual purifying selection (as for the majority of the genome), whereas the pN/pS ratio in Asia and Europe is higher than expected and consistent with positive Darwinian selection [28]. To date, we have no explanation for this observation. Within the 16p11.2 deletion, *PRRT2* seems to be the gene with the higher difference of selective pressure between Europe and Africa, but addition samples should be screened to ascertain if this difference is specific to *PRRT2* or is also true for other genes within the deletion. Considering this heterogeneous pattern of selective pressure, it would be interesting to see if there is a higher prevalence of *PRRT2* related disease in Asia and Europe compared to Africa. It would also be interesting to explore the genetic diversity of the binding partners of *PRRT2* in order to decipher whether this lower selective pressure is restricted to *PRRT2* or to other members of the same pathway.

Finally, we showed that whole genome amplification using multiple displacement amplification technology such as Genomi-Phi and Repli-G could lead to the appearance of the A217PfsX8 mutation. The genomic region surrounding the mutation is made of 4 guanines and 9 cytosines and seems therefore to be at risk for mutation both *in vivo* and *in vitro*. For this reason, we strongly suggest that *PRRT2* mutation screening should be restricted to native DNA and validate using Sanger sequencing. Interestingly, in the last release of the Exome Variant Server database, at the same location of the A217PfsX8 mutation (hg19, chr16: 29825015), 10% of the *PRRT2* allele contains an additional C (allele A1 in EVS) and 10% have a deletion of a C (allele A2 in EVS), but with very low average sample read depth (N = 10). Given the very high penetrance of the A217PfsX8 mutation in PRRT2-related diseases, it is impossible that 20% of the *PRRT2* alleles carry a frame shift mutation at this position. Especially, since we found the A217PfsX8 mutation in only 1 individual out of 1990 (Allelic frequency = 0.025%). This high frequency of A217PfsX8 mutation in EVS could be related to the DNA amplification step required for whole exome sequencing. Studying the mechanism leading to the A217PfsX8 mutation was beyond the scope of our study, but our observation that a DNA amplification step through RCA could introduce this additional C/G might help in understanding the mechanism leading to A217PfsX8 mutation.

In summary, our study indicates that *PRRT2* mutations do not play a major role in the susceptibility to ASD and confirm that truncating mutations of *PRRT2* are not fully penetrant. We also provide an ascertainment of the genetic diversity of *PRRT2* in worldwide populations as well as important indication on the pitfalls for the mutation screening. All together, these results should help researchers and clinicians to better investigate the role of *PRRT2* in human diseases.

Supporting Information

Figure S1 Sequence coverage of PRRT2 in Exome Variants Serveur. Total number of sample sequenced (in blue) and average read depth (purple) for *PRRT2* in Exome Variant server. The nucleotide positions are according to PRRT2 from NCBI37/hg19. The average coverage of 10×, 20× and 40× are indicated in red, yellow and green respectively.

Figure S2 Multiple dimension scale (MDS) of the genetic distances between individuals from the Human Genome Diversity Pannel. Insert. MDS restricted to the African populations including the two individuals with ASD carrying the in frame deletion p.A361_P362del (triangles).

Table S1 Cohorts used in this study.

Table S2 Ethnicity of the cohorts.

Table S3 PRRT2 primers.

Table S4 PRRT2 nonsynonymous variants identified in the HGDP.

Table S5 PRRT2 synonymous variants identified in the HGDP.

Table S6 PRRT2 coding variants present in dbSNP, Exome variant Server (EVS) and the 1000 genome project (1KG).

Table S7 Identity by state (IBS) values for the 2 individuals with ASD carrying the mutation p.A361_P362del compared with the IBS from different African populations.

Table S8 Evolutionary analysis of all genes located within the 16p11.2 deletion.

Acknowledgments

We thank the DNA and cell bank of Cochin hospital and of the CRICM, the Plateforme de Ressource Biologique (B. Ghaleh), the Clinical Investigation Centers of Mondor-Chenevier and Robert Debré hospitals for their assistance, and the Psychiatric Genetics team (Stéphane Jamain) of Inserm U955 for collection and management of DNAs. We thank D. diMoreno for careful reading of the manuscript. We thank C. Bouchier for the use of sequencing facilities and B. Regnault and L. Lemée for the Illumina genotyping arrays at the Institut Pasteur Génopole.

Author Contributions

Conceived and designed the experiments: GH NL EE CN TB PS CD. Performed the experiments: GH CN NL. Analyzed the data: GH TB EP GL. Contributed reagents/materials/analysis tools: AB ML CG CD RD. Wrote the paper: GH RD TB.

References

1. Association AP (1994) Diagnostic and Statistical Manual of Mental Disorders, Fourth Edition. Washington, DC: APA.
2. Baio J (2012) Prevalence of autism spectrum disorders–Autism and Developmental Disabilities Monitoring Network, 14 sites, United States, 2008. MMWR Surveill Summ 61: 1–19.
3. Huguet G, Ey E, Bourgeron T (2013) The Genetic Landscapes of Autism Spectrum Disorders. Annu Rev Genomics Hum Genet 14: 191–213.
4. Pinto D, Pagnamenta AT, Klei L, Anney R, Merico D, et al. (2010) Functional impact of global rare copy number variation in autism spectrum disorders. Nature 466: 368–372
5. Sanders SJ, Ercan-Sencicek AG, Hus V, Luo R, Murtha MT, et al. (2011) Multiple recurrent de novo CNVs, including duplications of the 7q11.23 Williams syndrome region, are strongly associated with autism. Neuron 70: 863–885.
6. Toro R, Konyukh M, Delorme R, Leblond C, Chaste P, et al. (2010) Key role for gene dosage and synaptic homeostasis in autism spectrum disorders. Trends Genet 26: 363–372.
7. Jacquemont S, Reymond A, Zufferey F, Harewood L, Walters RG, et al. (2011) Mirror extreme BMI phenotypes associated with gene dosage at the chromosome 16p11.2 locus. Nature 478: 97–102.
8. Barge-Schaapveld DQ, Maas SM, Polstra A, Knegt LC, Hennekam RC (2011) The atypical 16p11.2 deletion: a not so atypical microdeletion syndrome? Am J Med Genet A 155A: 1066–1072.
9. Crepel A, Steyaert J, De la Marche W, De Wolf V, Fryns JP, et al. (2011) Narrowing the critical deletion region for autism spectrum disorders on 16p11.2. Am J Med Genet B Neuropsychiatr Genet 156: 243–245.
10. Ballif BC, Hornor SA, Jenkins E, Madan-Khetarpal S, Surti U, et al. (2007) Discovery of a previously unrecognized microdeletion syndrome of 16p11.2-p12.2. Nat Genet 39: 1071–1073.
11. Kumar RA, KaraMohamed S, Sudi J, Conrad DF, Brune C, et al. (2008) Recurrent 16p11.2 microdeletions in autism. Hum Mol Genet 17: 628–638.
12. Weiss LA, Shen Y, Korn JM, Arking DE, Miller DT, et al. (2008) Association between microdeletion and microduplication at 16p11.2 and autism. N Engl J Med 358: 667–675.
13. McCarthy SE, Makarov V, Kirov G, Addington AM, McClellan J, et al. (2009) Microduplications of 16p11.2 are associated with schizophrenia. Nat Genet 41: 1223–1227.
14. Walters RG, Jacquemont S, Valsesia A, de Smith AJ, Martinet D, et al. (2010) A new highly penetrant form of obesity due to deletions on chromosome 16p11.2. Nature 463: 671–675.
15. Kumar RA, Marshall CR, Badner JA, Babatz TD, Mukamel Z, et al. (2009) Association and mutation analyses of 16p11.2 autism candidate genes. PLoS One 4: e4582.
16. Konyukh M, Delorme R, Chaste P, Leblond C, Lemiere N, et al. (2011) Variations of the candidate SEZ6L2 gene on Chromosome 16p11.2 in patients with autism spectrum disorders and in human populations. PLoS One 6: e17289.
17. Najmabadi H, Hu H, Garshasbi M, Zemojtel T, Abedini SS, et al. (2011) Deep sequencing reveals 50 novel genes for recessive cognitive disorders. Nature 478: 57–63.
18. Chen WJ, Lin Y, Xiong ZQ, Wei W, Ni W, et al. (2011) Exome sequencing identifies truncating mutations in PRRT2 that cause paroxysmal kinesigenic dyskinesia. Nat Genet 43: 1252–1255.
19. Cloarec R, Bruneau N, Rudolf G, Massacrier A, Salmi M, et al. (2012) PRRT2 links infantile convulsions and paroxysmal dyskinesia with migraine. Neurology 79: 2097–2103.
20. Gardiner AR, Bhatia KP, Stamelou M, Dale RC, Kurian MA, et al. (2012) PRRT2 gene mutations: from paroxysmal dyskinesia to episodic ataxia and hemiplegic migraine. Neurology 79: 2115–2121.
21. Lee HY, Huang Y, Bruneau N, Roll P, Roberson ED, et al. (2012) Mutations in the novel protein PRRT2 cause paroxysmal kinesigenic dyskinesia with infantile convulsions. Cell Rep 1: 2–12.
22. Cann HM, de Toma C, Cazes L, Legrand MF, Morel V, et al. (2002) A human genome diversity cell line panel. Science 296: 261–262.
23. Librado P, Rozas J (2009) DnaSP v5: a software for comprehensive analysis of DNA polymorphism data. Bioinformatics 25: 1451–1452.
24. Kelley JL, Swanson WJ (2008) Positive selection in the human genome: from genome scans to biological significance. Annu Rev Genomics Hum Genet 9: 143–160.
25. McDonald JH, Kreitman M (1991) Adaptive protein evolution at the Adh locus in Drosophila. Nature 351: 652–654.
26. Golzio C, Willer J, Talkowski ME, Oh EC, Taniguchi Y, et al. (2012) KCTD13 is a major driver of mirrored neuroanatomical phenotypes of the 16p11.2 copy number variant. Nature 485: 363–367.
27. Becker F, Schubert J, Striano P, Anttonen AK, Liukkonen E, et al. (2013) PRRT2-related disorders: further PKD and ICCA cases and review of the literature. J Neurol 260: 1234–1244.
28. Tennessen JA, Bigham AW, O'Connor TD, Fu W, Kenny EE, et al. (2012) Evolution and functional impact of rare coding variation from deep sequencing of human exomes. Science 337: 64–69.

16

Soy Infant Formula and Seizures in Children with Autism

Cara J. Westmark*

Department of Neurology, University of Wisconsin, Madison, Wisconsin, United States of America

Abstract

Seizures are a common phenotype in many neurodevelopmental disorders including fragile X syndrome, Down syndrome and autism. We hypothesized that phytoestrogens in soy-based infant formula were contributing to lower seizure threshold in these disorders. Herein, we evaluated the dependence of seizure incidence on infant formula in a population of autistic children. Medical record data were obtained on 1,949 autistic children from the SFARI Simplex Collection. An autism diagnosis was determined by scores on the ADI-R and ADOS exams. The database included data on infant formula use, seizure incidence, the specific type of seizure exhibited and IQ. Soy-based formula was utilized in 17.5% of the study population. Females comprised 13.4% of the subjects. There was a 2.6-fold higher rate of febrile seizures [4.2% versus 1.6%, OR = 2.6, 95% CI = 1.3–5.3], a 2.1-fold higher rate of epilepsy comorbidity [3.6% versus 1.7%, OR = 2.2, 95% CI = 1.1–4.7] and a 4-fold higher rate of simple partial seizures [1.2% versus 0.3%, OR = 4.8, 95% CI = 1.0–23] in the autistic children fed soy-based formula. No statistically significant associations were found with other outcomes including: IQ, age of seizure onset, infantile spasms and atonic, generalized tonic clonic, absence and complex partial seizures. Limitations of the study included: infant formula and seizure data were based on parental recall, there were significantly less female subjects, and there was lack of data regarding critical confounders such as the reasons the subjects used soy formula, age at which soy formula was initiated and the length of time on soy formula. Despite these limitations, our results suggest that the use of soy-based infant formula may be associated with febrile seizures in both genders and with a diagnosis of epilepsy in males in autistic children. Given the lack of data on critical confounders and the retrospective nature of the study, a prospective study is required to confirm the association.

Editor: Stephen D. Ginsberg, Nathan Kline Institute and New York University School of Medicine, United States of America

Funding: This work was supported by FRAXA Research Foundation (www.fraxa.org) and National Institutes of Health (NIH) (www.nih.gov) [1UL1RR025011 and 9U54TR000021]. The funders had no role in study design, data collection and analysis, decision to publish, or preparation of the manuscript.

Competing Interests: The author has declared that no competing interests exist.

* E-mail: westmark@wisc.edu

Introduction

Autism is a cluster of complex neurobiological disorders known as autism spectrum disorders. The core features include impairments in social interaction and communication, and repetitive stereotyped behavior. Autism is estimated to occur in 1 in 88 children with prevalence 4.7-fold higher in males [1]. The etiology of autism is not known but genetic as well as environmental factors likely affect the severity of symptoms [2–4]. Our findings in rodent models of neurological disease demonstrate that soy ingestion during a critical period of sensory development significantly increases seizure activity [5]. Mouse colonies are typically maintained on Purina-type lab chows, which are grain-based with their protein content derived from soybeans [6]. Soybeans are rich in phytoestrogens, "plant estrogens", which are transferred to offspring through the placenta as well as maternal milk [7]. The steady-state level of phytoestrogens found in serum (2,338±531 ng/mL) of Purina-fed mice is greater than endogenous estrogen levels by at least 30,000-fold and has immense potential to affect development [8]. The soy phytoestrogen daidzein was identified as a seizure-promoting ingredient in mice [5]. Thus, we hypothesized that the use of soy-based infant formulas could be contributing to seizure incidence in autism and other neurodevelopmental disorders.

While there are many health benefits for adults that are associated with the consumption of soy products in terms of prevention of age-related cardiovascular disease and osteoporosis [9,10], there is a paucity of studies on the effects of phytoestrogens on fetal and early childhood development [11–16]. Nearly a quarter of infant formulas are based on soy protein and have high phytoestrogen levels approaching 4.5–8 mg/kg/day [17,18]. Considering body weight, these infants are getting six to 11 times the dose of phytoestrogens necessary to exert hormone-like effects in adults [17]. In placental mammals, the fetus is continuously exposed to high levels of estrogen from the placenta and the mother. Studies in pregnant rats demonstrate that the placenta acts as a sink for phytoestrogens, and that while transport of phytoestrogens across the placenta is inefficient, low levels are found in the fetus and are sufficient for activation of estrogen receptor beta [19]. Thus, environmental exposure to phytoestrogens or synthetic estrogens during gestation and/or postnatal development could disrupt the function of the natural steroid hormones and contribute to the incidence of idiopathic disorders such as autism. The aim of this retrospective study was to determine if there was an association between seizure incidence and the use of soy-based infant formula by utilizing medical record data available through the Simons Foundation Autism Research Initiative (SFARI) Simplex Collection, which is a medical record database and biological specimen resource for the identification of genetic risk factors for autism. We present data below suggesting a potential association between the use of soy-based infant formula and increased incidence of febrile seizures, simple partial seizures and epilepsy in autistic children.

Results

Demographics

The population for this study was defined as all probands in the Simons Simplex Collection who had non-null medical record data for the type of infant formula used. Demographics indicate that there were 86.6% males and 13.4% females in a population size of 1,949 autistic children. The 6.5-fold increase in the number of male subjects is supported by epidemiological data indicating that autism is 4.7-fold more prevalent in boys than girls [1]. Soy-based infant formula was used by 17.6% of the male and 17% of the female probands (Table 1). The cohorts have similar population characteristics regarding ethnicity, age at evaluation, birth weight, and scores on the ABC, ADI-R and ADOS.

Seizure and epilepsy rates

There was a 2.6-fold higher rate of febrile seizures in the soy-fed cohort (4.2% seizures with soy and 1.6% seizures without soy) (odds ratio = 2.6, 95% confidence interval 1.3–5.3; $P = 0.003$) (Table 2). The results were statistically significant for females (9% seizures with soy and 1.4% seizures without soy) (odds ratio = 7.2, 95% confidence interval 1.3–42; $P = 0.02$) with a Bonferroni correction for gender comparisons, but were not statistically significant in males (3.4% seizures with soy and 1.7% seizures without soy) (odds ratio = 2.1, 95% confidence interval 0.92–4.7; $P = 0.050$). The prevalence of childhood epilepsy in the general population is 0.63% [21]. In this autism cohort, epilepsy prevalence ranged from 1.6–3.8% dependent on gender and diet (Table 2). A comorbid diagnosis of autism and epilepsy was more prevalent in males fed soy-based formula (odds ratio = 2.4, 95% confidence interval 1.1–5.2; $P = 0.02$) than females (odds ratio = 1.4, 95% confidence interval 0.056–14; $P = 0.8$). Febrile seizures are associated with an increased incidence of epilepsy [22]. In this study population, there was no overlap between subjects that reported epilepsy and febrile seizures. However, there were only 39 subjects reporting febrile seizures. Epilepsy developed by seven years of age in 2% of children who had experienced at least one febrile seizure [22]; thus, we would predict less than one subject in our study population with both epilepsy and febrile seizures.

The soy-based formula was not associated with statistically significant higher rates of infantile spasms, atonic (drop attack), generalized tonic clonic (grand mal), absence (petit mal), or complex partial seizures for either gender albeit many of these seizure types were very infrequent (Table 2). Although not statistically significant, infantile spasms (three cases total) were only observed in the males and were higher in soy-fed infants (odds ratio = 9.5, 95% confidence interval 0.68–265; $P = 0.08$). Simple partial seizures (eight cases total) were higher with soy-based formula for both genders but only reached statistical significance when combining the data (odds ratio = 4.8, 95% confidence interval 1.0–23; $P = 0.04$). Thus, a larger study population is necessary to confirm whether the use of soy-based infant formula is associated with higher rates of infantile spasms and simple partial

Table 1. Characteristics of the Autistic Population.

		Soy Formula	Non-Soy Formula
Population Size, % (N)	**Male**	17.6 (297)	82.4 (1391)
	Female	17 (44)	83.1 (217)
Ethnicity Males, %	**African American**	5.1	3.4
	Asian	2.4	4.2
	Other[a]	13.5	13.8
	White	79.1	78.6
Ethnicity Females, %	**African American**	9	3.2
	Asian	5	3.2
	Other[a]	9	11.1
	White	77	82.5
Age at Evaluation, Years (SD)	**Male**	9.2 (3.8)	8.9 (3.6)
	Female	8.3 (3.4)	9.0 (3.7)
Birth Weight, Pounds (SD)	**Male**	7.1 (1.2)	7.3 (1.2)
	Female	6.7 (1.1)	7.0 (1.2)
ABC Score, Mean (SD)	**Male**	48.3 (25.4)	46.2 (26.2)
	Female	49.0 (28.0)	46.1 (24.0)
ADI-R Score[b], Mean (SD)	**Male**	36.6 (8.9)	35.9 (9.3)
	Female	36.5 (9.7)	36.1 (10.0)
ADOS Score[c], Mean (SD)	**Male**	28.2 (8.9)	28.4 (9.0)
	Female	28.8 (8.5)	29.3 (9.8)

[a]Other in the Ethnicity category includes other, not specified, more than one race, Native American, and Native Hawaiian.
[b]ADI-R total score is the sum of the Reciprocal Social Interaction, Nonverbal and Repetitive Behavior/Stereotyped Patterns scores. The Verbal score was omitted in order to include both verbal and nonverbal participants.
[c]ADOS total score is the sum of the Communication and Social Interaction, Restricted and Repetitive Behavior, and Social Affect scores.

Table 2. Prevalence of Seizures in Autistic Subjects Dependent on Soy Formula.

	Male		Female		Combined	
Phenotype, % (N)	**Soy**	**Non-Soy**	**Soy**	**Non-Soy**	**Soy**	**Non-Soy**
Febrile Seizures	3.4[a] (290)	1.7 (1368)	9[b] (43)	1.4 (213)	4.2[c] (333)	1.6 (1581)
Epilepsy Diagnosis	3.8[d] (291)	1.6 (1352)	3 (39)	1.9 (211)	3.6[e] (330)	1.7 (1563)
Infantile Spasms	0.7 (292)	0.1 (1377)	0 (42)	0 (215)	0.6 (334)	0.1 (1592)
Atonic Seizures	0.3 (291)	0.2 (1377)	0 (42)	0 (215)	0.3 (333)	0.1 (1592)
Tonic Clonic Seizures	1.4 (291)	1.7 (1378)	0 (42)	3.7 (216)	1.2 (333)	1.9 (1594)
Absence Seizures	3.4 (291)	2.0 (1378)	2 (42)	2.3 (216)	3.3 (333)	2.0 (1594)
Simple Partial Seizures	1.0 (292)	0.3 (1377)	2 (42)	0 (215)	1.2[f] (334)	0.3 (1592)
Complex Partial Seizures	0.3 (291)	0.4 (1377)	2 (42)	0.4 (215)	0.6 (333)	0.4 (1592)

N = number of subjects in cohort.
[a]$P = 0.050$ as determined by the Pearson's uncorrected chi-squared test, OR = 2.1, 95% CI = 0.92–4.7.
[b]$P = 0.02$ as determined by Fisher's exact test (two-tail), OR = 7.2, 95% CI = 1.3–42.
[c]$P = 0.003$ as determined by the Pearson's uncorrected chi-squared test, OR = 2.6, 95% CI = 1.3–5.3.
[d]$P = 0.02$ as determined by the Pearson's uncorrected chi-squared test, OR = 2.4, 95% CI = 1.1–5.2.
[e]$P = 0.02$ as determined by the Pearson's uncorrected chi-squared test, OR = 2.2, 95% CI = 1.1–4.7.
[f]$P = 0.04$ as determined by Fisher's exact test (two-tail), OR = 4.8, 95% CI = 1.0–23.

seizures in both boy and girls with autism. The age of seizure onset (Table 3) and IQ (Table 4) were not statistically different dependent on infant formula (Student T-test, $P = 0.9$ for soy versus non-soy in both males and females for age of onset of febrile seizures; $P = 0.3$ for soy versus non-soy in both males and females for age of onset of non-febrile seizures; $P = 0.4$–0.5 for soy versus non-soy in both males and females for full-scale IQ and non-verbal IQ; $P = 0.6$–0.8 for soy versus non-soy in males and females for verbal IQ). In summary, our results suggest that soy-based infant formula may be associated with higher rates of febrile seizures, epilepsy and simple partial seizures in autistic children.

Discussion

In this autism-based population study, febrile seizures were 2.6-fold more prevalent in children fed soy-based formula. Febrile seizures are convulsions brought on by a fever in infants or small children. They are the most common type of childhood convulsive events occurring in 2–5% of children in Europe and North America and in 6–9% in Japan [23], an Asian country with a soy-rich diet. A diagnosis of epilepsy was also significantly elevated in association with the consumption of soy. The prevalence of epilepsy in autism is 21.4% in subjects with intellectual disability and 8% in subjects without intellectual disability [24]. Our study indicates a comorbidity of autism and epilepsy of 1.6–3.8% dependent on gender and diet. This is significantly higher than the general population, but lower than published reports of epilepsy in autism likely due to the inclusion criteria of probands with relatively little intellectual disability. The 2-fold difference in epilepsy comorbidity between soy (3.6%) and non-soy (1.7%) groups was statistically significant ($P = 0.02$). The 2.6-fold difference in febrile seizure rates between soy (4.2%) and non-soy (1.6%) cohorts was highly statistically significant ($P = 0.003$). These may be considered by some readers as small percentages in each group who had seizures, but the two-fold or greater differences between soy and non-soy diets are statistically significant. Pharmaceutical interventions that reduced the incidence of febrile seizures or epilepsy by 2-fold would be in demand, and we consider a possible dietary intervention equally relevant.

Table 3. Age of Seizure Onset with Soy-Based Formula.

		Febrile Seizures			Non-Febrile Seizures		
		Years	**SD**	**N**	**Years**	**SD**	**N**
Males	**Soy**	2.0	1.5	16	3.6	2.5	22
	Non-Soy	2.0	1.5	43	4.4	3.3	71
Females	**Soy**	2.0	1.7	5	2.1	1.3	3
	Non-Soy	1.9	1.1	7	4.0	3.0	11

Seizures are a serious and common phenotype in many neurological disorders besides autism and epilepsy including fragile X syndrome [25], Alzheimer's disease [26], Down syndrome [27], tuberous sclerosis [28] and Rett syndrome [29]. According to the Epilepsy Foundation, ten percent of the American population will experience a seizure in their lifetime; however, the underlying molecular mechanisms that cause seizures are not well understood. Seizure severity is likely a combination of both genetic and environmental factors. Our hypothesis is that the effects of an underlying genetic mutation that lowers seizure threshold may be exacerbated, for example, by dietary exposure to high concentrations of phytoestrogens. This would be particularly significant for individuals whose diet is solely soy-based, for example, soy-based infant and gastric tube feeding formulas. Nearly a quarter of infant formulas are soy-based; yet, there is no epidemiological data examining the incidence of seizures, autism, or the severity of fragile X syndrome and other developmental disorders in children fed soy-based versus non-soy-based formula.

The strength of this study design includes a large sample size of autistic children with comprehensive medical record histories. An autism diagnosis was based on ADI-R and ADOS scores. The limitations of the study include: (1) it is based on retrospective data regarding the type of formula, (2) the quality of the epilepsy data is declarative, (3) there is low statistical power regarding the gender comparison analyses, and (4) there is lack of data regarding confounding issues. Data regarding the type of formula consumed was based on parental recall, which is expected to decrease in accuracy as the length of recall increases. A diagnosis of epilepsy

Table 4. IQ with Soy-Based Formula.

		Full-Scale IQ			Non-Verbal IQ			Verbal IQ		
		Mean	SD	N	Mean	SD	N	Mean	SD	N
Males	**Soy**	80.1	27.8	293	83.3	25.8	294	77.1	31.6	294
	Non-Soy	81.5	28.1	1364	84.8	26.4	1366	78.2	31.3	1366
Females	**Soy**	72.0	28.7	41	74.8	25.1	41	72.3	35.0	41
	Non-Soy	75.5	27.7	212	78.2	26.1	212	74.1	31.2	212

was defined as either a specific report of epilepsy on the ADI-R or at least two seizures on the medical history report, which are also based on parental recall. This study is a retrospective analysis of an existing data set and a neurologist did not verify the diagnoses. However, according to NINDS, detailed medical history reports of seizure history are considered one of the best methods available to determine if a person has epilepsy and what kind of seizures he/she has (http://www.ninds.nih.gov/disorders/epilepsy/detail_epilepsy.htm#242093109). There were significantly less female subjects than males in accordance with current autism prevalence statistics. Despite this limitation, our results suggest that the use of soy-based infant formula may be associated with febrile seizures in females and with epilepsy in males. A larger female cohort is necessary to confirm whether the use of soy-based infant formula may be associated with epilepsy comorbidity in girls with autism. Data regarding critical confounders such as the reasons the subjects used soy formula, age at which soy formula was initiated and the length of time on soy formula are not available. It is possible that sick children who were fed soy-based formula for various diagnosed or undiagnosed health complications are somehow predisposed to seizures; thus, soy could be a surrogate marker for an underlying condition that lowers seizure threshold. If soy is the causative agent in seizure induction, it would be expected that infants fed soy formula at younger ages and/or for longer periods of time would exhibit an increased incidence of seizures. A prospective study will be required to address these confounding issues. A possible criticism is that subjects, who were fed soy-based infant formula because they were allergic to cow's milk, had allergies that made them vulnerable to illnesses associated with fever-induced convulsions. Though the retrospective nature of the data does not allow us to make definitive conclusions regarding this point, we found that 2.7% of females and 1.7% of males in the study population reported allergies, but no subjects reported both allergies and febrile seizures suggesting that this criticism may not be valid.

We found that the use of soy-based formula was a potential risk factor for increased seizure incidence and epilepsy in autism. Independent studies in other infant populations (typically developing, fragile X and Down syndrome) are necessary before a general association between increased seizure risk and soy-based formula can be established. Of note, the SFARI autism database is not representative of all ASD because of exclusion criteria that bar important genetic causes of both seizures and ASD. For example, fragile X syndrome is the leading genetic cause of autism and accounts for approximately 5% of autism cases [30]. The studied population exhibited moderate to severe autistic symptoms with relatively little intellectual disability. The excluded population would be expected to be much lower functioning and perhaps more affected by environmental factors such as soy phytoestrogens. We did not observe statistically significant differences in the age of seizure onset or IQ with the use of soy-based infant formula, albeit there was a trend for a younger age of non-febrile seizure onset and lower IQ. The mean age of non-febrile seizure onset was 2.1–4.4 years dependent on gender and diet. These data raise the questions - can soy ingestion during infancy alter brain development such that seizure threshold, IQ and/or behavior are affected later in life? The data collection strategy for the SFARI Simplex Collection was not designed to answer these types of questions. The findings described herein are suggestive of a link between soy exposure and seizures, and prospective evaluation is needed.

Methods

Ethics statement

The institutional review protocol governing the Simons Simplex Collection was approved by the Institutional Review Board at Columbia University Medical Center. Written informed consent was provided by all guardians or research subjects. The privacy of participants was protected by using global unique identifiers. The research protocol for using the Simons Simplex Collection in this study was approved by the Human Research Protection Program at the University of Wisconsin-Madison, which determined that the study qualified for exemption.

Participants

SFARI in collaboration with medical centers across North America collected high quality phenotype data and biospecimens from 2,644 autism simplex families beginning in 2008. A simplex family is one in which only one child (the proband) is on the autism spectrum, while both biological parents and all siblings are not. All collection sites used the same inclusion and exclusion criteria, administered the same instruments and followed the same protocols in collecting biospecimens. Families were recruited from a coalition of clinics located at Baylor College of Medicine, Children's Hospital of Boston, Columbia University, Emory University, McGill University, University of California-Los Angeles, University of Illinois at Chicago, University of Michigan, University of Missouri, University of Washington, Vanderbilt University and Yale University.

The inclusion criteria included proband age and a diagnosis of autism spectrum disorder. The proband in the family was between four years and 17 years and 11 months of age when the phenotype measures were administered and the data collected. On the Autism Diagnostic Interview-Revised (ADI-R), the proband was required to meet one of the following criteria: (1) standard cutoff on the social and communication domains, (2) standard cutoff on the social domain and within two points of communication cutoff, (3) standard cutoff of the communication domain and within two points of social cutoff, or (4) within one point of the standard cutoffs for both the social and communication domains. On the

Autism Diagnostic Observation Schedule (ADOS), the proband must have received a valid and reliable administration and must have met the cutoffs for autism spectrum disorders or autism. On the Mullen Scales of Early Learning, the Differential Ability Scales-II, the Wechsler Intelligence Scale for Children-IV or the Wechsler Abbreviated Scale of Intelligence, the proband must have had a nonverbal deviation or ratio IQ score greater than or equal to 60 (four years of age) or greater than or equal to 40 (between five and eight years of age). Participants eight years of age or older must have had a nonverbal mental age of 36 months or older. The proband was also required to have a clinical "Best Estimate Diagnosis" of autistic disorder, Asperger's disorder, or pervasive developmental disorder not otherwise specified made by a psychologist or physician.

The exclusion criteria included: (1) pregnancy and birth issues for probands including fewer than 36 weeks gestation and less than 2,000 grams at birth, or a history of maternal pregnancy or birth complications; (2) other disorders or limitations in the proband including a positive diagnosis for fragile X syndrome or Down syndrome, sensory or motor difficulties that would preclude valid use of diagnostic instruments, or a history of severe nutritional or psychological deprivation; (3) sibling diagnosed with an autism spectrum disorder, mental retardation (except Down syndrome), schizophrenia, or a psychiatric disorder requiring treatment with more than one psychotropic medication; (4) sibling with an Adaptive Behavior Standard score on the Vineland-II that was 70 or below or an Individualized Education Plan for extensive special education services; (5) parent diagnosed with an autism spectrum disorder, mental retardation, or schizophrenia; or (6) any second- or third-degree relative diagnosed with an autism spectrum disorder

Simons Simplex Collection: Medical record data for the autistic probands and family members were available through an interactive database that facilitated correlations between clinical, genetic, and neurobiological data [20]. The dataset utilized for this study was from the Simons Simplex Complex version 14 Public Cohort, released March 21, 2012 (http://sfari.org/resources/sfari-base). The proband study participants exhibited moderate to severe autistic symptoms with relatively little intellectual disability. Data regarding the use of soy-based infant formula and the type of seizures were obtained from the medical history form, a questionnaire regarding the proband and administered to the parent by the clinical research staff. Specific questions regarding seizures included: (1) Has the proband ever been diagnosed with febrile seizures (no, yes, not sure)? (2) What was the age of diagnoses/onset (years or months)? (3) Has the proband ever been diagnosed with seizures (no, yes, not sure)? If Yes, (4) what was the age of onset (years, months, not sure), type (grand mal/generalized tonic clonic, petit mal/absence, infantile spasms, atonic/drop attacks, complex partial, simple partial/focal), frequency (times per day, week, month or year) and date of last seizure? A diagnosis of epilepsy was defined as either a specific report of epilepsy on the ADI-R or at least 2 seizures on the medical history form.

Data Coding & Analyses

The febrile and non-febrile seizure variables in the SFARI database combined information about the presence of seizures from the ADI-R (question 85) and the medical history form. In the database the variables were labeled "Febrile Seizures :: Proband CDV" and "Non Febrile Seizures :: Proband CDV", respectively. Coding of the febrile seizure data included scores of 0, 1 and 2 where 0 indicated there was no evidence of the presence of febrile seizures, 1 indicated the possible presence of febrile seizures or the caregiver reported that they were "not sure" if the child had experienced febrile seizures, and 2 indicated the presence of febrile seizures reported. The non-febrile seizure data coding included scores of 0, 1, 2 and 3 where 0 indicated that there was no evidence for the presence of non-febrile seizures, 1 indicated the possible presence of non-febrile seizures or the caregiver report that they were "not sure" if the child had experienced non-febrile seizures, 2 indicated the likely presence of non-febrile seizures and 3 indicated that a diagnosis of epilepsy was reported. We did not include subjects with scores of 1 in our analysis. Scores of 0 were counted as seizure negative and scores of 2 or 3 were counted as seizure positive.

Data were analyzed in accordance with STROBE guidelines (Figure S1). Percentages, means, standard deviations and 95% confidence intervals were computed to describe the population. To statistically test for differences in seizure incidence across groups, Pearson's uncorrected chi-squared approximation and Fisher's exact test (two-tail) were used. The Pearson's uncorrected chi-squared approximation was only utilized in cases where there were at least five expected outcomes per cell. Statistical significance for age of seizure onset and IQ were determined by Student t-test analyses. Statistical significance was defined as $P<0.050$. For multiple comparisons (male versus female), a Bonferroni correction was applied and statistical significance was defined as $P< 0.025$. The number of subjects at each stage of the study is reported in the corresponding tables (Tables 1–4) as well as in a flow chart (Figure S2).

Conclusions

Published estimates of formula intolerance range from 2%–7.5% [31]; yet, nearly a quarter of infant formulas are soy-based suggesting that they are used excessively. The current position of the American Academy of Pediatrics is, "There is no conclusive evidence from animal, adult human, or infant populations that dietary soy isoflavones may adversely affect human development, reproduction, or endocrine function [32]." The data presented herein provide evidence that the use of soy-based formula may be associated with reduced seizure threshold in a vulnerable population of children diagnosed with autism. Given the lack of data on critical confounders in this retrospective study, a prospective study is required to confirm this association.

Supporting Information

Figure S1 Completed checklist of items included in reports of observational studies as recommended by STROBE guidelines and PLOS ONE editorial staff.

Figure S2 Flowchart of SFARI subject numbers per analysis as recommended by STROBE guidelines and PLOS ONE editorial staff.

Acknowledgments

The author thanks Drs. Elizabeth Berry-Kravis, Dan Bolt, Rick Chappell, Chris Ikonomidou, Pamela Westmark and Robert Wong for critical reading of the manuscript.

Author Contributions

Conceived and designed the experiments: CW. Performed the experiments: CW. Analyzed the data: CW. Contributed reagents/materials/analysis tools: CW. Wrote the paper: CW.

References

1. Autism and Developmental Disabilities Monitoring Network Surveillance Year 2008 Principal Investigators, Centers for Disease Control and Prevention (2012) Prevalence of autism spectrum disorders–autism and developmental disabilities monitoring network, 14 sites, United States, 2008. MMWR Surveill Summ 61: 1–19.
2. Hessl D, Dyer-Friedman J, Glaser B, Wisbeck J, Barajas RG, et al. (2001) The influence of environmental and genetic factors on behavior problems and autistic symptoms in boys and girls with fragile X syndrome. Pediatrics 108: E88.
3. Newschaffer CJ, Croen LA, Daniels J, Giarelli E, Grether JK, et al. (2007) The epidemiology of autism spectrum disorders. Annu Rev Public Health 28: 235–258.
4. Spencer CM, Alekseyenko O, Hamilton SM, Thomas AM, Serysheva E, et al. (2011) Modifying behavioral phenotypes in Fmr1KO mice: Genetic background differences reveal autistic-like responses. Autism Res 4: 40–56.
5. Westmark CJ, Westmark PR, Malter JS (2013) Soy-based diet exacerbates seizures in mouse models of neurological disease. J Alzheimers Dis 33: 797–805.
6. Ricci MR, Ulman EA (2005) Laboratory animal diets: A critical part of your research. Animal Lab News 4: 1.
7. Weber KS, Setchell KD, Lephart ED (2001) Maternal and perinatal brain aromatase: Effects of dietary soy phytoestrogens. Brain Res Dev Brain Res 126: 217–221.
8. Brown NM, Setchell KD (2001) Animal models impacted by phytoestrogens in commercial chow: Implications for pathways influenced by hormones. Lab Invest 81: 735–747.
9. Shukla SK, Gupta S, Ojha SK, Sharma SB (2010) Cardiovascular friendly natural products: A promising approach in the management of CVD. Nat Prod Res 24: 873–898.
10. Wei P, Liu M, Chen Y, Chen DC (2012) Systematic review of soy isoflavone supplements on osteoporosis in women. Asian Pac J Trop Med 5: 243–248.
11. Bernbaum JC, Umbach DM, Ragan NB, Ballard JL, Archer JI, et al. (2008) Pilot studies of estrogen-related physical findings in infants. Environ Health Perspect 116: 416–420.
12. Gilchrist JM, Moore MB, Andres A, Estroff JA, Badger TM (2010) Ultrasonographic patterns of reproductive organs in infants fed soy formula: Comparisons to infants fed breast milk and milk formula. J Pediatr 156: 215–220.
13. Jing H, Gilchrist JM, Badger TM, Pivik RT (2010) A longitudinal study of differences in electroencephalographic activity among breastfed, milk formula-fed, and soy formula-fed infants during the first year of life. Early Hum Dev 86: 119–125.
14. Li J, Dykman RA, Jing H, Gilchrist JM, Badger TM, et al. (2010) Cortical responses to speech sounds in 3- and 6-month-old infants fed breast milk, milk formula, or soy formula. Dev Neuropsychol 35: 762–784.
15. Adgent MA, Daniels JL, Edwards LJ, Siega-Riz AM, Rogan WJ (2011) Early-life soy exposure and gender-role play behavior in children. Environ Health Perspect 119: 1811–1816.
16. Andres A, Cleves MA, Bellando JB, Pivik RT, Casey PH, et al. (2012) Developmental status of 1-year-old infants fed breast milk, cow's milk formula, or soy formula. Pediatrics 129: 1134–1140.
17. Setchell KD, Zimmer-Nechemias L, Cai J, Heubi JE (1997) Exposure of infants to phyto-oestrogens from soy-based infant formula. Lancet 350: 23–27.
18. Setchell KD, Zimmer-Nechemias L, Cai J, Heubi JE (1998) Isoflavone content of infant formulas and the metabolic fate of these phytoestrogens in early life. Am J Clin Nutr 68: 1453S–1461S.
19. Soucy NV, Parkinson HD, Sochaski MA, Borghoff SJ (2006) Kinetics of genistein and its conjugated metabolites in pregnant Sprague-Dawley rats following single and repeated genistein administration. Toxicol Sci 90: 230–240.
20. Fischbach GD, Lord C (2010) The Simons Simplex Collection: A resource for identification of autism genetic risk factors. Neuron 68: 192–195.
21. Russ SA, Larson K, Halfon N (2012) A national profile of childhood epilepsy and seizure disorder. Pediatrics 129: 256–264.
22. Nelson KB, Ellenberg JH (1976) Predictors of epilepsy in children who have experienced febrile seizures. N Engl J Med 295: 1029–1033.
23. Nakayama J, Arinami T (2006) Molecular genetics of febrile seizures. Epilepsy Res 70 Suppl 1: S190–8.
24. Amiet C, Gourfinkel-An I, Bouzamondo A, Tordjman S, Baulac M, et al. (2008) Epilepsy in autism is associated with intellectual disability and gender: Evidence from a meta-analysis. Biol Psychiatry 64: 577–582.
25. Berry-Kravis E, Raspa M, Loggin-Hester L, Bishop E, Holiday D, et al. (2010) Seizures in fragile X syndrome: Characteristics and comorbid diagnoses. Am J Intellect Dev Disabil 115: 461–472.
26. Irizarry MC, Jin S, He F, Emond JA, Raman R, et al. (2012) Incidence of new-onset seizures in mild to moderate Alzheimer disease. Arch Neurol 69: 368–372.
27. Lott IT (2012) Neurological phenotypes for Down syndrome across the life span. Prog Brain Res 197: 101–121.
28. Yates JR, Maclean C, Higgins JN, Humphrey A, le Marechal K, et al. (2011) The tuberous sclerosis 2000 study: Presentation, initial assessments and implications for diagnosis and management. Arch Dis Child 96: 1020–1025.
29. Brooks-Kayal A (2010) Epilepsy and autism spectrum disorders: Are there common developmental mechanisms? Brain Dev 32: 731–738.
30. McCary LM, Roberts JE (2012) Early identification of autism in fragile X syndrome: A review. J Intellect Disabil Res,Epub Ahead of Print doi: 10.1111/j.1365-2788.2012.01609.x.
31. Polack FP, Khan N, Maisels MJ (1999) Changing partners: The dance of infant formula changes. Clin Pediatr (Phila) 38: 703–708.
32. Bhatia J, Greer F, American Academy of Pediatrics Committee on Nutrition (2008) Use of soy protein-based formulas in infant feeding. Pediatrics 121: 1062–1068.

17

The Potential of Accelerating Early Detection of Autism through Content Analysis of YouTube Videos

Vincent A. Fusaro[1], Jena Daniels[1,3], Marlena Duda[1,3], Todd F. DeLuca[1], Olivia D'Angelo[1], Jenna Tamburello[1], James Maniscalco[1], Dennis P. Wall[1,2,3]*

1 Center for Biomedical Informatics, Harvard Medical School, Boston, Massachusetts, United States of America, **2** Department of Pathology, Beth Israel Deaconess Medical Center, Boston, Massachusetts, United States of America, **3** Department of Pediatrics, Division of Systems Medicine, Stanford University, Stanford, California, United States of America

Abstract

Autism is on the rise, with 1 in 88 children receiving a diagnosis in the United States, yet the process for diagnosis remains cumbersome and time consuming. Research has shown that home videos of children can help increase the accuracy of diagnosis. However the use of videos in the diagnostic process is uncommon. In the present study, we assessed the feasibility of applying a gold-standard diagnostic instrument to brief and unstructured home videos and tested whether video analysis can enable more rapid detection of the core features of autism outside of clinical environments. We collected 100 public videos from YouTube of children ages 1–15 with either a self-reported diagnosis of an ASD (N = 45) or not (N = 55). Four non-clinical raters independently scored all videos using one of the most widely adopted tools for behavioral diagnosis of autism, the Autism Diagnostic Observation Schedule-Generic (ADOS). The classification accuracy was 96.8%, with 94.1% sensitivity and 100% specificity, the inter-rater correlation for the behavioral domains on the ADOS was 0.88, and the diagnoses matched a trained clinician in all but 3 of 22 randomly selected video cases. Despite the diversity of videos and non-clinical raters, our results indicate that it is possible to achieve high classification accuracy, sensitivity, and specificity as well as clinically acceptable inter-rater reliability with nonclinical personnel. Our results also demonstrate the potential for video-based detection of autism in short, unstructured home videos and further suggests that at least a percentage of the effort associated with detection and monitoring of autism may be mobilized and moved outside of traditional clinical environments.

Editor: Vishnu Chaturvedi, California Department of Public Health, United States of America

Funding: Work was supported in part by funds to DPW from the Simons Foundation, Nancy Lurie Marks Family Foundation, the Harvard Catalyst Program, and grant 1R01MH090611-01A1 from the National Institutes of Health. VAF was supported by grant 1K99LM011020-01 from the National Library of Medicine. The funders had no role in study design, data collection and analysis, decision to publish, or preparation of the manuscript.

Competing Interests: The authors have declared that no competing interests exist.

* E-mail: dpwall@stanford.edu

Background

In the United States, autism spectrum disorder (ASD) is typically diagnosed in children at four years of age with an estimated 27% undiagnosed by eight years of age [1]. Yet, the majority of parents of ASD children report developmental concerns before one year of age [1–3]. To better understand the developmental progression of ASD and identify distinguishing behaviors between ASD and non-ASD children, a number of studies focused on retrospective home video analysis [4–12]. Previous home video studies showed that ASD and non-ASD children differ in frequency of responding to name [10], gaze [13], smiling [14], and stereotypic motor behaviors [15]. It is important to note that home videos generally will not reflect all aspects of the clinical evaluation and can present challenges to proper diagnosis such as not clearly capturing eye contact, capturing context-dependent behaviors that may not exemplify routine, and poorly demonstrating social behavior with unfamiliar person(s). Nevertheless, home videos are considered a more accurate representation of early events than parental recall [10], and could be of value in future efforts focused on lowering the average age of diagnosis in the Unites States and abroad.

Significant prior work has focused on creating structured questions and standardized approaches to evaluate home videos by retrospectively examining early videos of children later diagnosed with ASD. This allows researchers to combine additional clinical features, such as age and IQ, with the video to develop a more complete representation of behavioral development. To standardize the home videos, most research focuses on a common event such as first or second birthday, and/or pivotal developmental milestones (such as not pointing, not responding to name calling, or not playing [stereotypically or pretend]).

We sought to expand the concept and feasibility of home video analysis by applying the Autism Diagnostic Observation Schedule (ADOS) [16] questions, not the full exam, to ASD and non-ASD videos from YouTube, the largest public video-sharing Internet website. The ADOS is widely considered a gold standard and is one of the most common behavioral instruments used to aid in diagnosis of ASD [16–18]. Clinical application of the ADOS requires a clinician trained in administrating the exam in order to elicit specific types of responses during structured activities. The exam is divided into four modules that correspond to an

Table 1. Characteristics of ASD and Non-ASD videos on YouTube.

Characteristic	ASD (n = 55)	Non-ASD (n = 45)
Gender[a], % (M/F)	37/18	23/22
Age[a], mean (range)	4.35 (1.5–15)	2.89 (0.92–6)
Race[a]		
White, %	89.1	82.2
Black, %	1.8	3.6
Other, %	9.0	13.3
Video length (min), mean (range)	3:19 (0:31–9:16)	2:37 (0:36–6:09)
YouTube views[b], mean (range)	17,661 (17–96,469)	4,107,244 (146–102,871,735)
Date posted on YouTube, range	03/21/07–06/19/12	06/25/06–11/04/12
Appearance of other people[c], %		
One person	20.0	33.3
Two or more people	18.2	17.8
Interacting with adult, %	96.4	95.6
Interacting with peer, %	16.4	17.8
Types of videos[d], %		
Exhibiting a talent	5.5	33.3
Having a conversation	60.0	80.0
Playing	49.0	42.2
Inside	85.5	77.8
Outside	9.0	13.3
In a car	0.0	6.7
Party or birthday	1.8	8.9
Eating	10.9	22.2

[a]If not explicitly stated in metadata associated with the video value was estimated based on consensus of two or more investigators.
[b]The number of views on YouTube accessed on 12/10/13.
[c]Number of additional people in the video excluding the child and person recording the video.
[d]Videos were broadly categorized, after initial identification, to illustrate the diversity of videos evaluated.

individual's language and developmental level, ensuring coverage for a wide variety of behavioral manifestations. We used module 1, which contains 10 activities and 29 questions, for assessment because this module is largely focused on the behavioral characteristics most appropriate for characterizing the younger children found in a majority of the YouTube videos collected for this study, and also because this age group serves to benefit most from early detection and early intervention. Our aims were first to test the feasibility of answering the ADOS module 1 questions when viewing short (<10 min) unstructured videos, and second to test the accuracy of non-clinical raters to distinguish videos containing children with autism from videos of children who have no signs of autism.

Methods

Human Subjects

The use of videos from YouTube was approved for exemption by the Institutional Review Board at Beth Israel Deaconess Medical Center (protocol #2012P-000307), under exemption number 4 ("research involving the collection or study of existing data, documents, records, pathological specimens, or diagnostic specimens, if these sources are publicly available or if the information is recorded by the investigator in such a manner that subjects cannot be identified, directly or through identifiers linked to the subjects") of the Code of Federal Regulations, 45 CFR 46.101(b).

Video Selection

We searched YouTube (www.youtube.com) for videos of ASD and non-ASD children using the following keywords in the video title or description: autism, ASD, autism spectrum disorder, Asperger's, autistic child, autistic kid, autistic behavior, PDD-NOS, son, daughter, child, birthday party. We required each video to be under 10 minutes long, have clear audible sound quality, have continuous activity, and to contain a majority of footage on a child between the ages of 1 and 15. When age was not provided it was estimated based on a consensus from two or more investigators (pertinent to 7 of the 100 videos collected). In total, we identified 100 unique subject videos, 45 ASD and 55 non-ASD. We identified non-ASD videos as controls by matching age, gender, and race as closely as possible. Videos were labeled as ASD if the video title, video description, or meta-tag included autism, ASD, Asperger's, or hand-flapping/stimming; otherwise, the video was labeled non-ASD. The full list of videos is provided in **Table S1**.

Raters and ADOS Scoring

ADOS scoring instruments were purchased from Western Psychological Services (http://www.wpspublish.com/). Four non-clinical raters independently scored the 29 questions on ADOS

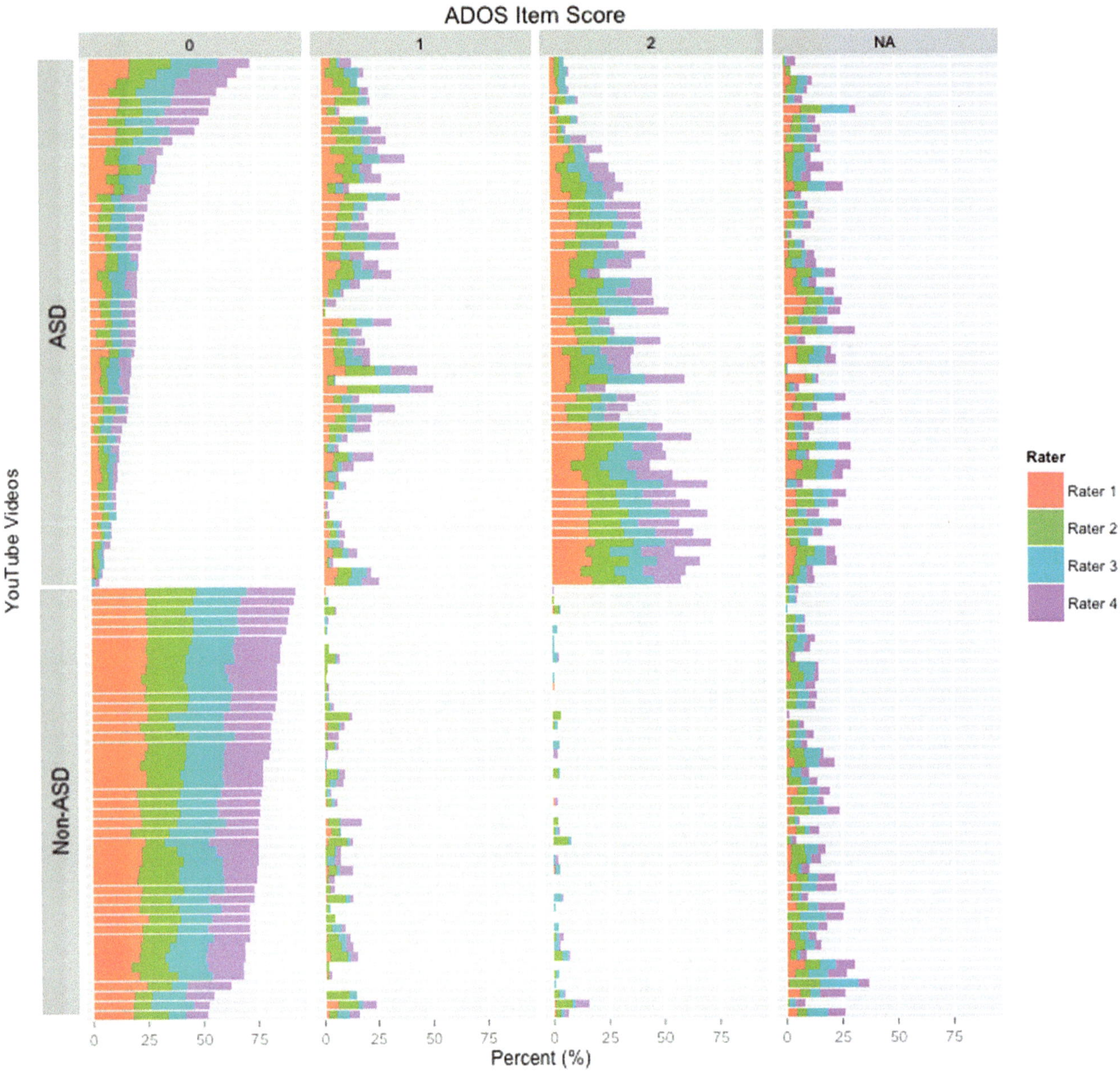

Figure 1. Inter-rater variability among cases previously diagnosed with autism and controls with no known diagnosis of autism. While subjectivity shifts did occur among the four independent raters, these shifts in qualitative judgment did not significantly impact the agreement among the reviewers. Both the inter-rater classification agreement (>90%) and classification accuracy (>95%) were found to be high in this analysis.

module 1 for each video. Raters were purposely given minimal instructions to code only when the video clearly depicted a behavior and/or contained opportunities for the child to exhibit the behavior in question, and otherwise to code the behavioral item as not applicable (N/A). Two of the four raters participated in the acquisition of the home videos from YouTube, and thus were not naïve to videos titles. An ADOS-certified clinical practitioner performed a blinded evaluation of a random subset of 22 videos (13 ASD and 8 non-ASD) that we used as a clinical standard for comparison to outcomes from the four non-clinical raters. We calculated the typical ADOS score as indicated in the exam instructions for the ADOS algorithm and followed the convention of converting all scores of three to two [19]. Videos were labeled ASD if the score was ≥7 and otherwise labeled as non-ASD. Any item that was scored N/A was removed from scoring and statistical analysis.

Statistical Analysis

We computed intra-class correlations across pairs of raters for the communication and social domains and overall for the ADOS module 1. We computed the mean item-level agreement across all raters and compared the mean item-level agreement between the four non-clinical raters to the clinical rater. We calculated the accuracy, sensitivity and specificity for classifications only if the majority of raters agreed (3 out of 4). For videos where there was no majority (2 out 4) we did not make a classification and labeled it "no call." We performed all such analyses in R [20,21] using the "IRR" package.

Table 2. Video Scoring Performance.

Characteristic	Total (n = 100)
Accuracy, %	96.8
Sensitivity, %	94.1
Specificity, %	100
No call (ASD/non-ASD)[a]	4/1
Interrater classification agreement (ASD vs. non-ASD), % mean (range)	92.2 (89–95)
Intraclass correlation across items	
Communication	0.84
Social	0.83
Total	0.88
Rater item-level mean agreement[b], % mean (range)	73.3 (58.1–95.3)
Rater vs. Expert item-level mean agreement[c], % mean (range)	71.3 (37.5–100)

[a]We required majority rater agreement (3 out of 4) for classification.
[b]Item-level agreement shown is the mean and range of 29 item agreements across four non-clinical raters.
[c]Clinical evaluation compared to four non-clinical raters for item-level agreement. All 29 items across a subset of 22 videos were considered.

Results

We identified and analyzed 100 videos on YouTube that met our criteria for ASD (45 videos) and non-ASD (55 videos). A complete summary of video characteristics is provided in **Table 1**. The average age of children with ASD was 4.35 and 2.89 for children without an ASD. The age of the child was available in the metadata associated with the video in all but 7 of the 100 videos. For these 7, age was estimated by 2 raters independently. We found more male videos (n = 37) than female (n = 18) for ASD, which is consistent with the higher percentage of autism found in males. The most common types of video were of a child playing inside with his/her collection of toys. Nearly all videos (91%) included interaction with an adult.

The high classification accuracy (96.8%) supported the feasibility of applying ADOS module 1 questions to videos on YouTube (**Table 2**). In addition, the high sensitivity (94.1%) and perfect specificity suggested that home video classification could yield both high positive and negative predictive value. While all behavioral items on the ADOS could be addressed by at least 1 rater in all 100 videos, 7 behaviors, including imagination and functional play, had 30% or higher N/A answer codes indicating that they were not adequately captured in the videos (**Table 3**). The intraclass correlation among raters for specific questions on ADOS module 1 were consistent with previous results [22] and ranged from 0.83–0.88. The mean rater agreement was high (73.3%) despite the diversity of environmental contexts represented in the videos. The lowest mean rater agreement was 58.1% for item B9 ("showing") possibly due in part to the fact that it had the a relatively high frequency of N/A codes across the raters (**Table 3**). The highest mean rater agreement was 95.3% for item D3 ("self-injurious behavior") as the children in the videos rarely exhibited this behavior. The distribution of raters' scores for all videos is shown in **Figure 1** which provides additional insight into the classification accuracy and inter-rater agreement.

Because two of the raters helped to locate videos appropriate for this study, they were not always naïve to the diagnoses. To address this possible bias, we recruited a research reliable and professionally trained ADOS clinical practitioner (blinded to the diagnosis) to score 22 randomly selected videos to ensure the non-clinical raters were not unduly influenced by their prior knowledge [23] or lack of clinical experience. The raters agreed with classification provided by the clinical expert in all but 3 of the 22 randomly selected videos. In each of these 3 cases, the classification provided by the clinician did not agree with the self-reported diagnosis of ASD. The mean agreement between each non-clinical and clinical rater was 71.3%, which was consistent with the mean among non-clinical raters (73.3%) indicating that prior knowledge did not obviously bias the non-clinical rater's scoring.

Conclusions

The absence of any reliable molecular, neurological or physical features to characterize ASD means the best-estimate behavioral diagnosis is still the gold standard. For this reason, previous studies focused on identifying a core set of primary deficits from home videos for early age detection, to allow behavioral intervention at key stages in child development. Here, we take a different approach and apply standard diagnostic questions from ADOS module 1 to a diverse collection of videos of children in a non-clinical environment using non-clinical raters. Our results show high classification accuracy and inter-rater reliability and together demonstrate that the ADOS module 1 questions can be used by non-clinicians on unstructured videos to effectively distinguish behavioral differences among children with and without ASD.

While not all questions on the ADOS were expected to be relevant to the YouTube videos, we did find that a majority of the questions could be applied. In particular, questions regarding vocalization, use of words or phrases, unusual eye contact, responsive social smile, and repetitive interests or behaviors were the most relevant to the broad assortment of videos. Adding even a limited set of criteria to meet when capturing home videos for prospective studies may increase the likelihood that the less detectable behaviors identified in this study are captured. We observed the length of time to screen a video was never more than one minute over the length of the video and that the average assessment times were ~4 min for ASD and ~3:30 min for non-ASD. These results could have important implications for faster screening approaches in the future.

There are important limitations to this proof-of-concept study. First, because we did not contact the individuals, we cannot confirm the diagnosis, gender, age, and race. Second, although by

Table 3. Scorability of each behavior across the ASD and non-ASD video collections.

	ASD		Non-ASD	
Behaviors (Code)	**Code**	**%N/A**	**Code**	**%N/A**
Anxiety (E3)	E3	0	D3	0
Facial Expressions (B3)	B3	0.0045	E2	0
Gaze to Initiate Interaction (B4)	B4	0.0045	E3	0
Repetitive Interests (D4)	D4	0.0045	A3	0.0056
Overactivity (E1)	E1	0.0045	D1	0.0056
Tantrums/Aggression (E2)	E2	0.0045	D4	0.0056
Spontaneous Expressive Language (A2)	A2	0.0091	E1	0.0056
Social Overtures (B12)	B12	0.0091	A1	0.01
Complex Mannerisms (D2)	D2	0.0091	A5	0.01
Gestures (A8)	A8	0.0182	D2	0.01
Self-Injurious Behavior (D3)	D3	0.023	B12	0.017
Eye Contact (B1)	B1	0.023	A4	0.02
Sensory Interest (D1)	D1	0.023	A8	0.028
Shared Enjoyment (B5)	B5	0.045	B1	0.028
Intonation (A3)	A3	0.086	B4	0.028
Responsive Smile (B2)	B2	0.1	A2	0.033
Idiosyncratic Use of Words (A5)	A5	0.12	B5	0.039
Pointing (A7)	A7	0.14	B3	0.044
Initiation of Joint Attention (B10)	B10	0.24	A6	0.061
Response to Name (B6)	B6	0.24	B2	0.14
Requesting (B7)	B7	0.27	B7	0.17
Showing (B9)	B9	0.29	B6	0.22
Spontaneous Expressive Language (A1)	A1	0.3	A7	0.3
Functional Play (C1)	C1	0.35	B11	0.34
Giving (B8)	B8	0.38	B10	0.35
Use of Other's Body to Communicate (A6)	A6	0.44	B9	0.38
Echolalia (A4)	A4	0.49	C1	0.57
Imagination/Creativity (C2)	C2	0.60	B8	0.65
Social Overtures (B11)	B11	0.62	C2	0.79

The frequency of N/A (not applicable) answer codes per video over all video raters is listed in descending order for both video collections. The lowest values correspond to the most readily scored behaviors. A large majority of items were readily detectable and resulted in only a small fraction of N/As.

design, our raters were not trained clinicians, were not certified as research-reliable to perform ADOS and were not professionally qualified to confirm a diagnosis. Third, we applied ADOS module 1 to all the videos despite the typical recommendation that it be applied to children with single word vocabulary and mental age less than 3 years of age. However, the high agreement among the non-clinical raters, as well as the agreement of the raters to a research-reliable ADOS practitioner suggests that these limitations did not heavily bias the results.

In conclusion, we demonstrate the feasibility of applying a standard diagnostic questions to ASD and non-ASD videos from YouTube. Our results show that despite the short length (<4 minutes), home-quality, and diversity of scenarios captured within the videos it is possible to achieve good inter-rater reliability and high classification accuracy, sensitivity, and specificity. Our results also indicate that it is possible for non-clinical raters to correctly detect the presence of autism with high inter-rater reliability and >94% accuracy. These results support the potential role for short home videos in rapidly screening for a potential autism diagnosis. Based on these results, we hypothesize that it may be possible to apply other testing modules, including highly abbreviated approaches [24] to home videos to further reduce the complexity of detecting autism outside of clinical settings, without appreciable loss of accuracy in comparison to the current standard of care. Our future efforts will focus on testing this and other related hypotheses, including the potential of combining a video-based classification with brief parent-directed classification systems [25] to increase accuracy. Our results also suggest a potential larger role for public video repositories such as YouTube in the detection of other human conditions that have behavioral symptomatology.

Supporting Information

Table S1 Details on the 100 YouTube videos. Forty-five autism spectrum disorder (ASD) and 55 non-ASD samples were collected in total. The Table contains the original download URL, the self-reported diagnosis, the gender and age of the subject, length of video, and the total number of YouTube views (as of 12/10/13).

Acknowledgments

We would like to thank the families with autism who contributed videos and who made this study possible. We would also like to thank Amy Gates for clinical interpretation of the videos.

Author Contributions

Conceived and designed the experiments: DPW. Performed the experiments: DPW. Analyzed the data: DPW VAF JD MD TFD OD JT JM. Wrote the paper: DPW VAF. Participated in experiment design: VAF.

References

1. Zwaigenbaum L, Bryson S, Lord C, Rogers S, Carter A, et al. (2009) Clinical assessment and management of toddlers with suspected autism spectrum disorder: insights from studies of high-risk infants. Pediatrics 123: 1383–1391.
2. Dawson G, Rogers S, Munson J, Smith M, Winter J, et al. (2010) Randomized, controlled trial of an intervention for toddlers with autism: the Early Start Denver Model. Pediatrics 125: e17–23.
3. Shattuck PT, Durkin M, Maenner M, Newschaffer C, Mandell DS, et al. (2009) Timing of identification among children with an autism spectrum disorder: findings from a population-based surveillance study. J Am Acad Child Adolesc Psychiatry 48: 474–483.
4. Freuler A, Baranek GT, Watson LR, Boyd BA, Bulluck JC (2012) Precursors and trajectories of sensory features: qualitative analysis of infant home videos. Am J Occup Ther 66: e81–84.
5. Baranek GT, Barnett CR, Adams EM, Wolcott NA, Watson LR, et al. (2005) Object play in infants with autism: methodological issues in retrospective video analysis. Am J Occup Ther 59: 20–30.
6. Maestro S, Muratori F, Cavallaro MC, Pei F, Stern D, et al. (2002) Attentional skills during the first 6 months of age in autism spectrum disorder. J Am Acad Child Adolesc Psychiatry 41: 1239–1245.
7. Stronach S, Wetherby AM (2012) Examining restricted and repetitive behaviors in young children with autism spectrum disorder during two observational contexts. Autism.
8. Ozonoff S, Iosif AM, Young GS, Hepburn S, Thompson M, et al. (2011) Onset patterns in autism: correspondence between home video and parent report. J Am Acad Child Adolesc Psychiatry 50: 796–806 e791.
9. Mahdhaoui A, Chetouani M, Cassel RS, Saint-Georges C, Parlato E, et al. (2011) Computerized home video detection for motherese may help to study impaired interaction between infants who become autistic and their parents. Int J Methods Psychiatr Res 20: e6–18.
10. Goldberg WA, Thorsen KL, Osann K, Spence MA (2008) Use of home videotapes to confirm parental reports of regression in autism. J Autism Dev Disord 38: 1136–1146.
11. Jameson R, Lorence D, Lee J (2012) Integrating computerized primitives and annotated video patterns: a proposed model for autism diagnosis and research. J Med Syst 36: 2037–2045.
12. Osterling J, Dawson G (1994) Early recognition of children with autism: a study of first birthday home videotapes. J Autism Dev Disord 24: 247–257.
13. Elsabbagh M, Volein A, Csibra G, Holmboe K, Garwood H, et al. (2009) Neural correlates of eye gaze processing in the infant broader autism phenotype. Biol Psychiatry 65: 31–38.
14. Key AP, Stone WL (2012) Same but different: 9-month-old infants at average and high risk for autism look at the same facial features but process them using different brain mechanisms. Autism Res 5: 253–266.
15. David FJ, Baranek GT, Wiesen C, Miao AF, Thorpe DE (2012) Coordination of precision grip in 2–6 years-old children with autism spectrum disorders compared to children developing typically and children with developmental disabilities. Front Integr Neurosci 6: 122.
16. Lord C, Rutter M, Goode S, Heemsbergen J, Jordan H, et al. (1989) Autism diagnostic observation schedule: a standardized observation of communicative and social behavior. J Autism Dev Disord 19: 185–212.
17. American Psychiatric A (2000) Diagnostic and Statistical Manual of Mental Disorders DSM-IV-TR. Washington, DC: American Psychiatric Association.
18. Lord C, Petkova E, Hus V, Gan W, Lu F, et al. (2012) A multisite study of the clinical diagnosis of different autism spectrum disorders. Arch Gen Psychiatry 69: 306–313.
19. Gotham K, Pickles A, Lord C (2009) Standardizing ADOS scores for a measure of severity in autism spectrum disorders. J Autism Dev Disord 39: 693–705.
20. Kim SH, Lord C (2012) Combining information from multiple sources for the diagnosis of autism spectrum disorders for toddlers and young preschoolers from 12 to 47 months of age. J Child Psychol Psychiatry 53: 143–151.
21. van Daalen E, Kemner C, Dietz C, Swinkels SH, Buitelaar JK, et al. (2009) Inter-rater reliability and stability of diagnoses of autism spectrum disorder in children identified through screening at a very young age. Eur Child Adolesc Psychiatry 18: 663–674.
22. Gotham K, Risi S, Pickles A, Lord C (2007) The Autism Diagnostic Observation Schedule: revised algorithms for improved diagnostic validity. J Autism Dev Disord 37: 613–627.
23. Clifford S, Young R, Williamson P (2007) Assessing the early characteristics of autistic disorder using video analysis. J Autism Dev Disord 37: 301–313.
24. Wall DP, Kosmicki J, Deluca TF, Harstad E, Fusaro VA (2012) Use of machine learning to shorten observation-based screening and diagnosis of autism. Transl Psychiatry 2: e100.
25. Wall DP, Dally R, Luyster R, Jung JY, Deluca TF (2012) Use of artificial intelligence to shorten the behavioral diagnosis of autism. PLoS One 7: e43855.

18

Structural Alterations of the Social Brain: A Comparison between Schizophrenia and Autism

Daniel Radeloff[1]*, Angela Ciaramidaro[1], Michael Siniatchkin[1], Daniela Hainz[1], Sabine Schlitt[1], Bernhard Weber[2,5], Fritz Poustka[1], Sven Bölte[1,3], Henrik Walter[2,4], Christine Margarete Freitag[1]

1 Department of Child and Adolescent Psychiatry, Psychosomatics and Psychotherapy, Johann Wolfgang Goethe-Universität, Frankfurt/Main, Frankfurt/Main,Germany, **2** Department of Psychiatry, Psychosomatics and Psychotherapy, Johann Wolfgang Goethe Universität Frankfurt/Main, Frankfurt/Main, Germany, **3** Department of Women's and Children's Health, Center of Neurodevelopmental Disorders at Karolinska Institutet (KIND), Stockholm, Sweden, **4** Division of Mind and Brain Research, Department of Psychiatry and Psychotherapy, Charité-Universitätsmedizin Berlin, Berlin, Germany, **5** Psychiatric University Clinics, University of Basel, Basel, Switzerland

Abstract

Autism spectrum disorder and schizophrenia share a substantial number of etiologic and phenotypic characteristics. Still, no direct comparison of both disorders has been performed to identify differences and commonalities in brain structure. In this voxel based morphometry study, 34 patients with autism spectrum disorder, 21 patients with schizophrenia and 26 typically developed control subjects were included to identify global and regional brain volume alterations. No global gray matter or white matter differences were found between groups. In regional data, patients with autism spectrum disorder compared to typically developed control subjects showed smaller gray matter volume in the amygdala, insula, and anterior medial prefrontal cortex. Compared to patients with schizophrenia, patients with autism spectrum disorder displayed smaller gray matter volume in the left insula. Disorder specific positive correlations were found between mentalizing ability and left amygdala volume in autism spectrum disorder, and hallucinatory behavior and insula volume in schizophrenia. Results suggest the involvement of social brain areas in both disorders. Further studies are needed to replicate these findings and to quantify the amount of distinct and overlapping neural correlates in autism spectrum disorder and schizophrenia.

Editor: Valerie W Hu, The George Washington University, United States of America

Funding: The study was partly supported by the Swedish Research Council (grant nr. 523-2009-7054) and by the LOEWE-Program 'Neuronal Coordination Research Focus Frankfurt' (NeFF). The funders had no role in study design, data collection and analysis, decision to publish, or preparation of the manuscript.

Competing Interests: The authors have declared that no competing interests exist.

* Email: daniel.radeloff@kgu.de

Introduction

Autism spectrum disorder (ASD) and schizophrenia (SCZ) are biologically based psychiatric disorders that share a substantial number of etiologic factors and phenotypic characteristics. For instance, rare and partly overlapping copy number variants have been identified to be a strong genetic risk factor for both disorders [1], and relatives of individuals with ASD are more likely to have a family history of SCZ [2].

Both disorders are influenced by deficits of the social brain [2,3], a specialized neural network dedicated to social cognition comprising in particular the medial prefrontal cortex (MPFC), the posterior temporal sulcus, and the adjacent temporo-parietal junction, the anterior cingulate cortex (ACC), the insula, the amygdala, the inferior frontal gyrus, and the interparietal sulcus [4,5]. Social cognition refers to psychological processes that benefit social exchanges, in particular, a specific cognitive ability, called "Theory of mind" (ToM) or mentalizing, allows humans to explain and predict the behavior of conspecifics by inferring their mental states [6]. FMRI studies have shown aberrant activation in SCZ and ASD using mentalizing and basic emotional tasks. In SCZ aberrant neural activation in fronto-temporo-parietal regions and in amygdala were found [7–13]. Also, in ASD reduced activation in regions of the social brain during processing of social information has been described in the right pSTS, amygdala and fusiform gyrus [14–21].

Moreover, in both disorders abnormalities in global brain volume measures have been reported when compared to typically developing subjects (TD). In ASD, a greater total brain volume is present mainly in early childhood, rarely in adults [22]. In SCZ, smaller global GM and WM volumes have been reported in meta-analytic studies [23–25]. Meta-analyses of voxel-based morphometry (VBM) studies reported volume alterations of social brain areas in both disorders. In ASD smaller grey matter (GM) volumes were found in the temporal lobe, MPFC, amygdala/hippocampus, and precuneus [26,22,27], instead larger GM volumes have been reported in the lateral prefrontal cortex and temporo-occipital regions [26,22,27]. Structural alterations in ASD seem to be age-related, as in adults with ASD structural alterations in fusiform gyrus, cingulum, amygdala and insula were less often reported compared to children/adolescents [22,27,1]. Similar to ASD, in SCZ structural alterations have been found in the social brain and meta-analyses have described smaller GM volumes in fronto-temporal regions, ACC, hippocampus/amygdala, and the insula [28–31,23]. GM alterations were more extensive in patients with long illness duration possibly indicating a neurodegenerative process [29,30,32,28]. A recent meta-analysis implemented anatomical likelihood estimation (ALE) to compare VBM studies on both SCZ and ASD [33]. Lower GM volumes in the limbic-striato-thalamic circuitry compared to controls were found as a structural overlap between SCZ and ASD. Distinct volumetric alterations were observed in the amygdala, caudate, frontal, and medial gyrus (SCZ) and putamen (ASD).

In summary, studies on structural alterations in ASD and SCZ compared to TD have shown GM volume alteration in social brain areas with a high diversity of brain volume changes within the social brain network, which are in part contradictory. The contradictions may be explained by the phenotypic differences within disorders, age and IQ effects, or by different methods used for data acquisition and analysis [32,31,27]. Therefore, a direct comparison of both disorders within a unitary methodological framework is necessary to clearly describe overlapping and disorder specific alterations of brain volume [34]. In the present VBM-study, ASD, SCZ, and TD were compared directly with respect to global and regional brain volume. Moreover, structural alterations were correlated with differences in mentalizing abilities and disorder specific symptom severity.

This study aims to address three hypotheses: First, in global brain measures, a slightly lower total GM and total white matter volume is expected in SCZ compared to TD. No differences in global brain measures are expected between ASD and TD, as greater total GM volume was found mainly in ASD children, but not in adults. Second, we hypothesize that in both disorders compared to TD, lower GM volumes are present social brain areas, reflecting impairments in social cognition. As ASD and SCZ show different and in part contrary deficits in social cognition (i.e. in ASD the ability to attribute mental states to others is deficient, while in paranoid SCZ these attributions are intensified), we expect distinct volume alterations comparing SCZ with ASD. Third, associations between the extent of volume alterations in these areas and behavioral data (symptom severity and mentalizing abilities) are expected.

Methods

Participants

Thirty-four patients with ASD (3 females, age range 14 to 33 years, mean age 19.06, SD 5.12; mean IQ 105.73, SD 12.92), 21 patients with SCZ (5 females, aged 14 to 33 years, mean age 24.67, SD 5.20; mean IQ 103.33, SD 11.21), and 26 TD (4 females, aged 14 to 27 years, mean age 19.54, SD 3.46; mean IQ 107.75, SD 11.97) were investigated. The ASD sample consisted of 16 patients with Asperger Syndrome, 11 patients with childhood autism and 7 with atypical autism. The study was approved by the local ethical committee of the medical faculty, JW Goethe-University, Frankfurt am Main, and was carried out according to the declaration of Helsinki. All subjects (and their parents in case of underage subjects) gave their written informed consent for participation in the study.

The following inclusion criteria were met by the clinical groups: 1) diagnoses according to ICD-10 (F84.0, F84.1, F84.5; F20.0); 2) no additional neurological or chronic medical disorder; 3) no other comorbid psychiatric disorder; 4) IQ >70. The diagnosis of paranoid hallucinatory schizophrenia (ICD-10: F20.0) was done by thorough clinical examination and validation by at least 2 experienced psychiatrists. The diagnoses of childhood autism, Asperger Syndrome or atypical autism (ICD-10: F84.0, F84.1, F84.5) was additionally confirmed by the Autism Diagnostic Interview - Revised (ADI-R, German version; [35,36]) and Autism Diagnostic Observation Schedule (ADOS, German version; [37,38]). In order to provide additional information on positive and negative symptoms, the Positive and Negative Syndrome Scale (PANSS, [39]) was obtained from SCZ. In SCZ, mean duration of illness was 67 months (SD: 45 months), ranging from 2 months to 144 months. Given the age at examination and the illness duration, 40% to 50% of the patients were considered as adolescent onset schizophrenia and 50% to 60% as adult onset schizophrenia (missing data in 2 datasets).

To exclude additional psychiatric disorders, all subjects were explored by experienced psychiatrists. In addition, participants filled in the youth or young adult self-report (YASR/YSR; [40,41]), a screening instrument to assess self-rated psychopathology. Also, the child behavior checklist/young adult behavior checklist (CBCL/YABCL; [42,41]) was completed by a parent, where possible. All TD subjects showed YASR/YSR and CBCL/YABCL subscales T-scores <67 (below borderline clinical cut-off). SCZ were older than ASD and TD. Therefore, age was controlled as a covariate in all further analyses.

Psychological assessment

IQ was measured by the Raven Standard Progressive Matrices (SPM, [43]). Handedness was determined by the Edinburgh handedness inventory [44]. To characterize deficits in mentalizing abilities, all subjects were investigated using the 'reading the mind in the eyes' test (RME) [45]. In this test, participants were asked to identify complex emotional and non-affective states in images presenting human eyes.

Demographic data, clinical characteristics, and dosage of daily neuroleptic treatment chlorpromazine equivalent doses according to Woods [46] are shown in Table 1. Within the SCZ sample, 21 patients were treated with at least one of the following substances: Risperidone/Paliperidone (7), Quetiapine (5), Olanzapine (2), Clozapine (4), Aripiprazole (2), Haloperidol (1), Benperidol (2), Chlorprothixen (2); Escitalopram (1), Fluvoxamine (1), Ziprasidone (1); (missing data in 2 datasets); within the ASD sample 7 patients were treated with at least one of the following substances: Risperidone (2); Methylphenidate (5); Sertraline (2), Escitalopram (1).

Data acquisition and voxel-based-morphometry analysis

Structural magnetic resonance images were acquired using a 3 Tesla Siemens Allegra scanner (Erlangen, Germany) with a 1-channel head coil. Data were recorded using a T1-weighted MDEFT-sequence [47] with parameters as follows: TR: 10.55 ms, TE: 3.06 ms; TI: 680 ms; flip angle: 22°. One dataset consisted of 176 axial images with an inplane resolution of 1 mm^3, field of view: 256 mm; slice thickness: 1 mm.

Imaging data pre-processing

All datasets were manually reviewed for head motion and image quality. Datasets with low image quality or motion artefacts were excluded from analysis. Structural images underwent pre-processing using optimized VBM as implemented in SPM8 (http://www.fil.ion.ucl.ac.uk/spm/software/spm8) according to the standardized procedure [48]. Images were segmented into GM and white matter (WM). Global GM, global WM, and total brain volume (TBV) were calculated. Subsequently, images were normalized by creating a DARTEL-template to provide an increased accuracy of inter-subject alignment. The images were resampled to $1.5\times1.5\times1.5$ mm^3 voxel size. Images were smoothed (using an 8 mm FWHM isotropic Gaussian kernel) and normalized to MNI space. Data were corrected for differences in global GM/WM volume. As treatment with neuroleptic medication differed

Table 1. Sociodemographical and clinical parameters of ASD, SCZ and TD.

Parameter		ASD	SCZ	TD	P<0.05
		(N = 34)	(N = 21)	(N = 26)	
		Mean (SD)	Mean (SD)	Mean (SD)	
age [years]		19.06 (5.12)	24.67 (5.20)	19.54 (3.46)	SCZ>TD,ASD
gender (m/f)		31/3	16/5	22/4	–
IQ		105.73 (12.92)	103.33 (11.21)	107.75 (11.97)	–
PANSS[a]	Ps	–	14.43 (5.35)	–	
	Ns	–	17.33 (6.03)	–	
	Gps	–	30.90 (9.95)	–	
	T	–	62.67 (17.74)	–	
ADOS[b]	C	3.65 (1.41)	–	–	
	Si	7.76 (2.84)	–	–	
	T	11.41 (3.82)	–	–	
ADI-R[c]	Si	21.96 (5.96)	–	–	
	Cl	14.04 (4.61)	–	–	
	Rb	5.87 (2.50)	–	–	
RME[d]		16.74 (4.25)	20.57 (2.27)	21.15 (2.74)	TD, SCZ>ASD
Medication (mean CPZ-eq [mg])[e]		300 (N = 2)	478.7 (367.6) (N = 15)	–	

Significance threshold was defined as P<0.05.
[a]PANSS = Positive and Negative Syndrome Scale; p = positive scale; ns = negative scale; gps = general psychopathology scale; t = total;
[b]ADOS = Autism Diagnostic Observery Scale; missing data in 2 cases; c = communication; si = social interaction; t = total;
[c]ADI-R = Autism Diagnostic Interview - Revised; missing data in 2 cases; si = social interaction; cl = communication and language; rb = restricted and repetitive behaviours;
[d]RME = 'Reading the Mind in the Eyes' test,
[e]CPZ-eq = Chlorpromazine equivalents.

between groups, daily chlorpromazine-equivalents were tested for association with local volume alterations in SCZ.

Statistical analysis

Total tissue volumes were calculated by summing the partial volume estimates multiplied by the voxel volume across the entire brain. Between-group differences in global brain measures were examined using an ANOVA with factor group including age as a covariate. Subsequent comparisons between means were performed using Bonferroni's post hoc test. Individual GM and WM segments were subjected to a voxel-wise multiple regression analysis. The differential effects of the three groups (ASD, SCZ and TD) were assessed within an ANCOVA model including age and global GM or global WM volume as covariates. ANCOVA was followed by between group comparisons. Significance threshold was set at $P<0.001$, uncorrected ($K>20$). Anatomical regions and denominations are reported according to the atlas of Talairach [49,50]. Coordinates are provided as maxima in given clusters according to the standard MNI-template. To identify brain abnormalities in ASD und SCZ associated with illness severity and social cognition, individual peak voxel data were extracted from the regions resulting from between groups comparison and associated with RME, ADOS, and PANSS using Pearson's correlation. Results reported as significant were defined as $P<0.05$ and $r>0.4$. Data were analysed using SPSS Statistics version 17.0.

Results

Global brain measures

Global brain measures were calculated in ASD (global GM [mean, SD]: 790.26 ml, 52.32 ml; global WM: 535.93 ml, 41.28 ml; TBV: 1326.19 ml, 94.87 ml), SCZ (global GM [mean, SD]: 731.69 ml, 85.63 ml; global WM: 518.96 ml, 59.08 ml; TBV: 1250.65 ml, 142.79 ml), and TD (global GM [mean, SD]: 777.48 ml, 52.31 ml; global WM: 537.50 ml, 42.53 ml; TBV: 1314.98 ml, 92.43 ml). No differences were found between groups in global GM ($F_{2,77} = 2.365$; $P = 0.101$), WM ($F_{2,77} = 0.894$; $P = 0.413$) or TBV ($F_{2,77} = 1.640$; $P = 0.201$) (Figure 1).

Voxel based morphometry

As results did not survive a FWE/FDR correction, they are given on a $P<0.001$ level, uncorrected. A main effect of group was observed for GM volume in the left anterior insula (AI), left amygdala and occipital medial area (Table 2). No main effect of group was found for WM volume. Thus, between groups analysis was performed for GM only. In the contrast SCZ vs. ASD, GM volume in left AI was smaller in ASD (Figure 2). In the contrast ASD vs. TD, smaller GM volumes were found in ASD in left amygdala, left AI and additionally in the anterior MPFC and right amygdala (Figure 2). In the medial occipital area, GM volume was larger in ASD. The contrast SCZ vs. TD did not reveal any significant GM alterations.

Antipsychotic treatment must be considered as a potential bias on regional brain volume. No association was observed with amygdala, insula, or MPFC volume and chlorpromazine-equivalents.

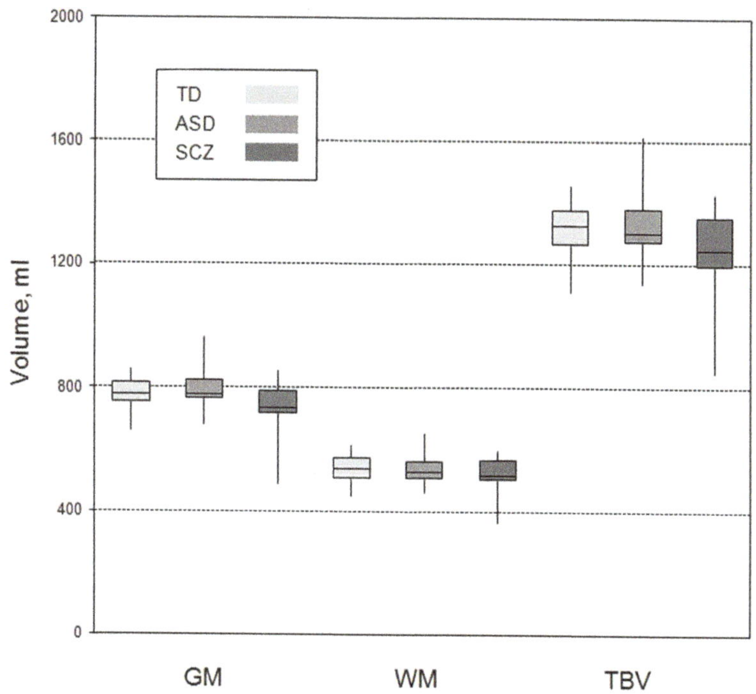

Figure 1. Box plots of global brain measures. Box plots are given for autism spectrum disorder (ASD), schizophrenia (SCZ) and typically developed control subjects (TD) each with global gray matter (GM), global white matter (WM) and total brain volume (TBV). The horizontal line in each box indicates the median, while the top and bottom borders of the box mark the 25th and 75th percentile, respectively. The vertical lines above and below the box mark the range of distribution.

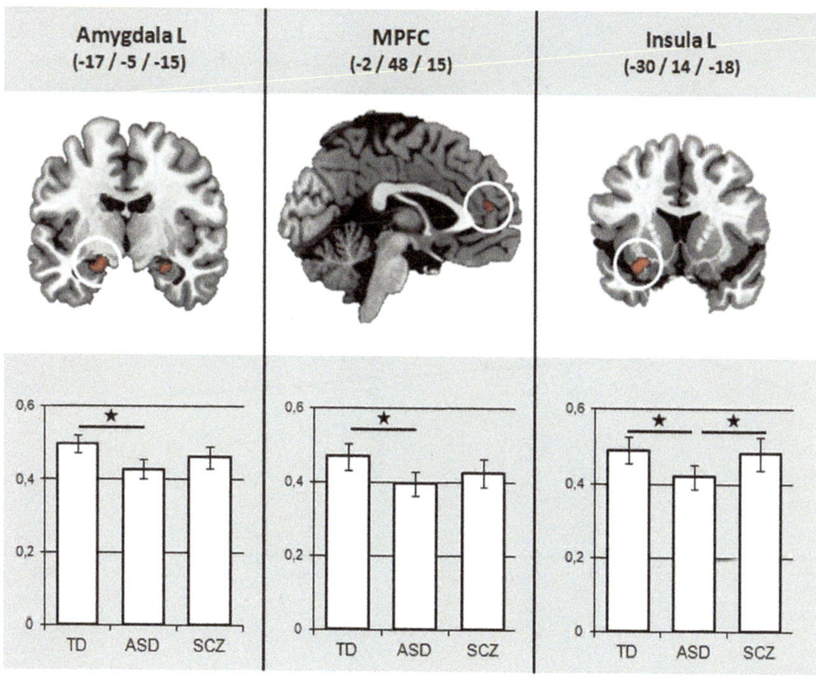

Figure 2. Results of conjunctional VBM analysis of T contrasts. All statistical parametric maps were thresholded at P<0.001 with a cluster level K>20, age was added as a covariate. In column diagrams, beta-values are given for each cluster. Significant contrasts (P<0.05) are marked with star (*). *Left:* contrast TD>ASD in a coronal view (Y = −5); *Middle:* contrast TD>ASD in a saggital view (X = −2); *Right:* contrast SCZ>ASD in a coronal view (Y = 14).

Table 2. Summary of main effect results and between group analyses in MNI space on a p<0.001 level.

Brain region	MNI Coordinates			Z-score	Cluster size
	x	Y	z		[voxels]
main effects					
Insula L	−30	14	−18	3.98	88
Amygdala L	−17	−5	−15	3.58	72
Occipital medial area	38	−74	23	3.43	29
TD>ASD					
Amygdala L	−17	−5	−15	4.10	319
Amygdala R	27	−9	−18	3.37	39
MPFC	−2	48	15	3.56	28
Insula L	−30	15	−18	3.54	22
ASD>TD					
Occipital medial area	39	−75	23	3.95	118
SCZ>ASD					
Insula L	−30	14	−18	4.22	224

Correlations between volumetric and behavioral data

In SCZ, a positive correlation was found between left AI GM volume and the PANSS hallucinatory behavior score ($r = 0.56$; $P = 0.008$). No correlation was found between GM alterations and illness duration. In ASD, a positive correlation was found between left amygdala volume and the RME-score ($r = 0.41$; $P = 0.015$) (Figure 3). As one peripheral data point (Figure 3, data point (0.37/7)) was suspect being an outlier, a second analysis was performed with the remaining data. The correlation persisted on a trend level.

Discussion

To our knowledge, this is the first structural MRI study that compared ASD and SCZ directly. The following main findings were revealed: 1) No global GM or WM alterations were present between groups. 2) In VBM analysis, GM alterations were present mainly in regions associated with social cognition (amygdala, MPFC and insula). Direct comparison of both disorders demonstrated a smaller GM volume in the left anterior Insula (AI) in ASD compared to SCZ. ASD showed smaller local GM volumes compared to TD in the bilateral amygdala, left AI and anterior MPFC. No differences were found between SCZ and TD. 3) Alterations in GM volume correlated significantly with specific parameters of psychopathology and social abilities: hallucinatory

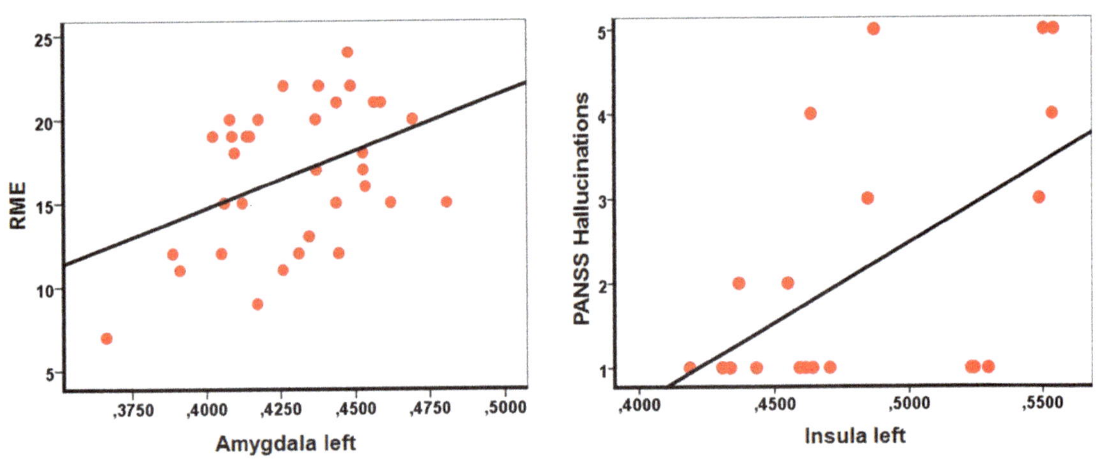

Figure 3. Correlation plots. Left: Correlation between left amygdala GM volume (beta-values) and the 'reading the mind in the eyes'-score (RME) in autism spectrum disorder ($r = 0.41$; $P = 0.015$). The RME-score represents the number of correctly identified emotions of pictures depicting facial expressions (maximum score = 28). Right: Correlation between left insular GM volume (beta-values) and the PANSS hallucinatory behaviour score in schizophrenia ($r = 0.56$; $P = 0.008$). The hallucinatory behaviour score represents the degree of a patient's verbal report or behaviour indicating perceptions which are not generated by external stimuli. The score ranges between 1 (absent) and 7 (extreme).

behavior with AI volume in SCZ, and mentalizing abilities with amygdala volume in ASD.

Global brain measures

No alterations in global GM/WM were found between groups. Although meta-analytic studies in SCZ reported alterations in global brain parameters such as smaller global GM, global WM and TBV [23,51,52] original data reported contradicting results. Out of 32 cross-sectional studies, that were included in meta-analytic studies on first episode SCZ [24,53], only 7 studies reported significant results. As alterations are subtle [54], large samples are needed to detect these differences. Thus, it is not surprising, that in our study, no differences between groups regarding global brain measures were detected. In ASD compared to TD, previous studies reported larger GM, WM and TBV predominantly in children, but not in the adult population [22]. This is in accordance with results of this study.

Voxel based morphometry

1. Direct comparison of ASD and SCZ. This study suggests a dysfunctional involvement of the AI in both disorders. ASD patients showed a smaller GM volume in the left AI compared to SCZ, whereas a positive correlation was found between insular GM volume in SCZ and PANSS hallucinatory behavior score.

In ASD and SCZ, the insula was consistently affected in structural and functional MRI studies [30,55–57,29,58,28]. Similar, smaller insular GM volumes were found in SCZ and ASD in a study using an anatomical likelihood estimation (ALE) approach [33].

The AI is an extensively connected, multifaceted brain region that is involved in numerous brain functions [59]. This brain region is highly involved in processing sensory stimuli with a unique role in interoception, monitoring the physiological reaction like heartbeat frequency, skin conductance, pain and touch [60–63] and also the emotional component of interoceptive awareness [64,65]. The interceptive awareness of the body as an independent entity that is distinct from external environment, is a precondition for self and non-self discrimination [66,59]. Furthermore, AI has been implicated in empathic abilities [67,68,62] and is involved in auditory and facial affect processing [69–71]. One theory, the salience network hypothesis [72–74] conceptualizes the disparate AI functions using a comprehensive "network perspective". According to this model, the AI is the integral hub of the salience network, and represents a multimodal salience detector that identifies the most relevant among several internal and external stimuli. It is associated with segregate functions (i.e. processing of sensory information like pain, social cues like facial expressions, and the analysis of own emotional state) which all facilitate subjectively relevant information.

A salience network dysfunction has been proposed to play a major role in ASD and SCZ [72,75–78]. In ASD the smaller insular GM volume found in this study fits well with AI hypo-activity reported by fMRI studies on tasks of social cognition [58]. A structural insular abnormality might lead to a disconnection between the AI and sensory and limbic structures, resulting in limited ability to identify salient stimuli necessary for adapting adequately to the social environment [72]. Due to this dysfunction, social cues might not be identified as salient and thus not labelled as emotionally rewarding in the insula. In contrast, sensory stimuli might be considered as salient, which may underlie sensory interests, repetitive behavior, or even anxiety and avoidance in ASD.

In SCZ, brain regions underlying the salience network are consistently changed, in example the insular cortex [79,29,80,77]. Studies on high-risk individuals show, that smaller GM volume of ACC and Insula, both major regions of the salience network, are associated with transition to psychosis [81,82]. Salience network dysfunction has been proposed to play a key role in positive and negative symptoms in SCZ [75,83,77]. In this study, we found a significant relation between insula volume and PANSS hallucinatory behavior score. Hallucinations can be conceptionalized as a failure to differentiate an internally generated from an externally sensory experience [84,85]. Functional and structural studies revealed that the insula, along with regions traditionally known as language areas, seem to play a key role in auditory hallucinations in SCZ [86–92]: A Insula dysfunction might cause a confusion of the two sources, resulting in internal sensory information being attributed to external sources [93]. Audible thoughts, thought insertions, and hallucinations might be the consequence. Still, a positive correlation between insula volume and PANSS hallucinatory behaviour score was surprising as it stays in contrast to reports of insular GM volume loss in SCZ [29]. Further studies are needed to investigate significance of these alterations in more detail and to resolve the mentioned inconsistencies.

2. Direct comparison of ASD and TD. The ASD group was characterized by significantly smaller GM volumes in bilateral amygdala, left AI and anterior MPFC compared to TD. Hence, only areas involved in social cognition were significantly smaller. Smaller GM volume in the amygdala-hippocampal complex represents a common finding in VBM-studies in ASD [53,94–97]. The amygdala is involved in emotion recognition and affective Theory of Mind and is thus a key player in social cognition [98]. The association of social impairment and abnormalities of the amygdala have been reported across many different scientific fields [99–101]. In a meta-analysis of functional neuroimaging studies in ASD, hypoactivation of the amygdala has been found in different social cognitive tasks [102,103]. Because a smaller cortical GM volume has been frequently associated with a reduced function in the affected structure [104], the smaller GM volume in the amygdala in ASD fits well to the lower amygdala activation in functional neuroimaging studies. This is supported by the positive correlation we found between mentalizing abilities and amygdala volume in ASD.

In agreement with results of this study, Mc Alonan found a significantly smaller insular GM volume in ASD [105]. Greater insular surface area is associated with poorer social behaviour in ASD [106] and a meta-analysis of functional MRI studies examining social processing identified the AI as a consistent locus of hypo-activity in autism [58]. Altered functional connectivity of AI with Amygdala and somatosensory regions were also present in ASD [107]. These structural and functional findings could underlie typical ASD symptoms like altered emotional experiences and impaired social abilities.

In MPFC, we found a smaller GM volume in ASD. According to a functional division of the MPFC this area is located in the anterior MPFC [108]. The MPFC, in particular its anterior part, is a key region of mentalizing abilities. It is involved during communicative intention [109–112] and triadic interactions [113]{Amodio 2006 #141 [114,115]. Different lines of evidence imply alterations of MPFC in ASD. For example, injuries of the MPFC have led to deficient mentalizing abilities and autism-like behavior [116]; histologic abnormalities in this region have been found in animal models of autism [117,118], and in postmortem-studies of ASD patients [119]. Different neuroimaging techniques have revealed a reduced activity in the MPFC in ASD patients using MEG [120], PET [121], and functional MRI during Theory of Mind tasks [122,14]. The reduced activity in the MPFC corresponds well with the smaller GM volume across ages described in previous meta-analyses [27]. This study provides an additional confirmation for this finding.

3. Direct comparison of SCZ and TD. No structural alterations were found in SCZ compared to TD. This is in disagreement with our hypothesis, as brain volume alterations were expected in areas encoding social cognition in SCZ. Smaller regional brain volumes were consistently reported in meta-analyses [55,31,29]. However, these results are highly heterogeneous, as age of onset and illness duration influence results of VBM analyses causing different alterations in regional GM volume [28,31]. In this study, three aspects might explain the lack of observed differences between SCZ and TD: First, SCZ comprised the smallest group of participants. Thus, the study has lacked power to find smaller volumetric changes [123], which must be considered as a limitation. Second, with a mean age of 24.7 years (range 14 to 33 years) the SCZ patients in our study were relatively young. In SCZ, GM alterations are more pronounced in samples with rising illness duration and age [51]. Third, the examined population was a mixed sample of adolescent-onset SCZ and adult-onset SCZ. A heterogeneous sample in terms of age of onset might have contributed to a lack of alterations in GM volume in this contrast.

Study limitations

Some aspects must be considered as limitations of this study. (1) The study was designed to detect only large volume differences; due to limited sample size and a lack of power, possibly existing smaller volume alterations were not detected. We can therefore only interpret the differences detected in our study but not the lack of differences. Results need to be considered preliminary, as they were reported given on a $p<0.001$ level and did not withstand a more stringent and conservative correction for multiple comparisons across the brain. (2) The SCZ sample was heterogeneous in regards of disease onset comprising both adolescent and adult onset schizophrenia.

Conclusion

In summary, this study compared ASD and SCZ patients directly for global and regional alterations in brain structure. Results emphasize distinct brain substrate in both disorders, as GM alterations of the social brain were prominent in ASD only. Still, we found that disturbances in the insula may play an important role in both conditions. As a morphologic correlate, this study revealed a lower insular GM volume in ASD; in SCZ individuals, a positive correlation of insular GM volume and PANSS hallucinatory behavior score was found, which contrasts to smaller insular volume frequently reported in SCZ. Further studies are needed to replicate the described findings and investigate neurophysiological significance of these alterations for ASD and SCZ in more detail.

Author Contributions

Conceived and designed the experiments: AC MS DH SS BW SB FP HW. Performed the experiments: AC DH SS BW SB FP HW. Analyzed the data: DR AC MS HW CMF. Contributed reagents/materials/analysis tools: DR AC MS DH SS SB FP HW CMF. Contributed to the writing of the manuscript: DR AC MS DH SS BW SB FP HW CMF.

References

1. Guilmatre A, Dubourg C, Mosca A, Legallic S, Goldenberg A et al. (2009) Recurrent rearrangements in synaptic and neurodevelopmental genes and shared biologic pathways in schizophrenia, autism, and mental retardation. Arch Gen Psychiatry 66 (9): 947–956.
2. Pelphrey KA, Shultz S, Hudac CM, Vander Wyk BC (2011) Research Review: Constraining heterogeneity: the social brain and its development in autism spectrum disorder. J Child Psychol Psychiatry 52 (6): 631–644.
3. Burns J (2006) The social brain hypothesis of schizophrenia. World Psychiatry 5 (2): 77–81.
4. Adolphs R (2003) Cognitive neuroscience of human social behaviour. Nat Rev Neurosci 4 (3): 165–178.
5. Frith CD, Frith U (2007) Social Cognition in Humans. Curr Biol 17 (16): R724–32.
6. Frith CD, Frith U (2006) How we predict what other people are going to do. Brain Res 1079 (1): 36–46.
7. Brunet E, Sarfati Y, Hardy-Baylé M, Decety J (2003) Abnormalities of brain function during a nonverbal theory of mind task in schizophrenia. Neuropsychologia 41 (12): 1574–1582.
8. Brüne M, Abdel-Hamid M, Sonntag C, Lehmkämper C, Langdon R (2009) Linking social cognition with social interaction: Non-verbal expressivity, social competence and "mentalising" in patients with schizophrenia spectrum disorders. Behav Brain Funct 5 (1): 6.
9. Das P, Lagopoulos J, Coulston CM, Henderson AF, Malhi GS (2012) Mentalizing impairment in schizophrenia: A functional MRI study. Schizophr Res 134 (2–3): 158–164.
10. Pedersen A, Koelkebeck K, Brandt M, Wee M, Kueppers KA et al. (2012) Theory of mind in patients with schizophrenia: Is mentalizing delayed. Schizophr Res 137 (1–3): 224–229.
11. Walter H, Ciaramidaro A, Adenzato M, Vasic N, Ardito RB, Erk S, Bara BG (2009) Dysfunction of the social brain in schizophrenia is modulated by intention type: An fMRI study. Soc Cogn Affect Neurosci 4(2): 166–76.
12. Pinkham AE, Hopfinger JB, Pelphrey KA, Piven J, Penn DL (2008) Neural bases for impaired social cognition in schizophrenia and autism spectrum disorders. Schizophr Res 99 (1–3): 164–175.
13. Johnston PJ, Stojanov W, Devir H, Schall U (2005) Functional MRI of facial emotion recognition deficits in schizophrenia and their electrophysiological correlates. Eur J Neurosci 22 (5): 1221–1232.
14. Castelli F (2002) Autism, Asperger syndrome and brain mechanisms for the attribution of mental states to animated shapes. Brain 125 (8): 1839–1849.
15. Kana RK, Libero LE, Hu CP, Deshpande HD, Colburn JS (2012) Functional Brain Networks and White Matter Underlying Theory-of-Mind in Autism. Soc Cogn Affect Neurosci 9(1): 98–105.
16. Lombardo MV, Chakrabarti B, Bullmore ET, Baron-Cohen S (2011) Specialization of right temporo-parietal junction for mentalizing and its relation to social impairments in autism. Neuroimage 56 (3): 1832–1838.
17. Critchley HD, Daly EM, Bullmore ET, Williams SC, van Amelsvoort T et al. (2000) The functional neuroanatomy of social behaviour: changes in cerebral blood flow when people with autistic disorder process facial expressions. Brain 123 (Pt 11): 2203–2212.
18. Wang AT, Dapretto M, Hariri AR, Sigman M, Bookheimer SY (2004) Neural correlates of facial affect processing in children and adolescents with autism spectrum disorder. J Am Acad Child Adolesc Psychiatry 43 (4): 481–490.
19. Suzuki K, Sugihara G, Ouchi Y, Nakamura K, Tsujii M et al. (2011) Reduced acetylcholinesterase activity in the fusiform gyrus in adults with autism spectrum disorders. Arch Gen Psychiatry 68 (3): 306–313.
20. Kleinhans NM, Richards T, Johnson LC, Weaver KE, Greenson J et al. (2011) fMRI evidence of neural abnormalities in the subcortical face processing system in ASD. Neuroimage 54 (1): 697–704.
21. Pelphrey KA, Morris JP, McCarthy G (2005) Neural basis of eye gaze processing deficits in autism. Brain 128 (Pt 5): 1038–1048.
22. Stanfield AC, McIntosh AM, Spencer MD, Philip R, Gaur S et al. (2008) Towards a neuroanatomy of autism: A systematic review and meta-analysis of structural magnetic resonance imaging studies. Eur Psychiatry 23 (4): 289–299.
23. Wright IC, Rabe-Hesketh S, Woodruff PW, David AS, Murray RM et al. (2000) Meta-analysis of regional brain volumes in schizophrenia. Am J Psychiatry 157 (1): 16–25.
24. Steen RG, Mull C, McClure R, Hamer RM, Lieberman JA (2006) Brain volume in first-episode schizophrenia: systematic review and meta-analysis of magnetic resonance imaging studies. Br J Psychiatry 188: 510–518.
25. Vita A, Peri L de, Silenzi C, Dieci M (2006) Brain morphology in first-episode schizophrenia: A meta-analysis of quantitative magnetic resonance imaging studies. Schizophr Res 82 (1): 75–88.
26. Nickl-Jockschat T, Habel U, Maria Michel T, Manning J, Laird AR et al. (2011) Brain structure anomalies in autism spectrum disorder-a meta-analysis of VBM studies using anatomic likelihood estimation. Hum Brain Mapp 33(6): 1470–89.
27. Duerden EG, Mak-Fan KM, Taylor MJ, Roberts SW (2012) Regional differences in grey and white matter in children and adults with autism spectrum disorders: an activation likelihood estimate (ALE) meta-analysis. Autism Res 5 (1): 49–66.
28. Chan RCK, Di X, McAlonan GM, Gong Q (2010) Brain Anatomical Abnormalities in High-Risk Individuals, First-Episode, and Chronic Schizophrenia: An Activation Likelihood Estimation Meta-analysis of Illness Progression. Schizophr Bull 37 (1): 177–188.

29. Ellison-Wright I, Glahn DC, Laird AR, Thelen SM, Bullmore E (2008) The Anatomy of First-Episode and Chronic Schizophrenia: An Anatomical Likelihood Estimation Meta-Analysis. Am J Psychiatry 165 (8): 1015–1023.
30. Shepherd AM, Laurens KR, Matheson SL, Carr VJ, Green MJ (2012) Systematic meta-review and quality assessment of the structural brain alterations in schizophrenia. Neurosci Biobehav Rev 36(4): 1342–56.
31. Honea R, Crow TJ, Passingham D, Mackay CE (2005) Regional deficits in brain volume in schizophrenia: a meta-analysis of voxel-based morphometry studies. Am J Psychiatry 162 (12): 2233–2245.
32. Olabi B, Ellison-Wright I, McIntosh AM, Wood SJ, Bullmore E et al. (2011) Are there progressive brain changes in schizophrenia? A meta-analysis of structural magnetic resonance imaging studies. Biol Psychiatry 70 (1): 88–96.
33. Cheung C, Yu K, Fung G, Leung M, Wong C et al. (2010) Autistic Disorders and Schizophrenia: Related or Remote? An Anatomical Likelihood Estimation. PLoS ONE 5 (8): e12233.
34. Sasson NJ, Pinkham AE, Carpenter KLH, Belger A (2011) The benefit of directly comparing autism and schizophrenia for revealing mechanisms of social cognitive impairment. J Neurodevelop Disord 3 (2): 87–100.
35. Le Rutter M, Couteur A., Lord C. (2003) Autism Diagnostic Interview - Revised (ADI-R). Los Angeles, CA: Western Psychological Services.
36. Bölte S, Rühl D., Schmötzer G., Poustka F. (2006) Diagnostisches Interview für Autismus – revidiert. Bern: Huber.
37. Lord C, Rutter M., DiLavore P., Risi S. (2001) Autism Diagnostic Schedule (ADOS). Los Angeles, CA: Western Psychological Services.
38. Rühl D, Bölte S., Feineis-Matthews S., Poustka F. (2004) Diagnostische Beobachtungsskala für Autistische Störungen (ADOS). Bern: Huber.
39. Kay SR, Opler LA, Lindenmayer JP (1989) The Positive and Negative Syndrome Scale (PANSS): rationale and standardisation. Br J Psychiatry Suppl (7): 59–67.
40. Achenbach T (1991) Manual for the Youth Self-Report and 1991 profile.: University of Vermont, Departement of Psychiatry.
41. Achenbach T (1997) Manual for the Young Adult Self-Report and Young Adult Behavior Checklist.: University of Vermont, Departement of Psychiatry.
42. Achenbach T (1991) Manual for the Child Behavior Checklist and 1991 profile.: University of Vermont, Departement of Psychiatry.
43. Kratzmeier H, Horn R (1988) Standard Progressive Matrices. Weinheim: Beltz.
44. Oldfield RC (1971) The assessment and analysis of handedness: the Edinburgh inventory. Neuropsychologia 9 (1): 97–113.
45. Baron-Cohen S, Wheelwright S, Hill J, Raste Y, Plumb I (2001) The "Reading the Mind in the Eyes" Test revised version: a study with normal adults, and adults with Asperger syndrome or high-functioning autism. J Child Psychol Psychiatry 42 (2): 241–251.
46. Woods SW (2003) Chlorpromazine equivalent doses for the newer atypical antipsychotics. J Clin Psychiatry 64 (6): 663–667.
47. Deichmann R, Schwarzbauer C, Turner R (2004) Optimisation of the 3D MDEFT sequence for anatomical brain imaging: technical implications at 1.5 and 3 T. Neuroimage 21 (2): 757–767.
48. Ashburner J (2010) VBM Tutorial. Available: http://www.fil.ion.ucl.ac.uk/~john/misc/VBMclass10.pdf.
49. Talairach J TP (1988) Co-Planar Stereotactic Atlas of the Human Brain: 3-Dimensional Proportional System: An Approach to Cerebral Imaging. New York: Thieme Medical Publishers.
50. Duvernoy HM (1991) The Human Brain: Surface, Three-Dimensional Sectional Anatomy and MRI. New York: Springer.
51. Hulshoff Pol HE, Kahn RS (2008) What happens after the first episode? A review of progressive brain changes in chronically ill patients with schizophrenia. Schizophr Bull 34 (2): 354–366.
52. Shenton ME, Dickey CC, Frumin M, McCarley RW (2001) A review of MRI findings in schizophrenia. Schizophr Res 49 (1–2): 1–52.
53. Via E, Radua J, Cardoner N, Happé F, Mataix-Cols D (2011) Meta-analysis of gray matter abnormalities in autism spectrum disorder: should Asperger disorder be subsumed under a broader umbrella of autistic spectrum disorder. Arch Gen Psychiatry 68 (4): 409–418.
54. Harrison PJ, Freemantle N, Geddes JR (2003) Meta-analysis of brain weight in schizophrenia. Schizophr Res 64 (1): 25–34.
55. Bora E, Fornito A, Radua J, Walterfang M, Seal M et al. (2011) Neuroanatomical abnormalities in schizophrenia: a multimodal voxelwise meta-analysis and meta-regression analysis. Schizophr Res 127 (1–3): 46–57.
56. Glahn DC, Laird AR, Ellison-Wright I, Thelen SM, Robinson JL et al. (2008) Meta-Analysis of Gray Matter Anomalies in Schizophrenia: Application of Anatomic Likelihood Estimation and Network Analysis. Biol Psychiatry 64 (9): 774–781.
57. Fornito A, Yücel M, Patti J, Wood S, Pantelis C (2009) Mapping grey matter reductions in schizophrenia: An anatomical likelihood estimation analysis of voxel-based morphometry studies. Schizophr Res 108 (1–3): 104–113.
58. Di Martino A, Ross K, Uddin LQ, Sklar AB, Castellanos FX et al. (2009) Functional Brain Correlates of Social and Nonsocial Processes in Autism Spectrum Disorders: An Activation Likelihood Estimation Meta-Analysis. Biological Psychiatry 65 (1): 63–74.
59. Craig ADB (2009) How do you feel-now? The anterior insula and human awareness. Nat Rev Neurosci 10 (1): 59–70.
60. Ochsner KN, Zaki J, Hanelin J, Ludlow DH, Knierim K et al. (2008) Your pain or mine? Common and distinct neural systems supporting the perception of pain in self and other. Soc Cogn Affect Neurosci 3 (2): 144–160.
61. Critchley HD, Wiens S, Rotshtein P, Öhman A, Dolan RJ (2004) Neural systems supporting interoceptive awareness. Nat Neurosci 7 (2): 189–195.
62. Singer T, Seymour B, O'Doherty J, Kaube H, Dolan RJ et al. (2004) Empathy for pain involves the affective but not sensory components of pain. Science 303 (5661): 1157–1162.
63. Lovero KL, Simmons AN, Aron JL, Paulus MP (2009) Anterior insular cortex anticipates impending stimulus significance. Neuroimage 45 (3): 976–983.
64. Craig ADB (2003) Interoception: the sense of the physiological condition of the body. Curr Opin Neurobiol 13 (4): 500–505.
65. Critchley HD (2002) Volitional Control of Autonomic Arousal: A Functional Magnetic Resonance Study. Neuroimage 16 (4): 909–919.
66. Devue C, Collette F, Balteau E, Degueldre C, Luxen A et al. (2007) Here I am: The cortical correlates of visual self-recognition. Brain Res 1143: 169–182.
67. Jabbi M, Swart M, Keysers C (2007) Empathy for positive and negative emotions in the gustatory cortex. Neuroimage 34 (4): 1744–1753.
68. Saarela MV, Hlushchuk Y, Williams ACC de, Schürmann M, Kalso E et al. (2007) The compassionate brain: humans detect intensity of pain from another's face. Cereb Cortex 17 (1): 230–237.
69. Wicker B, Keysers C, Plailly J, Royet JP, Gallese V et al. (2003) Both of us disgusted in My insula: the common neural basis of seeing and feeling disgust. Neuron 40 (3): 655–664.
70. Carr L, Iacoboni M, Dubeau M, Mazziotta JC, Lenzi GL (2003) Neural mechanisms of empathy in humans: a relay from neural systems for imitation to limbic areas. Proc Natl Acad Sci U S A 100 (9): 5497–5502.
71. Quadflieg S, Mohr A, Mentzel H, Miltner WHR, Straube T (2008) Modulation of the neural network involved in the processing of anger prosody: the role of task-relevance and social phobia. Biol Psychol 78 (2): 129–137.
72. Uddin LQ, Menon V (2009) The anterior insula in autism: Under-connected and under-examined. Neurosci Biobehav Rev 33 (8): 1198–1203.
73. Menon V, Uddin LQ (2010) Saliency, switching, attention and control: a network model of insula function. Brain Struct Funct 214 (5–6): 655–667.
74. Toyomaki A, Murohashi H (2013) "Salience network" dysfunction hypothesis in autism spectrum disorders. Jpn Psychol Res 55 (2): 175–185.
75. Manoliu A, Riedl V, Zherdin A, Muhlau M, Schwerthoffer D et al. (2013) Aberrant Dependence of Default Mode/Central Executive Network Interactions on Anterior Insular Salience Network Activity in Schizophrenia. Schizophr Bull 40(2): 428–37.
76. Manoliu A, Riedl V, Doll A, Bäuml JG, Mühlau M et al. (2013) Insular Dysfunction Reflects Altered Between-Network Connectivity and Severity of Negative Symptoms in Schizophrenia during Psychotic Remission. Front Hum Neurosci 7: 216.
77. Palaniyappan L (2012) Does the salience network play a cardinal role in psychosis? An emerging hypothesis of insular dysfunction. J Psychiatry Neurosci 37 (1): 17–27.
78. Lee S, Chun JW, Lee JS, Park H, Jung Y et al. (2014) Abnormal Neural Processing during Emotional Salience Attribution of Affective Asymmetry in Patients with Schizophrenia. PLoS ONE 9 (3): e90792.
79. Shepherd AM, Matheson SL, Laurens KR, Carr VJ, Green MJ (2012) Systematic Meta-Analysis of Insula Volume in Schizophrenia. Biological Psychiatry 72 (9): 775–784.
80. Ellison-Wright I, Bullmore E (2009) Meta-analysis of diffusion tensor imaging studies in schizophrenia. Schizophr Res 108 (1–3): 3–10.
81. Borgwardt SJ, Riecher-Rössler A, Dazzan P, Chitnis X, Aston J et al. (2007) Regional gray matter volume abnormalities in the at risk mental state. Biol Psychiatry 61 (10): 1148–1156.
82. Pantelis C, Velakoulis D, McGorry PD, Wood SJ, Suckling J et al. (2003) Neuroanatomical abnormalities before and after onset of psychosis: a cross-sectional and longitudinal MRI comparison. Lancet 361 (9354): 281–288.
83. Palaniyappan L, Simmonite M, White TP, Liddle EB, Liddle PF (2013) Neural Primacy of the Salience Processing System in Schizophrenia. Neuron 79 (4): 814–828.
84. Frith CD, Done DJ (1988) Towards a neuropsychology of schizophrenia. Br J Psychiatry 153: 437–443.
85. Ford JM, Mathalon DH (2004) Electrophysiological evidence of corollary discharge dysfunction in schizophrenia during talking and thinking. J Psychiatr Res 38 (1): 37–46.
86. Palaniyappan L, Balain V, Radua J, Liddle PF (2012) Structural correlates of auditory hallucinations in schizophrenia: A meta-analysis. Schizophr Res 137 (1–3): 169–173.
87. Copolov DL, Seal ML, Maruff P, Ulusoy R, Wong MT et al. (2003) Cortical activation associated with the experience of auditory hallucinations and perception of human speech in schizophrenia: a PET correlation study. Psychiatry Res: Neuroimage 122 (3): 139–152.
88. Diederen KMJ, Neggers SFW, Daalman K, Blom JD, Goekoop R et al. (2010) Deactivation of the parahippocampal gyrus preceding auditory hallucinations in schizophrenia. Am J Psychiatry 167 (4): 427–435.
89. Hoffman RE, Anderson AW, Varanko M, Gore JC, Hampson M (2008) Time course of regional brain activation associated with onset of auditory/verbal hallucinations. Br J Psychiatry 193 (5): 424–425.

90. Jardri R, Pouchet A, Pins D, Thomas P (2011) Cortical activations during auditory verbal hallucinations in schizophrenia: a coordinate-based meta-analysis. Am J Psychiatry 168 (1): 73–81.
91. Shergill SS, Brammer MJ, Williams SC, Murray RM, McGuire PK (2000) Mapping auditory hallucinations in schizophrenia using functional magnetic resonance imaging. Arch Gen Psychiatry 57 (11): 1033–1038.
92. Shergill SS, Brammer MJ, Amaro E, Williams SCR, Murray RM et al. (2004) Temporal course of auditory hallucinations. Br J Psychiatry 185: 516–517.
93. Wylie KP, Tregellas JR (2010) The role of the insula in schizophrenia. Schizophr Res 123 (2–3): 93–104.
94. Brieber S, Neufang S, Bruning N, Kamp-Becker I, Remschmidt H et al. (2007) Structural brain abnormalities in adolescents with autism spectrum disorder and patients with attention deficit/hyperactivity disorder. J Child Psychol Psychiatry 48 (12): 1251–1258.
95. Dziobek I, Fleck S, Rogers K, Wolf OT, Convit A (2006) The 'amygdala theory of autism' revisited: Linking structure to behavior. Neuropsychologia 44 (10): 1891–1899.
96. Aylward EH, Minshew NJ, Goldstein G, Honeycutt NA, Augustine AM et al. (1999) MRI volumes of amygdala and hippocampus in non-mentally retarded autistic adolescents and adults. Neurology 53 (9): 2145–2150.
97. Pierce K, Müller RA, Ambrose J, Allen G, Courchesne E (2001) Face processing occurs outside the fusiform 'face area' in autism: evidence from functional MRI. Brain 124 (Pt 10): 2059–2073.
98. Siegal M, Varley R (2002) Neural systems involved in "theory of mind". Nat Rev Neurosci 3 (6): 463–471.
99. Bauman ML, Kemper TL (2005) Neuroanatomic observations of the brain in autism: a review and future directions. Int J Dev Neurosci 23 (2–3): 183–187.
100. Baron-Cohen S, Ring HA, Bullmore ET, Wheelwright S, Ashwin C et al. (2000) The amygdala theory of autism. Neurosci Biobehav Rev 24 (3): 355–364.
101. Machado CJ, Bachevalier J (2006) The impact of selective amygdala, orbital frontal cortex, or hippocampal formation lesions on established social relationships in rhesus monkeys (Macaca mulatta). Behav Neurosci 120 (4): 761–786.
102. Sugranyes G, Kyriakopoulos M, Corrigall R, Taylor E, Frangou S et al. (2011) Autism Spectrum Disorders and Schizophrenia: Meta-Analysis of the Neural Correlates of Social Cognition. PLoS ONE 6 (10): e25322.
103. Dickstein DP, Pescosolido MF, Reidy BL, Galvan T, Kim KL et al. (2013) Developmental meta-analysis of the functional neural correlates of autism spectrum disorders. J Am Acad Child Adolesc Psychiatry 52 (3): 279–289.e16.
104. May A, Gaser C (2006) Magnetic resonance-based morphometry: a window into structural plasticity of the brain. Curr Opin Neurol 19 (4): 407–411.
105. McAlonan GM, Suckling J, Wong N, Cheung V, Lienenkaemper N et al. (2008) Distinct patterns of grey matter abnormality in high-functioning autism and Asperger's syndrome. J Child Psychol Psychiatry 49 (12): 1287–1295.
106. Doyle-Thomas KAR, Kushki A, Duerden EG, Taylor MJ, Lerch JP et al. (2013) The Effect of Diagnosis, Age, and Symptom Severity on Cortical Surface Area in the Cingulate Cortex and Insula in Autism Spectrum Disorders. J Child Neurol 28 (6): 732–739.
107. Ebisch SJ, Gallese V, Willems RM, Mantini D, Groen WB et al. (2011) Altered intrinsic functional connectivity of anterior and posterior insula regions in high-functioning participants with autism spectrum disorder. Hum Brain Mapp 32 (7): 1013–1028.
108. Amodio DM, Frith CD (2006) Meeting of minds: the medial frontal cortex and social cognition. Nat Rev Neurosci 7 (4): 268–277.
109. Walter H, Adenzato M, Ciaramidaro A, Enrici I, Pia L et al. (2004) Understanding intentions in social interaction: the role of the anterior paracingulate cortex. J Cogn Neurosci 16 (10): 1854–1863.
110. Kampe KKW, Frith CD, Frith U (2003) "Hey John": signals conveying communicative intention toward the self activate brain regions associated with "mentalizing," regardless of modality. J. Neurosci 23 (12): 5258–5263.
111. Gallagher HL, Jack AI, Roepstorff A, Frith CD (2002) Imaging the Intentional Stance in a Competitive Game. Neuroimage 16 (3): 814–821.
112. Ciaramidaro A, Becchio C, Colle L, Bara BG, Walter H (2013) Do you mean me? Communicative intentions recruit the mirror and the mentalizing system. Social Cognitive and Affective Neuroscience [Epub ahead of print].
113. Schilbach L, Wilms M, Eickhoff SB, Romanzetti S, Tepest R et al. (2010) Minds made for sharing: initiating joint attention recruits reward-related neurocircuitry. J Cogn Neurosci 22 (12): 2702–2715.
114. Frith U, Frith CD (2003) Development and neurophysiology of mentalizing. Philos Trans R Soc Lond B Biol Sci 358 (1431): 459–473.
115. Saxe R (2006) Uniquely human social cognition. Curr Opin Neurobiol 16 (2): 235–239.
116. Umeda S, Mimura M, Kato M (2010) Acquired personality traits of autism following damage to the medial prefrontal cortex. Soc Neurosci 5 (1): 19–29.
117. Rinaldi TR (2008) Hyper-connectivity and hyper-plasticity in the medial prefrontal cortex in the valproic acid animal model of autism. Front Neural Circuits 2: 4.
118. Testa-Silva G, Loebel A, Giugliano M, Kock CPJ de, Mansvelder HD et al. (2012) Hyperconnectivity and Slow Synapses during Early Development of Medial Prefrontal Cortex in a Mouse Model for Mental Retardation and Autism. Cereb Cortex 22 (6): 1333–1342.
119. Courchesne E, Mouton PR, Calhoun ME, Semendeferi K, Ahrens-Barbeau C et al. (2011) Neuron number and size in prefrontal cortex of children with autism. JAMA 306 (18): 2001–2010.
120. Honaga E, Ishii R, Kurimoto R, Canuet L, Ikezawa K et al. (2010) Post-movement beta rebound abnormality as indicator of mirror neuron system dysfunction in autistic spectrum disorder: An MEG study. Neurosci Lett 478 (3): 141–145.
121. Nieminen-von Wendt T, Metsähonkala L, Kulomäki T, Alto S, Autti T et al. (2003) Changes in cerebral blood flow in Asperger syndrome during theory of mind tasks presented by the auditory route. Eur Child Adolesc Psychiatry 12 (4): 178–189.
122. Wang AT, Lee SS, Sigman M, Dapretto M (2007) Reading affect in the face and voice: neural correlates of interpreting communicative intent in children and adolescents with autism spectrum disorders. Arch Gen Psychiatry 64 (6): 698–708.
123. Steen R, Hamer R, Lieberman J (2007) Measuring Brain Volume by MR Imaging: Impact of Measurement Precision and Natural Variation on Sample Size Requirements. AJNR Am J Neuroradiol 28 (6): 1119–1125.

A Genome Wide Association Study of Mathematical Ability Reveals an Association at Chromosome 3q29, a Locus Associated with Autism and Learning Difficulties

Simon Baron-Cohen[1,2]*, Laura Murphy[1], Bhismadev Chakrabarti[1,3], Ian Craig[4], Uma Mallya[1], Silvia Lakatošová[1], Karola Rehnstrom[5], Leena Peltonen[5], Sally Wheelwright[1], Carrie Allison[1], Simon E. Fisher[6,7], Varun Warrier[1]*

1 Autism Research Centre, Department of Psychiatry, University of Cambridge, Cambridgeshire, United Kingdom, **2** CLASS Clinic, Cambridgeshire and Peterborough NHS Foundation Trust (CPFT), Cambridgeshire, United Kingdom, **3** School of Psychology and Clinical Language Sciences, Centre for Integrative Neuroscience and Neurodynamics, University of Reading, Reading, United Kingdom, **4** MRC Centre for Social, Genetic and Developmental Psychiatry, King's College London, Institute of Psychiatry, London, United Kingdom, **5** The Wellcome Trust Sanger Institute, Hinxton, Cambridgeshire, United Kingdom, **6** Max Planck Institute for Psycholinguistics, 6500 AH Nijmegen, The Netherlands, **7** Donders Institute for Brain, Cognition and Behaviour, Radboud University Nijmegen, Nijmegen, The Netherlands

Abstract

Mathematical ability is heritable, but few studies have directly investigated its molecular genetic basis. Here we aimed to identify specific genetic contributions to variation in mathematical ability. We carried out a genome wide association scan using pooled DNA in two groups of U.K. samples, based on end of secondary/high school national academic exam achievement: high (n = 419) versus low (n = 183) mathematical ability while controlling for their verbal ability. Significant differences in allele frequencies between these groups were searched for in 906,600 SNPs using the Affymetrix GeneChip Human Mapping version 6.0 array. After meeting a threshold of $p<1.5\times10^{-5}$, 12 SNPs from the pooled association analysis were individually genotyped in 542 of the participants and analyzed to validate the initial associations (lowest p-value 1.14 $\times10^{-6}$). In this analysis, one of the SNPs (rs789859) showed significant association after Bonferroni correction, and four (rs10873824, rs4144887, rs12130910 rs2809115) were nominally significant (lowest p-value 3.278 $\times$ 10^{-4}). Three of the SNPs of interest are located within, or near to, known genes (*FAM43A*, *SFT2D1*, *C14orf64*). The SNP that showed the strongest association, rs789859, is located in a region on chromosome 3q29 that has been previously linked to learning difficulties and autism. rs789859 lies 1.3 kbp downstream of *LSG1*, and 700 bp upstream of *FAM43A*, mapping within the potential promoter/regulatory region of the latter. To our knowledge, this is only the second study to investigate the association of genetic variants with mathematical ability, and it highlights a number of interesting markers for future study.

Editor: Momiao Xiong, University of Texas School of Public Health, United States of America

Funding: This work was funded by grants to SBC from the Nancy Lurie Marks Family Foundation, the Medical Research Council (MRC) UK, and the Autism Research Trust (ART). LM and SEF were supported by the Max Planck Society. The funders had no role in study design, data collection and analysis, decision to publish, or preparation of the manuscript.

Competing Interests: The authors have declared that no competing interests exist.

* E-mail: vw260@medschl.cam.ac.uk (VW); sb205@cam.ac.uk (SBC)

Introduction

Mathematics is the basis of science, technology, engineering, and at complex levels (e.g. number theory, algebra) is uniquely human. Despite its obvious importance, our understanding of what gives rise to individual differences in mathematical ability has not been widely studied. Mathematical talent clusters in families [1] and heritability studies indicate that this is in part due to genetic factors. A wide range of estimates have been reported for the proportion of variation in mathematical ability accounted for by genetic factors, from 0.2 up to 0.9 [2–5]. The large variance may be due to different phenotypic measures used, as mathematics is not unitary, so different phenotypic measures may tap distinct components. Academic achievement [5], standardized test scores [2] and teacher reported skills [4] have all been used to measure aptitude for mathematics in quantitative genetic studies.

To our knowledge, only one genetic association study with mathematical ability has been published thus far. DNA pooling was used in two separate sample sets to test for statistically significant differences in allele frequency using a microarray with 500 K SNPs. The comparison was between participants classified as having high or low mathematical ability (measured using a web-based test performance as well as teacher ratings) who were 10 years old at time of testing. The 43 SNPs that most highly differed in frequency between the phenotype groups in the pools were chosen for individual genotyping using a sample set representing the distribution of mathematical ability as a quantitative trait. Ten of these 43 were found to be nominally associated (p-value<0.05) [6].

In the present study we extended the search for genetic factors for mathematical ability by using pooled DNA from participants who all had excellent verbal ability but who differed in terms of having either high or low mathematical ability, to look for association with any of 906,600 SNPs across the genome. There were four key differences from the Docherty et al. (2010) study: 1) We controlled for verbal ability while taking high and low ends of mathematical ability; 2) the phenotypic measure was based on standardized school examination performance; 3) the number of SNPs in the initial exploratory phase was nearly double that of the previous study; and 4) the mean age of the participants was significantly higher than that of Docherty et al. (2010). Twelve SNPs exceeded our designated threshold for significance (p-value$<1.5\times10^{-5}$) at the pooling stage and were individually genotyped and analyzed in the sample to validate the associations. This step also allowed us to evaluate the efficacy of the DNA pooling method in predicting allele frequency.

Methods

Ethics Statement

Ethical approval was obtained from the University of Cambridge Psychology Research Ethics Committee, and all participants provided written informed written consent. All participants in this study were above 16 years of age and written informed consent was obtained from the participant.

Participants

602 participants from the U.K. were recruited by advertisement from local sixth form schools (n = 230) and universities (n = 372) between 2004 and 2008. Participants were included in the study if they reported Caucasian ancestry for 2 generations and had no psychiatric and/or neurological conditions. All individuals were at least 16 years old.

Each individual was classed as having high or low mathematical ability depending on their General Certificate Standard Examination (GCSE) results for Mathematics. To be included in the study the Mathematics GCSE result for the high maths group had to be an A or A* grade (n = 419, 216 males and 203 females). To be included in the low maths group the Mathematics GCSE result had to be a C grade or below (n = 183, 50 males and 133 females). For both of these ability groups, the person's GCSE English grade had to be an A or A*. This was included to control for verbal ability and to ensure we were not just testing for genetic associations with general academic aptitude. The high maths group included some university students, studying a 'hard' science or mathematical degree and had also obtained an A grade at GCE Advanced Level (A-level). The low maths group also included some university students but they were studying a Humanities degree courses had not taken mathematics at A- level or had received a C or below grade. In this way the two maths groups were matched for both age and proportion in university education. Verbal ability for all individuals was high as they all had an A grade or above in English.

Pooling stage

Genomic DNA from each individual was extracted from buccal swabs supplied by the individuals and then anonymized. The DNA was then suspended in Tris-ethylenediamineaacetic acid (EDTA) (TE) buffer (0.01 M tris-hCl, 0.001 M EDTA, pH 8.0) and quantified using PicoGreen double-stranded DNA quantification reagent (Invitrogen, USA). An equimolar amount of DNA (100 ng) from each individual was added to his or her respective pool. There were 10 high mathematical ability pools (5 female only and 5 male only) and 5 low mathematical ability pools (3 female only and 2 male only) with a mean of 40.1 (SD = 12.1) individuals per pool. These pools were interrogated using an Affymetrix GeneChip Human Mapping version 6.0 array (Affymetrix, California, USA) using the standard Affymetrix protocol. Washing and staining was performed using the Fluidics Station 450 and scanned using the GeneChip Scanner 3000 7G, which was controlled using GENCHIP operating software (GCOS) generating cell intensity (.cel) files. The files generated were converted into relative allele signal (RAS) scores using a custom-made statistical protocol in R, snpmap.R [7].

Independent t-tests on the mean RAS scores from the pools for each SNP were performed between the different groups (high mathematical ability and low mathematical ability) to test for significant allele frequency differences. To be chosen for validation by individual genotyping, the difference between allele frequencies for any one SNP was required to have a p-value below 1.5×10^{-5}. This is a relatively lenient p-value threshold in the context of a genome-wide screen, but it was chosen *a priori* in order to reduce the risk of false negatives. Due to the low power retained in DNA pooling of the sample [8] causative SNPs are likely to be missed when adopting a higher threshold for taking them forward to validation. SNPs were rejected for the individual genotyping stage if their minor allele frequency (MAF) in the Caucasian population was below 0.01 as the study did not have the power to pick up rare variants. Post-hoc power calculation was performed using genetic power calculator [9]. Power was calculated using case-control for threshold selected quantitative traits option. QTL variance explained by each SNP was assumed to be 0.01. The frequencies of the increaser allele and the marker allele was assumed at 0.2 each, and the LD (D′) between the marker and the increaser allele was 0.8. At $P < 0.05$, the power at this stage was 61% under an additive model. SNPs were also rejected depending on the calculated coefficient of variation (CV) of the RAS scores for the SNP. If 50% of the pools showed CV >20 for the SNP then it was rejected from analysis.

Individual genotyping stage

All genotyping was carried out by Geneservices UK Ltd using the Sequenom MassARRAY iPLEX platform (Sequenom, San Diego, USA). Out of the 592 individuals screened in the pooling stage, 542 were available for the individual genotyping stage (high maths group n = 375, 194 males, 181 females; low maths group n = 167, 40 males, 127 females). 60 individuals were not individually genotyped due to the lack of DNA. To check if the missing individuals significantly altered the composition of the groups between the pooling and the individual genotyping stage, a chi-square test was performed and the results were non-significant at three degrees of freedom (chi-sq = 6.89; P-value = 0.07). Four individuals were excluded for having over 10% genotyping data missing in the individual genotyping stage and two individuals were excluded due to uncertainty over phenotype status. However, since they were present in different pools during the pooling stage, it is unlikely that they greatly influenced the results of the pooling stage. Out of the 15 SNPs that were selected for individual genotyping, three SNPs had <90% genotyping success in this stage of work, and hence were excluded (noted in Table 1). For the remaining 12 SNPs, no marker deviated significantly from Hardy-Weinberg equilibrium (p<0.001).

Validation of association

To validate the results of association found in the pooling stage, association analysis was carried out on the individual genotype data using PLINK version 1.07 [10]. For each of the 12 SNPs that

Table 1. 15 SNPs chosen for individual genotyping with the P-values from the pooling stage.

rsID	Chr	Nearest gene	Pooling P-value	Chromosome Position	Allele1	Allele2	Allele 1 Frequency	Allele 2 Frequency
rs12130910	1	*RP11-815M8.1*	5.04×10^{-06}	222038372	G	A	0.647	0.353
rs11808800	1	*NTNG1*	9.41×10^{-06}	108040994	T	C	0.973	0.027
rs10873824	1	*HS2ST1*	1.42×10^{-05}	87688394	A	G	0.283	0.717
rs10179572[a]	2	*C2orf83*	1.31×10^{-05}	228504503	A	G	0.535	0.465
rs6546878	2	*DGUOK*	1.02×10^{-05}	74175324	C	A	0.248	0.752
rs12629229	3	*FRMD4B*	1.07×10^{-05}	69411222	T	C	0.765	0.235
rs789859	3	*FAM43A*	4.57×10^{-06}	194405888	G	T	0.611	0.389
rs9884781[a]	4	*AC007106.1*	9.80×10^{-06}	27989923	T	A	0.535	0.465
rs13355548	5	*RP11-152K4.2*	1.14×10^{-06}	31089349	G	A	0.875	0.125
rs2974097	5	*CTD-2036A18.2*	1.30×10^{-05}	85333953	T	A	0.58	0.42
rs9400442[a]	6	*RPF2*	3.42×10^{-06}	111298225	A	G	0.823	0.177
rs4144887	6	*SFT2D1*	3.19×10^{-06}	166747512	G	A	0.748	0.252
rs973582	8	*SGCZ*	1.50×10^{-05}	13909182	G	A	0.69	0.31
rs2138861	12	*RP11-25I15.3*	3.96×10^{-06}	43166458	A	T	0.704	0.296
rs2809115	14	*C14orf64*	6.89×10^{-06}	98406425	A	T	0.559	0.441

[a]Indicates SNPs that did not survive quality control measures to be included in the association validation analysis.

were successfully genotyped, a Cochran-Armitage trend test (1df) was performed, under the null hypothesis that the allele frequencies did not deviate significantly between the different ability groups. A Bonferroni correction was applied to correct for multiple testing of 12 different SNPs in this stage. Thus, we considered a result to be significant in this validation analysis if it yielded a p-value below 0.0042 (0.05/12).

Results

Analysis of the mean RAS scores from the DNA pools identified 15 SNPs with evidence of association that passed our pre-designated significance threshold of $p<1.5\times10^{-5}$ (see Figure 1). All 15 SNPs were taken forward to the next stage of individual genotyping (see Table 1).

To assess the ability of DNA pooling to accurately predict the allele frequency in these individuals, the real allele frequencies of 31 SNPs (the 12 SNPs that met our significance threshold as well as 19 other SNPs) individually genotyped were compared with the mean RAS scores calculated for these SNPs from the DNA pooling stage. Pearson's correlation coefficient for the correlation was $r = 0.8424$ (see Figure 2). The 31 SNPs and the rationale for choosing them is given in File S1.

Of the 15 SNPs chosen for individual genotyping, 12 survived quality control at the individual genotyping stage and were analyzed. Five SNPs were nominally significant, with one of them remaining significant after correcting for multiple comparisons of 12 SNPs in this stage (see Table 2). Three of these SNPs map near to, or within, known genes (*FAM43A, SFT2D1, C14orf64*). The most significant SNP in our study, rs789859 (p-value: 0.000328, Odds ratio: 1.629), is located 700 bp upstream of *FAM43A*.

Discussion

The present study involved a genome-wide screen for association with mathematical ability in a general population sample. In a pooling based genome-wide screen, 15 SNPs were associated with a $p < 1.5 \times 10^{-5}$, leading to follow up individual genotyping and analysis of 12 of these SNPS. This revealed five SNPs to be nominally significant ($p < 0.05$), one of which remained significant after Bonferroni correction for testing multiple markers in the individual genotyping stage. Three of these SNPs are located close to known genes (*FAM43A, SFT2D1, C14orf64*).

The SNP with the highest significance, rs789859, can have a G or T allele and is located in an intergenic region on chromosome 3q29. Microdeletions and duplications in this region have been associated with autism, schizophrenia as well as learning difficulties [11–14]. rs789859 is approximately 700 bp upstream of *FAM43A*,within its 5′ -regulatory region, and 1.3 kbp downstream of *LSG1*. The fact that rs789859 is located in a region that has been previously associated with neurological conditions affecting associative learning [12] is consistent with a putative contribution to mathematical ability. *FAM43A* is a plausible candidate gene, since the SNP maps within the potential promoter/regulatory region of this gene. rs789859 is in high LD with six other variants when queried in Haploreg. Two of these variants (rs150293579 and rs1675923) map within *LSG1*. Both these variants regulate chromatin states in various cell types from the human CNS. The remaining four variants map near *FAM43A* and also regulate chromatin states in brain cell types and alter TF binding sites. The web resource FASTSNP [15] predicts this SNP to be in a possible transcription-factor binding region. *FAM43A* has thus far only been characterized in cDNA assays and is predicted to encode a hypothetical protein, LOC131583, with little knowledge about its function. RNA expression assays have found *FAM43A* RNA in a variety of tissues including tissues from the brain, cerebellum and spinal cord. Since *FAM43A* is not a well-characterized gene at this stage, conclusions about its viability as a candidate, and its possible contributions to the phenotype are not easily reached.

There was no overlap between the SNPs associated in this study and those reported in the only previously published molecular screen of mathematics abilities. This is not surprising given that such abilities must have a complex genetic basis with multiple genetic factors of small effect size, and both studies involved relatively small sample sizes (further discussed below). Methodological differences between the studies may also have contributed to the lack of overlap. The phenotype in this investigation was standardized national exam performance at age 16–18 years old, where the previous published association study [6] employed a composite score based on web-based testing and teacher report of 10-year-olds. Heritability studies of mathematical ability and how

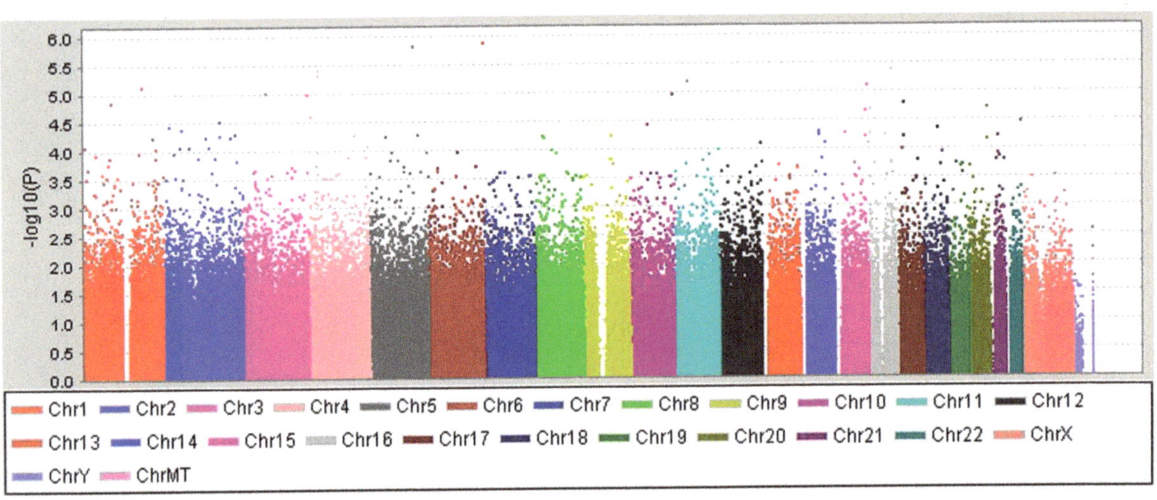

Figure 1. Graphical summary of association results from the genome-wide screen of pooled samples. X-axis represents the chromosome position; y-axis shows -log10 of the P-value obtained for each SNP.

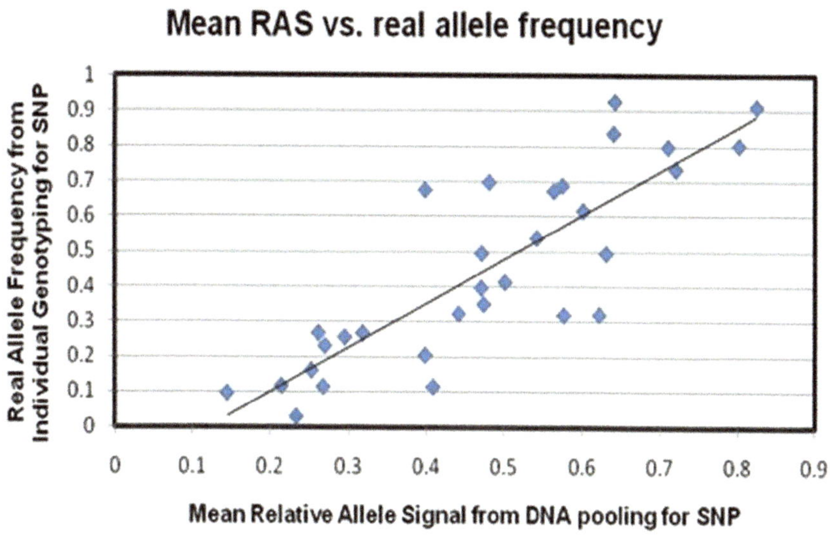

Figure 2. Pearson's correlation of real allele frequencies in total sample (calculated from individual genotyping,y-axis) and frequency estimates from pooled DNA (mean RAS-scores of the 15 pools, x-axis) of 32 SNPs (r = 0.8424).

it changes with age may indicate whether age should be an important issue in experimental design for future association studies.

A limitation of this study is its statistical power. The sample size is small to robustly detect causative loci for a complex trait. Due to the expected small effect sizes of the variants underlying mathematics ability, and complexity of the phenotype tested, larger samples will be needed to definitively identify causative variants. In addition, a previous study using a pooling method suggested the power retained is 68% of the sample [8]. Considering the relatively high correlation of the RAS scores from DNA pooling to real allele frequency demonstrated in this study, the failure of a majority of the SNPs chosen for individual genotyping to reach expected thresholds of significance reflects this lack of power. Quality control exclusions and the fact that a number of individuals from the pooled analysis were not available for individual genotyping are other issues affecting this. The correlation to compare pooling estimates to real allele frequencies was conducted by calculating means of the RAS scores for each SNP from all the pools and thus all the individuals together, so that the missing individuals would have a lesser effect on the numbers than if the correlations were conducted between the phenotype groups separately. These issues may have contributed to the weaker evidence for association observed in the validation step compared to the p-values seen in the DNA pooling GWA study.

In addition to pointing to genetic variation potentially linked to mathematical ability, this study also provides methodological insights for genetic association studies that use pooled DNA. To our knowledge, there is one other published DNA pooling study which used the same Affymetrix GeneChip Human Mapping version 6.0 array [16]. In contrast to the results obtained in this study, which reported a low correlation between allele frequency estimated by the pooled DNA analysis and the real allele frequency determined by individual genotyping (Pearson's r = 0.2734), we report a higher correlation of 0.8424, using the same technique (using DNA from buccal swabs). This improved correlation between estimated and real allele frequencies in this study could be due to a) higher DNA quality in this study, and b) the fact that 110 SNPs were individual genotyped by Schosser et al. 2010, while the current paper only included 32 SNPs. However, the higher correlation in the current analysis for the subset of 32 SNPs suggests that the inferences drawn about these 32 SNPs are reliable. Thus, is it suggested that this microarray may be more suitable for using a DNA pooling approach with buccal mucosa swab samples than previously reported.

Table 2. Association results of SNPs associated at a significance value of 0.05 or less in the individual genotyping stage, along with their pooling stage results.

Variation	Nearest Gene	DNA Pooling		Individual Genotyping	
		P-value	X2	P-value (additive)	Odds ratios (with 95% confidence intervals)
rs789859	*FAM43A*	4.57×10^{-6}	12.9	0.000328	1.629 (2.129–1.247)
rs4144887	*SFT2D1*	3.19×10^{-6}	6.66	0.009838	1.488 (2.014–1.099)
rs12130910	*RP11-815M8.1*	5.04×10^{-6}	4.57	0.03242	1.353 (1.785–1.044)
rs2809115	*C14orf64*	6.89×10^{-6}	4.27	0.03878	1.318 (1.714–1.014)
rs10873824	*HS2ST1*	1.42×10^{-5}	3.89	0.04848	1.343 (1.801–1.002)

SNPs written in bold are significant after correcting for multiple testing.

In conclusion, in this study we detect new candidate loci that might be associated with mathematical ability. The SNP showing the strongest association is located in a genetic region (3q29) that has been proposed to be associated with autism, schizophrenia and learning difficulties [12–14]. Potential future studies could explore the phenotypic overlap (or non-overlap) between mathematical ability and different psychopathological conditions. The known association between autism spectrum conditions and mathematical ability [17,18] suggests that these SNPs should also be tested for association with autism. We acknowledge that the sample size is small for robustly detecting loci with small effect sizes, and research in larger, independent samples should be conducted to further delineate the genetic architecture that contributes to mathematical ability in the general population.

Supporting Information

File S1 This file contains Table S1 and Table S2. Table S1 provides the results of the sex-stratified analyses for the pooling stage. Table S2 provides the list of SNPs used to assess the accuracy of the pooling stage.

Acknowledgments

We are grateful to Imre Leader, Lindsey Kent and Frank Dudbridge for advice and discussions.

Author Contributions

Conceived and designed the experiments: SBC BC IC UM SW CA. Performed the experiments: LM UM SL. Analyzed the data: VW LM. Contributed reagents/materials/analysis tools: IC KR LP. Wrote the paper: SBC LM BC SEF VW.

References

1. Wijsman EM, Robinson NM, Ainsworth KH, Rosenthal EA, Holzman T, et al. (2004) Familial aggregation patterns in mathematical ability. Behav Genet 34: 51–62.
2. Alarcón M, Knopik V, DeFries J (2000) Covariation of mathematics achievement and general cognitive ability in twins. J School Psychol 38: 63–77.
3. Kovas Y, Haworth CMA, Petrill SA, Plomin R (2007) Mathematical ability of 10-year-old boys and girls: genetic and environmental etiology of typical and low performance. J Learn Disabil 40: 554–567.
4. Oliver BR, Harlaar N, Hayiou-Thomas ME, Kovas Y, Walker S, et al. (2004) A Twin Study of Teacher-Reported Mathematics Performance and Low Performance in 7-Year-Olds. J Educ Psychol 96: 504–517.
5. Wadsworth SJ, DeFries JC, Fulker DW, Plomin R (1995) Cognitive ability and academic achievement in the Colorado Adoption Project: a multivariate genetic analysis of parent-offspring and sibling data. Behav Genet 25: 1–15.
6. Docherty SJ, Davis OS, Kovas Y, Meaburn EL, Dale PS, et al. (2010) A genome-wide association study identifies multiple loci associated with mathematics ability and disability. Genes Brain Behav 9: 234–47.
7. Davis OS, Plomin R, Schalkwyk LC (2009) The SNPMaP package for R: a framework for genome-wide association using DNA pooling on microarrays. Bioinformatics 25: 281–3.
8. Barratt BJ, Payne F, Rance HE, Nutland S, Todd J, et al.(2002) Identification of the sources of error in allele frequency estimations from pooled DNA indicates an optimal experimental design. Ann Hum Genet 66: 393–405.
9. Purcell S, Cherny SS, Sham PC (2003) Genetic Power Calculator: design of linkage and association genetic mapping studies of complex traits. Bioinformatics 19: 149–150.
10. Purcell S, Neale B, Todd-Brown K, Thomas L, Ferreira MA, et al. (2007) PLINK: a tool set for whole-genome association and population-based linkage analyses. Am J Hum Genet 81: 559–75.
11. Nava C, Keren B, Mignot C, Rastetter A, Chantot-Bastaraud S, et al. (2014) Prospective diagnostic analysis of copy number variants using SNP microarrays in individuals with autism spectrum disorders. Eur J Hum Genet22:71–8
12. Sagar A, Bishop JR, Tessman DC, Guter S, Martin CL, et al. (2013) Co-occurrence of autism, childhood psychosis, and intellectual disability associated with a de novo 3q29 microdeletion. Am J Med Genet. A161: 845–9.
13. Willatt L, Cox J, Barber J, Cabanas ED, Collins A, et al. (2005) 3q29 microdeletion syndrome: clinical and molecular characterization of a new syndrome. Am J Hum Gen 77: 154–60.
14. Mulle JG, Dodd AF, McGrath JA, Wolyniec PS, Mitchell AA, et al. (2010) Microdeletions of 3q29 confer high risk for schizophrenia. Am J Hum Genet 87: 229–36
15. Yuan HY, Chiou JJ, Tseng WH, Liu CH, Liu CK, et al. (2006) FASTSNP: an always up-to-date and extendable service for SNP function analysis and prioritization. Nucleic Acids Res 34: W635–41.
16. Schosser A, Pirlo K, Gaysina D, Cohen-Woods S, Schalkwyk LC, et al. (2010) Utility of the pooling approach as applied to whole genome association scans with high-density Affymetrix microarrays. BMC Res Notes 3: 274.
17. Baron-Cohen S, Wheelwright S, Skinner R, Martin J, Clubley E (2001) The Autism-Spectrum Quotient: Evidence from Asperger Syndrome/high-functioning autism, males and females, scientists, and mathematicians. J Autism Dev Disord 31: 5–17.
18. Baron-Cohen S, Wheelwright S, Burtenshaw A, Hobson E (2007) Mathematical talent is linked to autism. Human Nat 18: 125–131.

Progressively Increased M50 Responses to Repeated Sounds in Autism Spectrum Disorder with Auditory Hypersensitivity: A Magnetoencephalographic Study

Junko Matsuzaki[1], Kuriko Kagitani-Shimono[2,3]*, Hisato Sugata[4], Masayuki Hirata[4], Ryuzo Hanaie[2], Fumiyo Nagatani[1], Masaya Tachibana[1,2,3], Koji Tominaga[2,3], Ikuko Mohri[1,2,3], Masako Taniike[1,2,3]

1 Molecular Research Center for Children's Mental Development, United Graduate School of Child Development, Osaka University Graduate School of Medicine, Osaka, Japan, **2** United Graduate School of Child Development, Osaka University Graduate School of Medicine, Osaka, Japan, **3** Department of Pediatrics, Osaka University Graduate School of Medicine, Osaka, Japan, **4** Department of Neurosurgery, Osaka University Graduate School of Medicine, Osaka, Japan

Abstract

The aim of this study was to investigate the differential time-course responses of the auditory cortex to repeated auditory stimuli in children with autism spectrum disorder (ASD) showing auditory hypersensitivity. Auditory-evoked field values were obtained from 21 boys with ASD (12 with and 9 without auditory hypersensitivity) and 15 age-matched typically developing controls. M50 dipole moments were significantly increased during the time-course study only in the ASD with auditory hypersensitivity compared with those for the other two groups. The boys having ASD with auditory hypersensitivity also showed more prolonged response duration than those in the other two groups. The response duration was significantly related to the severity of auditory hypersensitivity. We propose that auditory hypersensitivity is associated with decreased inhibitory processing, possibly resulting from an abnormal sensory gating system or dysfunction of inhibitory interneurons.

Editor: Alexandra Key, Vanderbilt University, United States of America

Funding: This study was supported by a grant-in-aid for scientific research (No. 23591494) from Ministry of Education, Culture, Sports, Science and Technology (MEXT). The funders had no role in study design, data collection and analysis, decision to publish, or preparation of the manuscript.

Competing Interests: The authors have declared that no competing interests exist.

* Email: kuriko@ped.med.osaka-u.ac.jp

Introduction

Autism spectrum disorder (ASD) is a neurodevelopmental disorder characterized by qualitative impairments in social interaction and communication, as well as by restricted behavior and interests [1]. In the Diagnostic and Statistical Manual of Mental Disorders (5th edition), in addition to those classical features, sensory abnormalities were appended to the diagnostic criteria for ASD [2]. Unusual perceptual abilities are also common in ASD; for example, many individuals with ASD express extreme reactions to at least one sensory modality, such as auditory stimulation [3]. These individuals perceive innocuous sounds as painful and frightening noise; and in some cases, those sounds may be perceived as phobic stimuli and result in radical behavioral responses in autism spectrum individuals. There are very few clinical interventions available for the treatment of auditory hypersensitivity; and, also, the underlying physiological mechanism has yet to be elucidated. We recently reported that auditory hypersensitivity in ASD is strongly correlated with delayed M50/M100 peak latencies as well as with increased M50 dipole moments [4]. M50/M100 peak responses are activated by auditory stimuli, which responses reflect the process of sensory input and originate in or near the primary auditory cortex [5]. We concluded that these phenomena possibly resulted from neurological immaturity or functional abnormalities in the primary auditory cortex.

On the other hand, Guiraud *et al.* [6] reported that infants at high risk for autism show less habituation to repeated sounds compared with those at low risk; and they speculated that this reduced habituation could be associated with hyposensitivity or over-reactivity to repeated stimulation. Interestingly, in patients having schizophrenia with sensory abnormalities, P50 event-related potential responses are not diminished by repeated sound stimuli [7]. In order to clarify the differential time-course responses of the primary auditory cortex to repeated sounds, we examined M50/M100 responses in individuals with ASD and analyzed these responses in relation to those in patients with characteristic traits of auditory hypersensitivity.

Methods

Participants

Twenty-one male children diagnosed with ASD and 15 age-matched typically developing control males (TD) were recruited at the Osaka University Hospital (Table 1). The diagnosis for ASD was made according to the Diagnostic and Statistical Manual of Mental Disorders (4th edition) text revision (DSM-IV-TR) [1] and was made by an experienced clinician. Furthermore, the diagnosis was confirmed by the Japanese version of the Autism Screening Questionnaire (ASQ - J) [8,9] and Autism Diagnostic Observation Schedule - Generic (ADOS-G) [10]. The intelligence quotient (IQ) was assessed by the Wechsler Intelligence Scale for Children, 3rd version (WISC-III). We assessed the auditory hypersensitivity and behavioral problems by using the Sensory Profile (SP) [11] and the Japanese version of the Child Behavior Checklist (CBCL), respectively [12,13]. Children with ASD were divided into two groups based on the auditory item score of their SP: ASD individuals with auditory hypersensitivity were defined as those having a low SP score of under 30. TD participants were age-matched children without a history of neurological diseases or developmental disorders, and who also were not receiving special education services. In addition, all TD individuals were assessed by the ASQ-J and SP, and they showed no autism traits or sensory problems. Their hearing ability was normal according to available medical records or parent's report. Written informed consent was obtained from the parents of all participants in the study, which was approved by the Institutional Review Board of Osaka University Hospital.

Auditory Stimuli

Auditory stimuli, which were made by a presentation system (Presentation, Neurobehavioral System, Inc. San Francisco, CA), were delivered via a sound pressure transducer and sound conduction tubing to the participant's auditory canal via ear tip inserts. A 1,000- Hz sinusoidal tone pip of 200 msec' duration was binaurally presented (80 dB, with 10-msec rise and fall times). Stimuli were randomly presented with inter-stimulus intervals of 2,700 to 3,300 msec. The total number of stimuli was 100.

Measurements

Before recording by magnetoencephalography (MEG), we scanned the 3D facial surface of each participant (Fast SCAN Cobra, POLHEMUS, ARANTZ Scanning Limited, Christchurch, New Zealand), together with the five head-marker coils as fiduciary points (the external meatus of each ear, two points on the forehead, and nasion).

While lying down on a bed in a magnetically-shielded room, the participants were examined by a 160-channel whole-head MEG system equipped with SQUID gradiometers (PQ1160C, Yokogawa Electric Corporation, Tokyo, Japan). The positions of head marker coils were obtained before and after recording to evaluate head movement [14]. Data were acquired at a sampling rate of 1000 Hz, with an online band pass filter between 0.03 Hz and 200 Hz.

Individual anatomical magnetic resonance image (MRI) data were obtained with a 3.0-Tesla whole-body magnetic resonance scanner equipped with a standard whole-head coil (Signa Excite HD; GE Healthcare, Milwaukee, USA). A 3D-T1-weighted axial protocol was used. Imaging parameters for 3D-T1-weighted images were as follow: 3D-spoiled GRASS sequence, repetition time (TR) = 10.1 ms; echo time (TE) = 3.0 ms; flip angle = 18°; field of view (FOV) = 220×220 mm2; matrix size = 320×256; slice thickness = 1.4 mm; number of excitations (NEX) = 1.A 3D-T1 [15]. 3D facial surface data and fiduciary points were superimposed on the individual MRI data. The MEG data were superimposed on the individual MRI with an anatomical accuracy of a few millimeters.

Data analysis

The MEG data were analyzed by using standard analysis software (MEG Laboratory, Yokogawa Electric Corporation, Tokyo, Japan). The epochs were defined from 100 msec before stimulation to 1000 msec after it. This pre-stimulus period of 100 msec was used as the baseline for determination of ambient brain activity and noise of each epoch. Before analysis, all epochs for each participant were confirmed not to have included artifacts such as eye blinks or, head movements. To determine the M50/M100 peak, we calculated the root mean square (RMS) of half of all channels. The M50/M100 peak was determined as the peak in RMS value in the interval of 30–70 ms and 80–200 ms, respectively. The response duration of early auditory processing was determined as the interval between rising point of the M50 and the returning point to baseline of M100 (Fig. 1-B). For the time-course analysis of the M50/M100 component, we divided 100 epochs into five successive periods (a; 1–33, b; 15–47, c; 34–66, d; 48–80, e; 67–100), and analyzed the dipole moment and latency in each part. We calculated dipole moments (intensity) of the magnetic source by using the equivalent current dipole (ECD) estimation method [16]. Also, we accepted only those estimated ECDs that showed a goodness of fit (GOF) of over 80% [17]. The waveforms averaged in each epoch were high pass-filtered by using a cut-off frequency of 3 Hz and low pass-filtered by using one of 45 Hz. We evaluated responses of each hemisphere by using half of all channels.

All data analyses were performed by using SPSS statistics for Windows software, version 22.0 (IBM, Tokyo, Japan), and the level of significance was set at $p<0.05$. One-way analysis of variance (ANOVA) was used to compare age, IQ, SP, CBCL scores, and response duration. For M50/M100 measurements, we used a repeated measures linear model with five successive periods

Table 1. Demographic Information.

Groups	TD(N = 15)	ASD without auditory Hypersensitivity(N = 9)	ASD with auditory hypersensitivity(N = 12)
	Mean±SD	Mean±SD	Mean±SD
Age(years)	9.80±1.66	9.40±1.64	9.48±1.70
FIQ	–	99.22±11.38	97.58±18.06
ASQ	2.60±3.02*1,*2	15.11±4.73*1	14.58±6.05*2
SP score	38.73±1.83	31.78±2.44	21.67±5.60
CBCL	–	51.22±13.08	63.38±20.58

FIQ: Full-scale intelligence quotient of Wechsler Intelligence Scale for Children, 3rd version, ASQ: Autism Screening Questionnaire (cut-off ≥ 13). SP: Sensory Profile (cut-off ≥ 30). CBCL: Child Behavior Checklist.
For the ASQ, there were significant differences between TD and ASD with hypersensitivity (*1; $p<0.01$) and also between TD and ASD without hypersensitivity (*2; $p<0.01$).
There were significant differences in SP between TD and both ASD without/with hypersensitivity and also between ASD without and with hypersensitivity (all *; $p<0.01$).

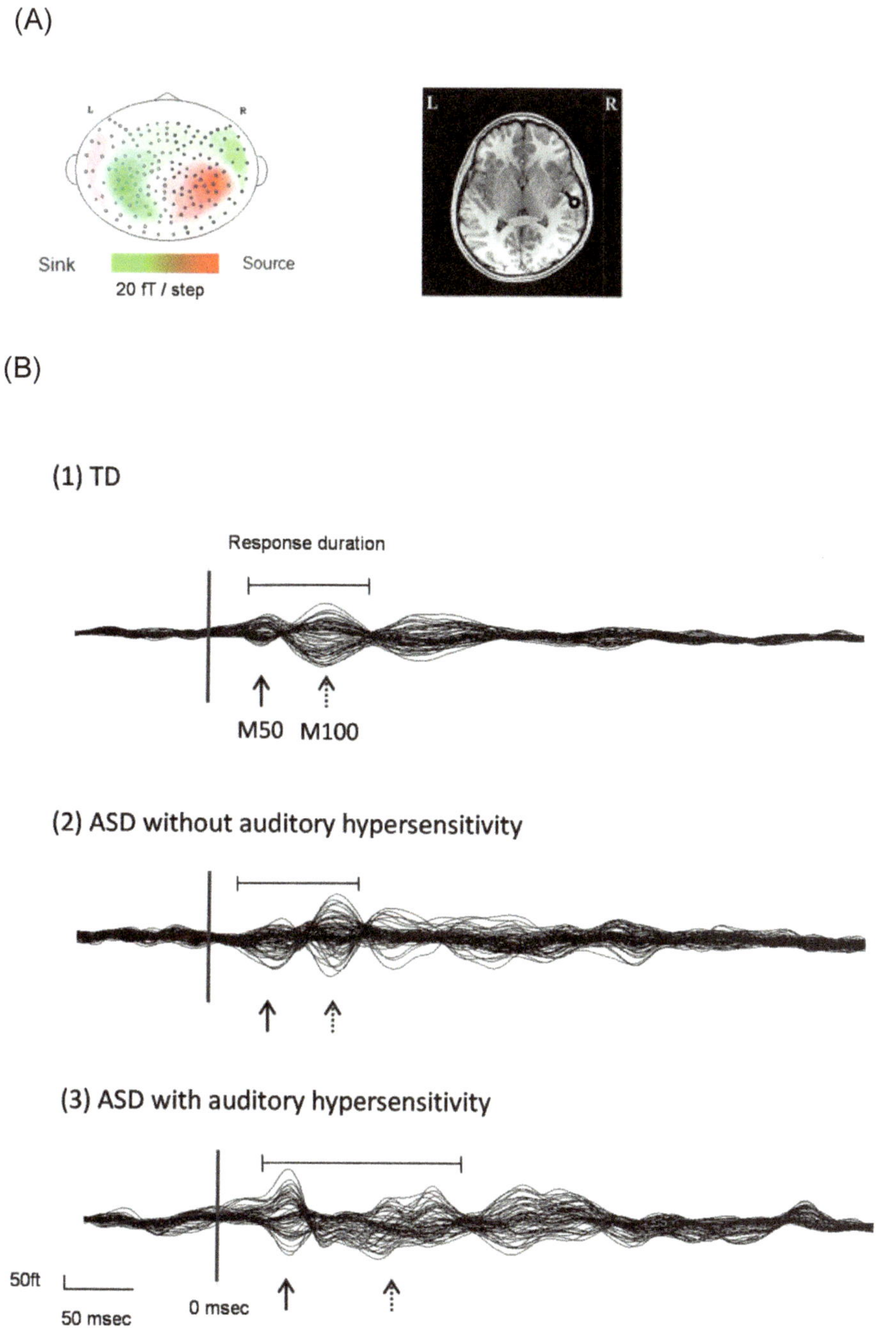

Figure 1. Magnetic isofield maps (A-left), and dipole sources (A-right), which were superimposed on the MRI of individual subjects, were selected; and examples from a TD individual are shown. M50, M100 average waveforms as examples from each of the 3 groups were selected and are shown (B). Vertical lines on the averaged waveform trace indicate stimulus onset (0 msec). Arrows point to M50; and dashed arrows, to M100. The response duration of early auditory processing was determined as the interval between the rising point of the M50 and the returning point to baseline of the M100.

(a/b/c/d/e) as within-subjects factor and the 3 different groups (TD/ASD without auditory hypersensitivity/ASD with auditory hypersensitivity) as between-subjects factor. We tested data for normality by using the Kolmogorov-Smirnov test. The Greenhouse-Geisser correction was applied to the data, if the Mauchly's test of sphericity was statistically significant. Bonferroni correction was applied for multiple comparison analysis. The Pearson test was used to examine the correlation.

Results

Demographics

There was no main effect of age [F (2, 33) = 0.202, p = 0.820, η^2 = .01]. In ASQ scores, there was a significant main effect of group [F (2, 33) = 30.372, p<0.001, η^2 = .65]. The ASQ scores of ASD with/without auditory hypersensitivity were significantly higher than those of the TD (p<0.001). The auditory score of the

SP revealed a significant main effect of group [F (2, 33) = 73. 058, $p<0.001$, $\eta^2 = .82$]. The ASD with auditory hypersensitivity group showed lower SP scores than those of the ASD without auditory hypersensitivity and TD groups [$p<0.001$, Table 1]. The CBCL scores of the patients having ASD with hypersensitivity were higher than those of the ones having ASD without hypersensitivity; however, the difference was not significant [F (1, 19) = 2.510, $p = 0.130$, $\eta^2 = .12$]. The scores of full intelligence quotient showed no difference between ASD groups with and without auditory hypersensitivity [F (1, 19) = 0.057, $p = 0.814$, $\eta^2 = .02$].

M50/M100 dipole moments

Magnetic isofield maps (Fig. 1-A-left) and dipole sources (Fig. 1-A-right), which were superimposed on the MRI of individual subjects, were prepared; and examples from a TD individual are shown (Fig. 1-A). M50, M100 average waveforms were selected as an example from each of the 3 groups (Fig. 1-B).

As shown in Fig. 2-A, significant interactions between group and periods were observed for M50 dipole moments [F (8,132) = 3.101, $p = 0.003$, $\eta^2 = .08$]. In addition, there were significant main effects of group [F (2, 33) = 6.395, $p = 0.004$, $\eta^2 = .11$] and periods [F (4,132) = 6.842, $p<0.001$, $\eta^2 = .08$]. From the simple effect analysis, we found significant differences between part a and b ($p = 0.022$), a and d ($p = 0.001$), a and e ($p<0.001$), and also b and e ($p = 0.001$) in the ASD with auditory hypersensitivity group. The M50 dipole moment showed a significant increase with time only in this group. In addition, there was a significant difference in part c ($p = 0.014$) between the ASD with auditory hypersensitivity group and ASD without auditory hypersensitivity one. There was a significant difference in part d between ASD with auditory hypersensitivity group and ASD without auditory hypersensitivity group ($p = 0.002$), and between ASD with auditory hypersensitivity group and TD group ($p = 0.004$). Also, in the case of part e, there was a significant difference between ASD with auditory hypersensitivity group and ASD without auditory hypersensitivity group ($p = 0.005$), and between ASD with auditory hypersensitivity group and TD group ($p<0.001$). The ASD with auditory hypersensitivity group showed significantly larger dipole moments than the other groups.

As was shown in Fig. 2-B, there were no significant interactions between groups and periods for M100 dipole moments [F (4.11, 67.816) = 0.882, $p = 0.482$, $\eta^2 = .03$]. Also, there was no significant main effect of periods [F (2.055, 67.816) = 1.023, $p = 0.367$, $\eta^2 = .02$]. In addition, there was a significant main effect of groups [F (2, 33) = 3.524, $p = 0.041$, $\eta^2 = .08$]. However, from the multiple comparison analysis, there were no significant differences between groups in any periods.

M50/M100 latencies

As shown in Fig. 2-C, there were no significant interactions between group and periods [F (8,132) = 0.276, $p = 0.973$, $\eta^2 = .01$] for M50 latencies. Also, there was no significant main effect of periods [F (4,132) = 0.999, $p = 0.410$, $\eta^2 = .01$]. However, there was a significant main effect of group [F (2, 33) = 7.418, $p = 0.002$, $\eta^2 = .21$]. From the multiple comparison analysis, M50 latencies were significantly delayed in the ASD with auditory hypersensitivity group than in the TD group in all periods ($p<0.03$).

As was shown in Fig. 2-D, there were no significant interactions between groups and periods for M100 latencies [F (5.102, 84.175) = 1.186, $p = 0.323$, $\eta^2 = .02$]. Also, there was no significant main effect of periods [F (2.551, 84.175) = 0.683, $p = 0.542$, $\eta^2 = .01$]. On the other hand, there was a significant main effect of groups [F (2, 33) = 6.597, $p = 0.004$, $\eta^2 = .21$]. From the multiple comparison analysis, there were significant differences between ASD with auditory hypersensitivity group and TD group for periods a, b, and c ($p<0.03$). The ASD with auditory hypersensitivity group showed delayed M100 latencies compared with those for the TD group. Also, the ASD with auditory hypersensitivity group showed latencies that were more delayed than the ASD without auditory hypersensitivity group; however, there were no statistically significant differences between these two groups.

Response duration

One-way ANOVA revealed a significant main effect of group for response duration [F (2, 32) = 32.84, $p<0.001$, $\eta^2 = .67$; Fig. 3]. From the multiple comparison analysis, individuals having ASD with auditory hypersensitivity showed a longer response duration than those in the other two groups ($p<0.001$). In addition, an obvious negative correlation was recognized between response duration and SP score ($r = -0.747$, $p<0.001$; Fig. 4). Also, there was positive correlation between response duration and CBCL score ($r = 0.522$, $p = 0.183$). There was no statistically significant correlation between response duration and FIQ score ($r = 0.1424$, $p = 0.549$).

Discussion

The results of our present study showed differential time-course responses of the auditory cortex to repeated auditory stimuli in individuals having ASD with auditory hypersensitivity compared with those responses in TD subjects or those having ASD without hypersensitivity. The main findings of our study were the following: 1) The ASD with auditory hypersensitivity group showed increased M50 dipole moments over time. 2) Their response duration was significantly longer than that of the other two groups; and this prolonged response duration also significantly correlated negatively with their auditory scores of SP (i.e., severity of hypersensitivity). 3) In all groups, responses of M50/M100 latencies were constant with time.

In our previous study, we reported delayed M50 and M100 latencies in ASD with auditory hypersensitivity. These results may have been due to abnormalities in the myelination process, thus resulting in slower transmission rates in the central auditory pathways [4,18]. In this present study, we found increased M50 dipole moments with time. However, there were no specific changes in M50 or M100 latency or in M100 dipole moments with time, in all groups.

Additionally, we found a significantly prolonged response duration in the ASD with auditory hypersensitivity group compared with that in the ASD without it or in the TD group. This prolonged response suggested the prolongation of convergence time, and reflected restoration of responses in the primary auditory cortex. In this study, we found that ASD with auditory hypersensitivity showed not only delayed M50/M100 peak latency, but also prolonged convergence time. Furthermore, this extension of the response duration correlated with the severity of auditory hypersensitivity. On the ground of the prolonged response duration, we speculate that the increased excitation and/or reduced inhibition might reflect hyperactivity in the primary auditory cortex, resulting in overlapped responses with time or increased M50 dipole moment responses in the ASD with auditory hypersensitivity group.

Recently, several studies have reported an aberrant white matter microstructure in ASD as compared with that in the controls [19,20]. As described previously, we suggest that those phenomena may be associated with slowed and/or prolonged activity of the neural circuitry of the auditory cortex, resulting

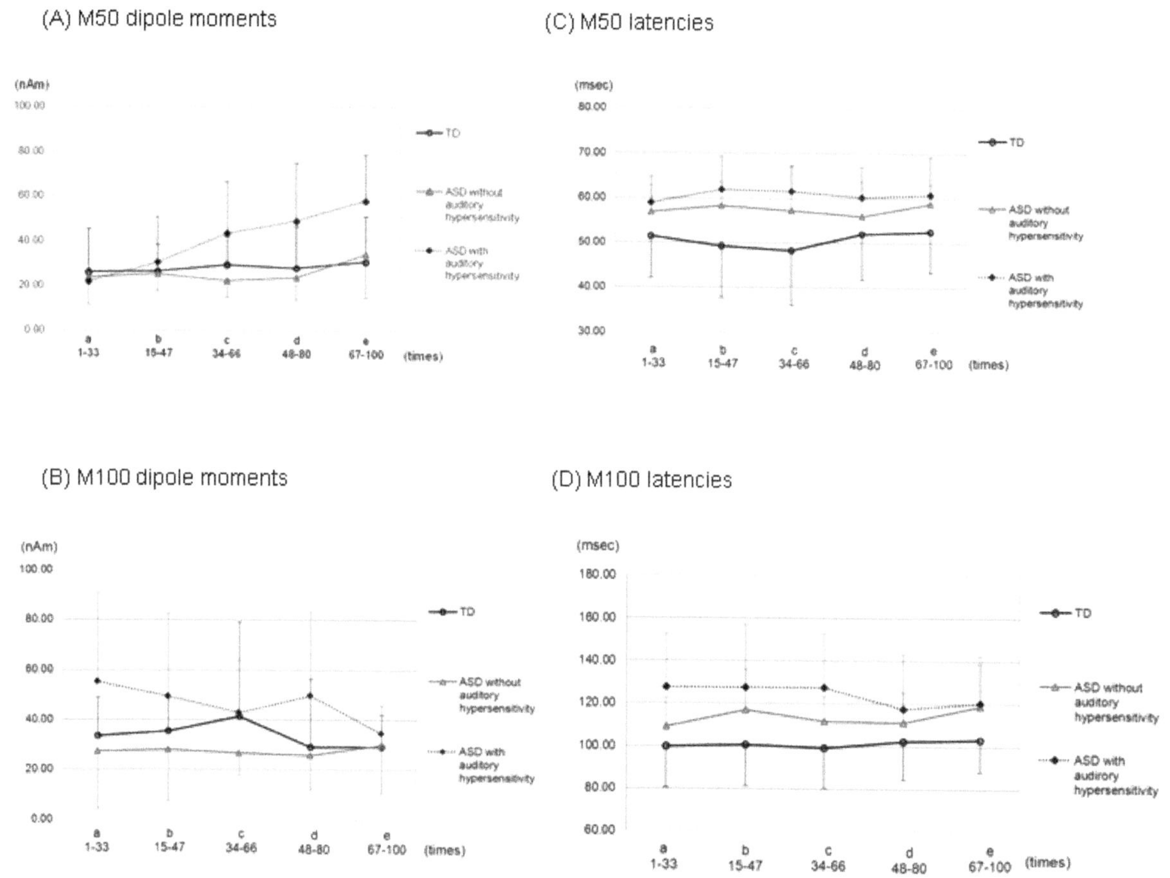

Figure 2. Data were divided into 5 successive periods consisting of a total of 100 epochs (a; 1–33, b; 15–47, c; 34–66, d; 48–80, e; 67–100). Error bars represent 1 standard error of the mean. A) Mean M50 dipole moments. The ASD with auditory hypersensitivity group showed a significant increase in the M50 dipole moment with time ($p<0.01$). B) Mean M100 dipole moments. The 3 groups did not show any significant differences among them in any of the successive periods. C) Mean M50 latencies. There were no significant differences among the groups in any of the successive periods. D) Mean M100 latencies. Again, no differences were noted.

from its abnormal maturation in ASD with auditory hypersensitivity.

Alternatively, Rotschafer and Razak reported that a mouse model of Fragile X Syndrome (FXS), which exhibits autistic features, shows expanded frequency tuning, enhanced response

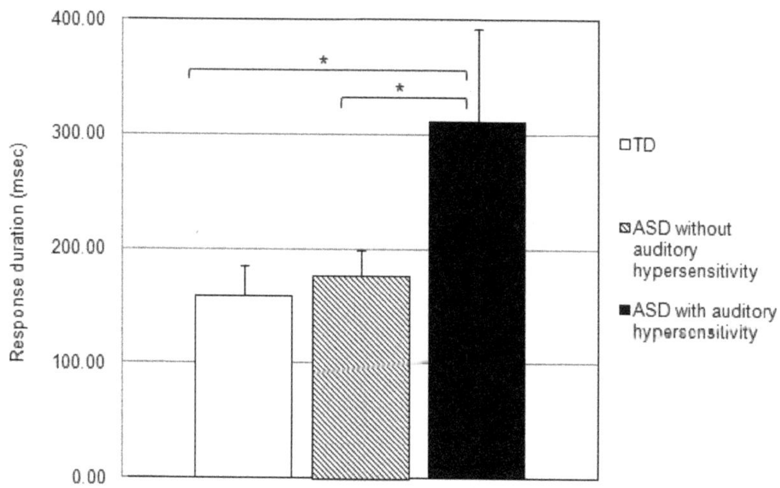

Figure 3. Mean response duration of each group. Error bars represent 1 standard error of the mean. The response duration in the ASD with auditory hypersensitivity group was significantly longer than that in the other 2 groups ($p<0.05$).

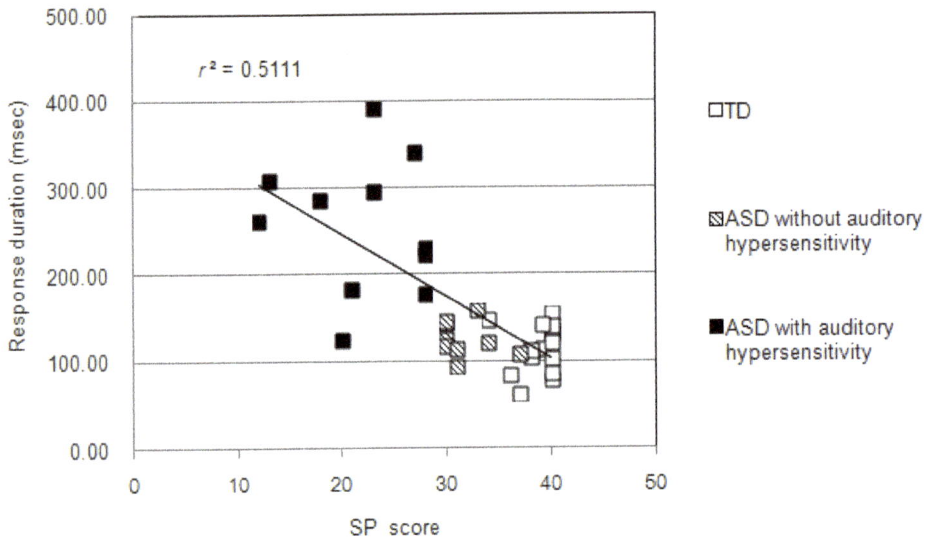

Figure 4. Scatter plot of response duration and auditory item scores of SP. Response duration was negatively correlated with auditory item scores of SP ($p<0.05$).

magnitude, and more variable first spike latencies compared to wild-type controls [21]. They concluded that these results may reflect the auditory processing deficits seen in FXS patients [21]. FXS patients are known to show autistic symptoms and also auditory abnormalities. We speculate that those phenomena may be related to the characteristics of auditory hypersensitivity in ASD.

On the other hand, according to a pathological study on autistic postmortem brain, the minicolumns in auditory cortex revealed less peripheral neuropil space, which is the conduit for the GABAergic inhibitory local circuit projection [22], leading to the speculation that abnormalities of GABAergic interneurons might induce cortical hypersensitivity in the auditory cortex.

As another possible neurochemical pathophysiology of auditory hypersensitivity, Curtin et al. [23] reported that the serotonin 5-HT5A receptor regulates excitability in the auditory startle circuit in the pre-pulse inhibition (PPI) paradigm. Serotonin 5-HT5A contributes to sensorimotor integration and decision-making by directly regulating excitability. Moreover, Medan and Preuss [24] found that dopaminergic modulation regulates the time course and magnitude of PPI, whereas 5-HT regulates tonic excitability. Many studies have found abnormalities in the serotonin/dopamine system in autism patients [25,26]. Therefore, we hypothesize that the auditory hypersensitivity in ASD could be related to dysfunctional regulation of the auditory startle circuit, a dysfunction resulting from abnormalities of serotonin 5-HT5A receptors or dopaminergic modulation.

Recently, some researchers have reported abnormal P50/M50 responses in the paired-click paradigm in patients with schizophrenia and other disorders, such as post-traumatic stress disorder [27,28], which is associated with thalamic sensory gating system [7]. Also, the similarities between schizophrenia and autism both in genetic and behavioral characteristics have also been reported [29–31]. Therefore, we speculate that the increased M50 dipole moment seen in ASD with auditory hypersensitivity may be related to impairment of the sensory filter mechanism resulting from abnormalities of the thalamic sensory gating system. Meanwhile, M100 dipole moment did not change with time in any of the groups. Although the M50/M100 responses arise from both the auditory cortex, their functional role might be different [5].

On the other hand, latencies were constant with time in all groups. We have already reported a delayed M50/M100 peak latency in ASD with auditory hypersensitivity. Therefore, delayed M50/M100 latencies resulting from abnormalities in the myelination processes might be unaffected by the stimulus frequency.

Based on the findings of this present study, we suggest that characteristics of auditory hypersensitivity may be associated with abnormalities in the early stages of auditory processing and that it involves multiple neural mechanisms.

Limitations of this study are as follow: 1) We focused on responses of the auditory cortex. It remains unclear whether any specific activation induced by sound occurred in any other brain region. 2) From the result showing an increased M50 dipole moment, we speculated that the abnormalities such as increased excitation/reduced inhibition and the thalamic sensory gating system were involved. However, in this study, we did not use the paired-click paradigm. Thus, future work will be needed to determine the validity of this speculation. 3) We have supposed that our results may be related to auditory hypersensitivity behavior in actual life. However, we used only a sinusoidal tone pip as auditory stimuli. Therefore, further work will be needed by using real-life sounds (e.g., baby crying, hair dryer, etc).

Even though auditory hypersensitivity tends toward maladaptation of patients with ASD, there is no effective therapeutic approach yet. At least, our study has provided objective assessments of clinical symptoms and also beneficial information for understanding the characteristics of ASD patients and for supporting their quality of life.

Conclusions

An increase in the M50 dipole moment with time and a prolonged response duration of the auditory cortex were found in our subjects having ASD with auditory hypersensitivity. In addition to the possibility of abnormalities of the maturational process, these phenomena might have occurred due to decreased inhibitory processing and an increase in the ratio of cortical excitation to inhibition, possibly resulting from an abnormal sensory gating system or dysfunction of inhibitory interneurons. Our findings suggest that auditory hypersensitivity may be associated with abnormalities in the early stages of auditory processing and that it involves multiple neural mechanisms. Understanding of the neurological basis of auditory hypersensitivity could have clinical benefits, resulting from validation of effective treatment for it in the future.

Acknowledgments

The authors gratefully acknowledge all participants and their parents.

Author Contributions

Conceived and designed the experiments: JM KKS. Performed the experiments: JM KKS HS MH. Analyzed the data: JM KKS HS FN RH KT. Contributed reagents/materials/analysis tools: JM KKS HS MH M. Taniike. Wrote the paper: JM KKS MH M. Tachibana IM M. Taniike. Assessment for autism: FN RH M. Tachibana. Diagnostic for autism: M. Tachibana KT IM M. Taniike.

References

1. American Psychiatric Association (2000) Diagnostic and statistical manual of mental disorders (4th edition) text revision (DSM-IV-TR). Washington, DC: American Psychiatric Association.
2. American Psychiatric Association (2013) Diagnostic and statistical manual of mental disorders (5th edition). Washington, DC: American Psychiatric Association.
3. Lane AE, Young RL, Baker AEZ, Angley MT (2010) Sensory processing subtypes in autism: Association with adaptive behavior. J Autism Dev Disord 40: 112–122.
4. Matsuzaki J, Kagitani-Shimono K, Goto T, Sanefuji W, Yamamoto T, et al. (2012) Differential responses of primary auditory cortex in autism spectrum disorder with auditory hypersensitivity. Neuro Report 23: 113–118.
5. Chait M, Simon J Z, Poeppel D (2004) Auditory M50 and M100 responses to broadband noise: functional implications. Neuroreport 15: 16.
6. Guiraud JA, Kushnerenko E, Tomalski P, Davies K, Ribeiro H, et al. (2011) Differential habituation to repeated sounds in infants at high risk for autism. Neuroreport 22: 845–849.
7. Faith MH, Gregory AM, Robert JT, Jessica I, Aaron J, et al. (2005) Distinct M50 and M100 auditory gating deficits in schizophrenia. Psychophysiology 42: 417–427.
8. Berument SK, Rutter M, Lord C, Pickles A, Bailey A (1999) Autism screening questionnaire: diagnostic validity. Br J Psychiatry 175: 444–451.
9. Dairoku H, Senju A, Hayashi E, Tojo Y, Ichikawa H (2004) Development of Japanese version of autism screening questionnaire. Kokuritsu Tokushu Kyoiku Kenkyusho Ippan Kenkyu Houkokusho 7: 19–34.
10. Di Lavore PC, Lord C, Rutter M (1995) The pre-linguistic autism diagnostic observation schedule. J Autism Dev Disord 25: 355–379.
11. Dunn W (2002) Infant/Toddler Sensory Profile. San Antonio, TX: Psychological Corporation.
12. Itani T, Kanbayashi Y, Nakata Y, Kita M, Fujii H, et al. (2001) Standardization of the Japanese version of the child behavior checklist/4–18. Psychiatra et Neurologia Pediatrica Japonica 41: 243–252.
13. Achenbach TM (1991) Manual for the child behavior checklist/4–18 and profile. Burlington, VT: University of Vermont.
14. Sugata H, Goto T, Hirata M, Yanagisawa T, Shayne M, et al. (2012) Neural decoding of unilateral upper limb movements using single trial MEG signals. Brain Res 1468: 29–37.
15. Hanaie R, Mohri I, Kagitani-Shimono K, Tachibana M, Azuma J, et al. (2013) Microstructural connectivity of the superior cerebellar peduncle is related to motor dysfunction in children with autistic spectrum disorders. The cerebellum 12: 645–656.
16. Uda T, Tsuyuguchi N, Okumura E, Sakamoto M, Morino M, et al. (2012) sLORETA-qm for interictal MEG epileptic spike analysis: Comparison of location and quantity with equivalent dipole estimation. Clin Neurophysiol 123: 1496–1501.
17. Yoshimura Y, Kikuchi M, Shitamichi K, Ueno S, Munesue T, et al. (2013) Atypical brain lateralization in the auditory cortex and language performance in 3- to 7 year-old children with high-functioning autism spectrum disorder: a child- customized magnetoencephalography (MEG) study. Mol Autism 4: 38.
18. Gage NM, Siegel B, Roberts TPL (2003) Cortical auditory system maturational abnormalities in children with autism disorder: an MEG investigation. Brain Res Dev Res 144: 201–209.
19. Shukla DK, Keehn B, Smylie DM, Muller RA (2011) Microstructural abnormalities of short-distance white matter tracts in autism spectrum disorder. Neuropsychologia 49: 1378–1382.
20. Cheng Y, Chou KH, Chen IY, Fan YT, Decety J, et al. (2010) Atypical development of white matter microstructure in adolescents with autism spectrum disorders. Neuroimage 50: 873–82.
21. Rotschater S, Razak K (2013) Altered auditory processing in a mouse model of fragile X syndrome. Brain Res 1506: 12–24.
22. Casanova MF, Buxhoeveden D, Gomez J (2003) Disruption in the inhibitory architecture of the cell minicolumn: implications for autism. Neuroschientist 9: 496–507.
23. Curtin PCP, Megan V, Neumeister H, Bronson DR, Preuss T (2013) The 5-HT_{5A} receptor regulates excitability in the auditory startle circuit: Functional implications for sensorimotor gating. J Neurophysiol 33: 10011–10020.
24. Medan V, Preuss T (2011) Dopaminergic-induced changes in mauthner cell excitability distrupt prepulse inhibition in the startle circuit of goldfish. J Neurophysiol 106: 3195–3204.
25. Nakamura K, Sekine Y, Ouchi Y, Tsujii M, Yoshikawa E, et al. (2010) Brain serotonine and dopamine transporter bindings in adults with high functioning autism. Arch Gen Psychiatry 67: 59–68.
26. Iwata K, Matsuzaki H, Tachibana T, Ohno K, Yoshimura S, et al. (2014) N-ethylmaleimide-sensitive factor interacts with the serotonin transporter and modulates its trafficking: implications for pathophysiology in autism. Mol Autism 5: 33.
27. Neylan TC, Fletcher DJ, Lenoci M, McCallin K, Weiss DS, et al. (1999) Sensory gating in chronic posttraumatic stress disorder: Reduced auditory P50 suppression in combat veterans. Biol Psychiatry 46: 1656–1664.
28. Thoma RJ, Hanlon FM, Moses SN, Edger C, Huang M, et al. (2003) Lateralization of auditory sensory gating and neuropsychological dysfunction in schizophrenia. Am J psychiatry 160: 1595–1605.
29. Burbach JPH, van der Zwaag B (2009) Contact in genetics of autism and schizophrenia. Trends Neurosci 32(2): 69–72.
30. Rapoport J, Chavez A, Greenstein D, Addington A (2009) Autism spectrum disorders and childhood-onset schizophrenia: Clinical and biological contributions to a relation revisited. J Am Acad Child Adolesc Psychiatry 48(1): 10–17.
31. Bore M de, Spek AA, Lobbestael J (2014) Comparing cognitive functioning in schizophrenia and autism using WAIS-III. Res Autism Spect Dis 8: 737–745.

21

Voxel-Wise Motion Artifacts in Population-Level Whole-Brain Connectivity Analysis of Resting-State fMRI

Tamás Spisák[1]*, András Jakab[2], Sándor A. Kis[1], Gábor Opposits[1], Csaba Aranyi[1], Ervin Berényi[3], Miklós Emri[1]

1 Department of Nuclear Medicine, Medical and Health Science Centre, University of Debrecen, Debrecen, Hungary, **2** Department of Radiology, Medical University of Vienna, Vienna, Austria, **3** Department of Biomedical Laboratory and Imaging Science, Medical and Health Science Center, University of Debrecen, Debrecen, Hungary

Abstract

Functional Magnetic Resonance Imaging (fMRI) based brain connectivity analysis maps the functional networks of the brain by estimating the degree of synchronous neuronal activity between brain regions. Recent studies have demonstrated that "resting-state" fMRI-based brain connectivity conclusions may be erroneous when motion artifacts have a differential effect on fMRI BOLD signals for between group comparisons. A potential explanation could be that in-scanner displacement, due to rotational components, is not spatially constant in the whole brain. However, this localized nature of motion artifacts is poorly understood and is rarely considered in brain connectivity studies. In this study, we initially demonstrate the local correspondence between head displacement and the changes in the resting-state fMRI BOLD signal. Than, we investigate how connectivity strength is affected by the population-level variation in the spatial pattern of regional displacement. We introduce Regional Displacement Interaction (RDI), a new covariate parameter set for second-level connectivity analysis and demonstrate its effectiveness in reducing motion related confounds in comparisons of groups with different voxel-vise displacement pattern and preprocessed using various nuisance regression methods. The effect of using RDI as second-level covariate is than demonstrated in autism-related group comparisons. The relationship between the proposed method and some of the prevailing subject-level nuisance regression techniques is evaluated. Our results show that, depending on experimental design, treating in-scanner head motion as a global confound may not be appropriate. The degree of displacement is highly variable among various brain regions, both within and between subjects. These regional differences bias correlation-based measures of brain connectivity. The inclusion of the proposed second-level covariate into the analysis successfully reduces artifactual motion-related group differences and preserves real neuronal differences, as demonstrated by the autism-related comparisons.

Editor: Jerzy Bodurka, Laureate Institute for Brain Research and The University of Oklahoma, United States of America

Funding: The study was partially supported by the European Union and the European Social Fund through project "Supercomputer, the national virtual lab" (grant. no.: TÁMOP-4.2.2.C-11/1/KONV-2012-0010). The work was supported by the European Union and the State of Hungary, co-financed by the European Social Fund through project "Basic and applied research to assist the development of speech for the deaf" (TÁMOP 4.2.2.C-11/1/KONV). The project was supported by the State of Hungary through the National Brain Research Program ("Charting the normal and pathological macro-scale brain connectome by in vivo neuroimaging", KTIA_13_NAP-A-II/3). T.S. was supported by the European Union and the State of Hungary, co-financed by the European Social Fund in the framework of TÁMOP-4.2.4.A/2-11/1-2012-0001 'National Excellence Program'. A.J. was supported by the European Commission, 7th European Community Framework Programme, Marie Curie IEF Research grant FABRIC – "exploring the Formation and Adaptation of the Brain Connectome", 2012-PIEF-GA-33003. The funders had no role in study design, data collection and analysis, decision to publish, or preparation of the manuscript.

Competing Interests: The authors have declared that no competing interests exist.

* Email: tspisak@pet.dote.hu

Introduction

Background

Motion artifacts are problematic for all types of MRI including resting-state functional MRI (fMRI) and therefore motion correction is a vital step in every work-flow during fMRI analysis. According to population-level analysis and group comparisons, retrospective motion related artifact removal strategies can be performed at five different stages of the data processing pipeline: (i) motion correction of fMRI time-series by realignment to a reference image (using automatic co-registration approaches) [1]; (ii) censoring data to exclude periods of high motion (scrubbing, de-spiking) [2,3]; (iii) modeling the effect of motion-related nuisance parameters on blood oxygen level dependent (BOLD) signal [4–7]; (iv) temporal filtering of BOLD timecourses to discard frequencies encumbered by motion artifacts and (v) correct for subject-specific motion effects on population-level (descriptive summary statistics of subject-specific motion as second-level model regressors) [8–10].

Traditional realignment-based correction approaches ensure that different time-points of the BOLD signal correspond to the same location. However, such methods do not handle voxel-level intensity confounds originating from the establishment of magnetic gradients and subsequent readout of the BOLD signal [2,11]. Furthermore, automatic co-registration approaches may introduce spurious displacements in intervals of relatively low motion [12]. Nonetheless, subject movement is often measured with parameters based upon the resulting image realignment transformations.

Large BOLD intensity confounds (spikes) in time-frames with extreme, abrupt movement can be eliminated from the analysis by simply dropping the corrupted data ("scrubbing") [2] or by spike-regression [13]. However, the reduction in time points is associated with an increase in the likelihood of high correlation scores [8]; moreover, recent findings [8,14,15] suggest that in population-level functional connectivity studies, scrubbing can be omitted from the analysis when using proper second-level correction.

Intensity confounds originating from micro-movements (as small as 0.1 mm from one time point to the next) can also disrupt results, especially in case of correlation based connectivity analysis methods, where such small but temporally concordant noise leads to spurious increase in connectivity strength [2,9,16]. Nuisance signal regression approaches aim to eliminate the signal components of non-neuronal origin from the raw BOLD data utilizing linear regression. These confounder signals can be defined by dedicated physiological monitoring devices during the scan, calculated from motion parameters extracted during spatial realignment based motion correction or derived directly form the data itself, using a "noise ROI" [6,7,17].

Temporal filtering is also a crucial step in the reduction of fMRI brain connectivity artifacts, including motion confounds. Most connectivity studies apply a band-pass filter with a high-pass cutoff of 0.008–0.01 Hz and a low-pass threshold of 0.08–0.1 Hz [18]. While there is evidence that resting-state networks are present at a relatively broad band in the frequency spectra [19], slight modifications in the frequency band have been suggested [3].

Some of these techniques can effectively reduce not only motion-related effects, but also physiological noise (e.g. cardiac or respiratory confounds) or hardware drifts and instabilities. However, recent studies [3,8,20] report that clear artifacts remain in the data even after such regression and filtering approaches, and that these artifacts have systematic effects upon resting-state functional MRI connectivity (rs-fcMRI) patterns.

When performing group comparisons in functional connectivity studies, one can account for these motion-related residual artifacts during the second-level analysis by inclusion of motion-related, subject-specific covariates into the population-level model. A common choice is to include a measure of the average patient movement [8–10]. Alternatively, the value of global voxel-to-voxel correlation (GCOR) can be utilized as confounder, as in [20], although the latter quantity can also carry valuable neurological information.

Due to in-scanner head rotation, the effect of patient movements on the BOLD signal is not spatially constant in the whole brain; however, this local relationship is poorly understood and is rarely considered in brain connectivity studies. The pattern of voxel-wise motion not only varies among different loci of the same subject, but also among subjects. According to Satterthwaite et al. [9], between-subject differences of motion are stable and hence, in-scanner head motion should be considered as a trait. Thus, the effect of the subject-specific spatio-temporal motion pattern on the BOLD signal could bias group analysis when different groups have different tendencies in their spatio-temporal motion patterns. This is particularly problematic in studies when regional connectivity deficits are associated with a pathological condition, and thus, limits the usability of functional connectivity as a biomarker of disease. These biases in the functional connectivity pattern can lead to invalid conclusions regarding biomedical hypotheses, as denoted by [21] and demonstrated by [20], especially in patholological conditions associated with hyperkinetic patients (epilepsy, attention deficit hyperactiviy disorder, some forms of autism). Group-wise inconsistencies in motion patterns can arise from different patient positioning and multi-center studies are also challenging in this regard.

Purposes

Here, we hypothesize that at least some of the above-mentioned artifactual effects may originate from the complex voxel-wise spatio-temporal nature of head displacement, and can be modeled more efficiently using this information.

The possibilities for utilizing the voxel-wise nature of in-scanner motion in artifact removal approaches has not been intensively investigated, as yet. As recently reported by two studies [3,14] and confirmed by our preliminary analysis, including voxel-wise displacement parameters as voxel- or region-wise covariates in the appropriate nuisance signal regression model does not significantly improve motion artifact removal, compared to the usual technique, the regression of spatially averaged global displacement parameters. However, Yan et al. in [14] also brings up the possibility that an appropriate correction technique may have greater success in using the rich information encapsulated by voxel-specific indices.

Our study was designed to characterize the impact of voxel-wise head motion artifacts in population-level rs-fcMRI brain connectivity studies and investigate how this local information on displacement can be utilized for artifact removal.

We initially demonstrate the local correspondence between head displacement and the changes in the rs-fcMRI BOLD signal. We then aim to investigate how functional connectivity strength is affected by the deviations in the average regional spatial displacements on the population-level. We propose Regional Displacement Interaction (RDI), a novel modeling approach for second-level brain connectivity analysis, which provides the opportunity to incorporate voxel-wise motion information into the population-level model and to account for corresponding artifactual effects. The effectiveness of this motion artifact reduction technique is evaluated by investigating the variance explained by the proposed confound modeling covariates in the model. The method is than demonstrated in group comparisons of cohorts with differing average voxel-wise displacement patterns. Due to the disagreement [3,14,20,22] about the optimal first-level nuisance signal regression technique, we perform a comparison of prevailing first-level nuisance signal regression approaches and characterize their interference with the proposed method. Finally, to test whether the proposed method preserves group differences of neuronal origin, a comparison of autistic and control groups is performed.

Materials and Methods

Image acquisition

Analysis was performed on the resting-state fMRI data of 184 patients obtained from the Autism Brain Imaging Dataset Exchange database [15,23,24] (ABIDE). All of the images were acquired at the NYU Langone Medical Center using a 3 Tesla Siemens Magnetom Allegra syngo MR 2004A. A T1-weighted sagittal MP-RAGE structural image was obtained (TE = 3.25 ms, TR = 2530 ms, TI = 1100 ms, flip angle = 7, 256 slices with 1.3×1×1.3 mm voxels). Functional images were obtained using a BOLD contrast sensitive gradient echo echo-planar sequence (TE = 15 ms, flip angle = 90, in-plane resolution = 3×3 mm; volume TR = 2000 ms). Whole-brain coverage for the functional data was obtained using 33 contiguous interleaved 4 mm axial slices. During the resting-state fMRI scan, most participants were asked to relax with their eyes open, while a white cross-hair against a black background was projected on a screen. However, data were also included for some individuals who were asked to keep their eyes closed; and, in a few cases, participants closed their eyes regardless of instructions to keep them open.

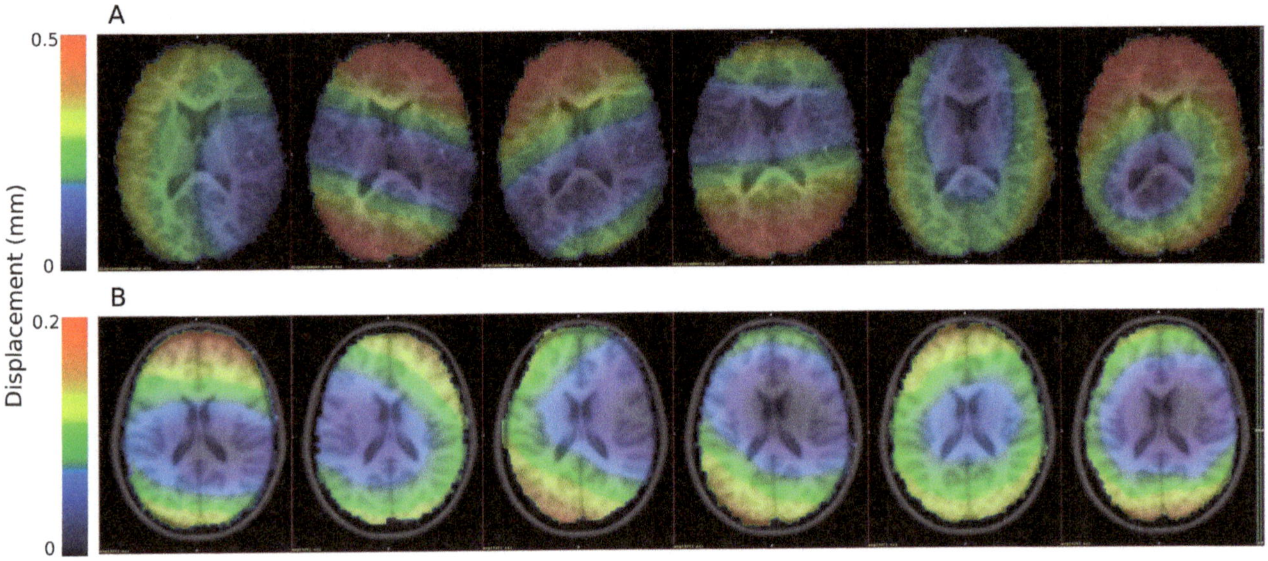

Figure 1. Voxel-wise characteristics of head motion during an fMRI scan. Examples of different patterns of voxel-wise displacement within the time frames of one illustrative subject (A) and temporally averaged voxel-wise displacement of six illustrative subjects (B).

The population sample consisted of 79 patients with autism spectrum disorders (7.1–39.1 years) (53 Autistic Disorder, 21 Asperger's Disorder, 5 Pervasive Developmental Disorder-Not Otherwise Specified) and an age and gender-matched group of 105 typical control subjects (6.5–31.8 years).

Data collection for the ABIDE dataset was approved by the institutional review boards of the New York University School of Medicine and New York University. Prior to participation, written informed consent and assent (for participants>18 years) were obtained from all participants and their parents/legal guardians (for participants<18 years). Participants received monetary compensation for completing the study. In this study, the patient data were analyzed anonymously.

Preprocessing

FMRI time series were co-registered and frame-wise estimation of head displacement was performed using FSL McFlirt [25,26]. Matrices defining the rigid-body (three translation and three rotation parameter) transformation that fit each frame to the reference frame (at the middle time-point) were saved for further use. The first five volumes of each dataset were discarded from further analysis to allow for T1 equilibration effects. BET was used to remove non-brain areas [27]. The resulting pre-processed fMRI data were nonlinearly co-registered to the brain-extracted anatomical image, and then, spatially standardized to the MNI152 space using the FLIRT and FNIRT utilities [28] of the FSL package, to achieve spatial correspondences for group analysis. Since further processing steps utilized averaged regional time courses, no smoothing was applied on the images.

Calculation of voxel-wise displacement

With an in-house-developed utility based on the m3i software library system [29], transformation matrices outputted by McFlirt were converted to world coordinate origin. The respective inverse transformations were applied to each frame of the fMRI time-series and the root mean squared voxel position change in world coordinates was calculated for each voxel of each frame. The first derivate of the resulting local displacement time-series was saved in NIfTI format dynamic images in the same space as the fMRI time-series (see Fig. 1 for demonstrative images), and then realigned to standard space.

ROI definition

In order to improve the signal-to-noise ratio and reduce the amount of data to analyze, all regional timecourses (regional BOLD signal, temporal derivate of its root mean squared variance, regional displacement) and corresponding correlation coefficients presented in this paper were drawn from a set of ROIs (M = 88) that were defined based on the Harvard-Oxford Cortical and Subcortical brain atlases [30]. Probability maps for all regions were accessed and region borders were delineated by retaining voxels with a probability greater than 25%. Voxels associated with multiple regions (in case of overlapping regions) were assigned to the region in which the underlying probability was higher. To avoid very small regions with poor signal-to-noise ratio, ROIs having a volume less than 30 cm^3 were merged into neighboring ROIs. A complete list of the brain regions and the modifications are summarized in Table 1. Fig. 2 presents the axial projection of brain regions in the glass-brain plot used to demonstrate results.

Calculation of regional and frame-wise displacement

We defined two metrics of displacement: regional and frame-wise displacement (RD and FD). RD time-courses were calculated as averaged voxel-wise displacements over ROIs, while FD is the analogous measurement for the entire brain. This method of calculating FD and RD is analogous to the parameter FD_{vox} described in [14].

Quantification of global and regional BOLD intensity change

While DVARS (D referring to temporal derivative of time-courses and VARS referring to RMS variance over voxels) [31] indexes the rate of change of BOLD signal across the entire brain at each time-point of the data, Regional DVARS (RDVARS) shows the same rate for each ROI:

Table 1. Brain atlas regions, left hemisphere.

id	long name	hemisphere	short name	H-O atlas regions merged
1	Left Caudate	left	l-caud	Caudate, Accumbens
2	Cingulate Gyrus anterior division	left	l-cinga	
3	Frontal Medial Cortex	left	l-fmedc	
4	Operculum	left	l-operc	frontal operc, central operc, parietal operc
5	Frontal Orbital Cortex	left	l-forbc	
6	Frontal Pole	left	l-front	
7	Inferior Frontal Gyrus pars opercularis	left	l-inffrontgop	
8	Inferior Frontal Gyrus pars triangularis	left	l-inffrontgtri	
9	Juxtapositional Lobule Cortex	left	l-juxlob	
10	Middle Frontal Gyrus	left	l-mfg	
11	Paracingulate Gyrus	left	l-parcing	
12	Pre-frontal	left	l-prefront	
13	Subcallosal Cortex	left	l-subcall	
14	Superior Frontal Gyrus	left	l-sfg	
15	Insular Cortex	left	l-ins	
16	Cuneal Cortex	left	l-cun	
17	Calcarine Cortex	left	l-calc	intracalcarine, supracalcarine
18	Lateral Occipital Cortex inferior division	left	l-latocinf	
19	Lingual Gyrus	left	l-ling	
20	Occipital Fusiform Gyrus	left	l-occfus	
21	Occipital Pole	left	l-occ	
22	Angular Gyrus	left	l-ang	
23	Cingulate Gyrus posterior division	left	l-cingpost	
24	Lateral Occipital Cortex superior division	left	l-latoccsup	
25	Postcentral Gyrus	left	l-postcent	
26	Precuneous Cortex	left	l-precun	
27	Superior Parietal Lobule	left	l-supparl	
28	Supramarginal Gyrus anterior division	left	l-smarga	
29	Supramarginal Gyrus posterior division	left	l-smargp	
30	Lentiform	left	l-lent	putamen, pallidum
31	Superior Temporal Gyrus	left	l-stg	sup.temp.g. post; sup.temp.g. ant; Heschl gyrus
32	Inferior Temporal Gyrus	left	l-itg	inf.temp.g. post; inf.temp.g. ant
33	Inferior Temporal Gyrus temporooccipital part	left	l-itgtempoc	
34	Amygdala	left	l-amyg	
35	Hippocampus	left	l-hip	
36	Middle Temporal Gyrus anterior division	left	l-mtgant	
37	Middle Temporal Gyrus posterior division	left	l-mtgpost	
38	Middle Temporal Gyrus temporooccipital part	left	l-mtgtempoc	
39	Parahippocampal Gyrus	left	l-parhipc	Parahippocampal Gyrus post.; Parahippocampal Gyrus ant.
40	Planum	left	l-plan	Planum Temporale, planum polare
41	Temporal Fusiform Cortex	left	l-tfus	fusiform ant, fusiform post
42	Temporal Occipital Fusiform Cortex	left	l-tofus	
43	Temporal Pole	left	l-temp	
44	Left Thalamus	left	l-thal	

Lateralization, and long and short names of brain atlas-based ROIs used for estimating regional BOLD and motion related measures. The sources of brain regions are the Harvard-Oxford Cortical and Subcortical brain atlases [30]. Probability maps for all regions were accessed and region borders were delineated by kretaining voxels with a probability greater than 25%. Voxels associated with multiple regions (in case of overlapping regions) were assigned to the region in which the underlying probability was higher. ROIs having a volume less than 30 cm^3 were merged into neighboring ROIs, as indicated by column five. The table lists only regions in the left hemisphere. The naming conventions and the region merging procedure was analogous for their contra-lateral pairs.

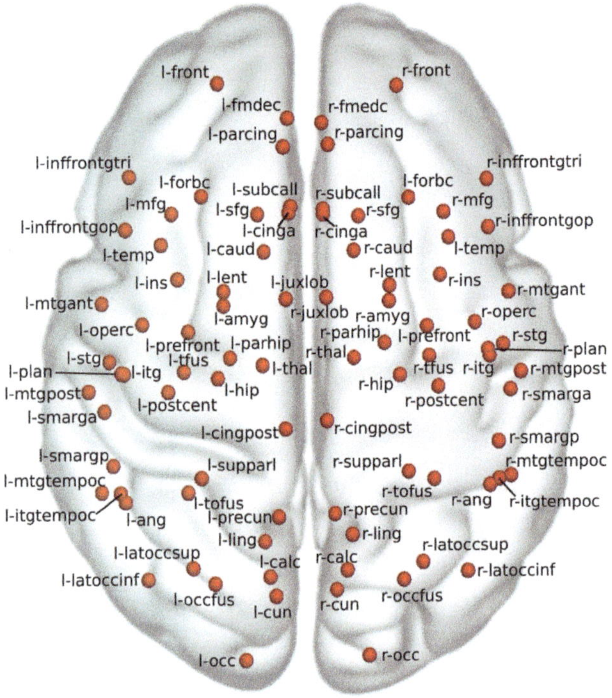

Figure 2. Brain atlas regions. Short names of atlas regions in the glass brain plot used to demonstrate results. Full names and additional information about regions can be seen in Table 1. Red spheres imply the axial projection of the center of mass of brain regions. Note that this plot does not indicate the axial depth of the regions.

$$DVARS(\Delta I)_i^R = \sqrt{\langle (I_i(x) - I_{i-1}(x))^2 \rangle^{(R)}} \quad (1)$$

where $I_i(x)$ is the image intensity at locus x on frame i, angle brackets $\langle \bullet \rangle^{(R)}$ denote the spatial average over all voxels x within ROI R ($R = 1 \ldots 88$) and $i = 2 \ldots N$ where N is the number of time-frames. In order to effectively relate RDVARS to RD, RDVARS was calculated on the timeseries following re-alignment, but prior to confound regression and filtering.

Investigating the effect of regional displacement on DVARS

We reproduced results showing global motion-related BOLD changes [2,14,16] by computing the correlation coefficient between FD and DVARS. Then, to distinguish global from local effects, we defined two measures, residual RD and residual RDVARS (denoted with ΔRD and $\Delta RDVARS$), as follows:

$$\Delta RD_i^{(R)} = RD_i^{(R)} - FD_i \quad (2)$$

and

$$\Delta RDVARS_i^{(R)} = RDVARS_i^{(R)} - DVARS_i \quad (3)$$

where $i = 2 \ldots N$, N is the number of time-frames and R ($R = 1 \ldots M$) identifies the region. After computing these measures for every subject and every ROI, we computed their correlation coefficient and investigated whether it depends on the degree of the global motion-BOLD relationship among subjects.

Functional connectivity processing and graph formation

For rs-fcMRI analysis, additional preprocessing steps were utilized on regional BOLD timecourses to reduce spurious variance that was unlikely to reflect neural activity. These steps included: (i) multiple regression of nuisance variables; and (ii) a temporal band-pass filter on residual data using a standard fourth-order Butterworth band-pass filter, retaining frequencies between 0.01 and 0.1 Hz.

The detailed data processing steps involved in the following strategies are discussed in the relevant works. Here, we only summarize the protocols based on basic criteria, such as the sources of nuisance signal, the number of such signal time-courses and whether global signal regression was performed.

1. NOREG: No nuisance regression,
2. WMCSF: average BOLD signals of eroded white matter and cerebrospinal fluid ROI-s, segmented using FAST [27],
3. GSREG: regression of whole-brain global signal as a covariate,
4. COMPCOR: Nuisance regression of five principal components of a noise ROI, defined based on the temporal signal-to-noise ratio, as proposed in [7],
5. NOREG+M6: NOREG + six motion parameters,
6. WMCSF+M6: WM+CSF regression + six motion parameters,
7. GSREG+M6: GSREG + six motion parameters,
8. COMPCOR+M6: COMPCOR + six motion parameters,
9. SAT36: A 36-parameter nuisance regression model proposed in [3] (incorporating global signal regression).

To ensure that neighboring regional BOLD time courses do not show spurious increase in connectivity strength, no smoothing was applied. Connectivity strength between pairs of preprocessed regional time series were calculated as the Fisher-Z transformed Pearson product moment ($z = atanh(\rho)$), and ordered into 88×88 correlation matrices for each subject (hitherto referred to as C_i for subject i) and for each nuisance regression technique, resulting in a total of 184*9 = 1656 matrices.

Group formation

One subject with extreme in-scanner motion (average FD greater than 0.7 mm) was excluded from further analysis. The remaining 183 subjects were arranged into various groups:

- Autistic and normal control groups. Based on the clinical neuropsychological diagnostic tests for autism, as detailed in the original study description of the ABIDE dataset [15]. A group of 49 autism subjects and a neurotypical control group (n = 105) were defined.
- Groups of healthy control patents with different average voxel-wise displacement patterns, based on the group mean voxel-wise displacement maps. The healthy control group was divided into two sub-groups randomly. Temporally averaged standard-space voxel-wise displacement maps were averaged across subjects of both sub-groups separately and the spatial Pearson correlation coefficients for the group-mean voxel-wise displacement maps were calculated between the sub-groups (hitherto referred to as ρ_{WD}). This random group formation was repeated 5000 times to generate groups-pairs with different between-group voxel-wise displacement correlation. The histogram of observed ρ_{WD} values can be seen in Fig. 3. Group-pairs were chosen so that the corresponding ρ_{WD} values are relatively low, meaning that the subjects in one sub-group tend to have different voxel-vise displacement patterns than in the other. We chose eight pairs of groups with ρ_{WD}

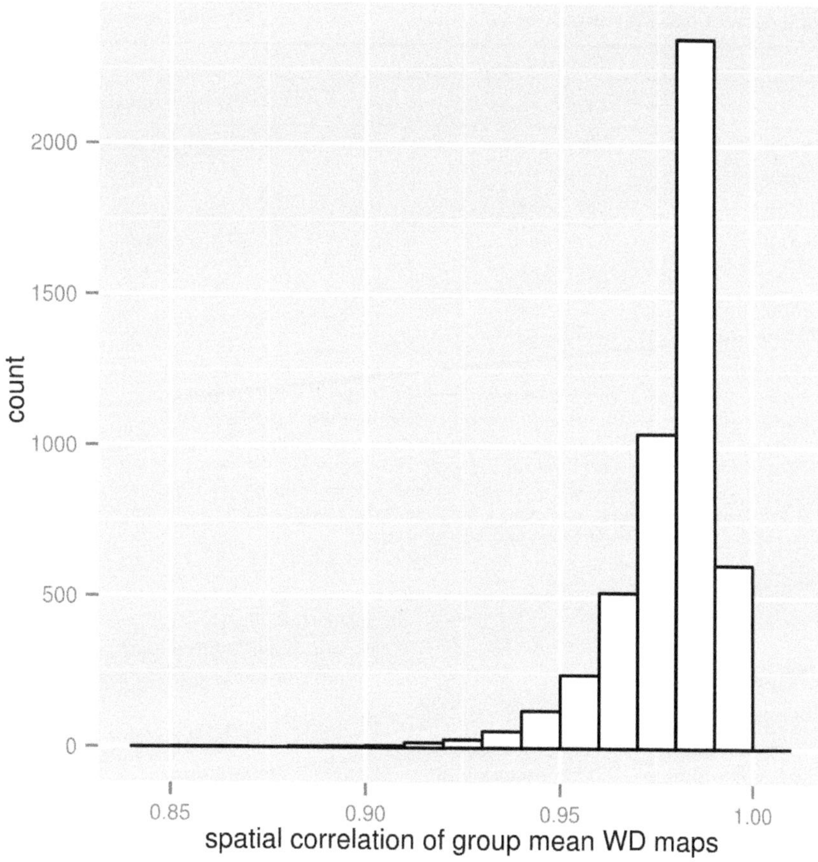

Figure 3. Histogram of group averaged voxel-wise displacement correlations based on 5000 random permutations. Temporally averaged standard-space voxel-wise displacement maps were averaged across the subjects of two randomly assigned groups. Spatial Pearson correlation was calculated between these group-mean voxel-wise displacement maps (ρ_{WD})). The histogram of this inter-group voxel-wise displacement correlation was computed based on 5000 random group formulation. Group-pairs with extrem inter-group differences in voxel-wise displacement were chosen for further analysis.

coefficients between 0.89–0.95 (Table 2). ρ_{WD} was also computed for the autism-related group-pair.

Group comparisons

Group comparisons were performed by fitting Generalized Linear Models (GLM) [32] and arranging statistical parameters into differential statistical parametric networks (SPNs) [33]. We investigated the effect of the grouping variable on functional connectivity strength. Additional covariates that might significantly influence functional connectivity, and thus, disturb comparison, were also included in the models. These are phenotypic covariates describing age, full-scale Wechsler Abbreviated Scale of Intelligence (full IQ), gender, and subject-specific mean FD. Connectivity strength is therefore modeled as:

$$y_i^{(A,B)} = \alpha + \beta GRP_i + \gamma_1 AGE_i + \gamma_2 FIQ_i + \gamma_3 SEX_i + \gamma_4 FD_i + \epsilon_i \quad (4)$$

where $y_i^{(A,B)}$ is the measured connectivity strength between regions A and B for subject i (element at the Ath row and B^{th} column of the C_i matrix), GRP_i is the dummy variable coding groups to compare, and AGE_i, FIQ_i, SEX_i and FD_i are the aforementioned subject-specific confounder variables, α, β and γ_is are the coefficients to estimate, and ϵ_i is the the ith independent identically distributed normal error. Models were fitted utilizing an iteratively reweighted least squares (IWLS) algorithm. T-scores and p-values of the effect of interest were obtained by dividing the β coefficient of interest by the estimated standard error.

Regional Displacement Interaction – RDI. According to our hypothesis, differences in the mean RDs of region-pairs A and B may have an important effect on the population-level distribution of correlation coefficients corresponding to the given connection. This can be tested by adding new terms to the linear model: the temporally averaged RDs of regions A and B and, furthermore, the interaction term between these two covariates. Since RDs are strongly correlated with each other and with the global FD, we introduced $\overline{\Delta RD}$ which is an alternative to the average RD, but with FD subtracted, in order to avoid multicollinearity in the model. Accordingly, $\overline{\Delta RD}$ can be defined as follows:

$$\overline{\Delta RD}_i^{(R)} = \frac{\sum_t^{1 \ldots T_i} RD_{i,t}^{(R)} - \sum_t^{1 \ldots T_i} FD_{i,t}}{T_i} \quad | \, i = 1 \ldots N \quad (5)$$

or using the terminology of equation (2):

Table 2. Voxel-vise displacement-dependent groups.

ρ_{WD}	FA_1	FA_2	$p_{FA_1=FA_2}$	maxVIF_{GRP}^{STD}	max$VIF_{GRP}^{STD+RDI}$
0.89	0.06 (±0.03)	0.08 (±0.04)	0.011	1.11	1.2
0.90	0.07 (±0.04)	0.07 (±0.03)	0.46	1.24	1.09
0.91	0,07 (±0.03)	0.07 (±0.04)	0.99	1.36	1.00
0.92	0.07 (±0.03)	0.07 (±0.04)	0.11	1.37	1.08
0.93	0.07 (±0.03)	0.08 (±0.04)	0.12	1.41	1.07
0.94	0.07 (±0.02)	0.07 (±0.04)	0.78	1.38	1.1
0.95	0.07 (±0.03)	0.07 (±0.04)	0.67	1.23	1.02
0.96	0.07 (±0.03)	0.07 (±0.03)	0.82	1.21	1.01

Formation of voxel-wise displacement related groups. N = 105 healthy control patients were divided into group-pairs randomly, 5000 times. Eight pairs of groups were chosen so that correlation between the group-mean voxel-wise displacement maps (ρ_{WD}) were 0.89, 0.9, 0.91, 0.92, 0.93, 0.94, 0.95 and 0.96. FA_1 and FA_2 denotes the mean (± standard deviation) FD of the group-pairs (in mm) and $p_{FA_1=FA_2}$ denotes the probability that the groups are identical regarding FD (obtained using permutation test). MaxVIF_{GRP}^{STD} and max$VIF_{GRP}^{STD+RDI}$ denotes the obtained maximal variance inflation factor (VIF) (throughout all connections) corresponding to the grouping factor, in models STD and STD+RDI, respectively. None of the groups introduce multicollinearity in the models. (however there is a slight difference between the FDs of the group-pairs with a spatial voxel-wise displacement correlation of 0.98).

$$\overline{\Delta RD}_i^{(R)} = \frac{\sum_t^{1\ldots T_i} \Delta RD_i^{(R)}}{T_i} \qquad (6)$$

where i denotes the subject, t the time frame, T_i the number of time frames in the fMRI time series of subject i (after exclusion of first five volumes).

Thus, in case of a GLM model for the connection between regions A and B, equation (4) extends to:

$$y_i^{(A,B)} = \alpha + \beta GRP_i + \gamma_1 AGE_i + \gamma_2 FIQ_i + \gamma_3 SEX_i + \gamma_4 FD_i + \\ + \gamma_5 \overline{\Delta RD}_i^{(A)} + \gamma_6 \overline{\Delta RD}_i^{(B)} + \gamma_7 \overline{\Delta RD}_i^{(A)} \overline{\Delta RD}_i^{(B)} + \epsilon_i \qquad (7)$$

Henceforward, we refer to the model specified in equation (4) as a standard (STD) model and, to the terms $\gamma_5 \overline{\Delta RD}_i^{(A)} + \gamma_6 \overline{\Delta RD}_i^{(B)} + \gamma_7 \overline{\Delta RD}_i^{(A)} \overline{\Delta RD}_i^{(B)}$ as *regional displacement interaction* (RDI) and, to the model defined by equation (7) as an STD+RDI model.

Characterization of the RDI effect. To investigate the RDI interaction effect on connectivity strength we utilized the following models:

$$y_i^{(A,B)} = \alpha + \gamma_1 AGE_i + \gamma_2 FIQ_i + \gamma_3 SEX_i + \gamma_4 FD_i \\ + \gamma_5 \overline{\Delta RD}_i^{(A)} + \gamma_6 \overline{\Delta RD}_i^{(B)} + \gamma_7 \overline{\Delta RD}_i^{(A)} \overline{\Delta RD}_i^{(B)} + \epsilon_i \qquad (8)$$

and

$$y_i^{(A,B)} = \alpha + \gamma_1 AGE_i + \gamma_2 FIQ_i + \gamma_3 SEX_i + \gamma_4 FD_i + \epsilon_i \qquad (9)$$

which are alternative versions of models (7) and (4), respectively, with GRP variable excluded. Since models (8) and (9) are nested, we can compare the reduction in deviance to residuals utilizing an F-test under the null hypothesis that none of the additional RDI covariates in the STD+RDI model is related to the measured connectivity strength. The resulting statistical parameters for each connection were ordered into nine differential SPNs for each nuisance regression model, showing connections significantly related to RDI. Model (8) was also used to demonstrate RDI in case of a single, representative connection.

We furthermore fitted a model defined as:

$$Y_j = \alpha + \gamma_1 AGE_j + \gamma_2 FIQ_j + \gamma_3 SEX_j + \gamma_4 FD_j \\ + \gamma_5 \overline{\Delta RD}_k + \gamma_6 \overline{\Delta RD}_l + \beta \overline{\Delta RD}_k \overline{\Delta RD}_l + \epsilon_j \qquad (10)$$

where $Y_j = Y_i^{(A,B)}$ so that $j = iM^2 + AM + B$ and $\overline{\Delta RD}_k = \overline{\Delta RD}_i^{(A)}$ so that $k = iM^2 + AM$ and $\overline{\Delta RD}_l = \overline{\Delta RD}_i^{(B)}$ so that $l = iM^2 + B$, or, in other words, the dependent and independent variables of model (8) are concatenated following the A and B ($A = 1\ldots M, B = 1\ldots M$) atlas regions. In contrast to the previously introduced models, here, we utilize one model for all connections of all subjects. The effect of interest is the RDI interaction term. This model was used to analyze the overall nature of the interaction term.

To avoid the disturbing effect of autistic differences when characterizing the interaction term, only the healthy control population was involved when applying models defined by Eqs. (8), (9) and (10).

Voxel-wise motion-related group comparison. Differences between low and high motion groups were investigated by two GLM models for every connection: STD (Eq. (4)) and STD+RDI (Eq. (7)) models were applied where GRP was a dummy variable that defined the motion-related groups as listed in Table 2. Results were ordered into 8*9*2 t-score SPNs, summarizing motion-related group differences (eight pairs of motion-related groups, nine first-level nuisance regression methods, and two second-level regression models [STD and STD+RDI]). Since, in these comparisons, the variable of interest (grouping factor) and the motion-related covariates (FD and the RDI covariates) are potentially related, we computed the variance inflation factor (VIF) [34] for each model. VIF values suggest that these modeling approaches are free from multicollinearity issues. (Maximal observed VIF values for the variable of interest are reported in Table 2.)

Autistic-control comparison. We tested the proposed RDI second-level interaction covariate set by comparisons of autistic and control groups defined by phenotypic information that was provided with the Autism Brain Imaging Dataset Exchange database. Results were arranged into 9*2 SPNs for nine nuisance regression methods and two second-level regression methods (STD and STD+RDI).

Computations and network visualization

Computations in this study, when not specified otherwise, were performed using R statistical programming language [35], using the packages "glm" [36], "fdrtool" [37,38], "HH" [39] and "visreg" [40]. Differential SPNs were thresholded and visualized with the in-house developed software BrainCON (www.minipetct.com/braincon) [29].

Results and Discussion

fMRI motion artifacts have spatial predisposition

As noted by Power et al. [2,41], the effect of motion appears to scale with the amplitude of the displacement over the whole brain: frames with greater amplitude displacements are associated with a greater change in BOLD signal. As a first step, we reproduced these results by observing a $\rho=0.485$ ($p<0.000001$) correlation between frame-wise displacement FD and DVARS.

Our results also show that this effect is not spatially constant. Although as also reported in [3], RD time courses a show high correlation in the entire brain of one subject, if the global effect is subtracted from the regional measures (FD from RD and DVRAS from RDVARS, respectively) the resulting residual measures $\Delta RD_i^{(R)}$ and $\Delta RDVARS_i^{(R)}$ (Eqs. (2) and (3)) still show a significant correlation of $\rho=0.278$ ($p<0.0001$). In addition, as presented in Fig. 4, the correlation of these residual regional measures increases with the global motion-BOLD relationship throughout subjects.

In-scanner head motion consists not only of translations. Rotational components make the displacement diverse in distinct locations: it becomes greater when moving further from the center of rotations. A plausible explanation of the reported regional relationship is that this complex spatio-temporal pattern of displacement implicitly affects local BOLD signal changes.

These results can also yield a potential explanation of the phenomenon that motion tends to increase connectivity for locally adjacent nodes, but reduces connectivity between distant nodes [2,8,9,14,16]: neighboring regions having more similar RD will share more similar motion artifacts than regions being far from each other and this effect biases the distance dependence of connectivity strength.

However, we should point out that all the discussed voxel-wise and regional displacement measures are only "apparent displacements": their estimated values may have been affected by phenomena other than head motion, including physiological noise, magnetic field inhomogeneities, instrumental instabilities, as well as BOLD activity of neuronal origin. This effect should be more pronounced for regional displacements than for the frame-wise displacements. Furthermore, the computation of RD implicitly include integrating of motion effects within each fMRI volume. Rapid head movements occurring on time scale shorter than the fMRI repetition time TR may affect different slices within an fMRI volume differently [42]. Effects of such rapid movements cause slice-specific image distortions that cannot be accurately taken into account by the volume realignment-based procedure, but can still affect fMRI functional connectivity results. Averaging over all time frames and within time frames is a simplification in modeling the spatial predisposition of head motion. However, as suggested by the significant correlation between $\Delta RD_i^{(R)}$ and $\Delta RDVARS_i^{(R)}$, this simplification seems to be reasonable. Nevertheless, sub-TR frequency components of in-scanner motion deserve more attention and their voxel-wise effect should be investigated in more detail in future publications.

The interaction of regional displacements affects measured connectivity strength

Evidences of a spatially non-constant motion artifact in brain connectivity analysis, like an increase in short-range and a decrease in long-range connectivity, or the special pattern of related changes in connectivity strength reported in [2,8,9,14,16], suggest that the reported local relationship between motion and BOLD signal changes should be considered when performing correction techniques. This is especially true for correlation-based functional connectivity analysis, where the similarity of two regional BOLD time courses can be increasingly affected by these small but systematic variations.

However, including voxel-wise motion parameters in nuisance signal regression does not seem to be efficient (as reported by [3,14] and also found in our preliminary analysis). Yan et al. [14] used voxel-wise displacement as a reference to evaluate the differential region-specific impact of motion on the BOLD signal. Although these authors presented significant correlations with a spatial pattern similar to that previously reported, it is still not clear whether those patterns can be explained only by locally differential BOLD answers to a global motion effect, or, alternatively, by a real local relationship with the spatio-temporal motion pattern.

To investigate this question, we defined RDI, a set of second-level regression covariates that models the interaction effect between the temporally averaged regional displacements of the regions involved in the connection. In regression analysis, an interaction effect is said to exist when the effect of the focal independent variable on the dependent variable differs depending on the value of a third variable [43], called the moderator variable. (Statistically, the choice of which of the two independent variables should be the moderator variable is unimportant.) The proposed RDI interaction term in the second-level GLM model defined by Eq. (10) was found to be significant ($p<0.000001$) for all first-level nuisance regression methods), which means that the effect of the average RD of one region on the dependent variable (connectivity strength) changes when the average RD of the other region changes. The effect is visualized in Fig. 5 by the filled contour plots. The predicted connectivity strength changes depending on the simultaneously varying values of $\overline{\Delta RD_i^{(A)}}$ and $\overline{\Delta RD_i^{(B)}}$, in case of all investigated first-level nuisance regression methods. These results imply that throughout the population, connectivity strength between two brain regions tends to increase if the average RD of the regions is similar (eg. both are larger or smaller than the average FD) and tends to decrease otherwise.

This effect is demonstrated for a representative connection (occipital fusiform gyrus - prefrontal gyrus) in Fig. 6. While the presented partial residual plot reveals no significant relationship between connectivity strength and ΔRD_A, the $\Delta RD_A \Delta RD_B$ interaction effect is significant implying that the effect of ΔRD_A on connectivity strength differs depending on the value of ΔRD_B. This is demonstrated by dividing the data into four groups based on the value of ΔRD_B and visualizing the corresponding cross-sectional CCPR (component and component-plus-residual) plots, which reveal that in each group the relationship between ΔRD_A and partial residual connectivity strength is significant in all cases but the regression lines have different slopes. Thus, this latent relationship is not observable without accounting for the interaction of the regional displacement covariates.

To characterize how this phenomenon is related to the spatial patterns of measured functional connectivity and to what extent it

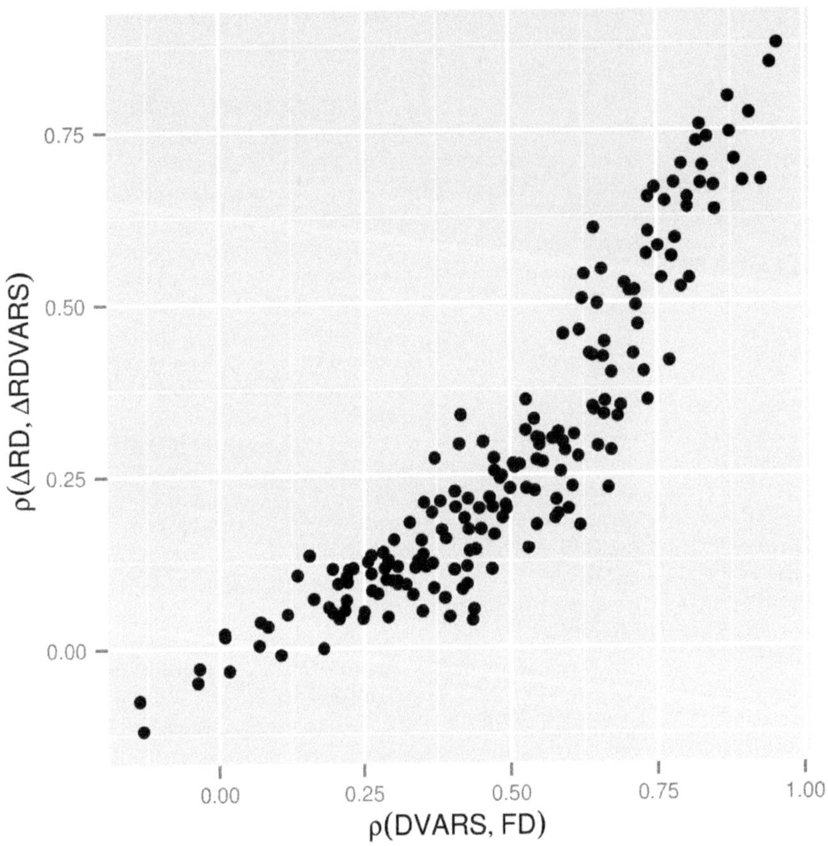

Figure 4. Regional motion-BOLD relationship scales with the global motion-BOLD relationship. Within-subject correlation of $\Delta RD_i^{(R)}$ and $\Delta RDVARS_i^{(R)}$ (horizontal axis) plotted against the correlation of FD and DVARS (vertical axis) for all brain regions and time frames of N = 183 subjects. The regional effect of motion on BOLD seems to scale with the global relationship which is correlated ($\rho = 0.485$ ($p < 0.000001$) with the mean FD.

is present in case of the applied first-level nuisance signal regression techniques, we performed a comparison of the STD (Eq. (8)) and STD+RDI (Eq. (9)) models. The model comparison was realized by F-tests between the models and resulted in the SPNs shown in Fig. 7. In this figure, connections are visualized, where the STD+RDI model explains significantly more variance than the STD model (the null hypothesis of the F-test can be rejected) with a false discovery rate of $q<0.05$. The proposed method, RDI proved to be the most efficient with nuisance signal regression methods NOREG, WMCSF, WMCSF+M6, GSREG, and COMPCOR+M6. The explanatory power added by RDI is most pronounced typically in case of middle- and long-range connections of the temporal poles.

The interaction of regional displacements may bias functional connectivity group comparisons

The correlation coefficient of two regional BOLD time courses can be sensitive to the regional displacement time course (RD) of both regions. Even if the motion-related artifactual component is small, it still can significantly affect correlations, depending on the degree to which it is shared between the time courses.

This phenomenon becomes even more problematic on the population-level. Satterthwaite et al. [9] reported that between-subject differences in head motion are stable: that subjects who tend to move on one occasion tend to move on another occasion. This means that analyses of functional connectivity needs to consider the possibility that *certain aspects of head motion behave as a trait*. Accordingly, even if the above-mentioned effect is otherwise small, it can disturb group comparisons and lead to erroneous conclusions, since it is of non-neural origin.

This assumption can be admitted easily by considering two patient cohorts where region A and B have similar RD within each subject of one group (e.g., due to relatively smaller rotations), and different RD in the subjects of the other (e.g., more prevalent rotations with a center to which A and B are located asymmetrically). The significant RDI interaction effect means that the corresponding correlation coefficient will be biased, and tends to be larger in the first group, even in the absence of a real functional difference. However, it is still not clear how different grouping conditions interfere with the tendency of motion patterns.

One can hypothesize that the spatio-temporal pattern of motion can be significantly different between groups that were defined by a factor in relation to motion. This could be the case in group comparisons in several physiological and pathological conditions co-occurring with hypo- or hyperkinetic signs.

Our results show that the spatio-temporal pattern of head motion biases measured connectivity strength on the population level, and, practically speaking, *the proposed second-level covariates (RDI) can be utilized as a method to incorporate these individual regional differences of in-scanner head motion into the model, and thus, reduce artifactual variance in the data.*

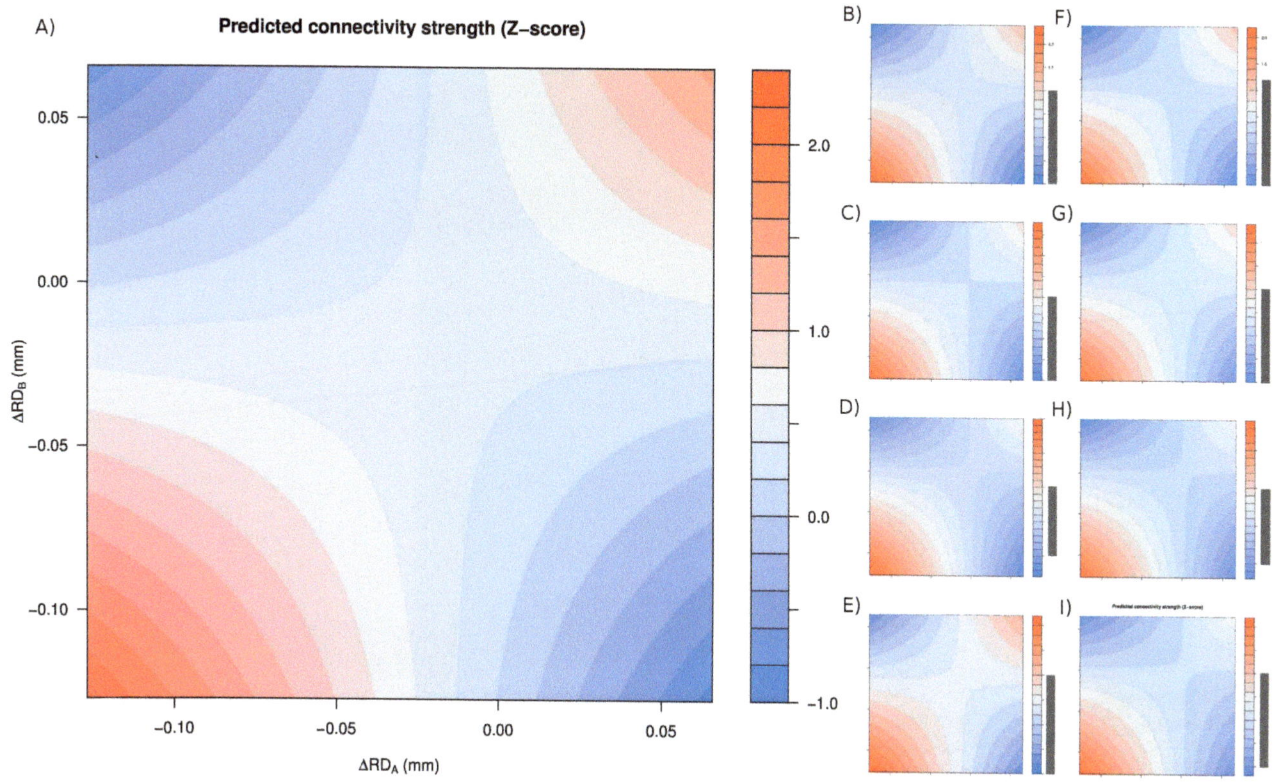

Figure 5. Filled contour plots visualizing the Regional Displacement Interaction (RDI) effect: how the predicted connectivity strength (color-coded) changes depending on the simultaneously varying values of $\overline{\Delta RD_i^{(A)}}$ and $\overline{\Delta RD_i^{(B)}}$, in case of no nuisance regression (A:NOREG) and all investigated first-level nuisance regression methods, i.e., NOREG+M6 (E), WMSCF (B), COMPCORR (C), GSREG (D), WMSCF+M6 (F), COMPCORR+M6 (G), GSREG+M6 (H), and SAT36 (I). Vertical and horizontal axes of plots B-I are the same as those of plot A. Gray bars next to the legends indicate the (−1,1) interval to ease interpretation of color-coded Z-score values.

Including RDI as a covariate in second-level regression efficiently reduces group differences caused by differences in voxel-wise motion

To demonstrate the reported confounding effect of voxel-wise motion on population-level analysis, we performed eight group comparisons (See Table 2) where the groups to compare have different average voxel-wise displacement patterns.

Results are summarized in Table 3. In Fig. 8, the number of significantly ($p<0.01$) differing connections is plotted against the group-defining mean FD threshold for each nuisance signal regression method. Results show that, for less extensive nuisance regression methods (NOREG, NOREG+M6, WMCSF, WMCSF+M6), when the voxel-wise displacement maps between groups are more different (lower between-group mean voxel-wise displacement map correlations), more group differences appear. These findings seem to confirm that group comparisons may be biased when groups show different tendencies in voxel-wise motion. Results, in conjunction with the results of the F-test based model comparisons Fig. 7, also show that *the inclusion of RDI covariates seems to decrease these artifuctual group differences, especially by moderate nuisance regression methods*.

The change in the corresponding connectivity pattern is visualized in Fig. 8 for the nuisance signal regression methods NOREG, COMPCOR, and GSREG, and for each motion-related group comparison defined by ρ_{WD}. Results with the STD and STD+RDI second-level regression models are presented in the upper and lower rows on each panel, respectively. Group differences with probability ($p>=0.01$) are not visualized.

As predicted by the F-test-based model comparisons (Fig 7), the reduction of false group differences caused by voxel-wise motion most markedly improved in the NOREG, WMCSF and COMPCOR methods. Regressing out six motion parameters did not seem to be highly efficient but may be beneficial when no other nuisance signal regression covariate is applied (NOREG+M6).

However, the small number of differences surviving the $q<0.05$ false discovery rate criterion implies that - when utilizing a proper second-level model - all the investigated methods are able to reduce motion-related group comparison artifacts to a decent extent. With the RDI correction, no FDR significant group differences remained in any of the comparison cases.

We note, that, in contrast to most prior studies, here, we performed more than a single pair of group comparisons, thus avoiding that results reflect only the random effects of the grouping condition.

Including RDI as a covariate in second-level regression preserves autism-related group differences

To test the efficiency of the proposed correction method, we performed group comparisons where both motion-related artifacts [20,21] and real neuronal differences [10,15,44] were expected to be present. We compared the functional networks of autistic and control patients.

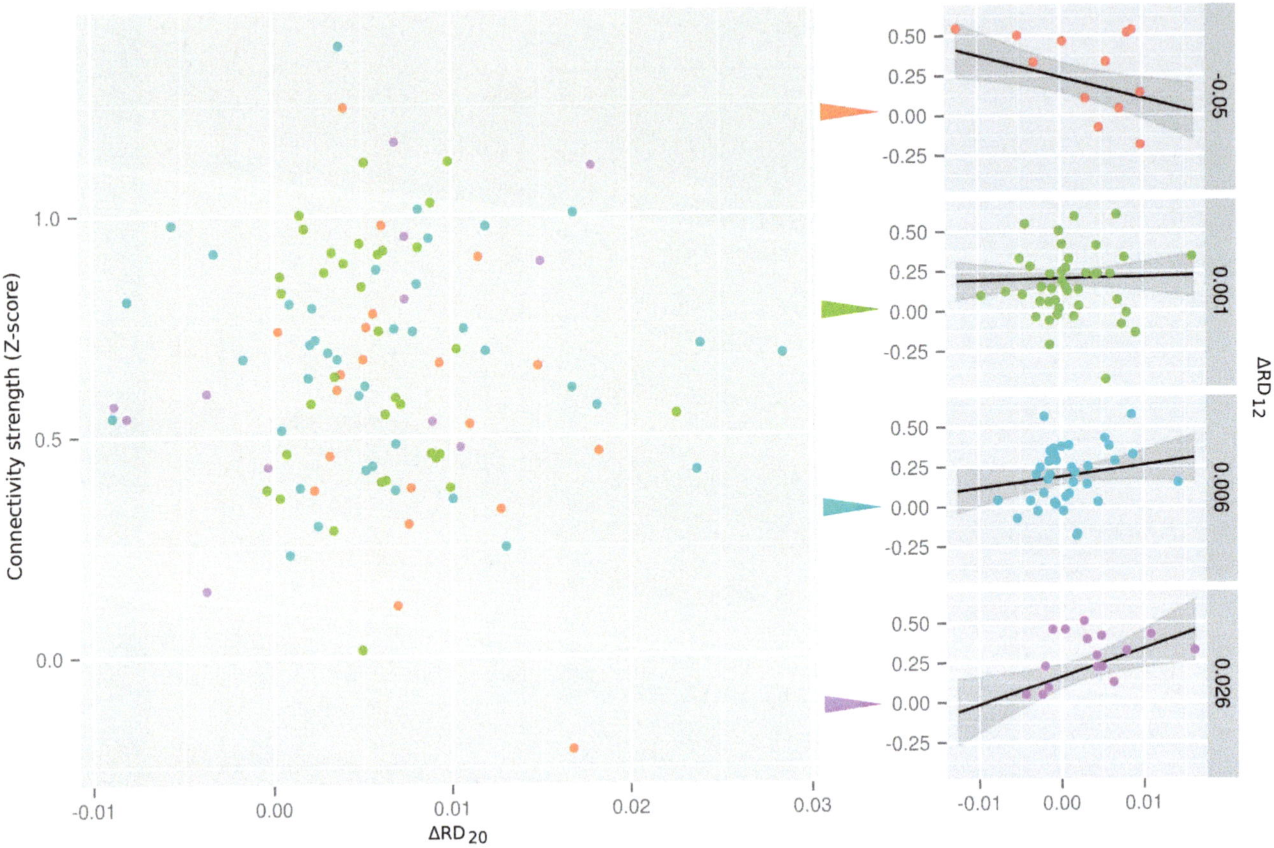

Figure 6. RDI effect in case of a demonstrative connection: occipital fusiform gyrus (A = 20) - prefrontal gyrus (B = 12). On the left, the partial residuals for ΔRD_A from the model defined by Eq. (8) (dependent variable: connectivity data of the healthy control population (N = 105), without nuisance signal regression (NOREG)) are plotted against ΔRD_A. Although the model reveals no significant relationship ($t = -1.46, p = 0.15$) between connectivity strength and ΔRD_A, the $\Delta RD_A \Delta RD_B$ interaction effect is significant ($t = 3.31$, $p = 0.0013$), implying that the effect of ΔRD_A on connectivity strength differs depending on the value of ΔRD_B. This is demonstrated by dividing the data into four groups based on the value of ΔRD_B (color-coded on the left plot) and visualizing the corresponding cross-sectional CCPR (component and component-plus-residual) plots (on the left). Mean value of ΔRD_B corresponding to the cross-section is indicated. Partial residuals are plotted with colored dots corresponding to the cross-section group. The corresponding regression line estimated from the full model fit and the corresponding 95% confidence interval is displayed in black and gray, respectively. The horizontal and vertical axes of the cross-sectional CCPR plots are the same as those of the partial residual plot on the left. Cross-sectional CCPR plots imply that in each group the relationship between ΔRD_A and partial residual connectivity strength is significant but the regression lines have different slopes, which makes this latent relationship not observable without accounting for the interaction of the regional displacement covariates.

The correlation between the group-mean voxel-wise correlation map (ρ_{WD}) between the autistic and the normal control groups was found to be 0.98. It suggests that this grouping condition should be only slightly biased by the effect of regional displacement on the measured connectivity strength. Thus, as predicted by voxel-wise displacement pattern-related group comparisons, utilizing the RDI correction method should introduce only minor changes in the differential connectivity patterns.

Results are presented in Fig. 9 and Tables 4 and 5.

More than 200 connectivity differences survived the $q<0.05$ false discovery rate criterion in NOREG and COMPCOR (both with and without RDI) and none survived in GSREG+RDI, GSREG+M6, GSREG+M6+RDI, SAT36 and SAT36+RDI. As predicted above, the inclusion of RDI introduces only slight changes in the pattern of autism-related group differences.

All the evaluated signal regression approaches revealed presumably autism-linked impairments of functional connectivity. Autism was mainly characterized by decreased synchronicity, i.e., under-connectivity. This finding is in line with the majority of intrinsic functional connectivity studies. The spatial predisposition, along with the 30 most significant differences, is presented in Fig. 9 and Table 4 and 5.

While including RDI significantly reduced (presumably artifactual) differences between voxel-wise displacement-related subject cohorts, differences in the autism-related comparison were more or less preserved. These results suggest that the proposed correction method, while effectively reducing motion artifacts in group comparisons, preserves the sensitivity to neural differences.

A critical interpretation of our autism-linked findings in this study is not directly possible. This mainly stems from the lack of ground truth information about the basic neuropathology of the disease. Furthermore, larger-scale, multi-centric comparisons would be optimal to test the reproducibility of any finding.

Contrasting the impact of head motion and nuisance signal regression strategies

The efficiency of nuisance signal regression techniques in the context of rs-fcMRI motion artifacts analysis has been intensively investigated in the last few years; however, a significant part of these studies did not apply second-level regression covariates

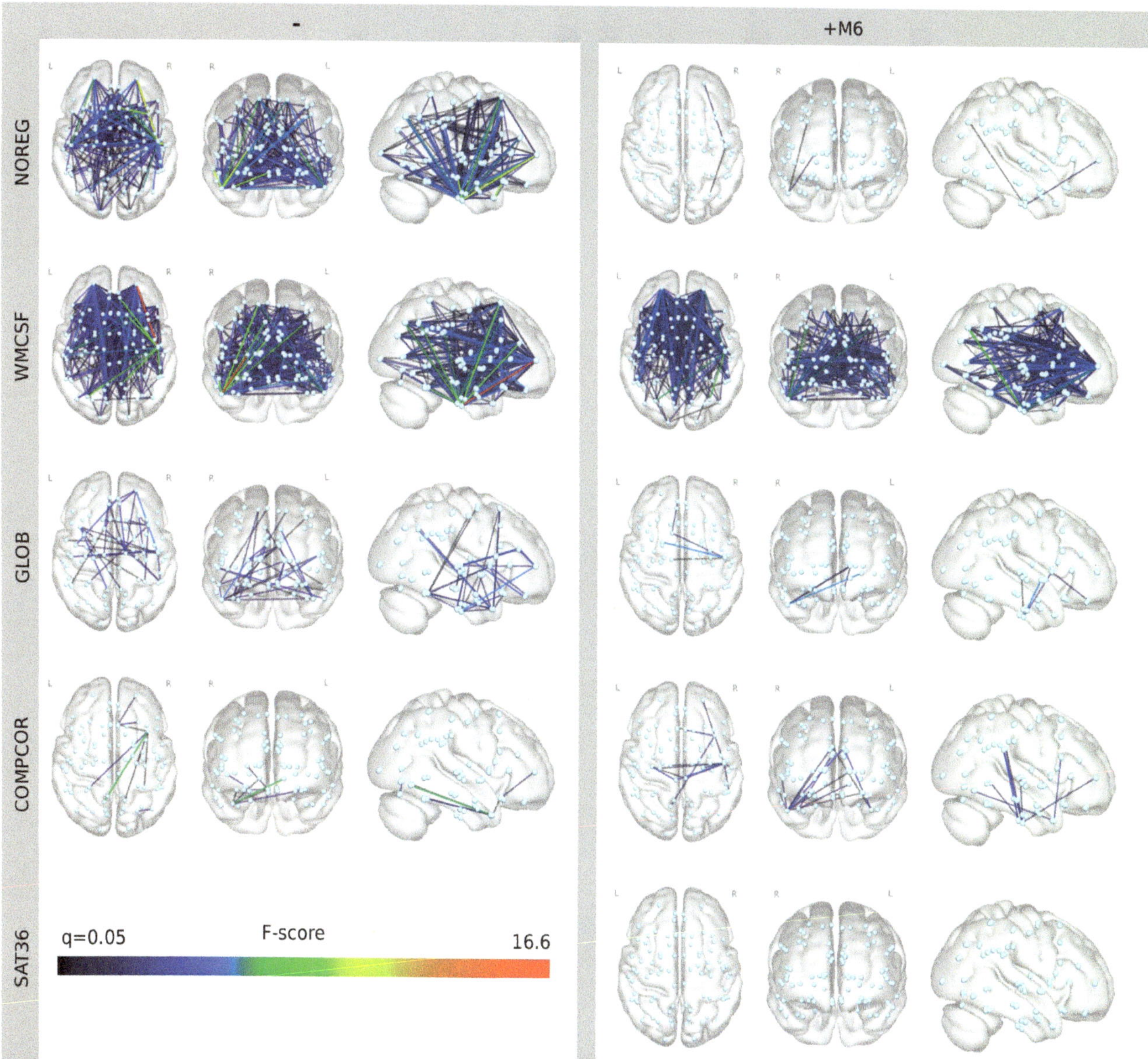

Figure 7. Network pattern of connections where utilizing RDI significantly improves second-level modeling. Statistical parametric networks presenting the model comparison performed by F-tests between the STD and STD+RDI models (Eq. (9) and (8)). Connections are only visualized, when the STD+RDI model explains significantly more variance than the STD model (the null hypothesis of the F-test can be rejected) with a false discovery rate of $q<0.05$. The proposed STD+RDI method proves to be most efficient with the nuisance signal regression methods NOREG, WMCSF, WMCSF+M6, GSREG, and COMPCOR+M6, and seems to demonstrate no significant improvement in case of SAT36, after correction for multiple comparison.

[2,3,9,16] in population-level analysis. Their overall conclusion was that global signal regression, high-parameter nuisance signal regression, scrubbing, and de-spiking are potentially beneficial. However, recent studies have questioned some of these conclusions. In the following, we summarize the latest findings in the literature in contrast to our results.

Effect of global signal regression. In our analysis, patterns of group differences become extremely different when regressing out the whole-brain signal from regional BOLD time courses (GSREG, GSREG+M6 and SAT36). Most of the above-mentioned studies, which did not utilize second-level correction, applied GSREG in their analysis pipeline. Recent studies using mean FD as a second-level regressor [14,45] also concluded that GSREG mitigates the effects of motion-related differences among subjects, but warns that investigators must weigh up the pros and cons of GSREG when deciding whether to employ it in the context of testing specific hypotheses.

Our results show that, after the correction of group-wise differences in head movement in the autism-control comparison, over-connectivity and under-connectivity can simultaneously appear. However, global signal regression in the processing pipeline appears to bias results toward over-connected differential networks. In addition to under-connectivity, many authors suggested short-distance over-connectivity (in the frontal lobe or globally) as a possible finding in autism spectrum disorders [46]. This theory was then questioned on the grounds that head-

Table 3. Motion-related group differences.

ρ_{WD}	0.89	0.90	0.91	0.92	0.93	0.94	0.95	0.96
NOREG	106 (1)	12	12	5	8	3	4	0
NOREG+RDI	63	3	6	3	3	2	0	0
WMCSF	139 (2)	5	26	9	5	11	17	1
WMCSF+RDI	84	2	15	8	1	4	2	0
GSREG	11	46	30	75 (1)	30	63	17	38
GSREG+RDI	11	29	33	58	29	40	12	33
COMPCOR	35	16	40	17	21	7	104 (2)	12
COMPCOR+RDI	8	8	26	11	12	7	46	10
NOREG+M6	121	5	20	3	3	2	9	0
NOREG+M6+RDI	54	1	13	3	1	1	1	0
WMCSF+M6	106	6	39	5	2	44	58	2
WMCSF+M6+RDI	37	4	25	7	1	26	4	1
GSREG+M6	20	32	31	108 (1)	23	52	16	29
GSREG+M6+RDI	19	15	29	94	19	53	20	22
COMPCOR+M6	59	5	39	66	25	5	62 (1)	13
COMPCOR+M6+RDI	17	4	37	41	9	6	30	12
SAT36	20	38	34	85	22	43	17	33
SAT36+RDI	21	15	39	69	20	44	13	34

Number of connections significantly ($p<0.01$) differing between groups. Voxel-wise displacement-related group comparisons corresponding to given ρ_{WD} are presented in columns. Rows correspond to the nine nuisance regression methods and their +RDI variants. Number of differences surviving the $q<0.05$ false discovery rate criterion (if any) is indicated in parentheses.

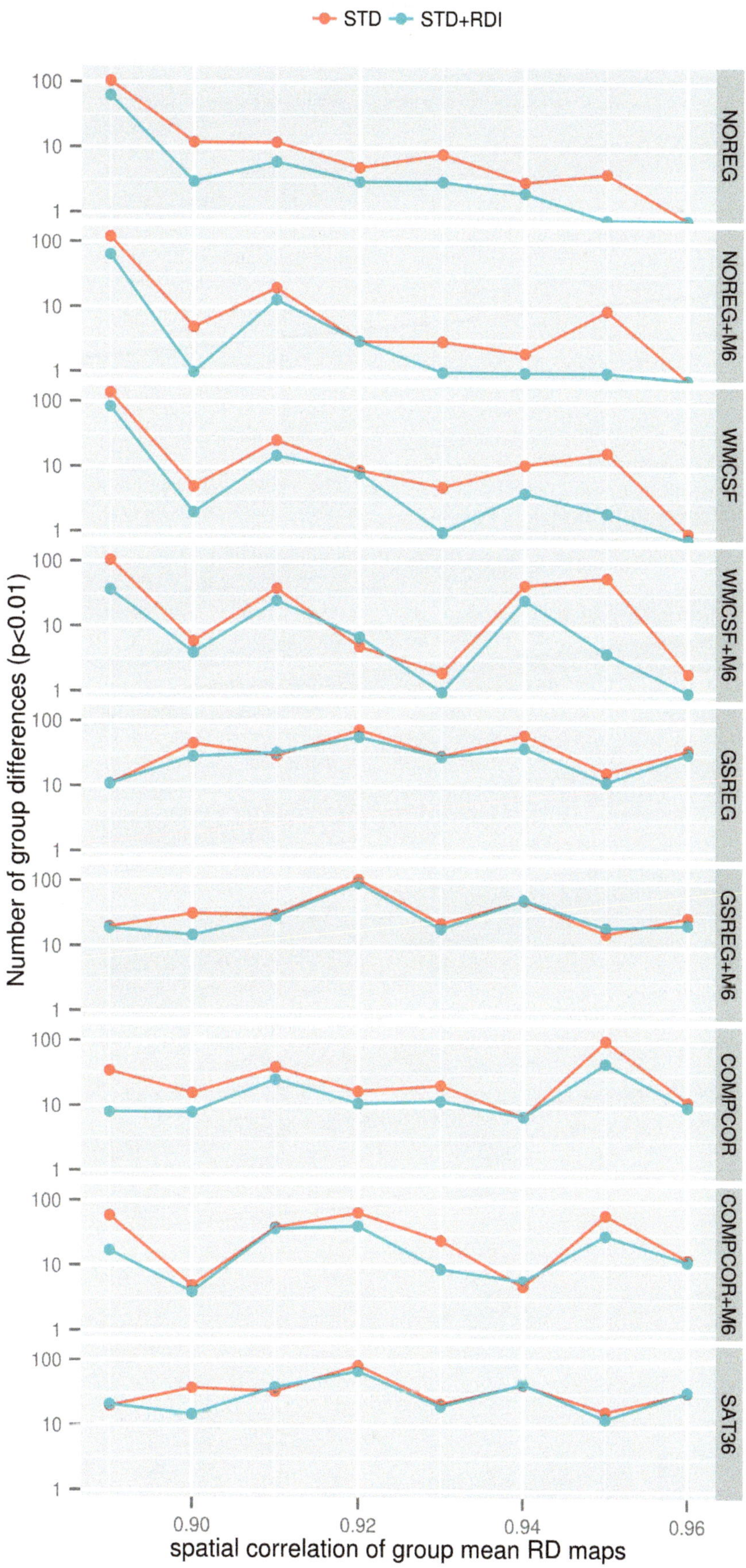

STD
STD+RDI
Number of group differences (p<0.01)
100
10
1
NOREG
NOREG+M6
WMCSF
WMCSF+M6
GSREG
GSREG+M6
COMPCOR
COMPCOR+M6
SAT36
0.90
0.92
0.94
0.96
spatial correlation of group mean RD maps

Figure 8. The effect of RDI on motion-related group differences. The number of significantly ($p<0.01$) differing connections is plotted against the spatial correlation coefficient of group-mean voxel-wise displacement maps for RD-based group-pairs for each nuisance signal regression method. The number of significant group differences is plotted on logarithmic axis. Improvement in the reduction of motion-related group differences was most pronounced for the NOREG, WMCSF and COMPCOR methods. Nuisance regression methods incorporating GSREG seem not to be sensible for differences in group-mean voxel-wise displacement patterns however, they show relatively high number of group differences by all group comparisons.

movement could induce similar effects [21]. As reported in [47], correlation estimates obtained after GSREG are more susceptible to the presence of motion and exacerbate distance-dependent bias. Moreover, as reported in [20,22], correlation patterns and group differences may become distorted after GSREG (depending on, e.g., region size or the underlying true connectivity structure). According to Müller et al. [48], pre-processing strategies greatly affect the spatial patterns of autism-linked connectivity traits, although under-connectivity is the most prevalent across studies. It is, therefore, safe to conclude that GSREG not only introduces anti-correlations in the functional connectome [49], but can also confound case-control comparisons in autism.

Effect of including motion parameters. In the case of voxel-wise motion pattern-related group comparisons, inclusion of the six motion parameters in first-level nuisance signal regression showed no obvious improvement in motion-artifact reduction. However, the inclusion of these parameters had a pronounced effect in autism-related group comparisons, especially in NOREG, WMCSF and COMPCOR techniques: the number of significant group differences decreased. Whether this phenomenon is due to improved motion-artifact reduction in the special case of autistic group comparisons, or due to overfitting and the removal of real brain signal, remains a question. However, evidence that spatial realignment-based estimation of motion parameters may yield poor results in periods of small movements [12] point toward the conclusion that motion parameter estimates should be applied carefully. As a possible solution, we suggest utilizing thresholded motion estimates and avoiding the use of motion parameters in periods of relatively small movements.

Optimal choice of individual-level motion-correction technique. In some cases, it is not clear whether various high-parameter nuisance regression techniques eliminate group differences due to increased specificity or decreased sensitivity. Considering most significant autism-related group differences, minimal nuisance regression techniques (NOREG, NOREG+M6) show a high consensus with moderate (WMCSF, WMSCF+M6) and more complex (COMPCOR, COMPCOR+M6) methods. This points to the conclusion that when analyzing a sufficiently large sample and utilizing an appropriate second-level model, the choice of individual-level signal nuisance regression technique becomes less crucial. However, when analyzing small samples and also with individual analysis, the role of these techniques is unquestionably important.

The role of confounds not related to subject motion. This article focused on motion-related artifacts, which are only one, although a conspicuous source of confounding effects in functional MRI. In thes context, the performance of NOREG and NOREG+M6 methods in motion-related comparisons deserves attention. One possible explanation is that, although artifacts of other sources are obviously present in the data, their individual spatio-temporal pattern is more constant and their population-level distribution is more similar among the investigated subpopulations compared to motion-related confounds. Thus, these artifacts may have only a moderate disturbing effect in large-sample group comparisons. However, by grouping conditions in relation to physiological conditions, like blood pressure and blood oxygenation (or artifacts of scanner-related sources in multi-center studies), non-motion originated artifacts can appreciably affect the results. Thus in such experimental designs, nuisance regression methods may have a more important role.

This is also suggested by the results of autism-related group comparisons, where pronounced differences were experienced among various nuisance signal regression techniques. A potential explanation for these deviations is that, although the proposed

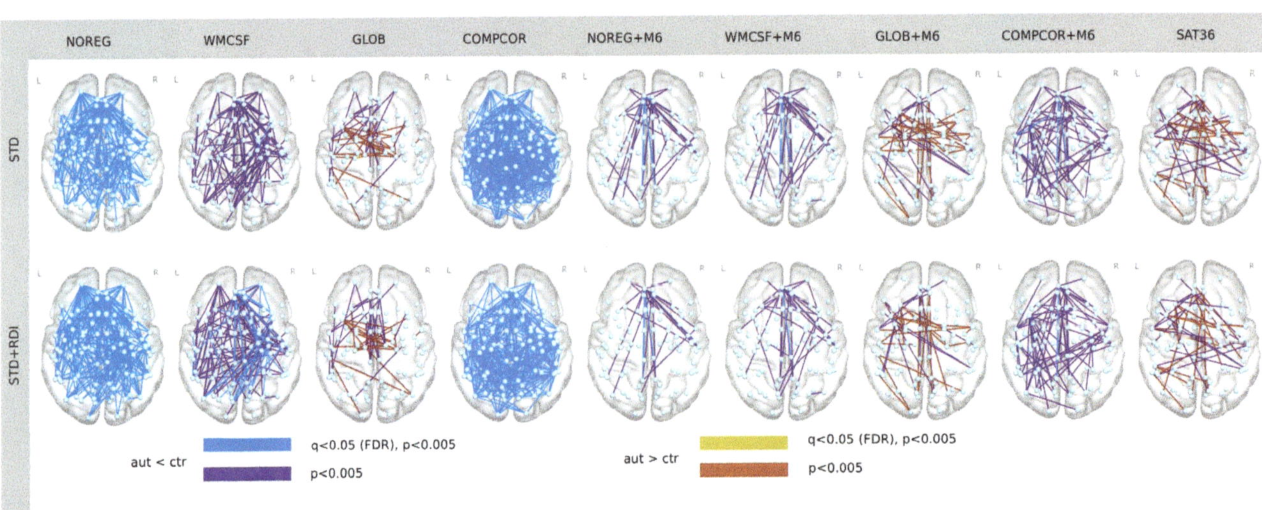

Figure 9. Autism related group comparisons. Autism related group differences for the investigated correction strategies. Colors denote significance levels as detailed in the legend.

Table 4. Autism-related group differences (without nuisance signal regression of six motion parameters).

Connection	NOREG	+RDI	WMCSF	+RDI	GSREG	+RDI	COMPCOR	+RDI
l-cun - l-stg	−3.73 ***	−3.52 ***	−2.79 *	−2.56	−2.67 *	−2.19	−5.03 ***	−4.57 ***
l-occfus - r-tfus	−3.64 ***	−3.98 ***	−3.88 **	−4.03 ***	−3.26 *	−3.17 *	−4.88 ***	−4.62 ***
l-fmedc - r-parcing	−4.30 ***	−4.11 ***	−4.16 **	−4.06 ***	−3.02 *	−3.09 *	−4.86 ***	−4.77 ***
l-fmedc - r-cingpost	−4.54 ***	−4.23 ***	−3.94 **	−3.86 ***	−1.92	−1.94	−4.83 ***	−4.55 ***
r-mfg - r-parhipc	−3.14 ***	−3.63 ***	−4.54 ***	−4.67 ***	−3.70 **	−3.85 **	−3.55 ***	−3.47 ***
l-smargp - l-mtgant	−3.38 ***	−3.54 ***	−2.66 *	−2.79 *	−2.48	−2.54	−4.65 ***	−4.49 ***
r-tfus - r-tofus	−3.35 ***	−4.13 ***	−2.92 *	−3.48 ***	−1.57	−1.75	−4.43 ***	−4.59 ***
l-fmedc - l-cingpost	−4.30 ***	−3.97 ***	−3.52 **	−3.40 ***	−1.83	−1.84	−4.19 ***	−3.95 ***
l-hip - l-thal	−0.28	−0.06	2.2	2.03	4.53 ***	4.21 **	−0.15	0.45
l-sfg - l-mtgant	−3.71 ***	−3.97 ***	−2.84 *	−3.00 *	−3.00 *	−2.97 *	−4.49 ***	−4.30 ***
l-fmedc - r-front	−4.49 ***	−3.98 ***	−4.03 **	−3.61 ***	−2.78 *	−2.45	−4.00 ***	−3.63 ***
l-cun - l-plan	−3.24 ***	−2.96 ***	−2.27	−2.01	−1.72	−1.18	−4.47 ***	−3.96 ***
l-stg - r-cun	−3.19 ***	−2.97 ***	−2.47	−2.24	−2.82 *	−2.45	−4.46 ***	−4.02 ***
l-temp - l-thal	0.28	0.48	2.03	2.16	4.45 ***	4.07 **	0.02	0.13
r-parhipc - r-hip	0.99	0.52	2.33	2.17	4.44 ***	4.29 **	0.34	0.29
l-mtgant - r-sfg	−3.33 ***	−3.50 ***	−2.82 *	−2.89 *	−1.85	−1.73	−4.44 ***	−4.25 ***
r-fmedc - r-precun	−4.43 ***	−4.35 ***	−3.12 *	−3.10 *	−0.89	−1.03	−3.55 ***	−3.67 ***
l-fmedc - l-precun	−4.02 ***	−3.83 ***	−3.54 **	−3.55 ***	−1.22	−1.35	−4.40 ***	−4.28 ***
l-fmedc - l-sfg	−4.16 ***	−3.87 ***	−3.51 **	−3.39 ***	−2.21	−2.31	−4.38 ***	−4.17 ***
l-fmedc - r-precun	−4.17 ***	−3.99 ***	−3.65 **	−3.62 ***	−1.1	−1.22	−4.34 ***	−4.29 ***
l-ins - r-mtgtempoc	−3.12 ***	−3.10 ***	−1.88	−2.02	−2.34	−2.36	−2.36	−1.84
l-fmedc - r-mtgant	−4.33 ***	−3.95 ***	−2.76 *	−2.45	−1.69	−1.47	−3.26 ***	−3.20 ***
l-ang - l-mtgant	−3.76 ***	−3.91 ***	−3.48 **	−3.68 ***	−3.02 *	−3.14 *	−4.29 ***	−4.26 ***
l-parhipc - r-sfg	−2.79 ***	−2.63 ***	−2.81 *	−2.51	−0.67	−0.89	−4.26 ***	−3.87 ***
l-fmedc - l-parcing	−3.93 ***	−3.62 ***	−3.59 **	−3.45 ***	−2.74 *	−2.74 *	−4.23 ***	−4.05 ***
r-sfg - r-parhipc	−3.03 ***	−3.59 ***	−3.47 **	−3.66 ***	−1.14	−1.34	−4.23 ***	−4.13 ***
l-occfus - l-tfus	−2.66 ***	−2.67 ***	−3.20 *	−3.14 *	−2.16	−2.3	−4.23 ***	−4.18 ***
l-fmedc - l-front	−4.23 ***	−3.49 ***	−3.33 *	−2.73 *	−1.83	−1.43	−3.41 ***	−2.79 ***
l-temp - r-sfg	−2.90 ***	−2.99 ***	−2.56	−2.44	−0.79	−0.78	−4.21 ***	−3.88 ***
r-occfus - r-tfus	−3.74 ***	−4.21 ***	−3.15 *	−3.49 ***	−2.14	−2.3	−3.66 ***	−3.57 ***

The overall 30 most significant autism-related group differences in order of significance level. The first column lists the short names of the region pairs (See Table 1 for full names and other information). The corresponding T-value estimated from the STD and STD+RDI models are shown for all investigated nuisance signal regression methods. Significance level is implied by asterisks: * $p<0.01$, ** $p<0.001$, *** FDR $q<0.05$.

Table 5. Autism-related group differences (with nuisance signal regression of 6 motion parameters).

Connection	NOREG+M6	+RDI	WMCSF+M6	+RDI	GSREG+M6	+RDI	COMPC+M6	+RDI	SAT36	+RDI
l-cun - l-stg	−2.88 *	−2.6	−2.54	−2.29	−2.93 *	−2.41	−3.57 **	−3.13 *	−2.14	−1.52
l-occfus - r-tfus	−1.98	−2.05	−2.16	−2.25	−2.33	−2.3	−2.96 *	−2.84 *	−2.35	−2.4
l-fmedc - r-parcing	−4.18 ***	−4.01 **	−3.98 **	−3.90 **	−2.82 *	−3.08 *	−3.86 **	−4.00 **	−2.24	−2.82 *
l-fmedc - r-cingpost	−4.61 ***	−4.31 ***	−4.63 ***	−4.54 ***	−2.93 *	−3.12 *	−4.21 ***	−4.16 **	−2.38	−2.63 *
r-mfg - r-parhipc	−1.55	−1.62	−2.25	−2.36	−1.35	−1.56	−1.8	−1.63	−1.21	−1.28
l-smargp - l-mtgant	−1.87	−1.99	−1.78	−1.97	−2.55	−2.65 *	−2.88 *	−2.86 *	−2.75 *	−2.82 *
r-tfus - r-tofus	−1.6	−2.1	−1.63	−2.18	−1.05	−1.5	−2.5	−2.95 *	−1.24	−1.66
l-fmedc - l-cingpost	−4.58 ***	−4.31 ***	−4.56 ***	−4.51 ***	−2.73 *	−3.01 *	−4.24 ***	−4.25 **	−2.27	−2.49
l-hip - l-thal	0.56	0.8	1.44	1.43	2.54	2.48	1.16	1.7	2.28	2.19
l-sfg - l-mtgant	−2.52	−2.58	−2.59	−2.75 *	−3.41 **	−3.41 **	−4.09 **	−4.13 **	−3.84 **	−3.83 **
l-fmedc - r-front	−3.89 **	−3.39 **	−4.04 **	−3.54 **	−2.15	−1.87	−3.23 *	−3.00 *	−2.09	−1.93
l-cun - l-plan	−2.56	−2.24	−2.13	−1.83	−2.06	−1.51	−3.10 *	−2.62 *	−1.28	−0.64
l-stg - r-cun	−2.61 *	−2.39	−2.34	−2.15	−3.15 *	−2.82 *	−3.40 **	−2.99 *	−2.5	−2.03
l-temp - l-thal	1.02	1.28	1.57	1.8	2.53	2.28	0.85	0.95	2.36	2.16
r-parhipc - r-hip	1.6	1.27	1.58	1.32	3.16 *	2.89 *	1.34	1.09	2.77 *	2.6
l-mtgant - r-sfg	−2	−1.99	−2.1	−2.17	−1.25	−1.23	−3.21 *	−3.10 *	−2.2	−2.15
r-fmedc - r-precun	−3.22 *	−3.05 *	−3.16 *	−3.03 *	−1.49	−1.56	−3.25 *	−3.35 *	−1.26	−1.38
l-fmedc - l-precun	−4.40 ***	−4.17 ***	−4.17 ***	−4.09 **	−2.52	−2.61	−4.37 ***	−4.32 **	−2.16	−2.2
l-fmedc - l-sfg	−3.98 ***	−3.73 **	−3.79 **	−3.54 **	−2.63 *	−2.64 *	−3.87 **	−3.77 **	−2.3	−2.14
l-fmedc - r-precun	−4.17 ***	−3.89 **	−4.02 **	−3.85 **	−2.19	−2.24	−3.91 **	−3.86 **	−2.02	−2.02
l-ins - r-mtgtempoc	−2.52	−2.58	−2.18	−2.56	−3.46 **	−3.86 **	−1.77	−1.64	−3.77 **	−4.33 **
l-fmedc - r-mtgant	−3.31 *	−3.25 *	−3.15 *	−3.27 *	−1.71	−2.05	−3.22 *	−3.49 **	−1.68	−1.77
l-ang - l-mtgant	−2.55	−2.71 *	−2.42	−2.67 *	−2.31	−2.58	−2.78 *	−2.88 *	−2.54	−2.83 *
l-parhipc - r-sfg	−2.19	−1.94	−2.24	−2.02	0.31	0.14	−2.85 *	−2.52	0.11	−0.15
l-fmedc - l-parcing	−4.03 ***	−3.81 **	−3.92 **	−3.77 **	−2.81 *	−2.90 *	−3.66 **	−3.72 **	−2.47	−2.80 *
r-sfg - r-parhipc	−1.93	−2.09	−2.2	−2.39	−0.06	−0.32	−2.80 *	−2.65 *	−0.37	−0.53
l-occfus - l-tfus	−1.66	−1.62	−1.78	−1.8	−1.08	−1.28	−2.13	−2.11	−0.75	−0.94
l-fmedc - l-front	−3.53 **	−2.93 *	−3.37 **	−2.66 *	−1.62	−1.09	−3.01 *	−2.39	−1.69	−1.22
l-temp - r-sfg	−1.84	−1.7	−1.98	−1.92	−0.32	−0.26	−3.57 **	−3.38 **	−1.26	−1.2
r-occfus - r-tfus	−1.97	−2.24	−2.38	−2.67 *	−2.19	−2.54	−3.01 *	−3.14 *	−1.89	−2.19

motion-correction technique successfully reduces motion-related erroneous group differences, artifacts of other physiological and scanner-related sources affect autism-related group comparisons and these phenomenon is handled differently by various signal regression techniques.

Conclusion

In this study, we demonstrated that small movements during scanning can cause different displacements in various locations of the brain, and, accordingly, motion-related BOLD signal changes also depend on location. We characterized the effect of this spatio-temporally complex BOLD artifact pattern on functional connectivity. We proposed RDI, a set of regression covariates for the population-level correction of motion artifacts arising from local head motion. As shown with comparisons of groups with differing average voxel-wise motion pattern, the proposed correction technique efficiently reduces artifacts caused by differences in voxel-wise motion patterns in population-based connectivity analysis; and meanwhile, as demonstrated by comparing autistic and control groups, preserves differences corresponding to neural origin. Our findings suggest that, especially by moderate nuisance correction methods, the inclusion of RDI as second-level nuisance covariates is generally appropriate and may become increasingly necessary when the variable of interest is interrelated with altered subject kinetics.

A limitation of the proposed method is that it cannot be effectively applied in case of individual studies or small sample sizes. Nevertheless, one should note that, in situations where the variable of interest is correlated with motion, second-level regression-based, motion-correction approaches can be conservative, as they remove common variation among regressors. Furthermore, the proposed method is based only on a simplified measure of motion and does not handle rapid sub-TR displacements, which may play an important role in regional motion artifact interactions.

The question of what is the optimal individual-level signal regression technique for motion correction remains open, but, seems less crucial for large-sample, group-level studies using a proper second-level correction method.

This article focused on motion-related artifacts, which are only one, although a conspicuous source, of confounding effects in functional MRI. In-scanner head motion is relatively easy to measure, and thus, corresponding artifacts are actively investigated. However, as suggested by the observed differences among nuisance signal regression techniques, physiological and scanner-related artifacts may also have an essential impact on fc-MRI studies.

Author Contributions

Conceived and designed the experiments: TS ME AJ EB. Analyzed the data: TS AJ CSA. Contributed reagents/materials/analysis tools: GO SK CSA. Wrote the paper: TS AJ ME.

References

1. Kim B, Boes JL, Bland PH, Chenevert TL, Meyer CR (1999) Motion correction in fmri via registration of individual slices into an anatomical volume. Magnetic Resonance in Medicine 41: 964–972.
2. Power JD, Barnes KA, Snyder AZ, Schlaggar BL, Petersen SE (2012) Spurious but systematic correlations in functional connectivity mri networks arise from subject motion. Neuroimage 59: 2142–2154.
3. Satterthwaite TD, Elliott MA, Gerraty RT, Ruparel K, Loughead J, et al. (2013) An improved framework for confound regression and filtering for control of motion artifact in the preprocessing of resting-state functional connectivity data. Neuroimage 64: 240–256.
4. Friston KJ, Holmes AP, Worsley KJ, Poline JP, Frith CD, et al. (1994) Statistical parametric maps in functional imaging: a general linear approach. Human brain mapping 2: 189–210.
5. Fox MD, Zhang D, Snyder AZ, Raichle ME (2009) The global signal and observed anticorrelated resting state brain networks. Journal of neurophysiology 101: 3270–3283.
6. Glover GH, Li TQ, Ress D (2000) Image-based method for retrospective correction of physiological motion effects in fmri: Retroicor. Magnetic Resonance in Medicine 44: 162–167.
7. Behzadi Y, Restom K, Liau J, Liu TT (2007) A component based noise correction method (compcor) for bold and perfusion based fmri. Neuroimage 37: 90–101.
8. Fair DA, Nigg JT, Iyer S, Bathula D, Mills KL, et al. (2012) Distinct neural signatures detected for adhd subtypes after controlling for micro-movements in resting state functional connectivity mri data. Frontiers in systems neuroscience 6: 80.
9. Satterthwaite TD, Wolf DH, Loughead J, Ruparel K, Elliott MA, et al. (2012) Impact of in-scanner head motion on multiple measures of functional connectivity: relevance for studies of neurodevelopment in youth. Neuroimage 60: 623–632.
10. Jakab A, Beres M, Berenyi E, Emri M, Spisak T, et al. (2013) Autistic traits in neurotypical adults: Correlates of graph theoretical functional network topology and white matter anisotropy patterns. PloS one 8: e60982.
11. Friston KJ, Williams S, Howard R, Frackowiak RS, Turner R (1996) Movement-related effects in fmri time-series. Magnetic resonance in medicine 35: 346–355
12. Freire L, Mangin JF (2001) Motion correction algorithms may create spurious brain activations in the absence of subject motion. NeuroImage 14: 709–722.
13. Lemieux L, Salek-Haddadi A, Lund TE, Laufs H, Carmichael D (2007) Modelling large motion events in fmri studies of patients with epilepsy. Magnetic resonance imaging 25: 894–901.
14. Yan CG, Cheung B, Kelly C, Colcombe S, Craddock RC, et al. (2013) A comprehensive assessment of regional variation in the impact of head micromovements on functional connectomics. Neuroimage 76: 183–201.
15. Di Martino A, Yan C, Li Q, Denio E, Castellanos F, et al. (2013) The autism brain imaging data exchange: towards a large-scale evaluation of the intrinsic brain architecture in autism. Molecular psychiatry 19: 659–667.
16. Van Dijk KR, Sabuncu MR, Buckner RL (2012) The influence of head motion on intrinsic functional connectivity mri. Neuroimage 59: 431–438.
17. Jo HJ, Saad ZS, Simmons WK, Milbury LA, Cox RW (2010) Mapping sources of correlation in resting state fmri, with artifact detection and removal. Neuroimage 52: 571–582.
18. Cordes D, Haughton VM, Arfanakis K, Carew JD, Turski PA, et al. (2001) Frequencies contributing to functional connectivity in the cerebral cortex in resting-state data. American Journal of Neuroradiology 22: 1326–1333.
19. Van Someren E, Van Der Werf YD, Roelfsema PR, Mansvelder HD, Lopes da Silva FH (2011) Spectral characteristics of resting state networks. Slow Brain Oscillations of Sleep, Resting State and Vigilance 193: 259.
20. Gotts SJ, Saad ZS, Jo HJ, Wallace GL, Cox RW, et al. (2013) The perils of global signal regression for group comparisons: a case study of autism spectrum disorders. Frontiers in human neuroscience 7: 356.
21. Deen B, Pelphrey K (2012) Perspective: brain scans need a rethink. Nature 491: S20–S20.
22. Saad ZS, Gotts SJ, Murphy K, Chen G, Jo HJ, et al. (2012) Trouble at rest: how correlation patterns and group differences become distorted after global signal regression. Brain connectivity 2: 25–32.
23. Imperati D, Colcombe S, Kelly C, Di Martino A, Zhou J, et al. (2011) Differential development of human brain white matter tracts. PloS one 6: e23437.
24. Koyama MS, Di Martino A, Zuo XN, Kelly C, Mennes M, et al. (2011) Resting-state functional connectivity indexes reading competence in children and adults. The Journal of Neuroscience 31: 8617–8624.
25. Jenkinson M, Beckmann CF, Behrens TE, Woolrich MW, Smith SM (2012) Fsl. NeuroImage 62: 782–790.
26. Jenkinson M, Bannister P, Brady M, Smith S (2002) Improved optimization for the robust and accurate linear registration and motion correction of brain images. Neuroimage 17: 825–841.
27. Smith SM (2002) Fast robust automated brain extraction. Human brain mapping 17: 143–155.
28. Jenkinson M, Smith S (2001) A global optimisation method for robust affine registration of brain images. Medical image analysis 5: 143–156.
29. Spisák T, Opposits G, Kis SA, Clemens B, Emri M (2012) Braincon: Software tool for graph theory based multimodal brain connectivity analysis and visualization. Magn Reson Mat Phys Biol Med 25: 616.
30. Desikan RS, Ségonne F, Fischl B, Quinn BT, Dickerson BC, et al. (2006) An automated labeling system for subdividing the human cerebral cortex on mri scans into gyral based regions of interest. Neuroimage 31: 968–980.

31. Smyser CD, Inder TE, Shimony JS, Hill JE, Degnan AJ, et al. (2010) Longitudinal analysis of neural network development in preterm infants. Cerebral Cortex 20: 2852–2862.
32. Dobson AJ (2010) An introduction to generalized linear models. CRC press.
33. Ginestet CE, Simmons A (2011) Statistical parametric network analysis of functional connectivity dynamics during a working memory task. Neuroimage 55: 688–704.
34. Stine RA (1995) Graphical interpretation of variance inflation factors. The American Statistician 49: 53–56.
35. R Core Team (2013) R: A Language and Environment for Statistical Computing. R Foundation for Statistical Computing, Vienna, Austria. URL http://www.R-project.org/. R package version 3.1.0.
36. Venables WN, Ripley BD, Venables W (1994) Modern applied statistics with S-PLUS, volume 250. Springer-verlag New York.
37. Klaus B, Strimmer K (2013) fdrtool: Estimation of (Local) False Discovery Rates and Higher Criticism. URL http://CRAN.R-project.org/package=fdrtool. R package version 3.1.0.
38. Strimmer K (2008) fdrtool: a versatile r package for estimating local and tail area-based false discovery rates. Bioinformatics 24: 1461–1462.
39. Heiberger RM, Holland B (2004) Statistical Analysis and Data Display: An Intermediate Course with Examples in S-Plus, R, and SAS. Springer-Verlag, New York, first edition. URL http://springeronline.com/0-387-40270-5.
40. Breheny P, Burchett W (2012) Visualization of Regression Models Using visreg. URL http://myweb.uiowa.edu/pbreheny/publications/visreg.pdf. R package version 3.1.0.
41. Power JD, Barnes KA, Snyder AZ, Schlaggar BL, Petersen SE (2012) Steps toward optimizing motion artifact removal in functional connectivity mri; a reply to carp. Neuroimage 76: 439441.
42. Zotev V, Yuan H, Phillips R, Bodurka J (2012) Eeg-assisted retrospective motion correction for fmri: E-remcor. NeuroImage 63: 698–712.
43. Allison PD (1977) Testing for interaction in multiple regression. American Journal of Sociology 83: 144.
44. Belmonte MK, Allen G, Beckel-Mitchener A, Boulanger LM, Carper RA, et al. (2004) Autism and abnormal development of brain connectivity. The Journal of Neuroscience 24: 9228–9231.
45. Yan CG, Craddock RC, He Y, Milham MP (2013) Addressing head motion dependencies for small-world topologies in functional connectomics. Frontiers in human neuroscience 7: 910.
46. Courchesne E, Pierce K (2005) Why the frontal cortex in autism might be talking only to itself: local over-connectivity but long-distance disconnection. Current opinion in neurobiology 15: 225–230.
47. Jo HJ, Gotts SJ, Reynolds RC, Bandettini PA, Martin A, et al. (2013) Effective preprocessing procedures virtually eliminate distance-dependent motion artifacts in resting state fmri. Journal of applied mathematics 2013: 9.
48. Müller RA, Shih P, Keehn B, Deyoe JR, Leyden KM, et al. (2011) Underconnected, but how? a survey of functional connectivity mri studies in autism spectrum disorders. Cerebral Cortex 21: 2233–2243.
49. Murphy K, Birn RM, Handwerker DA, Jones TB, Bandettini PA (2009) The impact of global signal regression on resting state correlations: are anti-correlated networks introduced? Neuroimage 44: 893–905.

22

Individuals with Autism Spectrum Disorders Do Not Use Social Stereotypes in Irony Comprehension

Tiziana Zalla[1]*, Frederique Amsellem[2], Pauline Chaste[2], Francesca Ervas[1], Marion Leboyer[2], Maud Champagne-Lavau[3]

1 Institut Jean Nicod, CNRS, UMR 8129, Institut d'Etude de la Cognition, Ecole Normale Supérieure, Paris, France, **2** INSERM U 955, IMRB & University Paris Est Creteil, AP-HP, Henri Mondor-Albert Chenevier Hospitals, Department of Psychiatry, Fondation FondaMental, French National Science Foundation, Creteil, France, **3** Aix-Marseille University, CNRS, LPL UMR 7309, 13100 Aix-en-Provence, France

Abstract

Social and communication impairments are part of the essential diagnostic criteria used to define Autism Spectrum Disorders (ASDs). Difficulties in appreciating non-literal speech, such as irony in ASDs have been explained as due to impairments in social understanding and in recognizing the speaker's communicative intention. It has been shown that social-interactional factors, such as a listener's beliefs about the speaker's attitudinal propensities (e.g., a tendency to use sarcasm, to be mocking, less sincere and more prone to criticism), as conveyed by an occupational stereotype, do influence a listener's interpretation of potentially ironic remarks. We investigate the effect of occupational stereotype on irony detection in adults with High Functioning Autism or Asperger Syndrome (HFA/AS) and a comparison group of typically developed adults. We used a series of verbally presented stories containing ironic or literal utterances produced by a speaker having either a "sarcastic" or a "non-sarcastic" occupation. Although individuals with HFA/AS were able to recognize ironic intent and occupational stereotypes when the latter are made salient, stereotype information enhanced irony detection and modulated its social meaning (i.e., mockery and politeness) only in comparison participants. We concluded that when stereotype knowledge is not made salient, it does not automatically affect pragmatic communicative processes in individuals with HFA/AS.

Editor: Marco Iacoboni, UCLA, United States of America

Funding: This research was supported by Fondation FondaMental and Fondation Orange to TZ and ML, and by a "Ville de Paris" research grant to FE, and by a Fonds de la Recherche en Santé du Québec grant and the Agence Nationale de la Recherche grant (ANR-11-BSH2-006-01) to MC-L. The funders had no role in study design, data collection and analysis, decision to publish, or preparation of the manuscript.

* E-mail: tiziana.zalla@ens.fr

Introduction

Social and communication impairments are part of the essential diagnostic criteria used to define Autism Spectrum Disorders (ASDs) [1,2]. These impairments are often related to a serious deficit in the capacity for mentalizing [3], the natural tendency to explain everyday actions in terms of mental states. High Functioning Autism (HFA) and Asperger Syndrome (AS) are widely acknowledged to be variants on this spectrum [1,2]. While HFA commonly refers to individuals with a history of speech and language delay, individuals with AS show no evidence of delayed language function. Moreover, differently from individuals with low-functioning autism, adults with HFA and AS (HFA/AS) do pass first- and second-order Theory-of-Mind or mindreading (i.e., the ability to attribute mental states to oneself and to others; ToM) tests [4–5], but they may fail in more 'advanced' ToM tasks, based on the detection of sarcasm, irony or bluff [6] or the recognition of Faux Pas [7,8].

Using a computer-mediated communication program, Rajendran, Mitchell and Rickards [9] examined non-literal language comprehension in children and adolescents with HFA/AS and found that they were able to make appropriate responses in a verbal irony comprehension task. More recently, using a computer-mediated communication procedure, Glenwright and Agbayewa [10] confirmed that when verbal and social demands are minimized, children with HFA/AS are able to perform as well as control participants on measures of verbal irony comprehension, such as judging the speaker's intentions and irony's social function of conveying humour.

However, Jolliffe and Baron-Cohen [11] reported that although adults with HFA are able to grasp the speaker's ironic intent (i.e., that the speaker meant something other than the literal meaning), they may encounter difficulties processing mental state information and are less able than control subjects to use contextual information to justify the speaker's utterance. Along the same lines, in a neuroimaging study, Wang and collaborators [12] found good accuracy at irony detection along with a different pattern of neural activity in children with HFA, as compared to the typically developed group, when trying to incorporate contextual information in order to make inferences about speaker ironic intent. Specifically, the authors interpreted the significantly greater activity observed in the right inferior frontal gyrus and in the temporal regions bilaterally as reflecting different strategies for irony comprehension and greater cognitive demands in children with HFA.

It has been shown that irony comprehension requires the acquisition of the shared knowledge and communicative strategies adopted by a social community [13]. Irony is regarded as a more polite, and indirect, way of expressing a speaker's criticisms [14–16]. In the case of an ironic insult, the most widespread form of sarcasm, the speaker's attitude is regarded as being more *positive* than it is for its literal counterpart [17]. Such positiveness, known as the "Tinge Effect" [17,18] would be induced by the obligatory processing of the literal (positive) interpretation of ironic statements in negative situations, which would attenuate the negativity expressed by these statements, when ironically interpreted.

Various sources of information might influence the modulation of the overall meaning of the ironic comment. Irony understanding depends in part on the strength of the social cues contextually available for inferring the speaker's intent. According to Colston [19], the degree of negativity expressed by an ironic comment would depend on how critical the situational context perceived by the listener is, relative to the positiveness of the comment, ironically intended by the speaker. Hence, as proposed by Fussell and Kreuz [20], both psycholinguistic processes (e.g., lexical retrieval, syntactic processing) and social-interactional factors affect irony interpretation. Stereotypes are energy-saving devices associated with an automatic, unintentional, and unconscious process [21]; they guide expectations, inferences, and impressions, and shape interpretations and memory retrieval [22].

Remarkably, Pexman and Olineck [23] showed that speaker characteristics conveyed by an occupation stereotype are integrated in the linguistic comprehension process and may cue ironic intent when other contextual cues are minimal. For example, the effect of occupation stereotype information on irony comprehension has been explained by what people imagined about target individuals [24]. Specifically, an occupation stereotype affects irony comprehension if that occupation is strongly consistent with speaker behaviour. Similarly, it has been shown that people recall information better and more readily when it is consistent with a preexisting stereotype than when it is inconsistent [25]. Speakers' propensities to be humorous, mocking, less sincere and more prone to criticism act as salient cues for ironic intent. Thus, such speaker characteristics facilitate irony detection by indicating that the speaker is likely to have a negative attitude and that such an attitude would be indirectly expressed through humour and insincerity. Conversely, if the speaker's occupational stereotype is consistent with sincerity and seriousness, the listener might be less likely to detect the speaker's ironic intent [26–28]. All these features contribute to setting up a specific "ironic context" and enhance the speaker's ironic attitude [29].

A speaker's social stereotype (e.g., occupation, gender and ethnic group) also influences memory for and interpretation of potentially ironic remarks at a very early stage in the process of sarcasm and irony comprehension [23,30]. Using online reading tasks, Pexman, Ferretti and Katz [28] reported that when speaker occupation was mentioned, reading times were longer at the statement's end indicating that speaker occupation knowledge is integrated with lexical and syntactic information relatively early, even in the absence of an explicit decision about speaker intent. By using a series of puppet show scenarios, Pexman and collaborators [13] reported that children with HFA exhibited spared competence for irony comprehension, though group differences in processing strategies, in terms of gaze behavior and response latencies, likely reflected a less elaborate understanding of others' communicative intents. Notably, they failed to detect the intended humor conveyed by ironic criticisms and failed to appreciate the broader social function of irony, such as the speaker's intent to be simultaneously critical and humorous.

Recently, Hirschfeld and collaborators [31] have showed that ToM abilities are not crucial for acquiring social stereotypes, but they might be used to overcome them. Individuals with ASDs who have diminished mindreading capacities might find it easier to understand others as group members using stable character traits rather than explaining human behaviour by processing the large variety of detailed information available during on-line social interaction. Indeed, according to White and collaborators [32], the propensity to make judgments based on race and gender stereotypes in adults with AS is similar to that for typically developed populations, suggesting that the use and acquisition of stereotype knowledge can proceed along with diminished social engagement and ToM abilities. However, while this study provides evidence about the ability to use stereotypic knowledge in explicit tasks, it does not tell us to what extent this knowledge is spontaneously used in everyday communication.

Rumsey and Hamburger [33] proposed that a core deficit of autism consists in a broad class of verbal and nonverbal conceptual reasoning disabilities. In the same line, Minshew and Goldstein [34] put forward a multiple primary cognitive deficit model that described the cognitive profile of individuals with autism spectrum disorder as a disorder of complex information processing across cognitive domains. Complexity is defined in terms of the number of elements contained in the stimulus material as well as the multiplicity of cognitive processes involved in task performance. Within a cognitive theory, complex information processing requires the integration of multiple features and the reliance on different component processes. Across domains, complex information processing theory provided an explanation for the particular constellation of deficits that define ASDs, including impairments in concept formation, complex memory, complex language, and skilled motor abilities. The consequences of impaired complex information processing in ASDs would be also manifested in real-world situations, as this population will experience difficulty in fast dynamic social interactions because of their inability to quickly process relevant information on line.

In the present study, we aimed to investigate whether, as has previously been shown for typically developed subjects [23], social stereotype information can be used to enhance irony detection in individuals with HFA and AS. Given their difficulties in using context information and integrating them during communication and on-line comprehension processing one might expect that stereotype information would not enhance the propensity in individuals with ASDs to interpret an utterance as ironic in those circumstances in which the stereotype would favour an ironic interpretation (i.e. a sarcastic occupation). To investigate whether individuals with HFA or AS can use and integrate occupational stereotype knowledge in an irony comprehension task, we used a series of verbally presented stories containing either a sarcastic-ironic or literal statement uttered by a speaker characterised as having a "sarcastic" (i.e., perceived as more prone to use sarcasm) or "non-sarcastic" occupation. As already reported [26], people perceive speakers with certain occupations as being more likely to use irony than speakers with other occupations.

Given that the ability to process and integrate different types of information on-line rapidly and efficiently might be impaired in this population, one could also expect a reduced effect of stereotype knowledge on pragmatic processes underlying irony comprehension. Verbal irony can serve many social functions: Speakers can temper the aggression conveyed by criticism, or praise conveyed by a compliment (the Tinge Hypothesis) [35], while bringing humour to a situation. A full understanding of ironic language requires one to make complex inferences about speaker intent, a task that can be challenging for individuals with ASDs who might have difficulties with mentalizing in social contexts or with the interpretation of ambiguous stimuli. According to Pexman and Olineck [18], the degree of perceived irony would be a way to assess listeners' ToM abilities while the degree of perceived politeness would be a way to assess their social competence more broadly. In the present study, we also assessed whether occupational stereotype would influence recognition and apprehension of the communicative (i.e., mocking) and social features of irony (i.e., politeness). It is possible that they would fail to fully appreciate the social function of irony, such as its mocking and positive dimensions, indicating difficulties with pragmatic processing. Such subtle differences in pragmatic understanding may underlie some of the social difficulties faced by individuals with ASDs.

Materials and Methods

Participants

Seventeen adults with a clinical diagnosis of High Functioning Autism (HFA) (N = 6) or Asperger Syndrome (AS) (N = 11) according to DSM-IV R (American Psychiatric Association, 2000) and ASDI (Asperger Syndrome Diagnostic Interview) [36], were recruited from Albert Chenevier Hospital in Créteil (Table 1). The inclusion and exclusion criteria for the clinical group were based on retrospective parental information about the early language development of their child. All diagnoses were made by experienced clinicians and were based on clinical observations of the participants. Interviews with parents or caregivers using the ADOS (The autism diagnostic observation schedule-generic) [37] and the ADI-R (Autism Diagnostic Interview) [38] confirmed the diagnoses. The cut-off points for the three classes of behaviour for the ADI are a score of 10 for reciprocal social interaction [B], 8 for communication [C], and 3 for stereotyped behaviours [D], respectively. All participants scored above the cut-off points.

Seventeen typically developed comparison participants (CP) volunteered to match the clinical group with respect to age, IQ and gender (Table 1). Prior to their recruitment, the comparison participants were screened to exclude any with a history of psychiatric or neurological disorders. All participants were native French speakers, and had normal/corrected to normal vision. All participants received basic neuropsychological screening, which included Verbal and Performance IQs (WAIS-III) [39]. All participants had an IQ above 70. Overall, individuals with HFA/AS did not differ from the comparison participants on gender, chronological age (t-test: $t(32) = 1.14$, $p = 0.26$), education (t-test: $t(32) = 0.17$, $p = 0.87$), Full-scale ($t(32) = 0.43$, $p = 0.7$), verbal ($t(32) = -0.12$, $p = 0.90$) and Performance ($t(32) = 1.1$, $p = 0.31$) (Table 1).

The present research has been approved by the local Ethical committee (Inserm, Institut Thématique Santé Publique; C07-33). All participants signed informed consent agreements before volunteering for this study, and all investigation complied with APA ethical standards.

Procedure

Before running the main experiment, a pilot study was conducted on a preliminary set of 45 occupations. Forty French native speakers were required to rate the probability that a person with a given occupation would make an ironic utterance using a 1 (low probability) to 7 (high probability) rating scale. All of these participants were chosen from the general population (mean age: 29, SD 4.2) and did not participate in the experiment. The following seven occupations were judged to have the highest probability of ironic remarks (sarcastic occupations): *comedian*, *talk show host*, *actress*, *artist*, *mechanic*, *plumber* and *insurance agent*. The following seven occupations were judged to have the lowest probability of ironic remarks ("non-sarcastic occupations"): *accountant*, *clergyman*, *scientist*, *librarian*, *waiter*, *bank teller* and *veterinarian*.

Participants in the experiment were individually tested in a quiet room at the Albert Chenevier Hospital in Créteil. In line with Pexman and Olineck' study [23], twenty-one pairs of stories, containing either an ironic or a literal utterance were visually presented on a computer screen with no time limit. Each statement (ironic or literal) was uttered by a speaker having either a sarcastic occupation or a non-sarcastic occupation within seven stories (see Table 2 for examples). A no occupation condition, in which the speakers were only identified by surname, was included to rule out the possibility that participants would adopt a response strategy of predicting job information for each story. Testing time varied from approximately 45 to 60 minutes. The test consisted of two separate sessions with a short interval in between (15 to 20 min). Additional breaks or refreshments were given when requested. Stories having the same context and the same speaker uttering an ironic or a literal statement were presented in different sessions. Within each session, stories were presented in randomized order to avoid order effect, and session presentation was counterbalanced across subjects. Stories were visually presented on a computer screen and were available throughout the experiment.

Table 1. Means (and standard deviations) of demographic and clinical data for participants with HFA/AS and the comparison participants.

	HFA/AS	Comparison
N (male:female ratio)	14:3	12:5
Age in years (mean, SD, range)	27.3 (7.3); 18–40	30.1 (9.7); 20–47
Education in years (mean, SD)	13.4 (3.8); 8–18	13.5 (2); 10–18
ADI [B,C,D]*	18.6 (6.8); 11.6 (6.6); 6.9 (3.2)	–
Full-scale IQ	93.7 (21.1); 70–137	96.2 (10.9); 80–116
Verbal IQ	99.3 (20.1); 70–143	98.7 (9.9); 85–123
Performance IQ	90.7 (18.4); 70–122	95.9 (10.3); 80–118

* [B] = reciprocal social interaction, [C] = communication, [D] = stereotyped behaviours.

Table 2. Examples of story types.

Stories	Context	Literal statement	Ironic statement
1. Stories with speakers having a sarcastic occupation	*Marie-Eve told his friend, an actor (sarcastic occupation), that she could memorize a poem of 20 lines in 5 minutes. Marie-Eve recited only half a poem and forgot the rest.* ***The day after, the actor says to Guillaume:***	*Marie-Ève has a mediocre memory.*	*Marie-Ève has a phenomenal memory.*
2. Stories with speakers having a non-sarcastic occupation	*A veterinarian (non-sarcastic job) sees Joannie arriving at work on Monday morning. Joannie seems to be a little bit more tired than usual.* ***At midday, the actor says to Pierre:***	*Joannie does not look well.*	*Joannie looks well.*
3. Control stories with speakers with no occupation	*Louise (no job) has moved house today and Michel has told her that he will come to help her all day. Michel comes to help Louise but just for a few minutes.* ***The following day, Louise says to Amélie:***	*Michel is uncooperative.*	*Michel is helpful.*

Participants were asked to read each story attentively before answering questions. There was no time limit.

The experimenter introduced the experiment as follows: 'Here, on this computer screen, you will be presented with a series of stories describing social situations with one person, the speaker, expressing a judgment about another person. You are to read each story presented on this computer screen for as long as you wish. When you are finished reading the whole story, you will be asked to answer some questions. If you think that everything is clear and feel ready to start, you should press the space bar on the computer keyboard". Participants were invited to ask clarification questions; if needed, the experimenter could also read the stories. The experimenter sat close to the subject. The computer screen was placed in front of the participant and each story remained available throughout the reading and questioning. A training session of five trials preceded the experiment, and allowed participants to familiarise themselves with the task and with the response measures. Specifically, participants were required to use the rating scales and ask for clarifications. The following definition of irony was given: *Verbal irony is a statement in which what the speaker means is different from what he/she ostensibly states.* The experimenter also provided a few examples of verbal irony (e.g. "The speaker says "It's a lovely day," in a downpour of rain). Consistency between responses to the first question ("Speaker Intent Question") and irony rating was also used to ensure that participants fully understood how to use the scales and the notion of "irony".

The first question, the "Speaker Intent Question" ("*What does the speaker actually mean?*") allowed us to assessed accuracy at irony detection, that is the ability to understand whether the last remark in the story had been intended as ironic or literal, by a forced choice question ("*Does he mean that Marie-Ève has a good memory?*" or "*Does he mean that Marie-Ève does not have a good memory?*").

Then, using four 7-point rating scales, participants had to judge whether the speaker was *ironic* (ranging from 1 = not at all ironic to 7 = extremely ironic), *mocking* (1 = not at all mocking and 7 = extremely mocking), and *polite* (1 = not at all polite and 7 = extremely polite). The last question, a control question, was specific to each story and allowed us to verify that participants had not gotten confused or forgotten important details of the story.

The story was placed in front of the participant and remained there throughout the reading and questioning so that participants did not have to remember it. This was done in order to minimize memory and attention requirements.

Data Collection and Analyses

Conformity to the assumptions of parametric statistics was assessed using the Komolgorov-Smirnov Normality test (χ^2(2, N = 39) = 1.42, p = 0.98), to check that the data came from normally distributed samples and the F-test was used for equality of variances (F(21,16) = 0.49, p = 0.14).

The data were analysed using repeated-measures ANOVAs with factors Groups (2: CPs, HFA/AS) X Statement (2: ironic, literal) X Speaker's occupation (2: non-sarcastic, sarcastic). Scheffe's tests were used for post-hoc analysis. Pearson product-moment correlation coefficients were calculated across all participants between clinical measures and test results. Measures of effect size were calculated for each effect of interest by providing the Partial Eta-squared for ANOVAs and Cohen's **d** for t-test. The level of significance was at <0.05.

Results

Speaker Intent

A forced choice question assessed whether participants correctly recognized that speakers made literal or ironic compliments within a given context. Overall, 80% of CP and 72.5% of HFA/AS correctly recognized the speaker's communicative intent, that is whether the utterance was to be interpreted as ironic or literal.

Repeated-measures ANOVA yielded a marginally significant main effect of Group (F(1,32) = 2.9; p = 0.09, $\eta_p^2 = 0.09$) and significant main effects of Statement (F(1,32) = 34.4; p<0.0001, $\eta_p^2 = 0.51$) and Occupation (F(1,32) = 22.6; $p<0.0001$, $\eta_p^2 = 0.41$). The effect of Statement was due to both groups performing significantly better in the literal condition than in the ironic one (mean difference = −1.7; $p<0.0001$), while the Occupation effect was due to the greater number of correct responses on the speakers' sarcastic occupation condition, as compared to the speaker's non sarcastic occupation condition (mean difference = −0.75; $p<0.0001$). These effects were qualified by a significant Statement X Occupation interaction ($F(1,32) = 10.9$; $p = 0.002$, $\eta_p^2 = 0.25$), and a significant Statement X Occupation X Group interaction ($F(3,96) = 6.6$; $p = 0.01$, $\eta_p^2 = 0.17$). The significant Statement X Occupation interaction was due to the greater number of correct responses for the sarcastic occupation as compared to the non-sarcastic occupation in the ironic statement condition (mean difference = −1.14; $p = 0.006$), while this difference was not significant in the literal condition (mean difference = −0.35; $p = 0.17$). The Statement X Occupation X Group interaction further revealed that this difference was significant only for the CPs ($p = 0.001$) and not for the group with HFA/AS

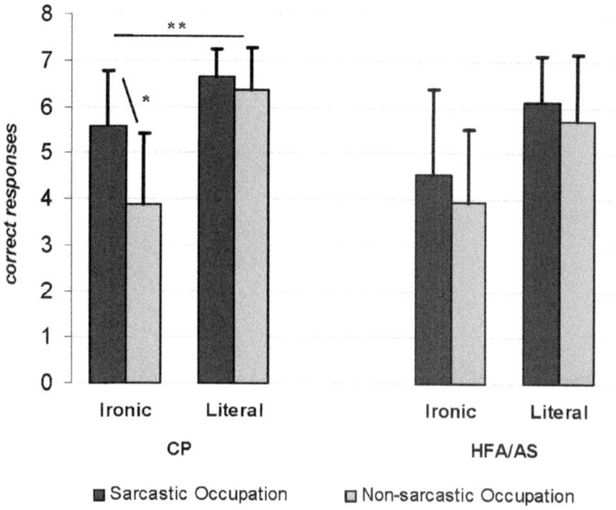

Figure 1. Number of correct responses produced by the two participant groups as a function of the statement (Ironic and Literal) and of the speaker (Sarcastic and Non-sarcastic). Error bars are standard deviations. * p<.0005; ** p<.0001.

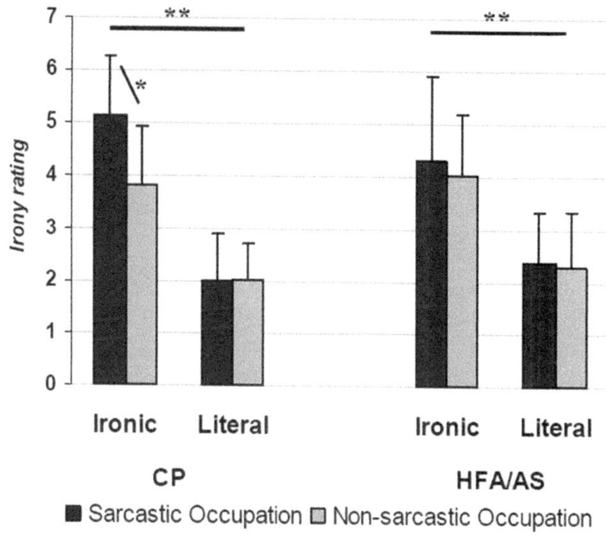

Figure 2. Irony ratings (1 = not at all ironic and 7 = extremely ironic) of the speaker statement by the two participant groups as a function of the statement (Ironic and Literal) and of the occupation (Sarcastic and Non-sarcastic). Error bars are standard deviations. * = p<.05; ** = p<.0001.

($p = 0.37$) (Figure 1). The Occupation X Group ($F(1,32) = 2.5$; $p = 0.12$, $\eta_p^2 = 0.07$) and the Statement X Group ($F(1,32) = 0.02$; $p = 0.88$, $\eta_p^2 = 0.0007$) interactions were not significant.

Irony Rating

Irony ratings were analyzed only for those trials on which participants correctly responded to the speaker's intended meaning. For ratings of the extent to which a speaker was being ironic, there were highly significant main effects of Statement ($F(1,32) = 87.7$; $p < 0.0001$, $\eta_p^2 = 0.72$) and Occupation ($F(1,32) = 13.5$; $p = 0.0009$, $\eta_p^2 = 0.30$), as well as a significant Statement X Occupation interaction ($F(1,32) = 8.2$; $p = 0.007$, $\eta_p^2 = 0.20$), a group X occupation interaction ($F(2,64) = 4.2$; $p = 0.047$, $\eta_p^2 = 0.11$) and a significant Statement X Occupation X Group interaction ($F(3,96) = 5.0$; $p = 0.032$, $\eta_p^2 = 0.13$). The main effect of Group ($F(1,32) = 0.3$; $p = 0.56$, $\eta_p^2 =$) and the Statement X Group interaction ($F(1,32) = 1.6$; $p = 0.21$, $\eta_p^2 = 0.04$) were not significant.

For both groups, irony ratings were higher when the statements were ironic as compared to literal (mean difference = 2.1; $p <$ 0.0001), while the Occupation effect was due to the higher irony ratings when the speakers had a sarcastic occupation as compared to speakers with non-sarcastic occupations (mean difference = − 0.42; $p = 0.0009$). As revealed by the significant Statement X Occupation interaction, this difference was only significant in the ironic statement condition ($p = 0.01$) and not in the literal one ($p = 0.89$). Moreover, the Statement X Occupation X Group interaction effect revealed that, in the irony statement condition, the irony ratings were higher for speakers with sarcastic occupations than for speakers with non-sarcastic occupations only for the CPs ($p = 0.001$), while the difference was not significant for the HFA/ASs ($p = 0.54$). Mean rating of ironic utterances pronounced by sarcastic speakers was higher for CPs than for participants with HFA/AS ($p = 0.05$) (Figure 2).

Mockery Rating

Mockery ratings were analyzed only for those trials on which participants correctly responded to the speaker's intended meaning. Repeated-measures ANOVA yielded a main effect of Statement ($F(1,32) = 36.2$; $p < 0.0001$, $\eta_p^2 = 0.55$) and Occupation ($F(1,32) = 14.5$; $p = 0.0006$, $\eta_p^2 = 0.34$), as well as significant interaction effects of Statement X Occupation ($F(1,1) = 8.7$; $p = 0.006$, $\eta_p^2 = 0.17$) and Occupation X Group ($F(2,64) = 5$; $p = 0.03$, $\eta_p^2 = 0.12$). The group difference was not significant ($F(1,32) = 1.5$; $p = 0.22$, $\eta_p^2 = 0.07$), nor were the Statement X Group ($F(1,32) = 2.6$; $p = 0.12$, $\eta_p^2 = 0.07$), and Statement X Occupation X Group ($F(3,96) = 1.3$; $p = 0.27$, $\eta_p^2 = 0.03$) interactions significant.

Ironic statements were rated as more mocking than the literal statements (mean difference = 1.3; $p < 0.0001$) and the statements uttered by the speakers with a sarcastic occupation were rated as more mocking than the statements uttered by speakers with a non-sarcastic occupation (mean difference = −0.41; $p = 0.0006$), However, as revealed by the Statement X Occupation and the Occupation X Group interactions, the difference between the mocking ratings produced by the two types of speakers was significant only for the ironic statement condition ($p = 0.004$), and for the comparison group ($p = 0.02$), but not for the HFA/AS group ($p = 0.28$). Mean rating of mockery for utterances pronounced by sarcastic speakers was significantly higher for CPs than for participants with HFA/AS ($p = 0.01$) (Figure 3).

Politeness Rating

Politeness ratings were analyzed only for those trials on which participants correctly responded to the speaker's intended meaning. Repeated-measures ANOVA yielded significant main effects of Statement ($F(1,32) - 70.9$; $p < 0.0001$, $\eta_p^2 = 0.56$) and Occupation ($F(1,32) = 25.7$; $p < 0.0001$, $\eta_p^2 = 0.34$), as well as a significant Occupation X Group interaction ($F(2,64) = 18.1$; $p = 0.0002$, $\eta_p^2 = 0.34$) and a Statement X Occupation X Group interaction ($F(3,96) = 4.5$; $p = 0.04$, $\eta_p^2 = 0.17$). No significant main effect of Group ($F(1,32) = 0.4$; $p = 0.50$, $\eta_p^2 = 0.02$) was found. Neither Statement X Occupation ($F(1,32) = 0.6$; $p = 0.4$, $\eta^2 = 0.02$) nor Statement X Group ($F(2,64) = 0.001$; $p = 0.97$, $\eta_p^2 = 0.0007$) interactions were significant.

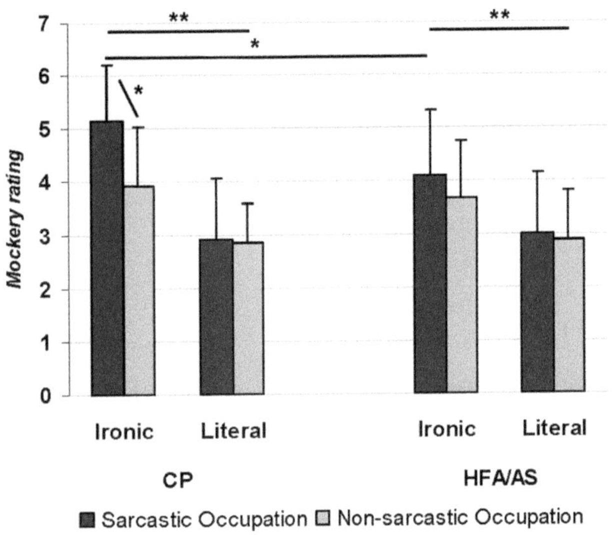

Figure 3. Mockery ratings (1 = not at all mocking and 7 = extremely mocking) of the speaker statement by the two participant groups as a function of the statement (Ironic and Literal) and of the occupation (Sarcastic and Non-sarcastic). Error bars are standard deviations. * = p<.05; ** = p<.0001.

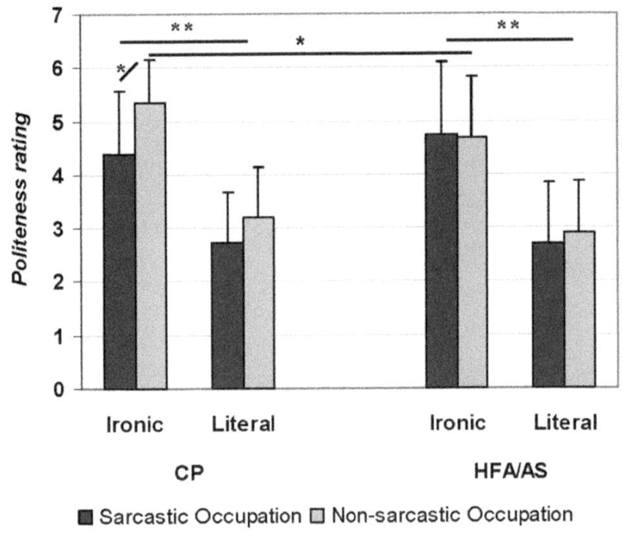

Figure 4. Politeness ratings (1 = not at all polite and 7 = extremely polite) of the speaker statement by the two participant groups as a function of the statement (Ironic and Literal) and of the occupation (Sarcastic and Non-sarcastic). Error bars are standard deviations. * = p<.05; ** = p<.0001.

The effect of Statement was due to the ironic statements being rated as more polite than the literal statements (mean difference = 1.9; $p<0.0001$), while the Occupation effect was due to the statements uttered by the speakers with non-sarcastic occupation being rated as more polite than the ones uttered by the speakers with sarcastic occupation (mean difference = 0.3; $p<0.0001$). Post-hoc Scheffe's tests revealed that this difference was significant only for the CPs ($p = 0.02$), while participants with HFA/AS rated ironic statements pronounced by the two types of speaker as equally polite ($p = 0.86$). Mean rating of politeness for ironic utterances pronounced by non-sarcastic speakers was significantly higher for CPs than for participants with HFA/AS ($p = 0.05$) while there was no significant group difference in the other conditions (Figure 4).

Control Questions

No group difference was found on the number of correct responses for the control questions on the two pairs of twenty-one stories ($t(1,30) = 0.7$, $p = 0.47$; Cohen's $d = -0.30$). Both participants with HFA/AS (mean = 41.5±0.8; range = 40–42) and comparison participants (mean = 41.7±0.5; range = 41–42) responded equally to the control questions. Overall, participants correctly understood the stories. The few errors committed concerned irrelevant details that did not crucially affect task performance (e.g., "*Samuel arrived two hours late at the meeting*" instead of "*Samuel arrived one hour late at the meeting*" or *"The first course was too salty" instead of "The main course was too salty"*).

Occupation Stereotype Judgment

To assess whether, like the comparison group, participants with HFA/AS possess acquired occupation stereotype knowledge or whether they are unable to use it in the context of irony understanding, in a subsequent session we asked participants with HFA/AS to rate the probability that persons with the occupations used in the experimental task would make a sarcastic utterance, a criticism, a mocking, or a polite remark by using a 1 (low probability) to 7 (high probability) rating scale. The sarcastic occupations (i.e., *comedian, talk show host, actress, artist, mechanic, plumber* and *insurance agent)* were judged as having a higher probability of sarcasm (mean rating = 4.2, ±0.2; $t(16) = 7.7$; $p< 0.0001$; Cohen's $d = 3.1$), criticism (mean rating = 4.4, ±0.8; $t(13) = 5.7$; $p<0.0001$; Cohen's $d = 1.8$), mocking (mean rating = 4.4, ±0.9; $t(13) = 8.4$; $p<0.0001$; Cohen's $d = 1.5$) and less polite (mean rating = 5.3±0.8; $t(13) = -4.6$; $p = 0.0004$; Cohen's $d = -1.2$) remarks than the non-sarcastic occupations (i.e., *accountant, clergyman, scientist, librarian, waiter, bank teller* and *veterinarian)* (Mean rating for sarcastic = 2.4, ±0.8; criticisms = 2.87, ±0.9; mocking = 2.6, ±1.4 and less polite = 6.1±0.5) remarks. The evaluation of each occupational category for irony propensity did not differ from that provided by a group of 17 age and gender matched subjects participating to the pilot study for both the sarcastic (mean rating = 4.4±0.6; $t(32) = 0.8$; $p = 0.41$ Cohen's $d = 0.4$) and non-sarcastic ones (mean rating = 2.5±0.4; $t(32) = 0.4$; $p = 0.7$; Cohen's $d = 0.1$).

Discussion

The present study aimed to investigate irony comprehension and understanding of social occupational roles in individuals with HFA/AS, and whether these two sources of knowledge would be processed in an integrated manner in communicative tasks. The results showed that participants with HFA/AS exhibited no difficulties understanding irony (i.e., utterances having a meaning that is the opposite of the literal meaning), confirming relatively preserved abilities to perform pragmatic reasoning tasks [10,40,41]. In fact, HFA/AS and comparison groups recognized a comparable number of ironic utterances and, accordingly, for both groups, the level of irony assigned to the ironic utterances was higher compared to the literal ones. Overall, participants performed significantly better in the literal condition than in the ironic one, confirming the claim that irony is more difficult to understand than literal language and makes greater cognitive demands [42,43].

Verbal irony plays an important role not only in conveying attitudes, but also as a reminder of moral, social and aesthetic norms tacitly shared by a culturally-defined social group [14, 35]. Importantly, a full understanding of irony requires some appreciation of why the speaker has chosen this communicative strategy to express her thought. Irony is generally perceived as a less negative, more humorous and polite manner of expressing criticism than its literal paraphrases [23,26,27,29,35]. According to the echoic account [44,45], the point of irony is not to commit the speaker to the truth of the proposition expressed by the statement, but rather to express a certain type of derisory or dissociative attitude to a tacitly attributed thought. In other words, the speaker in irony mode is *echoing* a thought she attributes to someone else, while she conveys her mocking, sceptical or contemptuous attitude to that thought. Processing such a *tacit* dissociative attitude requires metarepresentational and social abilities that, according to the present findings, appear to be preserved in our group of adults with HFA or AS.

In a recent study, Pexman and collaborators [13] showed unimpaired irony comprehension, but difficulties with the appreciation of the intended humor conveyed by ironic criticisms in children with HFA. These results are not in accordance with the present findings showing that adults with HFA were able to appreciate the social features of irony. However, the two experimental groups have different chronological ages and this might help explain the improvement in adults' performance. Indeed, it is likely that greater practice with social situations would play an important role in increasing the understanding of social norms in individuals with HFA/AS.

The present results reveal that occupation stereotype information modulates and improves irony detection only in comparison participants. As previously shown [18,28], the speaker's sarcastic occupation (e.g., *actor, talk show host*), which is associated with psychological traits and propensities consistent with irony, enhances detection of ironic intent, whereas a non-sarcastic occupation (e.g., *clergyman, scientist*) - being inconsistent with an ironic interpretation of that utterance - did not favor such an interpretation in comparison participants. Consistently, speaker's sarcastic occupation increased ratings of the speaker's ironic and mocking attitude with typically-developed adults. In contrast, for individuals with HFA/AS, speaker's occupation stereotype did not enhance accuracy performance in irony comprehension and did not modulate irony and mockery ratings as a function of the speakers' occupation. Given these expectations elicited by occupation stereotypes, typically-developed adults also regarded an ironic criticism expressed by a speaker with a sarcastic occupation as being less polite than the same insults expressed by speakers with a non-sarcastic occupation, showing that knowledge about the stereotypical traits associated with the speakers' occupation influenced other pragmatic and communicative processes related to the social function of irony. Such an effect seems to be absent in participants with HFA/AS who, despite their overall spared ability to understand irony and its social functions (i.e., irony is considered as being more mocking and polite than literal utterances), attributed equal level of mockery and politeness to both types of speakers. However, when explicitly asked to rate the probability that a person having one of the occupations used in the experimental task would make a sarcastic, a humoristic and a polite remark, participants with HFA/AS exhibited a propensity to perceive some occupations as being more ironic, sarcastic, mocking and polite than others, similarly to typically developed individuals. The present results point to a preserved ability to acquire and retrieve social occupational stereotypes in an explicit way, although such knowledge is not integrated in pragmatic reasoning in participants with HFA/AS to the same extent as in the comparison group.

Social stereotypes are cognitive structures (sets of associated beliefs) stored in long term semantic memory, containing large networks of abstract information about traits, attributes and expected behaviors of members of social groups. Stereotype information can be automatically activated in the presence of stimulus cues in the environment, such as a member of the stereotyped group or some symbolic equivalent. It does not require conscious effort when it exerts an influence on the encoding and interpretation of behaviour. This automatic stereotype processing involves unintentional or spontaneous activation of a well-learned set of associations or responses that have been acquired through repeated experience, while the controlled stereotype-related processes may exert a modulatory or inhibitory effect on automatically activated stereotypes [22]. Social stereotype knowledge might be part of a dedicated cognitive neural system, functionally dissociable from comparable classes of information in the brain, which stores and processes abstract person-based knowledge [46]. This dedicated knowledge memory system serve a fundamental aspect of social-cognitive functioning that might have evolved to deal with socially relevant information [47], since it allows making general prediction about people behaviours, when prior experience or on-line interaction are reduced.

Using a task of attribution of trustworthiness, attractiveness, socioeconomic status and age, White and collaborators [32] reported a preserved ability to make social stereotype judgments from photographs in participants with AS, despite their impairments in facial perception and mentalizing. Similarly, Hirschfeld and collaborators [31] showed intact reasoning about social groups in children with autism, since they performed like typically developing children in using race and gender stereotypes to predict behaviors in new contexts. Importantly, these studies focused on explicit measures to assess sensitivity to stereotypes in ASDs, such as asking the participants directly to make person judgments based on group membership.

Indeed, recent studies have shown that stereotype does not affect behaviour and attitudes only when one is required to make an explicit judgment about the speaker. There is substantial evidence that such information is automatically activated in the presence of a member or symbolic equivalent of the target group [22] and that the use of in social communicative tasks mostly relies on automatic and involuntary processes. As previously revealed [18], when participants were not asked to make an explicit decision about speaker intent, reading time measures showed that speaker occupation information is integrated at an early stage of statement processing. The same was likely the case in the present experiment in which the speaker's occupation is never overtly elicited during task completion.

Thus, the present findings show spared abilities to form and retrieve social stereotype knowledge, along with a reduced automatic effect of stereotype information upon pragmatic-inferential reasoning in participants with HFA/AS. It is possible that failure to integrate information from distinct special-purpose mechanisms, such as the "Naïve Sociology" system, implicated in processing knowledge about social groups, and the "Naïve Psychology" system responsible for mind-reading [39] might lead to longer response times in computing on-line pragmatic-inferential processes during social interaction, in people with ASDs. This explanation is consistent with the Minshew and Goldstein [34]'s cognitive model which regards ASDs as a complex information processing disorder affecting higher-order inferential cognitive ability.

It is noteworthy that depending on circumstances, as stereotype attitudes are simplified conceptions of persons and groups, they can also be maladaptive and originate prejudices. In accordance with our findings, a recent study using the Implicit Association Test [48], a computerized classification paradigm, showed that participants with ASDs are less affected by the influence of stereotypes than typically developed controls [49]. Therefore, since individuals with ASDs are less prone to use automatic stereotypes, one might expect a reduced conformity to social norms and reduced stereotype attitudes in these individuals, relative to typically developed individuals.

Conclusions

The present study confirms that stereotype knowledge is spontaneously activated during the psycholinguistic processing involved in irony comprehension and that information about ironic intent is combined with pragmatic and social information in typically developed subjects. In particular, stereotype knowledge exerts its influence on subjects' expectancies by enhancing irony detection and its social traits in an implicit manner. In contrast, although adults with HFA/AS possess a preserved ability to understand irony and exhibit a developed capacity for understanding social stereotypes, when this knowledge is not made salient, it is not integrated and used in pragmatic communicative processes. Therefore, while we conclude that irony comprehension is preserved in adults with HFA/AS, occupational stereotypes do not appear to engage those automatic processes that, in some circumstances, might enhance detection of the speaker's communicative intents and attitudinal features. Such reduced automaticity exerted by stereotype information might explain some of the impairments in rapid communication and on-line social interaction in individuals with HFA or AS. Hence, it is possible that the use of this information in social and communicative reasoning would occur only when it is previously activated through explicit and controlled processes.

Further studies are needed to investigate how different types of stereotypes are encoded and activated, as well as how this information covertly and overtly interacts with social reasoning and perception in individuals with ASDs.

Acknowledgments

We gratefully acknowledge the commitment of the participants and their families to the pursuit of research in autism.

Author Contributions

Conceived and designed the experiments: TZ MCL. Performed the experiments: FA FE. Analyzed the data: TZ MCL. Wrote the paper: TZ. Diagnosed and described participants: ML PC.

References

1. American Psychiatry Association (2000) Diagnostic and statistical manual of mental disorders (4th ed.). DSM-IV-TR (Text Revision). Washington, DC: American Psychiatry Association.
2. World Health Organisation (2004) International statistical classification and related health problems: Tenth revision. Geneva.
3. Baron-Cohen S, Leslie AM, Frith U (1985) Does the autistic child have a "theory of mind"? Cognition 21, 37–46.
4. Dahlgren SO, Trillingsgaard A (1996) Theory of mind in non-retarded children with autism and Asperger's syndrome: A research note. J Child Psychol Psyc 37, 759–763.
5. Ozonoff S, Rogers SJ, Pennington BF (1991) Asperger's syndrome evidence of an empirical distinction from high-functioning autism. J Child Psychol Psyc 32, 1107–1122.
6. Happé F (1994) An advanced test of theory of mind. J Autism Dev Disord 24, 129–154.
7. Baron-Cohen S, O'Riordan M, Stone V, Jones R, Plaisted K (1999) Recognition of faux pas by normally developing children and children with Asperger Syndrome or high-functioning autism. J Autism Dev Disord 29, 407–418.
8. Zalla T, Stopin A, Ahade S, Sav AM, Leboyer M (2009) Faux pas detection and intentional action in Asperger syndrome. A replication on a French sample. J Autism Dev Disord 39, 373–382.
9. Rajendran G, Mitchell P, Rickards H (2005) How do individuals with Asperger syndrome respond to nonliteral language and inappropriate requests in computer-mediated communication? J Autism Dev Disord 35(4), 429–442.
10. Glenwright M, Agbayewa AS (2012) Older children and adolescents with high-functioning autism spectrum disorder can comprehend verbal irony in computer-mediated communication. Res Autism Spect Dis 6, 628–638.
11. Jolliffe T, Baron-Cohen S (2000) Linguistic processing in high-functioning adults with autism or Asperger syndrome: Can global coherence be achieved? A further test of central coherence theory. Psychol Med 30, 1169–1187.
12. Wang AT, Lee SS, Sigman M, Dapretto M (2006) Neural basis of irony comprehension in children with autism: The role of prosody and context. Brain 129, 932–943.
13. Pexman PM, Rostad R, McMorris CA, Climie EA, Stowkowy J, et al. (2011) Processing of ironic language in children with autism spectrum disorders. J Autism Dev Disord 41, 1097–1112.
14. Kreuz RJ, Caucci GM (2009) Social Aspects of Verbal Irony Use. In H. Pishwa (Ed.), Language and Social Cognition: Expression of the Social Mind (pp. 325–345). Berlin: Mouton de Gruyter.
15. Wilson D, Sperber D (2012) Explaining irony in Meaning and Relevance, Cambridge UP, 123–145.
16. Sperber D, Wilson D (1986) Relevance: Communication and cognition. Oxford: Blackwell.
17. Dews S, Winner E (1995) Muting the meaning: A social function of irony. Metaphor symb act 10; 3–19.
18. Pexman PM, Olineck KM (2002) Does sarcasm always sting? Investigating the impact of ironic insults and ironic compliments. Discourse Process 33, 199–217.
19. Colston HL (1997) Salting a wound or sugaring a pill: The pragmatic functions of ironic criticism. Discourse Process 23(1), 25–45.
20. Fussell SR, Kreuz RJ (1998) Social and cognitive psychological approaches to interpersonal communication. Hillsdale, NJ: Erlbaum.
21. Macrae CN, Milne AB, Bodenhausen GV (1994) Stereotypes as energy-saving devices: A peek inside the cognitive toolbox. J Pers Soc Psychol 66, 31–41.
22. Devine PG (1989) Stereotypes and prejudice: Their automatic and controlled components. J Pers Soc Psychol 56, 5–18.
23. Pexman PM, Olineck KM (2002b) Understanding irony: How do stereotypes cue speaker intent? J Lang Soc Psychol 21, 245–274.
24. Slusher MP, Anderson CA (1987) When reality monitoring fails: The role of imagination in stereotype maintenance. J Pers Soc Psychol 52, 653–662.
25. Bodenhausen GV (1988) Stereotypic biases in social decision making and memory: Testing process models of stereotype use. J Pers Soc Psychol 55, 726–737.
26. Katz A, Pexman P (1997) Processing of figurative language: Occupation of speaker turns metaphor into irony. Metaphor Symbol 12, 19–41.
27. Katz A, Blasko DG, Kazmerski VA (2004) Saying what you don't mean: Social influences on sarcastic language processing. Curr Dir Psychol Sci 13, 186–189.
28. Pexman PM, Ferretti TR, Katz A (2000) Discourse factors that influence online reading of metaphor and irony. Discourse Process 29, 201–222.
29. Pexman PM (2005) Social factors in the interpretations of verbal irony: The roles of speaker and listener characteristics. In H.L. Colston and A.N. Katz (Eds.), Figurative language comprehension: Social and cultural influences. Mahwah, NJ: Erlbaum.
30. Heredia RR, Blumentritt TL (2002) On-line processing of social stereotypes during spoken language comprehension. Exp Psychol 49, 208–221.
31. Hirschfeld L, Bartmess E, White S, Frith U (2007) Can autistic children predict behavior by social stereotypes? Curr Biol 17, R451–R452.
32. White S, Hill E, Winston J, Frith U (2006) An islet of social ability in Asperger Syndrome: Judging social attributes from faces. Brain Cognition 61, 69–77.
33. Rumsey JM, Hamburger SD (1988) Neurophysiological findings in high-functioning men with infantile autism, residual state. J Clin Exp Neuropsychol 10: 201–221.
34. Minshew NJ, Goldstein G (1998) Autism as a disorder of complex information processing," Ment Retard Dev D R 4, no. 2, 129–136.
35. Dews S, Kaplan J, Winner E (1995) Why not say it directly? The social functions of irony. Discourse Process 19, 347–367.
36. Gillberg C, Gillberg C, Råstam M, Wentz E (2001) The Asperger Syndrome (and high-functioning autism) diagnostic interview (ASDI): A preliminary study of a new structured clinical interview. Autism, 5, 57–66.
37. Lord C, Risi S, Lambrecht L, Cook EH, Leventhal BL, et al. (2000) The autism diagnostic observation schedule-generic: a standard measure of social and communication deficits associated with the spectrum of autism. J Autism Dev Disord 30(3), 205–223.
38. Lord C, Rutter M, Le Couteur A (1994) Autism Diagnostic Interview-Revised: a revised version of a diagnostic interview for caregivers of individuals with possible pervasive developmental disorders. J Autism Dev Disord, 24(5), 659–685.
39. Wechsler D (1997) Wechsler Adult Intelligence Scale- Third edition. San Antonio, TX: The Psychological Corporation.

40. MacKay G, Shaw A (2004) A comparative study of figurative language in children with autistic spectrum disorders. Child Lang Teach The 20, 13–32.
41. Adachi T, Koeda T, Hirabayashi S, Maeoka Y, Shiota M, et al. (2004) The metaphor and sarcasm scenario test: A new instrument to help differentiate high functioning pervasive developmental disorder from attention deficit/hyperactivity disorder. Brain Dev 26, 301–306.
42. Giora R (1995) On Irony and Negation. Discourse Process 19, 239–64.
43. Champagne M, Virbel J, Nespoulous JL, Joanette Y (2003) Impact of right hemispheric damage on a hierarchy of complexity evidenced in young normal subjects. Brain Cognition 53, 152–157
44. Sperber D, Wilson D (1981) Irony and the use–mention distinction. In P. Cole (Ed.), *Radical Pragmatics* (pp. 295–318). New York: Academic Press.
45. Sperber D, Wilson D (2002) Pragmatics, Modularity and Mind-reading. Mind Lang 17, 3–23.
46. Caramazza A (2000) The organization of conceptual knowledge in the brain. In: The new cognitive neurosciences (Gazzaniga MS, ed.), 1037–1046. Cambridge, MA: MIT Press.
47. Sander D, Grafman J, Zalla T (2003) The human amygdala: an evolved system for relevance detection. Rev Neurosci 14, 303–316.
48. Greenwald AG, McGhee DE, Schwartz JLK (1998) Measuring individual differences in implicit cognition: the implicit association test. J Pers Soc Psychol 74(6), 1464–1480.
49. Kirchner JC1, Schmitz F, Dziobek I (2012) Brief report: stereotypes in autism revisited. J Autism Dev Disord 42(10), 2246–51.

The Cost of Autism Spectrum Disorders

Chiara Horlin[1], Marita Falkmer[1,2], Richard Parsons[1], Matthew A. Albrecht[3], Torbjorn Falkmer[1,4,5]*

1 School of Occupational Therapy & Social Work, CHIRI, Curtin University, Perth, Australia, **2** School of Education and Communication, CHILD Programme, Institute of Disability Research, Jönköping University, Jönköping, Sweden, **3** School of Psychology, CHIRI, Curtin University, Perth, Australia, **4** Rehabilitation Medicine, Department of Medicine and Health Sciences (IMH), Faculty of Health Sciences, Linköping University & Pain and Rehabilitation Centre, Linköping, Sweden, **5** School of Occupational Therapy, La Trobe University, Melbourne, VIC, Australia

Abstract

Objective: A diagnosis of an autism spectrum disorders is usually associated with substantial lifetime costs to an individual, their family and the community. However, there remains an elusive factor in any cost-benefit analysis of ASD diagnosis, namely the cost of *not* obtaining a diagnosis. Given the infeasibility of estimating the costs of a population that, by its nature, is inaccessible, the current study compares expenses between families whose children received a formal ASD diagnosis immediately upon suspecting developmental atypicality and seeking advice, with families that experienced a delay between first suspicion and formal diagnosis.

Design: A register based questionnaire study covering all families with a child with ASD in Western Australia.

Participants: Families with one or more children diagnosed with an ASD, totalling 521 children diagnosed with an ASD; 317 records were able to be included in the final analysis.

Results: The median family cost of ASD was estimated to be AUD $34,900 per annum with almost 90% of the sum ($29,200) due to loss of income from employment. For each additional symptom reported, approximately $1,400 cost for the family per annum was added. While there was little direct influence on costs associated with a delay in the diagnosis, the delay was associated with a modest increase in the number of ASD symptoms, indirectly impacting the cost of ASD.

Conclusions: A delay in diagnosis was associated with an indirect increased financial burden to families. Early and appropriate access to early intervention is known to improve a child's long-term outcomes and reduce lifetime costs to the individual, family and society. Consequently, a per symptom dollar value may assist in allocation of individualised funding amounts for interventions rather than a nominal amount allocated to all children below a certain age, regardless of symptom presentation, as is the case in Western Australia.

Editor: Jennifer Gladys Mulle, Emory University School Of Medicine, United States of America

Funding: This study was funded by the Department of Social Services (DSS), formerly the Department of Families, Housing, Community Services and Indigenous Affairs (FaHCSIA), with in-kind support of the Autism CRC, established and supported under the Australian Government's Cooperative Research Centres Program. The research was also conducted in collaboration with Disabilities Services Commission Western Australia (DSC). DSS had no active role in the design, implementation, data collection, analysis or interpretation of the study. DSC collaborated with the authors and assisted in data collection by in-kind contribution of its employee's time in some aspects of the study. Writing of the report and the decision to submit this manuscript were solely the role and responsibility of the authors. However, approval to submit this study for publication was sought from CRC Living with Autism Spectrum Disorders, DSS and DSC. All researchers are independent from both DSS and DSC and take full responsibility for the integrity of the data and the accuracy of the analyses. (DSS grant number - RES-HEA-CRD-TB-50940 http://www.dss.gov.au/)

Competing Interests: The authors have declared that no competing interests exist.

* Email: T.Falkmer@curtin.edu.au

Introduction

A diagnosis of an Autism Spectrum Disorder (ASD) results in an estimated annual national cost to Australia of $4.5–7.2 billion [1] that is borne by the individuals themselves, their families, their community, and by government. Costs of autism can peak during the periods when a diagnosis is being assessed and when treatments are being administered, but many costs are ultimately on-going and constitute a life-long burden. The accurate identification of ASDs necessarily relies on assessing observable behaviours using timely, accurate, reliable and valid diagnostic procedures. At present, the "gold standard" diagnosis of autism is a lengthy and time consuming process that requires a suitably qualified multi-disciplinary team (MDT) to assess behavioural, historical and parental report information to determine a definitive diagnosis [2–4]. This is discouraging since failing to accurately identify, or prolonging the identification of, children as having ASD will delay access to apposite intervention and support services [5,6]. This issue is compounded by the possible 25 fold increase in the recent diagnosis rates of ASD in Australia [1], and resultant pressing demand for delivery of diagnostic services and intervention.

It is possible that the delay in treatment and support for children with ASD results in significant costs. Recently, the estimated annual adjusted costs for an adult and a child with autism have been calculated as follows (all dollar values are in AUD and rounded to the nearest dollar):

$$(P+SP+S+M+C_{MD})\times 250$$

where, P = production loss of the individual and family with an ASD diagnosis, SP = support costs, S = school costs, mainly addition and specialist staff, M = medical costs, and C_{MD} = missed diagnosis. It is important to note that several assumptions are made regarding productivity costs that we do not feel fully encompass the impact of a child's diagnosis on parent employment resulting in what appears to be a very low estimate of the financial impact (e.g., time taken out from current employment for treatment visits is accounted for, but reduced employment of parents so that they can care for a child with ASD is not taken into account). Notably, estimates for the parameter C_{MD} (missed diagnosis) have not been made and, as a result, the true benefit of a diagnosis of ASD could not be calculated. It seems plausible that an early diagnosis of autism may reduce the cost of ASD because diagnosis leads to early intervention, which results in better outcomes [7,8], improved social behaviour [9,10], and less reliance on specialised education support classes [7,9]. These improvements may, in turn, have knock-on benefits to families and society more broadly, as well as increased productivity for parents and the individual themselves later in life. These gains are usually accomplished when intervention is commenced very early, between the ages of 2 and 4 [11,12].

However, the complication here is clear: those individuals remaining undiagnosed are, for that very reason, inaccessible to service providers and researchers alike. The next closest approximation that can be made for parameter C_{MD} is therefore the difference in costs between those children identified and treated early in their development and those not identified and/or treated until later in childhood or even adolescence and adulthood. One method of estimating this cost is to identify a subgroup of children who receive a diagnosis of ASD shortly after their parents suspect their child's development is atypical, and then compare costs for these children with a subgroup of children who had their diagnosis formally confirmed much later. However, one possible offset of the cost of early diagnosis is the long-term accumulated cost of interventions and special services. Therefore, the potential added cost associated with a later diagnosis may not be substantially higher than an earlier diagnosis.

Research into the impact of receiving an early diagnosis and on a family's financial burden is limited [4]. In Australia, state and territory governments are primarily responsible for supporting disability, including ASD, rather than the Commonwealth. However, families with a child diagnosed with an ASD receive a finite amount of Commonwealth funding up to the child's seventh birthday (the so-called "Helping Children with Autism "-funding) for the purposes of early intervention. From this point onwards, ongoing therapies and services outside of school are largely parent-funded on top of other medical and non-medical costs. Aside from the obvious cost to families of missing this early opportunity for government funding, the current study also seeks to determine whether a delayed diagnosis results in inflated costs, reduced incomes and increased financial stresses to families on a long-term basis when compared to families of individuals with a more immediate the immediate diagnosis. Thus it will be possible to estimate an accessible proxy of the parameter C_{MD}.

Methods

Participants and Procedures

With the assistance of the Disabilities Services Commission (DSC) Western Australia, a questionnaire was distributed to families with children registered as having an ASD on their client register. Only families with diagnosed children currently under the age of 18 years were included. This decision was made in line with recommendations from the DSC based on the likelihood of correct/valid information being extractable from the register. At the time of the mail out, 3,965 children were registered with DSC from 3,723 families. Of the packages mailed out, 3,494 were sent to families with one child with ASD, 217 packages sent to families with two diagnosed children, 11 packages sent to families with three diagnosed children and one package sent to a family with four children diagnosed with ASD. Families with more than one child under 18 received one questionnaire for each child with ASD. Of the 3,723 questionnaire packs (covering 3,965 children) sent out by DSC, 192 were returned as "address unknown". In total, 521 questionnaires were returned, resulting in a response rate of 15%.

Questionnaire Development. Development of the full parent-report questionnaire was informed by anecdotal reports from clinical experts and families, the current research literature and insurance reports. Firstly, the general areas of interest were listed and all financial aspects were itemised and categorised to cover as many potential expenses that were a consequence of having a child with ASD. The questionnaire also attempted to gather and summarise information on all possible direct medical, direct non-medical and indirect costs associated with having a child with an ASD. The areas of expense addressed in the questionnaire are listed in Table 1 and specific items relevant to each area are presented in the final questionnaire in the Appendix S1 in the provided Supporting Information.

Questions were then devised to gather the information conveniently and efficiently, which would lead to clear and relevant summary reports whilst taking into account the heterogeneity of families with ASD. A pilot version of the questions and response formats were sent for comments to a number of clinical psychologists, neuropsychologists, developmental psychologists, social workers, occupational therapists, and other clinicians and service providers.

A full version of the questionnaire was then piloted on three families who have children with ASD. Based on their comments and feedback the questionnaire was adjusted to its final version (Appendix S1) and comprised a total of 73 items on demographic information, the child's diagnosis, developmental history, treatment history, education, child care and qualitative questions about the child and families' quality of life.

The final page of the questionnaire included a diagnostic checklist of DSM-IV-TR/ICD-10 items [13]. The checklist consists of 20 symptom characteristics divided into 4 sections addressing the traditional symptom domains of;

-Impairments in social interaction (five symptom characteristics),
-Impairments in communication (seven symptom characteristics),
-Restricted, repetitive and stereotyped patterns of behaviour, interest or activities (seven symptom characteristics),
-The presence of impairments in at least one of the above before the age of three (one characteristic).

Parents were asked to indicate whether any of these characteristics currently previously applied to their child.

Data Collection. Questionnaire packs were prepared by the authors before being delivered to the DSC. To maintain confidentiality of the DSC's client register, all printing of cover letters and addressing of envelopes was handled by the DSC's staff and at no time did any of the researchers have access to this register. As per the DSC's records, packs were sent to the primary contact, the default for which was the diagnosed child's father.

Table 1. Areas of expense for families with children with ASD addressed in the questionnaire.

Direct Medical	Direct Non-Medical	Indirect
Physicians/dentists	Childcare	Caregiver lost productivity
Pharmaceuticals	Respite care	Family quality of life
Therapeutic services/interventions	Home improvement	
Alternative/complimentary therapies	Special education	
Emergency room/hospitals	Support services for other family members	
Home healthcare		
Treatment-related travel		

The questionnaire pack included the questionnaire itself and a reply paid return envelope. All questionnaires were de-identified and asked for no identifying information.

After a period of one month, reminders to complete the questionnaire were published online, in newspapers, DSC newsletters and on community radio. Upon receiving deidentified and completed questionnaires, a unique anonymous identifier was allocated to each questionnaire. Responses were then entered into a data file using IBM SPSS version 20 and analysed using the SAS version 9.2 statistical software.

Data analysis

Treatment-related travel costs. Direct costs associated with travel for medical, therapeutic and complimentary/alternative treatments were calculated as a function of the reported frequency of average visits per month (questions 19, 28 and 36 respectively) and distance from these services (questions 18, 27 and 35 respectively). Round trip costs were calculated based on doubling the median kilometre distance from services and the average per kilometre cost of running a small car (approximated at $0.65AUD per kilometre by the most recent Royal Automobile Club figures).

Individual cost estimates were calculated for medical visits relating to a child's ASD diagnosis, therapeutic visits relating to an ASD diagnosis and complimentary/alternative visits undertaken as part of ASD treatment. These were summed to create a monthly cumulative total, which was then adjusted to create an annual estimate of treatment related travel costs according to the following formula:

$$\text{Travel Cost (\$AUD)} = 12 \times \sum (0.65 \times (V_{Medical} \cdot D_{Medical} + V_{Therapy} \cdot D_{Therapy} + V_{Comp} \cdot D_{Comp}))$$

where V equals the number of visits per month, D equals the distance in km to the service. 'Medical', 'Therapy' and 'Comp' refer to medical professional services, other therapeutic services and complementary and alternative services respectively.

Out of pocket treatment costs. The reported annual out-of-pocket costs to families in relation to ASD- specific medical, therapeutic and complimentary/alternative treatment services (questions 22, 33 and 37) were summed to create a total direct treatment cost variable. All three questions had seven potential response options representing intervals of dollar amounts. These options were then converted to the mid-point of each interval to create a single dollar amount for analysis. These recoded variables were then summed to create a cumulative total of the out of pocket costs associated with ASD-specific medical, therapeutic and complimentary/alternative treatments.

Loss of income from employment reduction. The productivity loss associated with having a child diagnosed with ASD was calculated based on self-reported impact of their child's diagnosis on the parent/caregiver ability to work (question 51) and, if employment status was affected, the size of this reduction as a function of hours in the average work week (question 52). Those responding to question 51 by selecting options one, two or three, as presented in Table 2, then indicated the reduction in hours in question 52. This reduction was thereafter converted to a proportion of full-time equivalent (FTE) employment. Those indicating that either one or both parents could not work at all at this time due to the needs of their ASD child were converted to an FTE reduction of 1 or 2 units, respectively. Parents indicating that their employment status was unaffected were coded as 0. This variable was then multiplied with the median full-time income for 2010–2011 as reported by the Australian Taxation Office (the latest figures made available), which was $48, 864.

Cumulative cost of having a child diagnosed with ASD. To create a single estimate of direct and indirect expenses to each family that were specifically related to having a child diagnosed with ASD, the costs associated with treatment-related travel, out-of-pocket treatment expenses and loss of income/ productivity were summed.

'Immediate' versus 'delayed' diagnosis. A dichotomous 'immediate' versus 'delayed' diagnosis variable was created based on cross-tabulations between questions 10 (age at first suspicion of something not being quite right) and 12 (age at which a formal diagnosis was received). This variable was intended to capture the chronological difference between those receiving early or more immediate diagnosis (and presumably treatment and intervention) and a later or delayed diagnosis (often after the optimal developmental window for treatment and period at which early intervention would take place). Those children with a zero or one step chronological difference between questions 10 and 12 were coded as 'immediate' and those with a two or more step difference between these questions were coded as 'delayed'. A further, stricter, division of 'immediate' and 'delayed' was also conducted by retaining only those with a zero step difference between questions 10 and 12 ('immediate') and those with a three or more step difference ('delayed'). These divisions are delineated in Table 3.

Cumulative presence of ASD symptoms. The total number of ASD symptoms was estimated by a cumulative total of the positive indications from the presence of symptoms within the four domains listed on the DSM-IV/TR-ICD-10 checklist. Positive indications were coded as one and responses in domain one to

Table 2. Questions 51 and 52 and the coding of responses used to estimate proportions of FTE reductions.

Question 51: How much has your child's diagnosis affected the employment status of your household?		
1	Both parents must work less hours	
2	One parent (of a two-parent household) must work less hours	
3	Single parent must work less hours	
4	One parent cannot work at this time	**1** FTE reduction
5	Both parents cannot work at this time	**2** FTE reduction
6	Unaffected	**0** FTE reduction
Question 52: If your employment status has been affected, please estimate by how many hours in an average week your employment load has been reduced.		
−99	Not relevant	**0** FTE reduction
1	<7 hours	**.2** FTE reduction
2	7–14 hours	**.4** FTE reduction
3	15–21 hours	**.6** FTE reduction
4	22–28 hours	**.8** FTE reduction
5	29–35+hours	**1** FTE reduction

three were summed to create a total for each child. The fourth domain comprised one single developmental history question and was excluded from this total, since this characteristic was regarded as a prerequisite for receiving a diagnosis of ASD.

Analysis of non-respondents. Six months after the initial mail-out, a random sample of 405 families registered with the DSC were contacted for a telephone follow-up. Given the confidentiality of the DSC register and the de-identified nature of the returned questionnaires, it was not known which families on the register had or had not completed the long-form questionnaire. Thus, the random sample of 405 families would include those that had completed and returned a questionnaire and those that had not. Non-respondents were then asked to answer an abbreviated form of the questionnaire over the phone. This short-form phone questionnaire consisted of twenty questions taken from the original questionnaire for the purposes of a later drop-out analysis. Those questions included in the short-form are shown in italics in Appendix S1. For the purposes of comparisons between those that did and did not respond to the long-form questionnaire that was sent out via mail, independent samples *t*-tests were used to compare the ages of children, chi-square tests were used to compare categorical demographic variables and Mann-Whitney U tests were conducted to compare calculated cost variables. Due to the shortened nature of the short-form questionnaire, only the out of pocket treatment costs and the loss of income from employment reduction variables could be calculated for both respondents and non-respondents. The response categories of some demographic variables (question 10 and 12 specifically) were collapsed to ensure validity of the chi-square test.

Ethical approval

Ethical approval was obtained from the Curtin University Human Research Ethics Committee (HR 138/2012) and the internal ethical review board of the DSC in Western Australia. Questionnaire packs were sent to the DSC's clients with a cover letter from the Director General of DSC explaining the nature and purpose of the study as well as an information sheet inviting families to complete and return the questionnaire. Completed and returned questionnaires were taken as consent to participate in the study.

Results

The characteristics of the included 521 children with ASD are presented in Table 4. Descriptive statistics for all cumulative cost estimates and the cumulative presence of ASD symptoms are presented in Table 5. An additional total cost of ASD variable for families with only one child diagnosed with ASD was calculated to express the costs of ASD without the compounding effect of having multiple children with ASD and the implications this may have to

Table 3. Division of children receiving 'immediate' (N = 250) versus 'delayed' (N = 266) diagnoses.

		Q12: How old was your child when she/he was formally diagnosed with an ASD?				
		12–18 months*(2)*	**19–24 months***(3)*	**2–6 years***(4)*	**6–12 years***(5)*	**13–18 years***(6)*
Q10; How old	<12 months*(1)*	6	15	***65***	***34***	***6***
was your child	12–18 months*(2)*	***5***	22	91	***28***	***2***
when you or	19–24 months*(3)*	-	***7***	74	19	***3***
someone else noticed	2–6 years*(4)*	-	-	***93***	32	3
something was different	6–12 years*(5)*	-	-	-	***10***	-
or not quite right?	13–18 years*(6)*	-	-	-	-	***1***

Numbers in bold indicate the stricter division of 'immediate' (N = 116) versus 'delayed' (N = 138).

Table 4. Characteristics of the children with ASD and their families.

	N		%	
Total	521			
Male	431		83	
Female	90		17	
Age (months)	**Mean** (SD) 119 (50)		**Median** 113.5	
Respondent				
Biological mother	421		81	
Biological father	87		17	
Grandparent	5		.96	
Foster parent	4		.77	
Step parent	1		.2	
Other	1		.2	
ASD diagnosis				
Autism	272		52.60	
High-functioning autism	128		24.70	
Asperger Syndrome	36		7	
PDD-NOS	76		14.70	
CDD	2		.40	
Other	7		1.40	
How many children with ASD have one or more ASD sibling?				
0 (only child with ASD)	355		71	
1 sibling	121		24	
2 siblings	15		3	
3 siblings	9		2	
Presence of CD/ID				
Yes	371		72	
No	144		28	
Presence of other mental health/psychological conditions				
Yes	408		79	
No	108		21	
Presence of other medical conditions				
Yes	341		66.70	
No	170		33.30	
How old was your child when you first noticed something wasn't right?				
<12 months	126		24	
12–18 months	150		29	
19–24 months	103		20	
2–6 years	128		24.70	
6 12 years	10		2	
13–18 years	2		.3	
How old was your child when formally diagnosed?				
<12 months	0		0	
12–18 months	11		2.10	
19–24 months	44		8.50	
2–6 years	325		62.70	
6–12 years	123		23.70	
13–18 years	15		2.90	
Parent's highest education	**N**	**%**	**N**	**%**
	Mother		Father	
Completed year 10	72	14	74	15
Completed year 12	60	12	42	8.5

Table 4. Cont.

	N		%	
Completed certificate at TAFE (or similar)	135	26.40	87	17.60
Apprenticeship	13	2.50	94	19
Some university education but did not complete	46	9	36	7.60
Completed university undergraduate degree	103	20.10	85	17.20
Completed university postgraduate degree	82	16	75	15.20
Household composition	**N**		**%**	
Two-parent	396		76.90	
Single parent	72		14	
Only extended family (grandparents etc)	4		.80	
Two-parent plus extended	22		4.30	
Single parent plus extended	10		2	
Foster situation	3		.60	
Other	8		1.50	
Combined annual income				
<$25,000	55		10.50	
$25,000–$50,000	56		10.70	
$50,000–$75,000	68		13	
$75,000–$100,000	90		17.30	
$100,000–$125,000	59		11.30	
$125,000–$150,000	65		12.50	
$150,000–$200,000	57		11	
>$200,000	50		9.60	
Unknown	21		4	

Percentage values are rounded to two decimal places where possible.

reductions in FTE employment. The cumulative 'Cost of ASD' variable predominantly consisted of loss of income of the parents and caregivers (89%) with ASD-related travel costs (3%) and treatment costs (8%) making smaller contributions.

The cost of ASD as a function of 'immediate' versus 'delayed' diagnosis or frequency of ASD symptoms

A regression analysis was conducted with cost of ASD as the dependent variable. Independent variables included: 'immediate' (coded as 1) versus 'delayed' (coded as 2) diagnosis, ASD symptom frequency (as continuous numeric), age of child in years, number of siblings (0, 1, 2 or 3+), number of siblings with ASD (0, 1, or 2+), combined income (in $AUD), age of diagnosis of child with autism (1 = 0–12 months, 2 = 12–24 months, 3 = 2–6 years, 4 = 6–12 years, 5 = 12–18 years) and highest education of the mother and father (1 = year 10, 2 = year 12, 3 = TAFE, 4 = Apprenticeship, 5 = some university, 6 = Bachelor degree, 7 = postgraduate degree). The residuals from the regression analysis were plotted (histogram and density plots) and followed a normal distribution. The R^2 values for the two models evaluating the different criteria for immediate versus delayed diagnosis (i.e., loose and strict cut off) below were 21% and 31%, respectively, as shown in Table 6.

Table 5. Descriptive statistics for all estimated cost variables (rounded to nearest dollar) and cumulative presence of ASD symptomatology.

	N	Mean (SD)	Median	Quartiles		
				1st	2nd	3rd
ASD-related travel	521	$1,500 ($1,200)	$860	$620	$860	$2,000
Out of pocket treatment	370	$4,800 ($5,000)	$2,600	$1,000	$2,600	$7,500
Loss of income	474	$30,000 ($20,300)	$29,200	$19,500	$29,200	$48,700
Cost of ASD	**339**	**$37,60 ($21,700)**	**$37,800**	**$22,000**	**$37,800**	**$52,800**
Cost of ASD (1 ASD child per household)	**223**	**$35,100 ($20,300)**	**$34,900**	**$20,700**	**$34,900**	**$51,700**
Frequency of ASD symptoms	508	12.4 (4.2)	13	10	13	16

Table 6. Regression model of symptom frequency and delay from first identifying a problem to ultimate diagnosis and the total cost including covariates.

	Full available sample (final N = 332)						Strict immediate vs delayed sub-sample (final N = 152)					
	df	F	p^a	Contrast	Coefficient	95% CI	df	F	p^a	Contrast	Coefficient	95% CI
Immediate/Delayed diagnosis	1	0.13	0.72	1 vs 2	$-1500	−6000, 3100[b]	1	0.17	0.68	1 vs 2	$2100	−6200, 10500[b]
Cumulative symptom presence	**1**	**33.0**	**<0.0001**	**slope**	**$1400[c]**	**860, 1900**	**1**	**15.36**	**<0.0001**	**slope**	**$1500[c]**	**630, 2400**
Age group	**4**	**2.77**	**0.028**	**1 vs 5**	**$730**	**−15000, 16000**	4	1.58	0.18	1 vs 5	$-2200	−28300, 23900
				2 vs 5	**$720**	**−15000, 16000**				2 vs 5	$-80	−25300, 25200
				3 vs 5	**$-340**	**−16000, 15000**				3 vs 5	$-1900	−27400, 23600
				4 vs 5	**$-6900**	**−22000, 8300**				4 vs 5	$-9100	−34200, 15900
Number of Siblings	3	2.33	0.075	0 vs 3+	$4300	−4700, 13200	3	1.88	0.14	0 vs 3+	$15600	685, 30600
				1 vs 3+	$-4000	−11300, 3100				1 vs 3+	$2100	−8800, 13000
				2 vs 3+	$-4800	−12300, 2700				2 vs 3+	$1600	−9400, 12700
Number of Siblings with ASD	**2**	**5.34**	**0.005**	**0 vs 2+**	**$-29500**	**−46000, −13000**	**1**	**5.24**	**0.007**	**0 vs 2+**	**$-44500**	**−71700, −17400**
				1 vs 2+	**$-24600**	**−35600, −13600**				**1 vs 2+**	**$-35300**	**−52100, −18500**
Income	1	2.24	0.14	slope	$-800	−1900, 290	1	3.34	0.07	slope	$-1400	−3100, 270
Age of Diagnosis	4	0.18	0.95	1 vs 5	$9000	−12800, 30800	4	0.26	0.90	1 vs 5	$18800	−14100, 51800
				2 vs 5	$5300	−10800, 21500				2 vs 5	$12400	−15200, 39900
				3 vs 5	$5600	−9100, 20300				3 vs 5	$11200	−9500, 31900
				4 vs 5	$3900	−11300, 19100				4 vs 5	$9400	−11500, 30200
Education (Max of M/D)	7	0.31	0.95	1 vs 8	$17700	−5700, 41200	7	0.41	0.90	1 vs 8	$21600	−39300, 46000
				2 vs 8	$10300	−1100, 21700				2 vs 8	$8200	−5300, 27000
				3 vs 8	$1300	−7500, 10100				3 vs 8	$8800	−24200, 10500
				4 vs 8	$2800	−4300, 9800				4 vs 8	$5500	−12200, 9700
				5 vs 8	$2100	−5200, 9400				5 vs 8	$5900	−16500, 7000
				6 vs 8	$1400	−7200, 10000				6 vs 8	$7600	−15800, 14300
				7 vs 8	$1700	−4500, 8000				7 vs 8	$4900	−13300, 5900

[a]The p-value was obtained from a regression model using the square root of the total cost as dependent variable (because of skewness in this variable).
[b]This is the CI for the difference in cost between early and late.
[c]This is the amount by which the cost increases (dollars) per unit increase on the symptom score.

Regardless of whether the strict or loose definition of the 'immediate 'versus 'delayed' diagnosis variable was used, neither was found to be significantly associated with the of cost of ASD. However, in both regression models, the number of ASD symptoms present was a significant predictor. In both models, costs were increased by approximately $1,400 per ASD symptom reported for the loose and strict criteria models. Models with fewer covariates were also fitted yielding similar estimates for the cost of immediate versus delayed diagnosis and the cumulative presence of ASD symptoms.

Mediation analysis

A delay in diagnosis and treatment may have an indirect effect on costs associated with ASD by increasing the number of symptoms present. In order to test this hypothesis, a mediation analysis was conducted. Firstly, it was confirmed that a delay in diagnosis was statistically significantly associated with an increased number of symptoms (number of increased symptoms associated with delay $= 1.56$, $p = 0.001$, 95% CI = 0.63, 2.49). Following this, two models were constructed and contrasted: 1) total costs were modelled as a function of delay in diagnosis alone, with the direct effect of diagnostic delay denoted as c, and 2) total costs were modelled as a function of delay in diagnosis and cumulative symptom count, with the parameter estimate for delay in diagnosis with the effect attributable to cumulative symptom count partialled out denoted c'. The final mediated effect was calculated by subtracting c' from c (i.e., mediated effect $= c - c'$). To produce 95% CIs around the mediated effect, 10,000 bootstrapped samples were taken and the quantiles representing 2.5% and 97.5% of the c - c' distribution calculated. Bootstrapping the estimate of the mediated effect has been recommended for mediation analysis because the technique offers acceptable statistical power properties, directly estimates the mediated effect, and does not rely on many of the assumptions necessary for other tests [14,15].

The mediation analysis was supportive of this hypothesis. A statistically significant reduction in the effect associated with diagnostic delay of $2,110 (95% CI = 820, 3700) was observed when symptom count was included in the model. This was despite the delay in diagnosis not being statistically significantly associated with total cost directly (see above). The mediation analysis was repeated with all covariates included in the original model (age of child, number of siblings, number of siblings with ASD, combined income, age of ASD diagnosis, and highest education of mother and father) and a similar effect was found (mediated effect c-c' = $1,770, 95% CI = 360, 3340).

Analysis of non-respondents

Contact was established with 267 of the 405 families who did not return a completed questionnaire, and, of these, 148 agreed to complete the short-form questionnaire. Sixty-four families had already completed the long-form questionnaire. Fifty-two families (13%) declined to participate in the phone questionnaire. Incorrect phone numbers and no answer were the main reasons for failures to contact. A complete breakdown of the telephone sample is shown in Figure 1. Two of the 148 families that agreed to participate did not have a child with ASD. From the 146 families with children with ASD that agreed to complete the short- form questionnaire, data were collated for 171 individual children.

As shown in Table 7, there were few noteworthy differences between respondents and non- respondents. Demographically, respondents were slightly more likely to have a male child and to have noticed developmental atypicality earlier. Respondents also received a formal diagnosis of ASD earlier than non-respondents. Respondents reported higher treatment costs than non-respondents. However, there were no differences in reported income loss.

Discussion

ASD-related costs were strongly associated with the cumulative presence of the child's symptoms. This builds upon previous research that has found that having a child with ASD is associated with significant financial strain [16–19]. The association between increased costs and ASD symptom severity suggests that effective and early interventions that result in the reduction of expressed symptoms may have a significant impact on improving a family's productivity and their resultant financial situation.

Contrary to expectations, there was no statistically significant differences in costs related to receiving the diagnosis of ASD whether soon or late after suspicion. We suggest two possible reasons for this. Firstly, given the above finding that increasing symptomatology is directly related to the cost of ASD, the more immediate identification of ASD may create a situation where improvement in outcomes and the effect on associated symptomatology measures dwarfs the influence of delay to diagnosis on the final cost of ASD. This interpretation appears to be consistent with the mediation analysis, whereby an indirect effect of diagnostic delay on costs appeared to be mediated by an association between increased symptomatology and increased diagnostic delay. Secondly, families with a child with ASD may adapt their work-family balance regardless of whether the child has a diagnosis or not. This is reflected by the finding that the largest cost reported by parents was a loss of income from reduced working hours. This is consistent with a previous report stating that a loss of approximately 14% of family income is often the consequence of having a child with ASD [16], equalling $7,200 (based on the median income and average exchange rate of 2008). The results from the present study suggest a substantially higher (29%) loss of combined household income.

From a family and societal perspective, support that allows family members to work may more effectively assist families with children with ASD by lessening the financial burden and improving well-being of all family members. Furthermore, the long-term consequence of high costs associated with having a child who has a diagnosis of ASD is not well researched. A study reporting on the distribution of societal costs of ASD distributed throughout the lifespan estimated that fathers of children with moderate to severe autism were unemployed 20% of a full time equivalent [20], whereas 60% of mothers were unemployed and 30% worked part time of a full time equivalent [20]. If these estimates are indeed accurate, the family income may therefore be severely impacted through the lifespan as a result of having a child with ASD [20]. The largest direct life time cost is to provide care for adults with ASD [20,21]. Consequently, parents of adults with ASD may face an even larger financial strain when having to provide services for their adult children whilst having had less opportunity to save or accumulate superannuation funds due to reduced possibilities to work full time [20].

Limitations

There are several limitations to the cost analysis presented here: 1) The return rate of 15% observed in the present study is quite poor in comparison to similar studies. This may be because client details registered with the DSC are maintained sporadically and a number of records contained incomplete or inaccurate entries. Furthermore, distributed questionnaires were addressed only to the fathers of the registered child for some families due to a DSC database error. Given reports of higher than normal divorce rates

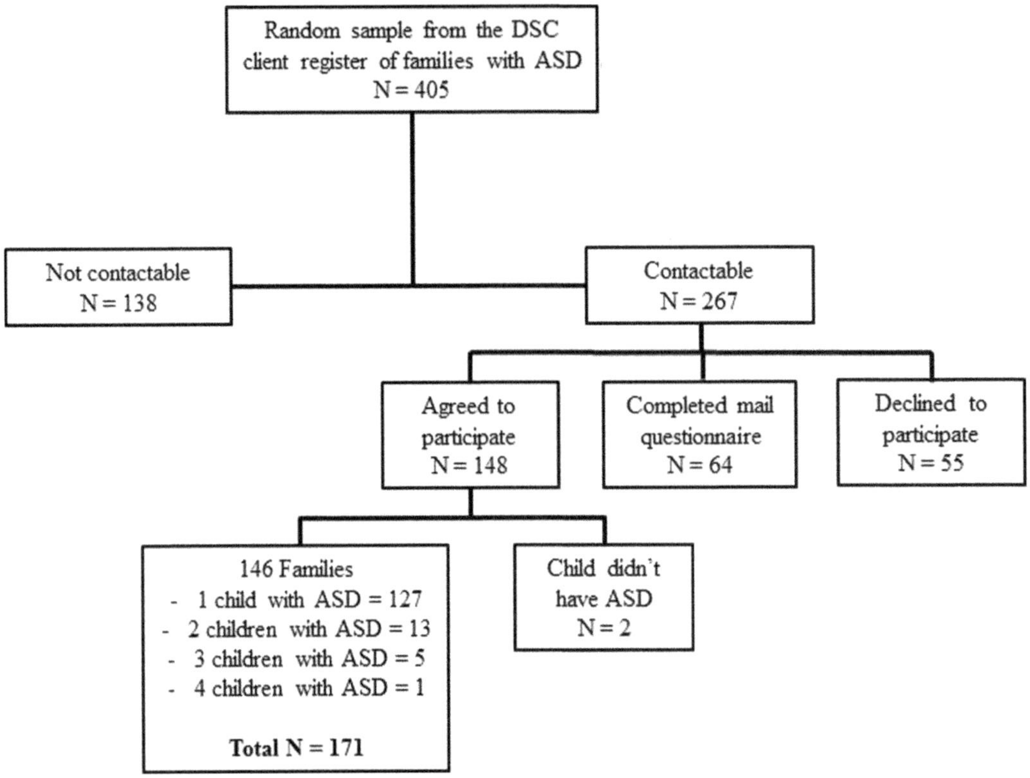

Figure 1. Breakdown of the non-respondent sample for the purposes of the short-form telephone questionnaire. A full representation of a random sample of families registered as having received or currently receiving service provision for the purposes of an analysis of non-respondents. From a random sample of 405 families, 146 families (totalling 171 children with ASD) agreed to participate in the telephone questionnaire

in families with children with ASD [22], this may be another reason for a lower than usual return rate reflected by the higher than expected number of respondents reporting being in two-parent households compared to non-respondents. 2) There are multiple reasons why a child might not be diagnosed until later in development, giving rise to a number of caveats with respect to the 'delayed' diagnostic group. For example, some of those diagnosed later in development may present with symptomatology that is either more complex or reduced in severity compared to those children with evident and more severe symptoms from an early age. However, this influence appeared to be relatively small as the effect of the variable "Age of diagnosis" was not a statistically significant contributor to cost, or may be reflected more by the cumulative presence of ASD symptomatology measure. 3) Requesting estimates of current costs may not be representative of historical costs as current expenses are dependent on the child's stage of development, time since diagnosis, and current stage of treatment or intervention. However, one aspect for which our estimates are robust is their specification of only ASD-related expenses for medical, behavioural or complimentary/alternative therapies. 4) In contrast to most parents that had reduced their hours due to the needs of their child with ASD, a small number of parents were seeking *more* work due to the expenses of having a child with ASD. This is not often considered when calculating the costs and productivity losses associated with a diagnosis of ASD. 5) A number of parents reported low treatment costs because they had exhausted all funded avenues and could not afford to independently fund treatment for their children. 5) Lastly, the present study does not address all aspects of how an immediate or delayed diagnosis may impact families and their financial situation. The processes that parents undergo in order to access a proficient diagnosis are reported as being extremely stressful [23] and may result in health related consequences difficult to estimate in any cost benefit analysis [18]. Consequently, health related consequences and costs for family members and society in relation to early/late diagnosis may warrant further scrutinising.

Conclusions

The median family cost of ASD was estimated to be AUD $34,900 per annum (IQR $20,700 - $51,700; based on median income from wages), with almost 90% of the sum ($29,200) due to loss of income from employment. While there was no statistically significant direct effect on the cost depending on the timeliness of the diagnosis (immediate versus delayed) the cumulative presence of ASD symptoms had a significant impact on the costs and a delay in diagnosis could indirectly increase costs by neglecting symptoms that may respond to more immediate intervention. For each additional symptom reported, a $1,400 cost for the family per annum was added. These findings take on a great deal of significance when considered within a regional context as funding amounts vary across states and countries. The financial burden of families of children with ASD is correlated with the existing societal financial safety net [17]. In an Australian context, families may miss out on the most widely available financial support for early intervention if the diagnosis is received after the age of six [24]. If the family is expected to carry a substantial share of the cost needed to support the development of children with ASD, this may have detrimental consequences for the wellbeing of the child

Table 7. Comparison between respondents (N = 521) and non-respondents (N = 171) on demographics and two main study variables that can be derived from the short-form telephone questionnaire.

	Non-Respondents (N = 171)	Respondents (N = 521)
Age (months)	Mean (SD) 122 (50)	Mean (SD) 119 (50)
	Median 120	Median 113.50
		t (678) = .53, p = .60
	Proportion (%)	**Proportion (%)**
Sex of diagnosed child		
Male	75.50	83
Female	24.50	17
		$\chi^2(1, N = 689) = 4.41, p = .04$
ASD diagnosis		
Autism	47.40	52.60
HFA	25.10	24.70
Asperger Syndrome	11.10	7
PDD-NOS	15.80	14.70
CDD	.60	.40
Other	-	1.40
		$\chi^2(6, N = 703) = 4.31, p = .64$
How old was your child when you first noticed something was not right?		
<12 months	24.10	24
12–18 months	17.10	29
19–24 months	18.20	20
2–6 years	35.30	24.70
6–18 years*	5.30	2.30
		$\chi^2(4, N = 704) = 15.38, p < .05$
How old was your child when formally diagnosed?		
<12–24 months*	10.30	10.60
2–6 years	50.10	62.70
6–18+ years*	38.70	26.60
		$\chi^2(2, N - 698) = 9.61, p < .01$
Household composition		
Two-parent	73.70	76.90
Single parent	22.20	14
Only extended family (grandparents etc)	.60	.80
Two-parent plus extended	2.30	4.3
Single parent plus extended	1.20	2
Foster situation	-	.6
Other	-	1.5
-		$\chi^2(6, N = 702) = 10.94, p = .09$
Out-of-pocket treatment costs	Mean (SD) $2,300 ($2,900)	Mean (SD) $4,800 ($5,000)
-	Median $1,000	Median $2,600
-		$Z = -16.95, p < .001, r = -.76$
Loss of income	Mean (SD) $25,400 ($21,000)	Mean (SD) $30,000 ($20,300)
-	Median $29,300	Median $29,200
-		$Z = -.94, p = .35, r = -.04$

Categorical demographic variables are presented as proportions due to missing data in some variables.
* These variables have been collapsed across categories for the purposes of chi-square analyses.

with ASD, as well as for other family members, especially for low income families that may not seek services at all for financial reasons [17].

Supporting Information

Appendix S1 The complete questionnaire. Those questions included in the short form are shown in italics.

Acknowledgments

Aoife McNally, Kirsty Oehlers, Mandy Richards, Geoff Cole, Susan Peden, staff at Disabilities Services Commission, Caitlin Axford, Fiona Choi, Helen Weldergergish, Rachel Owens, Rex Parsons, Stephen Lawrie, Gal Rose, Tim Parkin and the AIM employment AAWA.

Authorship statement& transparency declaration

The final manuscript has been seen and approved by all authors and they have taken due care to ensure the integrity of the work. The work is original and has not been published elsewhere and is currently not under consideration by another journal. All authors have had full access to the data, analysis and writing and editing has jointly been done.

The lead author affirms that this manuscript is an honest, accurate, and transparent account of the study being reported; that no important aspects of the study have been omitted; and that any discrepancies from the study as planned (and, if relevant, registered) have been explained.

Author Contributions

Conceived and designed the experiments: CH MF MA TF. Performed the experiments: CH MF. Analyzed the data: CH RP MA TF. Wrote the paper: CH MF RP MA TF.

References

1. Consulting SE (2007) Economic Costs of ASD in Australia. Synergies Economic Consulting.
2. Le Couteur A, Haden G, Hammal D, McComachie H (2008) Diagnosing Autism Spectrum Disorders in pre-school children using two standardised assessment instruments: The ADI-R and the ADOS. Journal of Autism and Developmental Disorders 38: 362–372.
3. Woolfenden S, Sarkozy V, Ridley G, Williams K (2012) A systematic review of the diagnostic stability of Autism Spectrum Disorder. Research in Autism Spectrum Disorders 6: 345–354.
4. Shattuck PT, Grosse SD (2007) Issues related to the diagnosis and treatment of autism spectrum disorders. Mental Retardation and Developmental Disabilities Research Reviews 13: 129–135.
5. Sikora D, Hall T, Hartley S, Gerrard-Morris A, Cagle S (2008) Does Parent Report of Behavior Differ Across ADOS-G Classifications: Analysis of Scores from the CBCL and GARS. Journal of Autism and Developmental Disorders 38: 440–448.
6. South M, Williams B, McMahon W, Owley T, Filipek P, et al. (2002) Utility of the Gilliam Autism Rating Scale in Research and Clinical Populations. Journal of Autism and Developmental Disorders 32: 593–599.
7. McEachin JJ, Smith T, Lovaas OI (1993) Long-term outcome for children with autism who received early intensive behavioral treatment. American Journal on Mental Retardation 97: 359–372.
8. Rogers S (1996) Brief report: Early intervention in autism. Journal of Autism and Developmental Disorders 26: 243–246.
9. Lovaas OI (1987) Behavioral treatment and normal educational and intellectual functioning in young autistic children. Journal of Consulting and Clinical Psychology 55: 3–9.
10. Remington B, Hastings RP, Kovshoff H, degli Espinosa F, Jahr E, et al. (2007) Early Intensive Behavioral Intervention: Outcomes for Children With Autism and Their Parents After Two Years. American Journal on Mental Retardation 112: 418–438.
11. Harris SL, Handleman JS (2000) Age and IQ at Intake as Predictors of Placement for Young Children with Autism: A Four- to Six-Year Follow-Up. Journal of Autism and Developmental Disorders 30: 137–142.
12. Fenske EC, Zalenski S, Krantz PJ, McClannahan LE (1985) Age at intervention and treatment outcome for autistic children in a comprehensive intervention program. Analysis and Intervention in Developmental Disabilities 5: 49–58.
13. Matson JL, Wilkins J, Boisjoli JA, Smith KR (2008) The validity of the autism spectrum disorders-diagnosis for intellectually disabled adults (ASD-DA). Research in Developmental Disabilities 29: 537–546.
14. Hayes AF (2009) Beyond Baron and Kenny: Statistical mediation analysis in the new millennium. Communication Monographs 76: 408–420.
15. MacKinnon DP, Fairchild AJ, Fritz MS (2007) Mediation analysis. Annual Review of Psychology 58: 593.
16. Montes G, Halterman JS (2008) Association of Childhood Autism Spectrum Disorders and Loss of Family Income. Pediatrics 121: e821–e826.
17. Parish SL, Thomas KC, Rose R, Kilany M, Shattuck PT (2012) State Medicaid Spending and Financial Burden of Families Raising Children with Autism. Intellectual and Developmental Disabilities 50: 441–451.
18. Phelps KW, Hodgson JL, McCammon SL, Lamson AL (2009) Caring for an individual with autism disorder: A qualitative analysis*. Journal of Intellectual and Developmental Disability 34: 27–35.
19. Sharpe D, Baker D (2007) Financial Issues Associated with Having a Child with Autism. Journal of Family and Economic Issues 28: 247–264.
20. Ganz ML (2007) THe lifetime distribution of the incremental societal costs of autism. Archives of Pediatrics & Adolescent Medicine 161: 343–349.
21. Ganz M (2006) The Costs of Autism. Understanding Autism: CRC Press. pp. 475–502.
22. Hartley SL, Barker ET, Seltzer MM, Floyd F, Greenberg J, et al. (2010) The Relative Risk and Timing of Divorce in Families of Children with an Autism Spectrum Disorder. Journal of Family Psychology 24: 449–457.
23. Keenan M, Dillenburger K, Doherty A, Byrne T, Gallagher S (2010) The Experiences of Parents During Diagnosis and Forward Planning for Children with Autism Spectrum Disorder. Journal of Applied Research in Intellectual Disabilities 23: 390–397.
24. Australian Government (2013) Helping Children with Autism. Department of Families, Housing, Community Services and Indigenous Affairs.

24

Gender-Dependent Effects of Maternal Immune Activation on the Behavior of Mouse Offspring

Ingrid C. Y. Xuan[1], David R. Hampson[1,2]*

1 Department of Pharmaceutical Sciences, Leslie Dan Faculty of Pharmacy, University of Toronto, Toronto, Canada, 2 Department of Pharmacology and Toxicology, Faculty of Medicine, University of Toronto, Toronto, Canada

Abstract

Autism spectrum disorders are neurodevelopmental disorders characterized by two core symptoms; impaired social interactions and communication, and ritualistic or repetitive behaviors. Both epidemiological and biochemical evidence suggests that a subpopulation of autistics may be linked to immune perturbations that occurred during fetal development. These findings have given rise to an animal model, called the "maternal immune activation" model, whereby the offspring from female rodents who were subjected to an immune stimulus during early or mid-pregnancy are studied. Here, C57BL/6 mouse dams were treated mid-gestation with saline, lipopolysaccharide (LPS) to mimic a bacterial infection, or polyinosinic:polycytidylic acid (Poly IC) to mimic a viral infection. Autism-associated behaviors were examined in the adult offspring of the treated dams. Behavioral tests were conducted to assess motor activity, exploration in a novel environment, sociability, and repetitive behaviors, and data analyses were carried independently on male and female mice. We observed a main treatment effect whereby male offspring from Poly IC-treated dams showed reduced motor activity. In the marble burying test of repetitive behavior, male offspring but not female offspring from both LPS and Poly IC-treated mothers showed increased marble burying. Our findings indicate that offspring from mothers subjected to immune stimulation during gestation show a gender-specific increase in stereotyped repetitive behavior.

Editor: Michel Baudry, Western University of Health Sciences, United States of America

Funding: This work was supported by the Canadian Institutes for Health Research (CIHR) and the CIHR Strategic Training Program in Biological Therapeutics. The funders had no role in study design, data collection and analysis, decision to publish, or preparation of the manuscript.

Competing Interests: The authors have declared that no competing interests exist.

* Email: d.hampson@utoronto.ca

Introduction

Autism spectrum disorders (ASDs) are a behaviorally defined class of neurodevelopmental disorders characterized by two core symptoms: 1) social and communication impairments, and 2) ritualistic repetitive behaviors [1]. The auxillary symptoms associated with ASDs are highly heterogeneous and vary in severity. Examples include hyperactivity, motor impairments, intellectual disability, and anxiety [2,3,4]. The diagnosis of ASD shows a marked male preponderance with incidence estimates of male-to-females ranging from 3-fold to 11-fold [5,6,7]. As noted by Kim et al., 2013, the male prevalence of ASD is similar to other early onset anti-social disorders such as developmental language disorder and attention-deficit hyperactivity disorder [8,9]. The reasons for this high male prevalence remain unclear.

About 10–20% of ASD cases can be attributed to genetic factors, while the causes of the other 80–90% are unknown [10]. Since ASD is typically diagnosed at 1–3 years of age, the prenatal environment may be particularly important for the pathogenesis of this disorder. Hallmayer et al., 2011 compared the incidence of ASD between monozygotic and dizygotic twins and found that approximately 58% of the liability to autism could be explained by environmental factors common to twins [11]. Environmental factors such as infection may trigger the maternal and/or fetal immune systems and alter the normal brain maturation process, resulting in brain pathologies and behavioral abnormalities. Epidemiological studies suggest that maternal immune activation (MIA) during pregnancy may be a risk factor for ASD. Based on a large Danish cohort (N = 1.6 million), Atladóttir et al., 2010 found that maternal viral and bacterial infection (specifically respiratory infection) during the first trimester increased the risk of ASD in the offspring by two and three-fold, respectively [12]. The same group also reported that a febrile episode lasting more than seven days increased the risk of infantile autism by three-fold in the first trimester and four-fold in the second trimester [13]. In a separate study based on a large Finnish cohort (N = 1.2 million), an increased level of maternal C-reactive protein, a biomarker for inflammation, was shown to be significantly associated with ASD diagnosis in the offspring [14].

The involvement of immune activation in ASD is further supported by reported increased serum cytokine levels in ASD patients [15], and by elevated expression of cellular markers for microglia and astrocytes in post-mortem brain tissue from persons with ASD [16,17,18,19]. Rodent-based MIA models of neurodevelopmental disorders were developed to mimic aspects of these phenomena in a laboratory setting. It is important to note however that in addition to ASD, the MIA paradigm has also been used to model schizophrenia, which has similarly been associated with prenatal immune disturbances in the patient population [20,21,22]. Maternal immune activation is typically induced by injecting lipopolysaccharide (LPS) or polyinosinic:polycytidylic acid (Poly IC) into pregnant female rats or mice during gestation to mimic a bacterial or viral infection, respectively [23]. ASD-like behaviors most often studied include measuring impairments in social interactions, increased repetitive behavior assessed using the marble burying test or quantitating self-grooming events, and the examination of anxiety levels in the open field test [24,25,26,27].

The objective of the present study was to compare the effects of MIA on the behavior of male vs. female mouse offspring. We examined the effects of MIA induced by either LPS, or by Poly IC. Our findings indicate that both the gender of the mouse, and the type of immune stimulus influence a subset of autistic behaviors of MIA offspring.

Experimental Procedures

Induction of MIA

All animal experiments were carried out in accordance with the guidelines set out by the Canadian Council on Animal Care and were approved by the University of Toronto Animal Care Committee. All experiments were carried out using C57BL/6 mice housed in cages containing 4 mice and with lights on at 6:00 a.m. and off at 8:00 p.m. The mice were mated overnight and checked for the presence of a vaginal plug at 9 a.m. each day; the day that the vaginal plug was observed was marked as embryonic day 0.5 (E0.5). A total of 5 litters were used from Poly IC-injected dams, 6 litters from LPS-injected dams, and 6 litters from saline-injected dams.

The LPS injection protocol used was a modification of the multiple injection procedure used in rats by Girard et al., 2010. For LPS treated mouse dams, two intra-peritoneal (i.p.) injections of 75 μg/kg LPS (5 μl/g lipopolysaccharide O127:B8; Sigma Cat. # L3129) were given on both days E11.5 and E12. For Poly IC, dams were injected i.p. with 20 mg/kg polyinosinic:polycytidylic acid (Poly IC) potassium salt (5 μl/g; Sigma Cat. #P9582) once on E12.5. Poly IC was dissolved in saline at 4 mg/mL (based on the weight of Poly IC itself, which was 10% of total weight of the salt). Separate groups of control female mice were injected with saline on E11.5 and E12.5 (LPS control), or only on E12.5 (Poly IC control).

Behavioral testing

All pups were housed with their mother until postnatal day (PND) 21 when they were weaned and ear tagged. After weaning, two to four pups of the same sex and treatment were housed together per cage. In cases where only a single female or male was born in one litter, it was housed with other mice of same sex and similar age (from a different treatment group). All animals were left undisturbed except for biweekly cage changes and behavior tests. The order of behavioral testing was as follows: 1) motor activity at postnatal 6–7 weeks; 2) modified 3-chamber paradigm social test at 7–8 weeks; 3) self-repetitive grooming at 7–8 weeks scored based on recorded videos during social testing; 4) marble burying test at 9–10 weeks. All behavioral testing with the exception of the social tests was conducted between 9 am and 2 p.m.; social testing was performed between 10 a.m. and 5 p.m.

Motor Activity

Motor activity was measured using an automated VersaMax animal activity monitoring system (AccuScan Instruments, Inc., U.S.A.) as previously described [28]. The detection system consisted of a 42×42×30 cm plexiglas box placed inside the activity monitor that emitted 16×16×16 laser beams, each separated by 2.5 cm; the system measured the animal's activity by tracking the number of beams that were broken. Two smaller plexiglas boxes (21×21×21 cm) were placed at diagonal corners inside the larger plexiglas box for activity measurement of each individual mouse. All animals were habituated under dim lighting (the room was evenly lit by three 14 W incandescent light fixtures) for at least one hour prior to testing. Before each test, the smaller box was wiped thoroughly with Virox (0.4% hydrogen peroxide) followed by water. The animal was gently placed in the center of the smaller box with a lid; the test was performed under dim lighting and the data generated by the monitor was tabulated every 5 minutes for an hour. The following parameters were analyzed: total distance travelled, horizontal movement number, vertical movement number, per cent of total distance travelled in the center zone (center defined as 10.5 cm×10.5 cm), and time spent in the center zone.

Social Interaction and Social Preference Tests

A modified three-chamber protocol was used based on that described by Ramsey et al., 2011 with some modifications [29]. The test was conducted under dim lighting (approximately 40 lux). A digital camera was mounted on the ceiling approximately one meter above the social apparatus to track the locomotion of the animal. Rather than physically separating the chambers, we virtually defined two identical circular zones (diameter: 19.8 cm) in a white plexiglas box (61.7×40.8×23 cm) using Viewer^2 software (BIOBSERVE GmbH, NJ). These two zones were side-by-side to each other and equidistant from the edge of the box (7.1 cm lengthwise, 10.5 cm widthwise). An empty white wire cage (top diameter 7.5 cm, bottom diameter 10 cm, height 10 cm) was placed at the center of each zone, covered by a white circular disk (diameter: 10 cm) and held down by a standard 400 ml glass beaker. The beaker prevented the test animals from climbing on top of the wire cages. Two removable, white cardboard dividers (40×23 cm) were inserted into the middle of the box to shield both zones. The activity of the animal in each zone was recorded every 2 minutes for 10 minutes.

The stimulus animals (untreated wild-type C57BL/6 mice age and sex matched with the test animal) were kept at the opposite corner from the test animal to ensure its novelty. Stimulus animals were habituated for 30–60 minutes in their respective home cage under dim lighting as previously described. Each animal was then allowed to habituate to the inside of a clean cylindrical wire cage placed inside the white plexiglas box. A maximum of six stimulus animals were habituated at the same time for two 15-minute sessions. The stimulus animals were used for subsequent social testing if no persistent aggressive behavior was observed (e.g. climbing and/or biting of the cage).

Test animals were habituated for at least one hour in their home cages under dim lighting as previously described. Before each test, all apparatus were wiped vigorously with Virox, followed by water. To begin, the test animal was gently placed between the dividers. Then the dividers were simultaneously lifted, exposing the animal to the two zones, each with an empty wire cage held down by a beaker as previously described. After the animal was allowed to habituate for 10 minutes, it was then isolated between the two dividers again, shielding it from the two zones. If side preference was present (i.e. the difference in time spent between the two zones was more than 30 seconds), the animal was returned to home cage and tested the next day. Otherwise, the social interaction test was performed. One stimulus animal (of same sex and similar age) was placed in one of the wire cages while a novel object was placed in the other cage. The designation of the zones was determined at random. The novel object used was a green Biobag tied into a knot placed on top of a roll of green tape (6 cm diameter). The dividers were then simultaneously lifted and the animal was allowed to

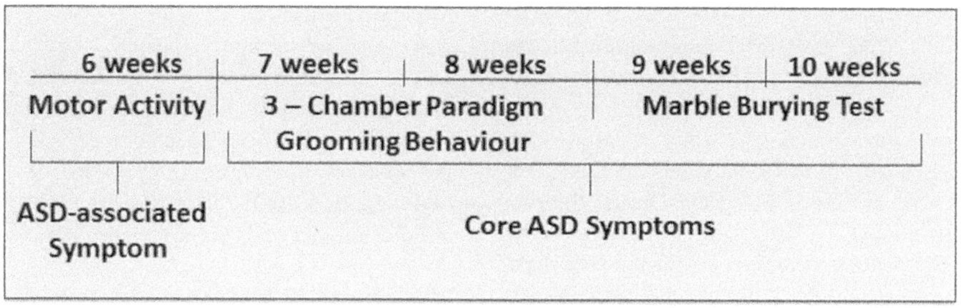

Figure 1. Timeline for behavioral testing. The age of the mice in weeks is indicated.

explore for 10 minutes. During this 10 minute period, the time spent in each zone was recorded. At the end of the social interaction test, the animal was again isolated between the dividers to shield it from both zones. Subsequently, the social preference test was performed where a novel stimulus mouse (of same sex and similar age) was placed in the non-social zone, replacing the novel object; this then became the non-familiar zone. The dividers were then lifted simultaneously and the animal was allowed to explore for 10 minutes while the time spent in each zone was recorded.

A t-test was performed to determine if there was a significant preference for one zone over the other in the social interaction and social preference tests; each treatment group was evaluated separately [30,31].

Marble Burying Assay

The marble burying assay, a test for repetitive/compulsive behavior, was conducted at 10 weeks of age as previously described [32]. Clean cages (29.5×17.5×12.5 cm) were filled 5 cm deep with corn cob bedding. Twenty identical navy blue marbles (1.2 cm diameter) were placed in a 4×5 rectangular matrix occupying 2/3 of the cage. The animals were first habituated in the biosafety cabinet class A/B for at least 30 minutes with the blower on as background noise. After habituation, the test mouse was gently placed into 1/3 of the cage without the marbles and a lid was immediately placed over the cage. Individual test animals were allowed to explore the cage for a 30 minute test period after which they were returned to the home cages. A marble was considered buried when more than 50% of its surface area was covered by the bedding. The marbles were cleaned with Virox and rinsed with water between each test.

Grooming analysis

Self-grooming behavior entails licking and scratching of any body parts of the mouse [33]. The total time spent grooming (in seconds) was recorded manually based on previously recorded video during the first 5 minutes of habituation in the three-chamber paradigm.

Statistical Analyses

Statistical analyses were performed using SPSS version 18. For thigmotaxis, marble burying, and grooming, a two-way ANOVA analysis was used to determine differences among multiple groups with two variables (i.e. gender and treatment), followed where appropriate by the Bonferroni post hoc test. For motor activity analysis, a three way ANOVA was carried out using treatment x gender x time interval. A two-tailed Student's t-test using GraphPad Prism was used for within group comparisons (e.g. saline social zone vs. saline non-social zone) in the social interaction and preference tests. Grubbs' test was used to eliminate outliers. For all statistical tests, $p<0.05$ was considered significant and $0.05<p<0.1$ was considered as a trend towards a significant effect.

Results

To avoid potential complications from analyzing mice during the period when the brain is rapidly maturing, behavioral testing began in late adolescent mice at 6 weeks of age (Fig. 1). This corresponds to an age just prior to brain maturation in the mouse at 7–8 weeks postnatal. To reduce the effects of repeated measures, behavioral analyses were conducted one week apart. Video recording of grooming was conducted during the habituation period of social testing as well as during the social preference test.

The effect of MIA on body weight

The body weights of MIA offspring were measured on PND 46 as an indicator of their overall health. Male saline, LPS, and Poly IC mice weighed 21.8±0.5, 23.0±0.2, 21.7±0.5 grams respectively; female saline, LPS, and Poly IC mice weighed 18.0±0.3, 17.6±0.4, and 17.8±0.6 grams (mean ± S.E.M; n = 7–17 per group). As expected, male mice were heavier than female mice (F (1, 68) = 160.9, $p<0.0001$). However, body weight was not affected by prenatal LPS or Poly IC infection (F (2, 68) = 1.14, $p = 0.3251$), and there was no significant interaction between treatment and gender (F (2, 68) = 2.45, $p = 0.0943$).

The effect of MIA on motor and open field activity

Locomotor and exploratory behaviors of MIA offspring were investigated by measuring horizontal activity, vertical activity, and thigmotaxis behavior in an automated activity box. All parameters were separately analyzed over three time intervals: 0 to 20, 20 to 40 and 40 to 60 minutes with the exception of thigmotaxis behaviour, which was analyzed only during the first time interval at 0 to 20 minutes. A summary of all statistical analyses is shown in Table S1.

The treatment x gender interaction effect was not significant for any of the three time intervals, and prenatal LPS treatment did not affect the horizontal activity of either female or male offspring during any of the three time intervals. However, in male offspring, a significant main effect of treatment was seen where the Poly IC mice displayed reduced total distance travelled (Fig. 2A) and reduced horizontal movement number (Fig. 2B) at 20–40 minutes (total distance travelled: F (2, 107) = 10.81, $p<0.001$, Bonferroni post hoc test $p<0.001$; horizontal movement number: F (2, 107) = 9.43, $p<0.001$, Bonferroni post hoc test $p<0.001$), and 40–60 minutes (total distance travelled: F (2, 107) = 4.35, $p<0.05$, Bonferroni post hoc test $p<0.01$; horizontal movement number: F (2, 107) = 5.41, $p<0.01$, Bonferroni post hoc test $p<0.01$). The gender effect was significant for total distance travelled only during the last two time intervals (20–40 min: F (1, 107) = 4.72, $p<0.05$; 40–60 min: F (1, 107) = 24.86, $p<0.001$) and significant for movement number during the last time interval (F (1, 107) = 13.30, $p<0.001$).

The effect of maternal immune activation on vertical activity, measured by vertical movement number, was gender-dependent (Figure S1). There was a significant gender effect during the first two time intervals (0–20 min: (F (1, 107) = 20.77, $p<0.001$) and 20–40 minutes (F (1, 107) = 6.40, $p<0.05$)). A significant treatment effect was observed for the middle time interval only (F (2, 107) = 4.91, $p<0.01$). However, further post-hoc test showed that neither LPS nor Poly IC offspring significantly differed from control. The treatment x gender interaction effect for vertical movement number was not significant for any of the three time intervals.

Thigmotaxis describes the animals' innate preference to stay near the walls rather than the center of the open field. Increased thigmotaxis is indicative of increased anxiety, which is an associated symptom of ASD. To investigate this behavior in the MIA mice, we measured the activity of the mice in the center zone of the motor activity box during the first 20 minutes of the exploration period (Figure S2). There was a significant gender effect for both time spent in center (F (1, 104) = 5.61, $p<0.05$) and per cent of total distance travelled in the center zone (F (1, 104) = 9.29, $p<0.01$). The treatment main effect and treatment x gender interaction were not statistically significant.

The effects of MIA on social behavior

Social impairment is one of the core symptoms of ASD and is often linked with deficits in communication. In rodents this behavior can be assessed using three-chamber testing paradigms [34]. The test is divided into two stages. In the social interaction test, sociability was measured by comparing the time the animal spent in the zone with a novel mouse (the social zone) versus a novel object (non-social zone; Fig. 3A). In the second stage,

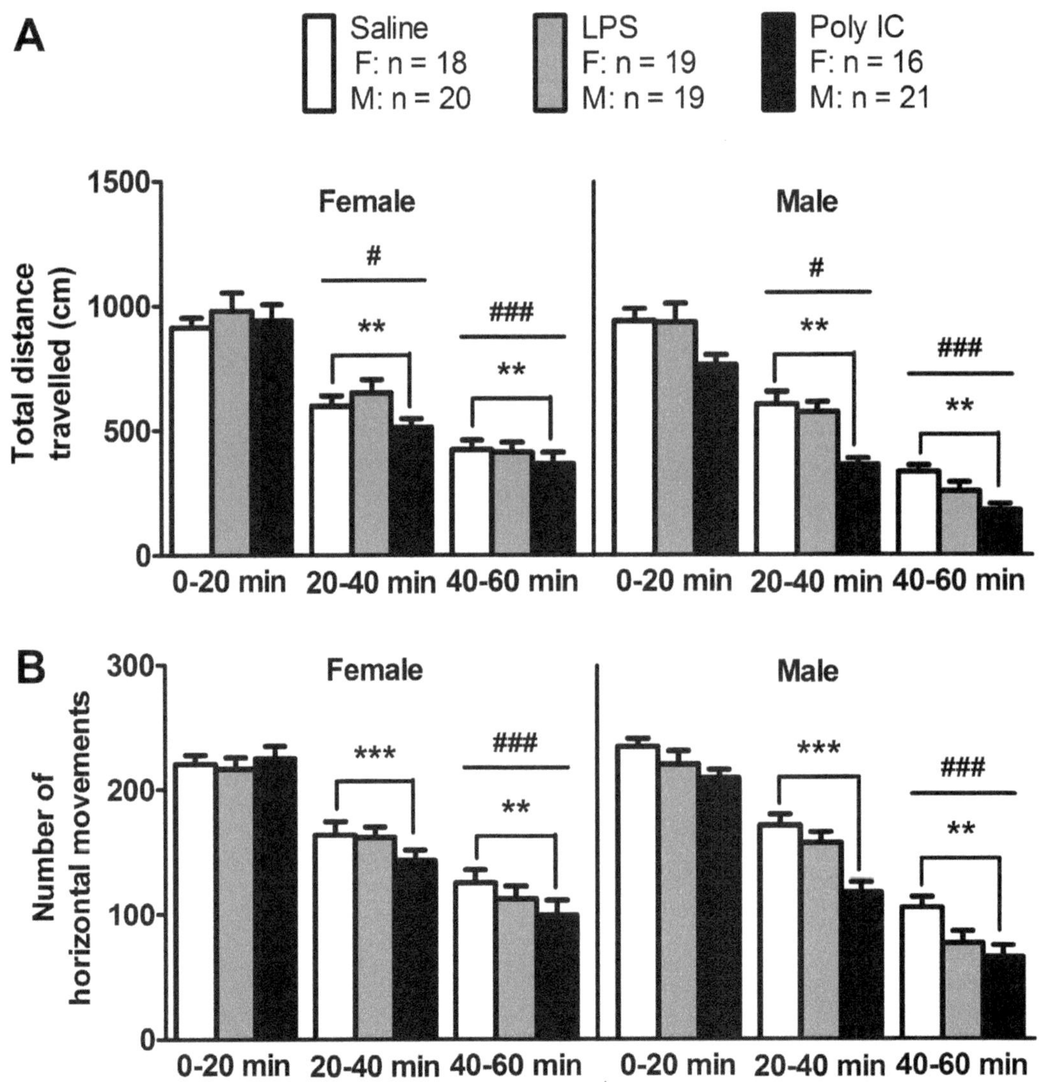

Figure 2. The effects of maternal immune activation on horizontal motor activity of adult offspring. Compared to saline offspring, Poly IC offspring, but not LPS offspring, showed significantly reduced (A) total distance travelled and (B) number of movements at 20–40 minutes and 40–60 minutes (**p<0.01, ***p<0.001; see Table S1 for a summary of statistical analyses). A significant gender effect was also observed at 20–40 minutes and/or 40–60 minutes (#p<0.05; ###p<0.001). Each column represents mean ± S.E.M. The number of mice tested (n) for males (m) and females (f) for each condition is indicated.

termed the social preference test, sociability was measured by comparing the time the animal spent in the zone with a familiar mouse (the familiar zone) versus a new non-familiar mouse (the non-familiar zone, Figure S3A). In both tests, normal social behavior entailed significant preference for the social and non-familiar zones over the non-social and familiar zones, respectively.

For the social interaction test, saline-treated offspring demonstrated normal social behavior by spending significantly more time in the social zone rather than the non-social zone (Fig. 3B; female: t (9) = 5.09, $p<0.001$; male: t (9) = 3.96, $p<0.01$). Prenatal LPS caused abnormal social behavior in female offspring where the mice did not show significant preference for the social chamber (LPS: t (10) = 1.79, $p = 0.1041$). In contrast, male LPS offspring demonstrated normal social behaviour (LPS: t (10) = 9.59, $p<0.0001$). Male mice from Poly IC injected mothers showed a strong trend towards normal behavior (Fig. 3B; t (6) = 2.38, $p = 0.0548$).

In the social preference test, neither female (saline: t (9) = 1.31, $p = 0.2222$, LPS: (t (10) = 1.14, $p = 0.2803$, Poly IC: (t (9) = 1.30, $p = 0.2261$) nor male offspring (saline: t (9) = 1.42, $p = 0.1893$, LPS: (t (10) = 1.59, $p = 0.1422$), Poly IC: (t (6) = 1.49, $p = 0.1870$) showed a significant preference for the non-familiar zone over the familiar zone (Figure S3B). A two-way ANOVA comparison of the time spent in the non-familiar zone between different treatment groups showed no significant treatment effect, gender effect, or interaction effect.

The effect of MIA on repetitive behaviors

Ritualistic and repetitive behavior is another core symptom of ASD. Such behavior can be assessed in rodents using the marble burying test where increased repetitive behavior is represented by more buried marbles (32). The results of the two-way ANOVA revealed a significant treatment effect (Fig. 4A; F (2, 89) = 5.72, $p<0.01$) where both male Poly IC (Bonferroni post-hoc test $p<0.001$) and male LPS offspring (Bonferroni post-hoc test $p<0.05$) buried significantly more marbles than compare to saline treated control male mice. The interaction between treatment x gender was significant (F (2, 89) = 4.09, $p<0.05$), and notably, neither LPS

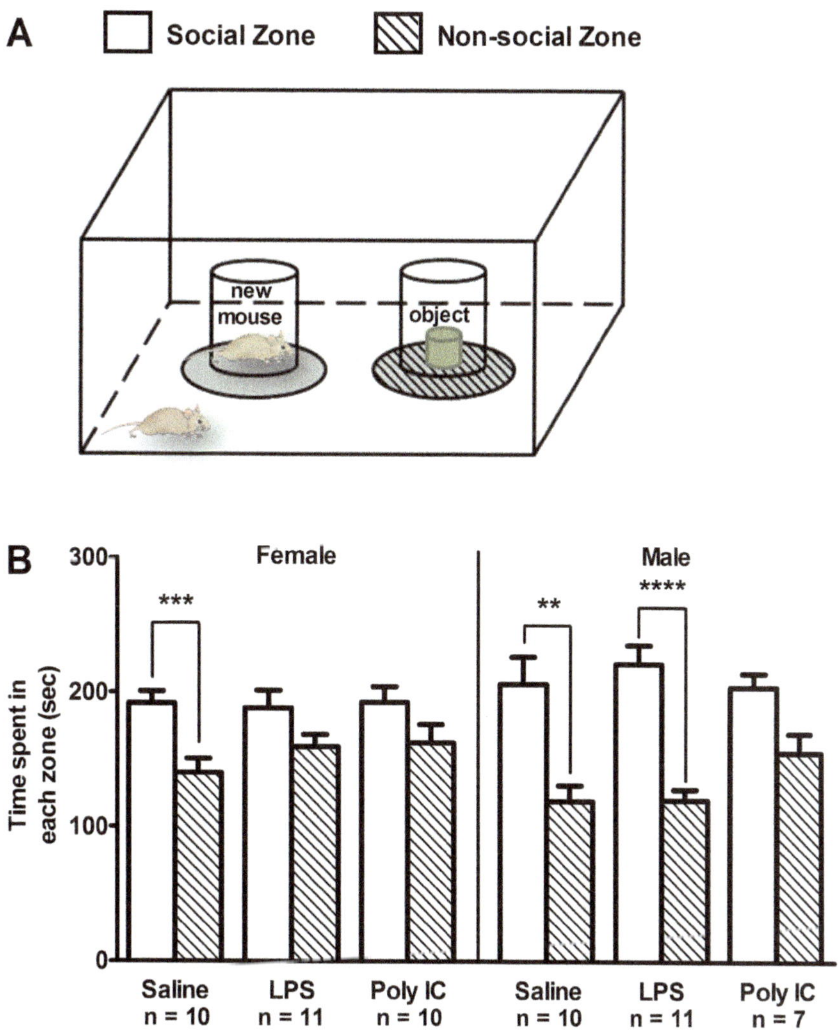

Figure 3. The effects of maternal immune activation on social behavior in the three-chamber social interaction test. (A) diagrammatic depiction of the experimental set-up for the social interaction test. (B) Male and female saline-treated mice showed the expected preference for the social zone (**$p<0.01$; ***$p<0.001$; ****p<0.0001). However, compared to saline-treated controls, female LPS and Poly IC offspring showed no significant preference for the social zone over the non-social zone. A loss of the normal social interaction behavior was also observed in male Poly IC mice, but not in male LPS mice compared to control mice. Each column represents mean ± S.E.M.

nor Poly IC female offspring displayed increased marble burying compared to controls (Fig. 4A).

Repetitive behavior was also evaluated by scoring the time the animal spent grooming during the first five minutes of the habituation period (i.e. exploration in open field box with two empty wire cages with no stimulus mice present) and the first five minutes of the social preference test (i.e. exploration in open field box with two wire cages, each with a stimulus mouse trapped inside) (Fig. 4B). There was a significant treatment effect for both grooming during habituation period (F (2, 51) = 3.76, $p<0.05$) and social preference test (F (2, 56) = 3.50, $p<0.05$). However, post-hoc analysis showed no statistical significance between saline and LPS or saline and Poly IC for both sexes. A significant gender effect was found only during the habituation period (F (1, 51) = 10.24, $p<$ 0.01). The treatment x gender interaction was not significant for the habituation period (F (1, 51) = 0.8205, p = 0.4459) or during social preference test (F (1, 56) = 0.2280, p = 0.7968).

Discussion

This study was designed to investigate gender differences in mice in response to immune activators administered to the mother during pregnancy. Whereas most (but not all, see below) previous studies on MIA have either examined only male rodents, or have combined male and females together, here we directly compared the behavioral effects of LPS and Poly IC in separate groups of male and female mice. Our findings indicate that male and female offspring from mothers injected with LPS or Poly IC during mid-gestation display disparate behaviors on tests of motor activity, social interactions, and repetitive or stereotyped behaviors.

Impairments in social interactions and communication are core symptoms of ASD. Our findings revealed modest social impairments in female LPS offspring. Kirsten et al. 2010; 2012 investigated sociability in rats prenatally treated with LPS by subjecting the offspring to a novel free moving stimulus animal in a

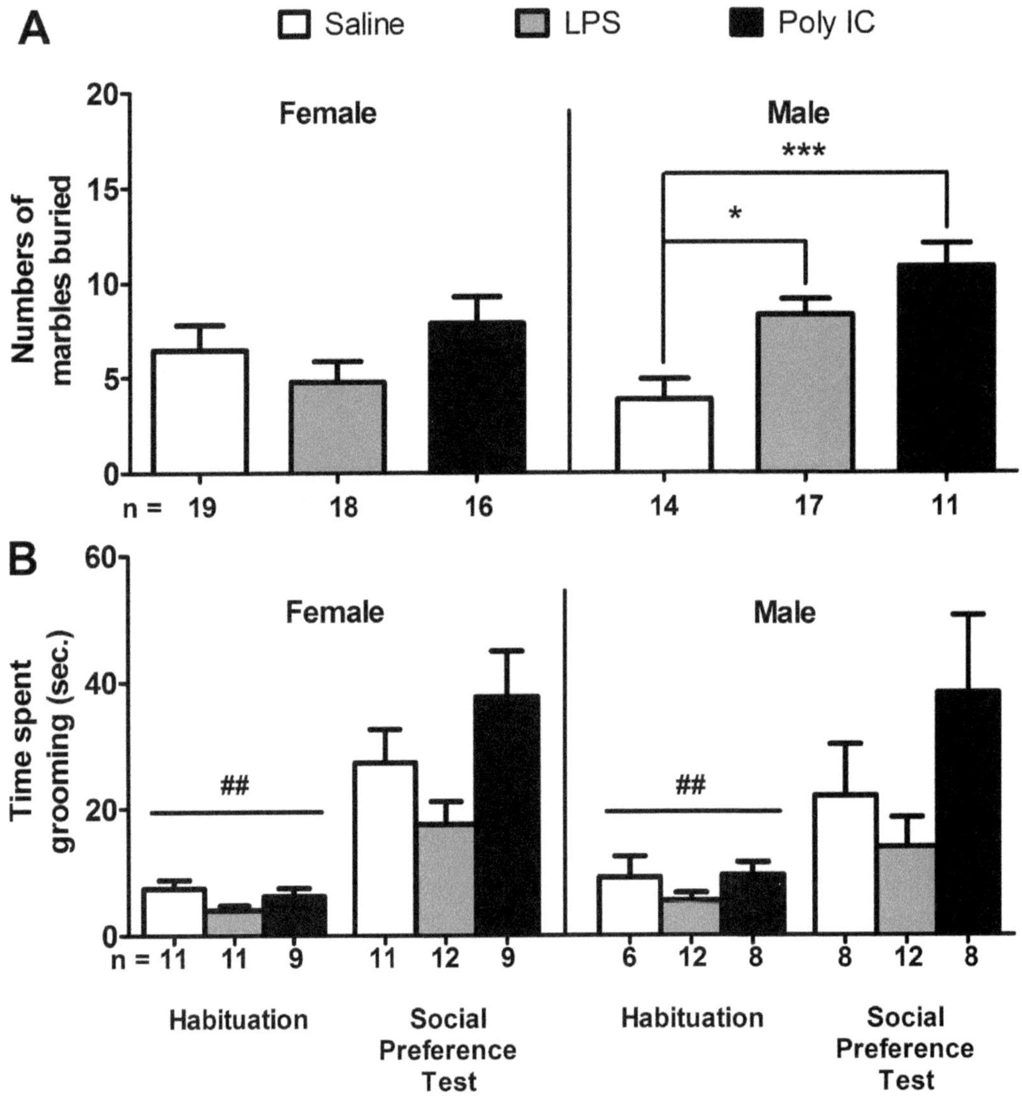

Figure 4. Analysis of repetitive behaviors. (A) In the marble burying test, both male LPS and male Poly IC offspring showed significantly increased repetitive behavior, whereas female LPS and female Poly IC offspring did not (*$p<0.05$, ***$p<0.001$, between treatments). (B) Self-grooming during the habituation period prior to social testing, and during the social preference test. During habituation, a significant gender main effect was observed (##$p<0.01$, between gender). During the social preference test, male Poly IC mice, and to a lesser extent female Poly IC mice, showed a non-significant elevation of grooming relative to saline-treated controls. Each column represents mean ± S.E.M.

cage, and manually scoring their play behavior including sniffing, following, crawling under/over, and mounting on the stimulus rat; they found male-specific deficits in the latter two parameters only [25,26]. These two parameters measure more aggressive behaviors that are usually more common in male rodents. Our test conditions were less aggressive because the stimulus mice were constrained in wire cups; this could have contributed to the differences that we observed between male and female animals. Importantly, Kirsten et al., 2010 were only able to detect deficits in social interaction when they isolated the rats (i.e. one rat per cage) for a week prior to testing in order to increase the rats' social motivation (not done in the present study) [25]. Therefore, due to the differences in experimental conditions, the lack of social interaction in female rats observed by Kirsten et al. 2012 does not necessarily contradict our results.

The presence of repetitive behavior remains one of the core criteria for the diagnosis of autism in the revised DMS-V manual used by many clinicians world-wide. One of the more striking results that we observed in terms of both the magnitude of the effect, and the gender divergence, was on the quantitation of repetitive and stereotyped behaviors. Although other groups have reported elevated repetitive behaviors after MIA in rodents [26,27,35,36,37], these and other studies most often used males only, or combined data from both sexes [38] for discussion on male bias in immune activation studies).

Our results highlight the male selectivity of this phenomenon in the MIA animal model. Male LPS and Poly IC offspring both showed robust increases in marble burying, whereas female LPS and Poly IC mice showed no significant increase. In addition to increased repetitive behaviors, the same group of male Poly IC-treated mice also showed decreased motor activity as measured by total distance traveled and the number of horizontal movements initiated. The decrease in movements is likely the result of more time spent engaging in stationary, stereotyped behavior.

Schwartzer et al., 2013 examined repetitive behaviors after Poly IC MIA in two strains of mice, the C57/BL6 as used here, and the BTBR mouse, an inbred strain reported to be predisposed to exhibit ASD-like behavior [35]. The Poly IC offspring of both strains showed significantly elevated marble burying compared to saline controls but male and female data were combined. In the grooming test where male and female data were reported separately, increased grooming was observed only in males for both strains (the effect was significant in BTBR mice). Moreover, in the present study, we also examined the offspring from a separate group of mice whose mothers were given a second injection of Poly IC during a second pregnancy after the first Poly IC litter was born. Again, male offspring from the second litter showed a significant increase in marble burying over saline controls, whereas the female mice did not (see Figure S4), further confirming the gender selectivity of stereotyped behavior in the Poly IC MIA model.

The strong sex-bias observed in marble burying and grooming in MIA mice is, in fact, reflected in human ASD patients. Several studies have demonstrated that male autistics have more repetitive and/or restricted interests compared to female autistics [39–44]. However, there are also a few published studies that found no gender differences in repetitive behavior in ASD in children and adolescents [45] and in pre-school children with suspected ASD [46]. Overall, we note that the lack of, or lower level of motor stereotypies generally reported in females with ASD, does not preclude the possibility that they may possess other forms of repetitive behavior, such as restricted interests or other forms of ritualistic behavior.

The question as to the nature of the underlying molecular and cellular mechanism(s) linking immune perturbations to ASD remains unanswered. Poly IC is a double-stranded RNA which mimics a viral infection and activates Toll-like Receptor 3 while LPS is a cell wall component of gram negative bacteria that activates Toll-like Receptor 4 [47,48]. Activation of Toll-like Receptors induces the production of immune proteins including cytokines, and also long non-coding RNAs which regulate the innate immune response [49]. The induction of MIA in rodents has been associated with elevated levels of pro-inflammatory cytokines in the maternal circulation, as well as in the placenta and fetal circulation [38,50,51]. It should be noted that another study in mice demonstrated that even in the absence of an immune stimulus, cytokines display dynamic changes in levels over the course of normal development and also that a widespread decrease was detected in several brain cytokines during peak periods of synaptogenesis and plasticity (PND 7–30) [51]. This group also reported low levels of some cytokines after induction of MIA and suggested that aberrantly low cytokine signaling might be a factor causing altered brain connectivity and ASD and/or schizophrenic-like behaviors in the offspring [51]. Finally, within the context of neurodevelopmental disorders, although the mechanisms by which cytokines (and chemokines) [15] might induce deleterious effects is not yet known, one working concept is that there is a disruption after MIA of the normal balance between pro- and anti-inflammatory influences that is critical for normal fetal brain development [23,52].

In summary, our findings indicate that immune stimulation during fetal development in mice causes differential effects in males vs. females. Intriguingly, our results reveal that MIA induces the selective induction of stereotyped, repetitive behavior in male mouse offspring but not female offspring. This finding is consistent with reports of a higher incidence of repetitive behaviors in male compared to female autistic patients. Although certain brain regions such as the cerebellum and basal ganglia have been associated with repetitive behaviors in both humans with autism and in animal models of autism, and alterations in cytokines could be a contributing factor, future studies should be directed towards further elucidating the molecular mechanisms underlying the gender-selective effects of *in utero* immune activation on repetitive and other autistic-like behaviors.

Supporting Information

Figure S1 The effects of maternal immune activation on vertical motor activity of adult offspring. ANOVA revealed a significant gender effect for first two time intervals (0–20 min: (F (1, 107) = 20.77, ###$p<0.001$) and 20–40 minutes (F (1, 107) = 6.40, #$p<0.05$). A significant treatment effect was observed in the middle time interval (F (2, 107) = 4.91, $p<0.01$), although a post-hoc Bonferroni test did not reveal a significance difference between groups. The treatment x gender interaction effect was not significant for any of the time intervals. Each column represents mean ± S.E.M. The number of mice tested (n) for males (m) and females (f) for each condition is indicated.

Figure S2 Analysis of thigmotaxis behavior of adult offspring. Total time in the center zone is shown in panel A, while the total distance travelled in the center zone of the activity box during the first 20 minutes of the exploration period is shown in panel B. No significant treatment effects were seen among the groups. However, a significant gender effect was observed for both tests (#p<0.05; ##p<0.01). Each column represents mean ±

S.E.M. The number of mice tested (n) for each condition is indicated.

Figure S3 The effects of maternal immune activation on social behavior of adult offspring during the three-chamber social preference test. (A) Diagrammatic depiction of the experimental set-up for the social preference test. (B) No significant preference for the non-familiar zone over the familiar zone was seen in any of the test conditions. Each column represents average ± S.E.M.

Figure S4 The effects of maternal immune activation on marble burying of adult offspring. Poly IC 2X offspring were produced from dams that have been injected with 20 mg/kg of Poly IC on E12.5 during two consecutive pregnancies. Two-way ANOVA revealed a significant treatment effect (F (1, 84) = 4.87, $p<0.05$), gender effect (F (1, 84) = 8.24, $p<0.01$), and treatment x gender interaction effect (F (1, 84) = 11.0, $p<0.01$, see Table S1 for statistical details). Further post-hoc test showed that male Poly 2X offspring buried significantly more marbles compared to the respective saline controls, while female Poly 2X offspring showed no significant difference. Each column represents mean ± S.E.M. ##$p<0.01$ (between gender); ***p<0.001 (between treatment).

Table S1 Summary of statistical analyses. 2-way ANOVA was conducted for Saline, LPS 1X, Poly IC 1X for all behavioural tests with the exception of Figure S4 where 2-way ANOVA analysis was performed for Saline and Poly 2X offspring only. 3-way ANOVA was performed for motor activity (i.e. Fig. 2 and Figure S1). In cases where the treatment effect was significant but the treatment x gender Interaction effect was not significant, a Bonferroni Post-hoc test was performed for treatment by combining male and female data. In cases where both the treatment effect and treatment x gender interaction effect were significant, a Bonferroni Post-hoc test was performed for treatment for each gender separately. Hor. – horizontal motor activity; Ver. – vertical motor activity; M – Male; F – Female. N/A – not applicable.

Acknowledgments

The authors thank Marija Milenkovic, Drs. Laurel Duquette, Nickolas Mitsakakis, Laura K. K. Pacey, and Amy Ramsey for advice on the behavioral tests and analysis of the data, and Dr. Dianne M. Broussard for helpful comments on the manuscript. This work was supported by the Canadian Institutes of Health Research.

Author Contributions

Conceived and designed the experiments: IX DRH. Performed the experiments: IX. Analyzed the data: IX DRH. Contributed to the writing of the manuscript: IX DRH.

References

1. American Psychiatric Association (2013) Diagnostic and statistical manual of mental disorders (5th ed.) http://dx.doi.org/10.1176/appi.books.9780890425596.910646.
2. Matson JL, Nebel-Schwalm MS (2007) Comorbid psychopathology with autism spectrum disorder in children: An overview. Res Dev Disabil 28: 341–352.
3. Charman T, Pickles A, Simonoff E, Chandler S, Loucas T, et al. (2011) IQ in children with autism spectrum disorders: Data from the special needs and autism project (SNAP). Psychol Med 41: 619–627.
4. Maski KP, Jeste SS, Spence SJ (2011) Common neurological co-morbidities in autism spectrum disorders. Curr Opin Pediatr 23: 609–615.
5. Gillberg C, Cederlund M, Lamberg K, Zeijlon L (2006) Brief report: the autism epidemic. The registered prevalence of autism in a swedish urban area. J Autism Dev Disord 36: 429–435.
6. Newschaffer CJ, Croen LA, Daniels J, Giarelli E, Grether JK, et al. (2007) The epidemiology of autism spectrum disorders. Annu Rev Public Health 28: 235–258.
7. Kim YS, Leventhal BL, Koh Y, Fombonne E, Laska E, et al. (2011) Prevalence of autism spectrum disorders in a total population sample. Am J Psychiatry 168: 904–912.
8. Kim KC, Kim P, Go HS, Choi CS, Park JH, et al. (2013) Male-specific alteration in excitatory post-synaptic development and social interaction in pre-natal valproic acid exposure model of autism spectrum disorder. J Neurochem 124: 832–843.
9. Zahn-Waxler C, Shirtcliff EA, Marceau K (2008) Disorders of childhood and adolescence: Gender and psychopathology. Annu Rev Clin Psychol 4: 275–303.
10. Abrahams BS, Geschwind DH (2008). Advances in autism genetics: On the threshold of a new neurobiology. Nature Rev Genet 9: 341–355.
11. Hallmayer J, Cleveland S, Torres A, Phillips J, Cohen B, et al. (2011) Genetic heritability and shared environmental factors among twin pairs with autism. Arch Gen Psychiatry 68: 1095–1102.
12. Atladóttir HÓ, Thorsen P, Østergaard L, Schendel DE, Lemcke S, et al. (2010) Maternal infection requiring hospitalization during pregnancy and autism spectrum disorders. J Autism Dev Disord 40: 1423–1430.
13. Atladóttir HÓ, Henriksen TB, Schendel DE, Parner ET (2012) Autism after infection, febrile episodes, and antibiotic use during pregnancy: An exploratory study. Pediatrics 130: e1447–e1454.
14. Brown AS, Sourander A, Hinkka-Yli-Salomäki S, McKeague IW, Sundvall J, et al. (2013) Elevated maternal C-reactive protein and autism in a national birth cohort. Mol Psychiatry In press.
15. Ashwood P, Krakowiak P, Hertz-Picciotto I, Hansen R, Pessah IN, et al. (2011) Associations of impaired behaviors with elevated plasma chemokines in autism spectrum disorders. J Neuroimmunol 232: 196–199.
16. Vargas DL, Nascimbene C, Krishnan C, Zimmerman AW, Pardo CA (2005) Neuroglial activation and neuroinflammation in the brain of patients with autism. Ann Neurol 57: 67–81.
17. Morgan JT, Chana G, Pardo CA, Achim C, Semendeferi K, et al. (2010) Microglial activation and increased microglial density observed in the dorsolateral prefrontal cortex in autism. Biological Psychiatry 68: 368–376.
18. Suzuki S, Kawamata J, Matsushita T, Matsumura A, Hisahara S, et al. (2013) 3-[(2,4-dimethoxy)benzylidene]-anabaseine dihydrochloride protects against 6-hydroxydopamine-induced parkinsonian neurodegeneration through α7 nicotinic acetylcholine receptor stimulation in rats. J Neurosci Res 91: 462–471.
19. Careaga M, Van de Water, J . Ashwood, P (2010) Immune dysfunction in autism: A pathway to treatment. Neurotherapeutics 7: 283–292.
20. Patterson PH (2009) Immune involvement in schizophrenia and autism: Etiology, pathology and animal models. Behav Brain Res 204: 313–321.
21. Piontkewitz Y, Assaf Y, Weiner I (2009) Clozapine administration in adolescence prevents postpubertal emergence of brain structural pathology in an animal model of schizophrenia. Biol Psychiatry 66: 1038–1046.
22. Harvey L, Boksa P (2012) Prenatal and postnatal animal models of immune activation: Relevance to a range of neurodevelopmental disorders. Dev Neurobiol 72: 1335–1348.
23. Patterson PH (2011) Maternal infection and immune involvement in autism. Trends Mol Med 17: 389–394.
24. Bakos J, Duncko R, Makatsori A, Pirnik Z, Kiss A, et al. (2004) Prenatal immune challenge affects growth, behavior, and brain dopamine in offspring, Ann N Y Acad Sci 1018: 281–287.
25. Kirsten TB, Taricano M, Flório JC, Palermo-Neto J, Bernardi MM (2010) Prenatal lipopolysaccharide reduces motor activity after an immune challenge in adult male offspring. Behav Brain Res 211: 77–82.
26. Kirsten TB, Chaves-Kirsten GP, Chaible LM, Silva AC, Martins DO, et al. (2012) Hypoactivity of the central dopaminergic system and autistic-like behavior induced by a single early prenatal exposure to lipopolysaccharide. J Neurosci Res 90: 1903–1912.
27. Malkova NV, Yu CZ, Hsiao EY, Moore MJ, Patterson PH (2012) Maternal immune activation yields offspring displaying mouse versions of the three core symptoms of autism. Brain Behav Immun 26: 607–616.
28. Pacey LKK, Doss L, Cifelli C, van der Kooy, DV, Heximer SP, et al. (2011) Genetic deletion of regulator of G-protein signaling 4 (RGS4) rescues a subset of fragile X related phenotypes in the FMR1 knockout mouse. Mol and Cell Neurosci 46: 563–572.
29. Ramsey AJ, Milenkovic M, Oliveira AF, Escobedo-Lozoya Y, Seshadri S, et al. (2011) Impaired NMDA receptor transmission alters striatal synapses and DISC1 protein in an age-dependent manner. Proc Natl Acad Sci USA 108: 5795–5800.
30. Ehninger D, Sano Y, De Vries PJ, Dies K, Franz D, et al. (2012) Gestational immune activation and Tsc2 haploinsufficiency cooperate to disrupt fetal survival and may perturb social behavior in adult mice. Mol Psychiatry 17: 62–70.

31. Lipina T V., Zai C, Hlousek D, Roder JC, Wong AHC (2013) Maternal immune activation during gestation interacts with Disc1 point mutation to exacerbate schizophrenia-related behaviors in mice. J Neurosci 33: 7654–7666.
32. Thomas A, Burant A, Bui N., Graham D, Yuva-Paylor LA, et al. (2009) Marble burying reflects a repetitive and perseverative behavior more than novelty-induced anxiety. Psychopharmacol 204: 361–373.
33. Kalueff AV, Tuohimaa P (2005) The grooming analysis algorithm discriminates between different levels of anxiety in rats: Potential utility for neurobehavioural stress research. J Neurosci Methods 143: 169–177.
34. Silverman JL, Yang M., Lord C, Crawley JN, 2010. Behavioural phenotyping assays for mouse models of autism. Nat Rev Neurosci 11: 490–502.
35. Schwartzer JJ, Careaga M, Onore CE, Rushakoff JA, Berman RF, et al. (2013) Maternal immune activation and strain specific interactions in the development of autism-like behaviors in mice. Transl Psychiatry 3: article number 240.
36. Hsiao EY, McBride SW, Chow J, Mazmanian SK, Patterson PH (2012). Modeling an autism risk factor in mice leads to permanent immune dysregulation. Proc Natl Acad Sci USA 109: 12776–12781.
37. Zager A, Mennecier G, Palermo-Neto J (2012). Maternal immune activation in late gestation enhances locomotor response to acute but not chronic amphetamine treatment in male mice offspring: Role of the D1 receptor. Behav Brain Res 232: 30–36.
38. Rana SA, Aavani T, Pittman QJ (2012) Sex effects on neurodevelopmental outcomes of innate immune activation during prenatal and neonatal life. Horm Behav 62: 228–236.
39. Hattier MA, Matson JL, Tureck K, Horovitz M (2011) The effects of gender and age on repetitive and/or restricted behaviors and interests in adults with autism spectrum disorders and intellectual disability. Res Dev Disabil 32: 2346–2351.
40. Sipes M, Matson JL, Worley JA, Kozlowski AM (2011) Gender differences in symptoms of autism spectrum disorders in toddlers. Res Autism Spect Disord 5: 1465–1470.
41. Mandy W, Chilvers R, Chowdhury U, Salter G, Seigal A, et al. (2012) Sex differences in autism spectrum disorder: Evidence from a large sample of children and adolescents. J Autism Dev Disord 42: 1304–1313.
42. Szatmari P, Liu X, Goldberg J, Zwaigenbaum L, Paterson AD, et al. (2012) Sex differences in repetitive stereotyped behaviors in autism: Implications for genetic liability. Am J Med Genet, Part B 159: 5–12.
43. Werling DM, Geschwind DH (2013) Sex differences in autism spectrum disorders. Curr Opin in Neurol 26: 146–153.
44. Zwaigenbaum L, Bryson SE, Szatmari P, Brian J, Smith IM, et al. (2012) Sex differences in children with autism spectrum disorder identified within a high-risk infant cohort. J Autism Dev Disord 42: 2585–2596.
45. Worley JA, Matson JL (2011) Psychiatric symptoms in children diagnosed with an autism spectrum disorder: An examination of gender differences. Res Autism Spectrum Disord 5: 1086–1091.
46. Andersson GW, Gillberg C, Miniscalco C (2013) Pre-school children with suspected autism spectrum disorders: Do girls and boys have the same profiles? Res Dev Disabil 34: 413–422.
47. Alexopoulou L, Holt AC, Medzhitov R, Flavell RA (2001) Recognition of double-stranded RNA and activation of NF-κB by toll-like receptor 3. Nature 413: 732–738.
48. Netea MG, Van Deuren M, Kullberg BJ, Cavaillon J, Van Der Meer JWM (2002) Does the shape of lipid A determine the interaction of LPS with toll-like receptors? Trends Immunol 23: 135–139.
49. Carpenter S, Aiello D, Atianand MK, Ricci EP, Gandhi P, et al. (2013) A long noncoding RNA mediates both activation and repression of immune response genes. Science 341: 789–792.
50. Ashdown H, Dumont Y, Ng M, Poole S, Boksa P, et al. (2006) The role of cytokines in mediating effects of prenatal infection on the fetus: Implications for schizophrenia. Mol Psychiatry 11: 47–55.
51. Garay PA, Hsiao EY, Patterson PH, McAllister AK (2013) Maternal immune activation causes age- and region-specific changes in brain cytokines in offspring throughout development. Brain Behav Immun 31: 54–68.
52. Jones KA, Thomsen C (2013) The role of the innate immune system in psychiatric disorders. Mol Cell Neurosci 53: 52–62.

An Inherited Small Microdeletion at 15q13.3 in a Patient with Early-Onset Obsessive-Compulsive Disorder

Carolina Cappi[1]*, Ana Gabriela Hounie[1,5], Daniel B. Mariani[2], Juliana Belo Diniz[1], Aderbal R. T. Silva[1], Viviane N. S. Reis[1], Ariane F. Busso[3], Amanda Gonçalves Silva[3], Felipe Fidalgo[3], Silvia Regina Rogatto[4], Euripedes C. Miguel[1], Ana C. Krepischi[3], Helena Brentani[1]

1 Institute and Department of Psychiatry, São Paulo University Medical School, São Paulo, Brazil, **2** Inter-institutional Grad Program on Bioinformatics, Institute of Mathematics and Statistics, São Paulo University, São Paulo, Brazil, **3** International Research Center, AC Camargo Cancer Center, São Paulo, Brazil, **4** School of Medicine, São Paulo State University, Botucatu, São Paulo, Brazil, **5** Federal University of São Paulo-UPIA-UNIFESP, São Paulo, Brazil

Abstract

Copy number variations (CNVs) have been previously associated with several different neurodevelopmental psychiatric disorders, such as autism, schizophrenia, and attention deficit hyperactivity disorder (ADHD). The present study consisted of a pilot genome-wide screen for CNVs in a cohort of 16 patients with early-onset obsessive-compulsive disorder (OCD) and 12 mentally healthy individuals, using array-based comparative genomic hybridization (aCGH) on 44K arrays. A small rare paternal inherited microdeletion (~64 kb) was identified in chromosome 15q13.3 of one male patient with very early onset OCD. The father did not have OCD. The deletion encompassed part of the *FMN1* gene, which is involved with the glutamatergic system. This finding supports the hypothesis of a complex network of several genes expressed in the brain contributing for the genetic risk of OCD, and also supports the glutamatergic involvement in OCD, which has been previously reported in the literature.

Editor: Chunyu Liu, University of Illinois at Chicago, United States of America

Funding: This study was supported by grants to Dras Cappi and Brentani from the Foundation for Research Support of the State of São Paulo (FAPESP); grant number: 2008/11537-7, and from the Brazilian National Council for Scientific and Technological Development (CNPq; protocol number MCT/CNPq 14/2008). The funders had no role in study design, data collection and analysis, decision to publish, or preparation of the manuscript.

Competing Interests: The authors have declared that no competing interests exist.

* Email: carolinacappi@gmail.com

Introduction

Twin and family studies provide strong evidence of the importance of genetic factors for the expression of obsessive-compulsive disorder (OCD) and other disorders in the obsessive-compulsive spectrum [1]. To date, more than 100 positional and functional candidate genes related to serotonin, dopamine, and glutamate transmission have been implicated in these disorders [2]. However, most of the findings have not been replicated. A recent meta-analysis of all genetic association studies of OCD, which provided sufficient information for data extraction, found that the disorder was associated with serotonin-related polymorphisms (*5-HTTLPR* and *HTR2A*) and that there may be significant sex differences in the genetic bases of the disease, with only male OCD patients carrying polymorphisms involved in catecholamine modulation (*COMT* and *MAOA*) [3]. Secondary analyses of polymorphisms examined in fewer than five data sets identified other candidate polymorphisms associated with trophic factors, neurotransmitters, and with an immunologic factor [3].

The first Genome-Wide Association Study (GWAS) of OCD, which was recently published, analyzed 400 trios, 1,465 cases and 5,557 controls having found no associations between any SNPs (single nucleotide polymorphisms) and OCD at a genome-wide significant level in the combined trio-case-control sample. It is worth mentioning, however, that the top-ranked SNPs were related to transcriptional regulation and to glutamatergic neurotransmission and signaling [4].

Recently, the original genetic model for psychiatric disorders, which explained these conditions as resulting from the effect of common genetic variants (>1% frequency), has been challenged by a model involving high impact variants which are individually rare, but collectively common [5]. Research has shown that, although SNPs outnumber CNVs (copy number variations) in the genome by three orders of magnitude, their relative contribution to genome variation is similar [6]. Therefore, as could be expected from these observations, the study of CNV has allowed a more comprehensive understanding of disease etiology, bringing rare variants to the forefront [7].

Early studies analyzed CNVs ranging from one kilobase (kb) to several megabases (Mb) in size, including large insertions or deletions in the genome. However, the increased accuracy of detection techniques has allowed the identification of smaller CNVs, so that many recent studies involve the analysis of fragments smaller than 1 kb [8].

CNVs are especially relevant to the study of mental disorders, as they have been causally associated with neurodevelopmental disorders and learning disabilities [9]. Specific rare CNVs have also been found to be associated with autism, schizophrenia, and attention-attention deficit hyperactivity disorder (ADHD) [10–14].

The current hypothesis for the etiology of mental disorders suggests that these conditions are polygenic, and that both common and rare variations contribute to their development. Therefore, rather than consisting of risk factors for specific conditions, CNVs are thought to confer broad susceptibility to a variety of neurodevelopmental disorders. Large, rare CNVs are more pathogenic, and are more likely to be under negative evolutionary selection [15]. Although CNVs with smaller effect sizes may also have an important role in the etiology of mental disorders, their individual influences and the impact of their interaction with other CNVs on the development of mental illnesses have been poorly studied [16].

To date, few studies have investigated CNVs in OCD patients. One study was conducted to search for CNVs in these individuals screened for 15q11-13 and 22q11.2 microrearrangements associated with Prader-Willi and DiGeorge Syndromes (DGS). The study was performed in 236 OCD probands using Multiplex Ligation-dependent Probe Amplification (MLPA), which allows the relative quantification of the copy number in at least 50 sequences in a single experiment. The study did not detect any CNVs in these regions, possibly due to the rare prevalence of these chromosomal anomalies in OCD and due to the exclusion of significant mental retardation in the samples studied [17]. Studies have shown that pathogenic CNVs are more prevalent among the individuals with moderate and severe intellectual disability, which are usually exclusionary criteria of research protocols [18].

Another study by Hooper et al., (2012) used cytogenetic analysis and fluorescence in situ hybridization (FISH) to identify an apparently balanced cytogenetic chromosome translocation t(6;22)(q16.2;p13) that segregated from the mother with OCD to her male son with Tourette Syndrome (TS) and OCD. Whole genome mate-pair sequencing and high resolution SNP array analysis was performed in the male proband to identify any related or additional sub-microscopic rearrangements. The largest heterozygous deletion identified in this secondary analysis was a 400 kb deletion located 1.3 Mb telomeric to the chromosome 6q breakpoint. This deletion caused heterozygous loss of all coding sequences of the *GPR63*, *NDUFA4* and *KLHL32* genes which are expressed in the brain [19]. In addition, this deletion coincides with a rearrangement previously reported in a girl diagnosed with Autism Spectrum Disorder (ASD) and developmental delay [20].

In a study of 136 cases of children and adolescents with OCD compared with 106 healthy age-matched controls, Walitza et al., (2011) reported that the deletion (one copy) of a small (100 bp) CNV localized near (68-bp upstream the rs 6311 in the promoter region of the *HTR2A* gene was associated to a very early-onset and to symptom severity of OCD. The frequency of this deletion was increased in the OCD group (n = 8) when compared to healthy controls (n = 1), and carriers of one copy (deletion) of the CNV were associated with a very-early-onset OCD and increased CY-BOCS scores [21].

The first genome-wide CNV analysis in OCD (1,613 patients) and the largest to date in Tourette Syndrome (TS) (1,086 patients) and 720 ancestry-matched controls was conducted to observe the effects of specific neurodevelopmental CNVs. The analyses were restricted to large (>500 kb an rare (<1% frequency in the Database of Genomic Variants-DGV) CNVs, using Illumina genotyping array. The results showed evidence for an increased burden of pathogenic neurodevelopmental deletions in OCD/TS patients compared with controls. Deletion at 16p13.11 was primarily associated with OCD, however 3 de novo CNVs in this region among 6 cases with OCD/TS point to the possibility of pleiotropic effect of this locus. These deletions at 16p13.11 have been extended to other neurodevelopmental disorders, including developmental delay, seizures, and autism [22].

In light of these findings and given our long-standing interest in the contribution of genetic variation to OCD, we conducted a preliminary study to identify rare CNVs in 16 patients with early-onset OCD and 12 controls, using array-based comparative genomic hybridization (aCGH).

Materials and Methods

The present study was approved by the Research Ethics Committees of the University of São Paulo School of Medicine, as well as by the Brazilian National Commission of Research Ethics (CONEP, process number: 16756). All participating subjects gave written informed consent.

The study was conducted in the Outpatient Clinic of the Obsessive-Compulsive Spectrum Disorders Program of the Institute of Psychiatry at the General Hospital of the University of São Paulo, School of Medicine.

Patients were referred from primary psychiatric services, or recruited through television, radio, and newspaper announcements. Healthy controls were recruited from university staff and students, hospital staff or by word of mouth.

Patients and healthy controls were assessed at baseline with the Structured Clinical Interview for DSM-IV Axis I Disorders and additional modules for tic and impulse control disorders, the ADHD and separation anxiety sections of the Kiddie Schedule for Affective Disorders and Schizophrenia (K-SADS), the Yale-Brown Obsessive- Compulsive Scale (Y-BOCS), the Dimensional Yale-Brown Obsessive- Compulsive Scale (DY-BOCS), the Yale Global Tic Severity Scale (YGTSS), and the Beck Depression (BDI) and Anxiety (BAI) Inventories [23,24]. Patients were included if they were aged between 18 and 65 years and had OCD as the primary diagnosis according to DSM-IV criteria. Healthy controls were included if they were aged between 18 and 65 years and did not have OCD, tic or impulse control disorders, ADHD, anxiety disorders or major depression according to the DSM-IV.

Subjects with a primary diagnosis of a psychotic disorder or with any other condition that could impair their understanding of the protocol questions were excluded. Patients with a clinical condition that could hamper the interpretation of the results, such as those whose OCD symptoms began after significant head trauma or were secondary to other neurological disorders and intellectual disability were also excluded.

Genomic DNA extraction

In those patients from whom it was possible to obtain blood samples, peripheral blood leukocytes were used as a source of DNA, which was extracted using the salting out method [25]. For the eight subjects from whom blood samples could not be drawn, DNA was extracted from saliva samples collected using the Oragene kit manufactured by Genotek according to the protocols available at http://www.dnagenotek.com/.

Comparative genomic hybridization based on microarray (aCGH)

Array-CGH analysis was performed using an oligonucleotide 44 K whole-genome microarray platform (design 14950, Agilent Technologies, Santa Clara, USA). The platform was composed of 44,290 60-mer oligonucleotide probes for mapped genes or unique DNA sequences with an average spatial resolution of ~30–35 kb. However, the platform does not cover the pseudoautosomal regions of the X and the Y chromosomes. The genomic DNA of patients and healthy controls was labeled with Cy3-fluorophores, while the reference DNA was labeled with Cy5-fluorophore. These were hybridized to the array in the presence of Cot-1 DNA, a blocking reagent which suppresses the nonspecific hybridization of repetitive sequences.

Test DNA samples were hybridized with gender matched reference DNA, which consisted of a pooled sample of human placenta DNA obtained from ten normal individuals. Purification, hybridization, and washing were carried out according to the manufacturer's instructions. Slides were read by a GenePix 4000B scanner, and the scanned images of the arrays were processed using the Feature Extraction software package (Agilent Technologies, Santa Clara, CA, USA). Fluorescence intensity was measured by the Feature Extraction software, version 9.5, using an Agilent whole human genome 4×44k microarray. Further details on the protocols used are available online (http://www.home.agilent.com/).

These analyses were performed in all patients, healthy controls and additionally, in the parents of one patient who had one rare CNV.

Selection of high-confidence copy number alterations

Constitutive or germline CNVs were identified using the Genomic Workbench software (Agilent Technologies, Santa Clara, CA, USA) with the statistical algorithm ADM-2, and a 6.7 sensitivity threshold. Poor quality hybridizations (QC>0.3) were discarded. For samples that passed quality control, CNV calling (deletions and duplications) was performed using the Nexus Copy Number 5.0 software, with a quality control threshold of < 0.18. CNVs were called in Nexus using the FASST2 segmentation algorithm; with at least three affected probes and default settings (threshold $\log_2$ ratio of 0.3 or 1.14 for gain or high copy gain, and −0.3 and −1.14 for loss and homozygous loss, respectively), and significance threshold set to 1.0E-6.

Samples that did not meet quality thresholds were excluded from further analysis, as were microarrays with low quality according to visual inspection. Although the initial sample was composed of 20 patients and 20 controls, 12 samples were subsequently excluded for quality reasons (4 patients and 8 controls).

CNVs were considered rare if they showed less than 50% overlap with CNVs predicted with frequency of at least 1% according to the March 2010 update of the Database of Genomic Variants (DGV). The confirmation of rare CNVs and determination of the parent of origin were conducted using 60 K SNP array analysis. Furthermore, rare CNVs were confirmed by quantitative PCR (qPCR).

Quantitative PCR (qPCR) validation

Rare CNVs were validated using the SYBR Green system from Applied Biosystems 7500 Real-Time PCR System. Two qPCR primers were designed and mapped against the NCBI reference sequence hg18 to obtain converging evidence for the detected CNVs. Primer sequences were as follows: *FMN1* forward primer: 5′ CAGGTTTGTCTGAAAGTCACC 3′, reverse primer: 5′ CTACTCTTTGTACCTGGGAGGAC -3′. The absolute number of gene copies was normalized using the *GAPDH* and *P2RX7* genes (control genes). Triplicates were analyzed using the comparative $2^{-}\Delta\Delta C^{t}$-cycle threshold method [26]. Values in the 0.8–1.2 range indicated duplication, <0.6 were indicative of deletions, and values>1.4 were considered duplications (Figure 1).

Statistical Analysis

We assessed the impact of CNVs in cases compared to controls using five measures: the number of CNVs per individual, the estimated CNV size, the percentage of CNVs that overlapped with CNVs in the DGV (overlap with>50% of length), and the percentage of CNVs in two different groups of CNV sizes (CNVs>1 Mb and CNVs>100 kb – 999 kb). *P*-values were calculated using two-tailed Fisher exact test and were shown for each comparison between cases and controls. The level of significance considered was alpha = 0.05 (Table 1).

We compared the proportion of subjects in each group harboring CNVs with sizes between 30 kb–500 kb and>500 kb. This last comparison was conducted to observe whether CNVs involved with neurodevelopment disorder were associated with the OCD group [6]. Pearson's Chi-square (two-tailed) p-values were calculated, using a pre-determined p-value threshold that corrected for 2 primary comparisons using a standard Bonferroni approach ($p<0.025$) [Table 2].

Results

After completing quality control and case-control matching, 12 samples were excluded (4 cases and 8 controls). Therefore, a total of 16 cases and 12 controls were included in the final analyses. The mean age at symptom onset in the patient group was 9.8 years (SD = 4.03) and the mean Y-BOCS score was 30.4 (SD = 4.93).

Characteristics of CNVs in patients and controls

The median CNV size in OCD patients was 435.4 kb and the median number of CNVs per individual was 3, with 11.3% of these events consisting of deletions (the remaining were all duplications). A total of 24.5% of CNVs in OCD patients were>1 Mb, while 67.9% of variants were in the 100-999 kb range. Patients and controls did not significantly differ with respect to these characteristics (Table 1).

Overall, no statistically significant differences in CNV size were found between cases and controls, even when a nominal uncorrected p-value of 0.05 was used. Similar results were obtained with regard to between-group differences in the frequency of CNV occurrence (Table 1 and Table 2).

Rare CNVs analyses

One OCD patient was found to carry a rare CNV consisting of an intragenic ~64 kb microdeletion at 15q13.3 encompassing part of the *FMN1* gene. Array CGH analyses of the patient's parents were performed to verify whether the CNV was *de novo* or inherited. The microdeletion was found to be inherited from a non-affected father (Figure 1).

Discussion

In this study an early-onset OCD patient (age of first obsessive-compulsive symptoms when he was 8 years old) was found to carry a rare intragenic ~64 kb microdeletion at 15q13.3. This microdeletion was present in the father who did not have OCD. The mother also did not have OCD, although his sister also had OCD. Unfortunately the sister did not agree to participate in the study.

This CNV encompasses two exons of the *FMN1* gene, which encodes the protein Formin1. The overexpression of Formin1b produces an increase in the number of primary dendrites in cultured hippocampal neurons and an increase in the number of glutamatergic synaptic inputs [27]. Additionally, it is thought that Formin1 may mediate the effect of the proneural transcription factor Ngn3, which regulates dendritogenesis and synaptogenesis [28].

The genetic findings in OCD has shown dysregulation in genes that are expressed in the brain and are involved in the

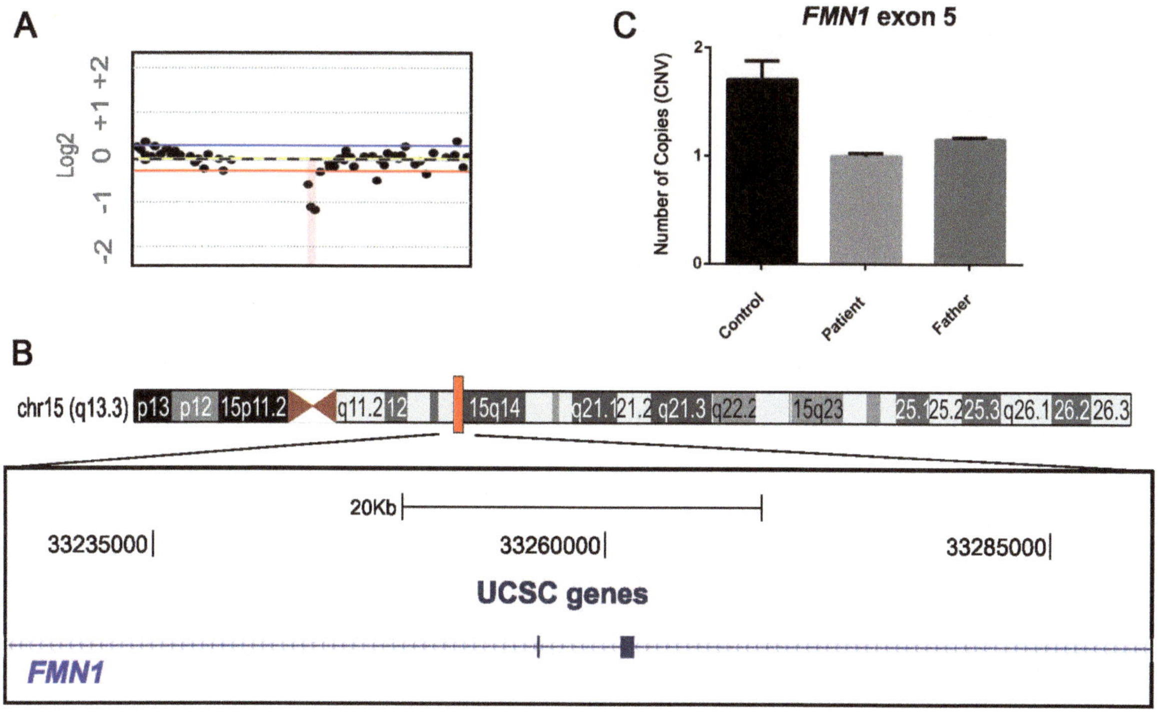

Figure 1. Chromosome 15q 13.3 after CNV and qPCR procedures. A. The microdeletion identified in the *FMN1* region of chromosome 15q13.3 using Genomic Workbench software (Agilent Technologies, Santa Clara, CA, USA). **B.** Genome browser image of the region containing the *FMN1* gene. One rare deletion was identified in the male proband (64 kb loss in OCD case 222_3). **C.** Rare CNVs were validated by SYBR Green-based real time PCR, and it was found that the father and son had only one copy of the exon while the gender-matched control had two copies.

glutamatergic, serotonergic and dopaminergic pathways playing an important part in the expression of OCD [2].

Recent evidence from a number of studies has highlighted the role of glutamatergic synaptic dysfunctions in the cortico-striatal-thalamo-cortical (CSTC) circuit in the etiology of OCD and related disorders [29]. According to a number of independent reports, one of the strongest candidate genes for OCD is the neuronal glutamate transporter gene *SLC1A1* (Solute Carrier, Family 1, Member 1) [30–32]. In fact, this is the only gene whose association with OCD has been replicated in independent samples [4]. However, it is interesting to note that the previously mentioned GWAS of OCD did not find any polymorphisms in the *SLC1A1* gene, although it did associate the disorder with a number of genes involved in glutamatergic processes. These findings corroborate the hypothesis that genes involved in the glutamatergic system may contribute to the pathophysiology of OCD [33,34].

The OCD Collaborative Genetics Study (OCGS) conducted a linkage analysis on 376 affected families using genetic association methods, and found that the SNPs most strongly associated with OCD were in chromosome 15q. Several of those SNPs are located in or near the *FMN1* gene. One SNP (rs2306277) in particular, located in exon 1 of the *FMN1* gene, was predicted by PolyPhen 2 (a tool which predicts the possible impact of an amino acid

Table 1. Characteristics of all copy number variations (CNVs) in obsessive-compulsive disorder (OCD) patients and controls.

	OCD patients (n = 16)	Controls (n = 12)	*P*-value
	All CNVs	All CNVs	
Samples with CNVs	16	12	0.4497
Number of CNVs	53	48	0.6188
Median number of CNVs per genome	3	2	0.6547
Median CNV size (kb)	435.4	389.8	0.1124
% Gain/Loss	88.6/11.3	85.4/14.5	0.8083/0.5287
Overlapping CNVs (%)[1]	58.4	68.7	0.3609
CNVs>1 Mb (%)	24.5	20.8	0.5825
CNVs>100 kb – 999 kb (%)	67.9	79.1	0.3556

P-values were calculated using two-tailed Fisher exact test.
[1]Overlapping CNVs = percentage of CNVs that overlap with CNVs in the DGV (overlap with>50% of length).

Table 2. Frequency of copy number variants of different sizes in patients with obsessive-compulsive disorder (OCD) and controls.

CNV Size				
Category	**Analysis**	**# OCD (N = 16)**	**# Controls (N = 12)**	***P*-value**
All 30–500 kb CNVs	CNVs	53	48	
	Samples	13	11	0.8151
	Proportion	81.2%	91.6%	
All>500 kb CNVs	CNVs	26	26	
	Samples	11	7	0.8644
	Proportion	68.7%	58.3%	

P-values were calculated using Pearson's Chi-square test; Bonferroni-adjusted significance of 0.025.

substitution on the structure and function of a human protein) to be a missense mutation with probable protein damage. The same study also found SNPs associated with OCD in the same chromosomal region (15q), but in the homeobox genes *MEIS2* and *NANOGP8*, which code for transcription factors or closely related proteins, all of which play an important role in neurodevelopment [35]. Other studies have also reported associations between OCD and the 15q region, although none has identified relevant SNPs in the region of the *FMN1* gene itself [36,37].

The main CNVs associated with psychiatric disorders have generally been rare variants in genes involved in synaptogenesis, neuronal and axonal mobility, protein degradation via the ubiquitin-proteasome system (ubiquitin signaling), protein complexes and postsynaptic signaling [11,12,38–48]. Studies have also suggested that the CNVs found in psychiatric probands are often in chromosomal regions associated with microdeletion syndromes, such as loci 16p11.2 and 7q11.23, both associated with Williams Syndrome, locus 15q11-13, associated with Prader-Willi and Angelman Syndromes, and, lastly, locus 22q11.2, which has been associated with DiGeorge syndrome [6].One of the most interesting observations in psychiatric genetic association studies has been the wide variability in the neuropsychiatric phenotype associated with one individual CNV or CNV region [49,50]. These findings are consistent with the hypothesis linking the known pleiotropic effects of these CNVs with shared abnormalities in early neural development [51].

Interestingly, a microduplication at 15q13.3 (including the first four exons of the CHRNA7 gene) was found in a proband with TS, ADHD and OCD and his mother who had subclinical ADHD. The other brother with TS and OCD (without ADHD) did not have this duplication. The authors suggest that this duplication may have an intermediate penetrance effect and may be involved with ADHD development [52].

Studies have described a broad variety of phenotypes associated with 15q13.3 deletion, including schizophrenia, epilepsy, autism, antisocial behaviors and mental retardation [36,37,53–56]. The frequency of these deletions in control individuals has been found to be much lower than in cases. Additionally, the types of deletions and duplications may vary between these individuals. The authors suggest that submicroscopic deletions and duplications in this region are associated with milder phenotypes, have less than 100% penetrance, and tend to be inherited in a larger fraction of cases. Environmental factors may also be important in explaining the lack of penetrance [57]. However, none of the studies cited herein have reported the microdeletion found in the present study. This may suggest a pleiotropic effect whereby multiple variants in the same region are associated with different phenotypes [58]. Perhaps the microdeletion found in the present study in conjunction with environmental factors or other genetic variants may contribute for the manifestation of OCD. The overall rate of *de novo* large CNVs (>500 kb) in OCD trio samples was 1.44%, which is intermediate between healthy controls and autism (1.8% multiplex and 3.9% simplex) and schizophrenia (2%–3%). This finding gives some support to the involvement of CNVs in OCD, despite this study was unable to call CNVs smaller than 500 kb due to technical limitations. There is still the possibility that smaller CNVs may be related to OCD [22].

Several limitations of the present study are worth mentioning. Firstly, the sample size was small, particularly for the purposes of the detection and analysis of rare CNVs. Although this association may have happened by chance alone, other possibilities such as incomplete penetration can be taken into account. Examining the affected sister could help understand this issue.

Furthermore, even though the 44 K platform allows for the observation of large and rare CNVs; the probe spacing may affect the accuracy of CNV length measurements. Future analyses should be conducted using larger sample sizes and a better platform resolution. However, regardless of these limitations, the present findings give further support to the hypothesis that many variations in genes that function in a brain network can be related with OCD, instead of single genes that simply cumulatively add risk.

Acknowledgments

We wish to thank the patients and heathy controls who volunteered to participate in this study.

Author Contributions

Conceived and designed the experiments: HB ACK SRR. Performed the experiments: CC AFB ARTS FF AGS VNSR. Analyzed the data: CC DBM. Contributed reagents/materials/analysis tools: SRR AFB ECM. Wrote the paper: CC AGH JBD ACK HB.

References

1. Pauls DL (2008) The genetics of obsessive compulsive disorder: a review of the evidence. Am J Med Genet C Semin Med Genet 148C: 133–139.

2. Pauls DL, Abramovitch A, Rauch SL, Geller DA (2014) Obsessive-compulsive disorder: an integrative genetic and neurobiological perspective. Nat Rev Neurosci 15: 410–424.

3. Taylor S (2012) Molecular genetics of obsessive-compulsive disorder: a comprehensive meta-analysis of genetic association studies. Mol Psychiatry.
4. Stewart SE, Yu D, Scharf JM, Neale BM, Fagerness JA, et al. (2012) Genome-wide association study of obsessive-compulsive disorder. Mol Psychiatry.
5. Coe BP, Girirajan S, Eichler EE (2012) A genetic model for neurodevelopmental disease. Curr Opin Neurobiol.
6. Malhotra D, Sebat J (2012) CNVs: harbingers of a rare variant revolution in psychiatric genetics. Cell 148: 1223–1241.
7. Conrad DF, Pinto D, Redon R, Feuk L, Gokcumen O, et al. (2010) Origins and functional impact of copy number variation in the human genome. Nature 464: 704–712.
8. Sebat J, Lakshmi B, Troge J, Alexander J, Young J, et al. (2004) Large-scale copy number polymorphism in the human genome. Science 305: 525–528.
9. Merikangas AK, Corvin AP, Gallagher L (2009) Copy-number variants in neurodevelopmental disorders: promises and challenges. Trends Genet 25: 536–544.
10. Sebat J (2007) Major changes in our DNA lead to major changes in our thinking. Nat Genet 39: S3–5.
11. Walsh T, McClellan JM, McCarthy SE, Addington AM, Pierce SB, et al. (2008) Rare structural variants disrupt multiple genes in neurodevelopmental pathways in schizophrenia. Science 320: 539–543.
12. Stefansson H, Rujescu D, Cichon S, Pietiläinen OP, Ingason A, et al. (2008) Large recurrent microdeletions associated with schizophrenia. Nature 455: 232–236.
13. Consortium GP (2010) A map of human genome variation from population-scale sequencing. Nature 467: 1061–1073.
14. Lesch KP, Selch S, Renner TJ, Jacob C, Nguyen TT, et al. (2011) Genome-wide copy number variation analysis in attention-deficit/hyperactivity disorder: association with neuropeptide Y gene dosage in an extended pedigree. Mol Psychiatry 16: 491–503.
15. Rucker JJ, McGuffin P (2012) Genomic structural variation in psychiatric disorders. Dev Psychopathol 24: 1335–1344.
16. Cook EH, Scherer SW (2008) Copy-number variations associated with neuropsychiatric conditions. Nature 455: 919–923.
17. Delorme R, Moreno-De-Luca D, Gennetier A, Maier W, Chaste P, et al. (2010) Search for copy number variants in chromosomes 15q11-q13 and 22q11.2 in obsessive compulsive disorder. BMC Med Genet 11: 100.
18. Engels H, Brockschmidt A, Hoischen A, Landwehr C, Bosse K, et al. (2007) DNA microarray analysis identifies candidate regions and genes in unexplained mental retardation. Neurology 68: 743–750.
19. Hooper SD, Johansson AC, Tellgren-Roth C, Stattin EL, Dahl N, et al. (2012) Genome-wide sequencing for the identification of rearrangements associated with Tourette syndrome and obsessive-compulsive disorder. BMC Med Genet 13: 123.
20. Derwińska K, Bernaciak J, Wiśniowiecka-Kowalnik B, Obersztyn E, Bocian E, et al. (2009) Autistic features with speech delay in a girl with an approximately 1.5-Mb deletion in 6q16.1, including GPR63 and FUT9. Clin Genet 75: 199–202.
21. Walitza S, Bové DS, Romanos M, Renner T, Held L, et al. (2012) Pilot study on HTR2A promoter polymorphism, -1438G/A (rs6311) and a nearby copy number variation showed association with onset and severity in early onset obsessive-compulsive disorder. J Neural Transm 119: 507–515.
22. McGrath LM, Yu D, Marshall C, Davis LK, Thiruvahindrapuram B, et al. (2014) Copy number variation in obsessive-compulsive disorder and tourette syndrome: a cross-disorder study. J Am Acad Child Adolesc Psychiatry 53: 910–919.
23. Miguel EC, Ferrão YA, Rosário MC, Mathis MA, Torres AR, et al. (2008) The Brazilian Research Consortium on Obsessive-Compulsive Spectrum Disorders: recruitment, assessment instruments, methods for the development of multicenter collaborative studies and preliminary results. Rev Bras Psiquiatr 30: 185–196.
24. Hoexter MQ, Shavitt RG, D'Alcante CC, Cecconi JP, Diniz JB, et al. (2009) The drug-naïve OCD patients imaging genetics, cognitive and treatment response study: methods and sample description. Rev Bras Psiquiatr 31: 349–353.
25. Miller SA, Dykes DD, Polesky HF (1988) A simple salting out procedure for extracting DNA from human nucleated cells. Nucleic Acids Res 16: 1215.
26. Livak KJ, Schmittgen TD (2001) Analysis of relative gene expression data using real-time quantitative PCR and the 2(-Delta Delta C(T)) Method. Methods 25: 402–408.
27. Simon-Areces J, Dopazo A, Dettenhofer M, Rodriguez-Tebar A, Garcia-Segura LM, et al. (2011) Formin1 mediates the induction of dendritogenesis and synaptogenesis by neurogenin3 in mouse hippocampal neurons. PLoS One 6: e21825.
28. Salama-Cohen P, Arévalo MA, Grantyn R, Rodríguez-Tébar A (2006) Notch and NGF/p75NTR control dendrite morphology and the balance of excitatory/inhibitory synaptic input to hippocampal neurones through Neurogenin 3. J Neurochem 97: 1269–1278.
29. Arnold PD, Macmaster FP, Hanna GL, Richter MA, Sicard T, et al. (2009) Glutamate system genes associated with ventral prefrontal and thalamic volume in pediatric obsessive-compulsive disorder. Brain Imaging Behav 3: 64–76.
30. Stewart SE, Mayerfeld C, Arnold PD, Crane JR, O'Dushlaine C, et al. (2013) Meta-analysis of association between obsessive-compulsive disorder and the 3′ region of neuronal glutamate transporter gene SLC1A1. Am J Med Genet B Neuropsychiatr Genet.
31. Veenstra-VanderWeele J, Xu T, Ruggiero AM, Anderson LR, Jones ST, et al. (2012) Functional studies and rare variant screening of SLC1A1/EAAC1 in males with obsessive-compulsive disorder. Psychiatr Genet 22: 256–260.
32. Ting JT, Feng G (2008) Glutamatergic Synaptic Dysfunction and Obsessive-Compulsive Disorder. Curr Chem Genomics 2: 62–75.
33. Shugart YY, Samuels J, Willour VL, Grados MA, Greenberg BD, et al. (2006) Genomewide linkage scan for obsessive-compulsive disorder: evidence for susceptibility loci on chromosomes 3q, 7p, 1q, 15q, and 6q. Mol Psychiatry 11: 763–770.
34. Ross J, Badner J, Garrido H, Sheppard B, Chavira DA, et al. (2011) Genomewide linkage analysis in Costa Rican families implicates chromosome 15q14 as a candidate region for OCD. Hum Genet 130: 795–805.
35. Nestadt G, Wang Y, Grados MA, Riddle MA, Greenberg BD, et al. (2012) Homeobox genes in obsessive-compulsive disorder. Am J Med Genet B Neuropsychiatr Genet 159B: 53–60.
36. Crespi B, Stead P, Elliot M (2010) Evolution in health and medicine Sackler colloquium: Comparative genomics of autism and schizophrenia. Proc Natl Acad Sci U S A 107 Suppl 1: 1736–1741.
37. Crespi BJ, Crofts HJ (2012) Association testing of copy number variants in schizophrenia and autism spectrum disorders. J Neurodev Disord 4: 15.
38. Sebat J, Lakshmi B, Malhotra D, Troge J, Lese-Martin C, et al. (2007) Strong association of de novo copy number mutations with autism. Science 316: 445–449.
39. Pinto D, Pagnamenta AT, Klei L, Anney R, Merico D, et al. (2010) Functional impact of global rare copy number variation in autism spectrum disorders. Nature 466: 368–372.
40. Sanders SJ, Ercan-Sencicek AG, Hus V, Luo R, Murtha MT, et al. (2011) Multiple recurrent de novo CNVs, including duplications of the 7q11.23 Williams syndrome region, are strongly associated with autism. Neuron 70: 863–885.
41. Glessner JT, Wang K, Cai G, Korvatska O, Kim CE, et al. (2009) Autism genome-wide copy number variation reveals ubiquitin and neuronal genes. Nature 459: 569–573.
42. Marshall CR, Noor A, Vincent JB, Lionel AC, Feuk L, et al. (2008) Structural variation of chromosomes in autism spectrum disorder. Am J Hum Genet 82: 477–488.
43. Gilman SR, Iossifov I, Levy D, Ronemus M, Wigler M, et al. (2011) Rare de novo variants associated with autism implicate a large functional network of genes involved in formation and function of synapses. Neuron 70: 898–907.
44. Consortium IS (2008) Rare chromosomal deletions and duplications increase risk of schizophrenia. Nature 455: 237–241.
45. Sebat J, Levy DL, McCarthy SE (2009) Rare structural variants in schizophrenia: one disorder, multiple mutations; one mutation, multiple disorders. Trends Genet 25: 528–535.
46. Kirov G, Grozeva D, Norton N, Ivanov D, Mantripragada KK, et al. (2009) Support for the involvement of large copy number variants in the pathogenesis of schizophrenia. Hum Mol Genet 18: 1497–1503.
47. Xu B, Woodroffe A, Rodriguez-Murillo L, Roos JL, van Rensburg EJ, et al. (2009) Elucidating the genetic architecture of familial schizophrenia using rare copy number variant and linkage scans. Proc Natl Acad Sci U S A 106: 16746–16751.
48. Malhotra D, McCarthy S, Michaelson JJ, Vacic V, Burdick KE, et al. (2011) High frequencies of de novo CNVs in bipolar disorder and schizophrenia. Neuron 72: 951–963.
49. Williams NM, Zaharieva I, Martin A, Langley K, Mantripragada K, et al. (2010) Rare chromosomal deletions and duplications in attention-deficit hyperactivity disorder: a genome-wide analysis. Lancet 376: 1401–1408.
50. Fernandez TV, Sanders SJ, Yurkiewicz IR, Ercan-Sencicek AG, Kim YS, et al. (2012) Rare copy number variants in tourette syndrome disrupt genes in histaminergic pathways and overlap with autism. Biol Psychiatry 71: 392–402.
51. Ahn K, Gotay N, Andersen TM, Anvari AA, Gochman P, et al. (2013) High rate of disease-related copy number variations in childhood onset schizophrenia. Mol Psychiatry.
52. Melchior L, Bertelsen B, Debes NM, Groth C, Skov L, et al. (2013) Microduplication of 15q13.3 and Xq21.31 in a family with Tourette syndrome and comorbidities. Am J Med Genet B Neuropsychiatr Genet 162B: 825–831.
53. Coppola A, Bagnasco I, Traverso M, Brusco A, Di Gregorio E, et al. (2013) Different electroclinical picture of generalized epilepsy in two families with 15q13.3 microdeletion. Epilepsia 54: e69–73.
54. Pagnamenta AT, Wing K, Sadighi Akha E, Knight SJ, Bölte S, et al. (2009) A 15q13.3 microdeletion segregating with autism. Eur J Hum Genet 17: 687–692.
55. Le Pichon JB, Yu S, Kibiryeva N, Graf WD, Bittel DC (2013) Genome-wide gene expression in a patient with 15q13.3 homozygous microdeletion syndrome. Eur J Hum Genet.
56. Barrett MT, Scheffer A, Ben-Dor A, Sampas N, Lipson D, et al. (2004) Comparative genomic hybridization using oligonucleotide microarrays and total genomic DNA. Proc Natl Acad Sci U S A 101: 17765–17770.
57. Ben-Shachar S, Lanpher B, German JR, Qasaymeh M, Potocki L, et al. (2009) Microdeletion 15q13.3: a locus with incomplete penetrance for autism, mental retardation, and psychiatric disorders. J Med Genet 46: 382–388.
58. Solovieff N, Cotsapas C, Lee PH, Purcell SM, Smoller JW (2013) Pleiotropy in complex traits: challenges and strategies. Nat Rev Genet 14: 483–495.

Impaired Perception of Facial Motion in Autism Spectrum Disorder

Justin O'Brien[1], Janine Spencer[1]*, Christine Girges[1], Alan Johnston[2], Harold Hill[3]

1 Centre for Research in Infant Behaviour, Department of Psychology, Brunel University, Uxbridge, United Kingdom, **2** Cognitive, Perceptual and Brain Sciences, Psychology and Language Sciences, University College London, London, United Kingdom, **3** School of Psychology, University of Wollongong, Wollongong, New South Wales, Australia

Abstract

Facial motion is a special type of biological motion that transmits cues for socio-emotional communication and enables the discrimination of properties such as gender and identity. We used animated average faces to examine the ability of adults with autism spectrum disorders (ASD) to perceive facial motion. Participants completed increasingly difficult tasks involving the discrimination of (1) sequences of facial motion, (2) the identity of individuals based on their facial motion and (3) the gender of individuals. Stimuli were presented in both upright and upside-down orientations to test for the difference in inversion effects often found when comparing ASD with controls in face perception. The ASD group's performance was impaired relative to the control group in all three tasks and unlike the control group, the individuals with ASD failed to show an inversion effect. These results point to a deficit in facial biological motion processing in people with autism, which we suggest is linked to deficits in lower level motion processing we have previously reported.

Editor: Galit Yovel, Tel Aviv University, Israel

Funding: The authors have no funding or support to report.

Competing Interests: The authors have declared that no competing interests exist.

* Email: janine.spencer@brunel.ac.uk

Introduction

The human body conveys an abundance of information necessary for mediating socio-emotional communication [1]. Bodily movements, facial expressions and eye gaze shifts allow us to extract information from others. We can then use this to understand their thoughts, intentions and moods [2]. Without the ability to perceive this information, social interaction would be difficult. Autism spectrum disorder (ASD) is a heterogeneous developmental disorder, characterised by a severe impairment in social communication and interaction. One factor may be due to abnormalities in the mechanisms responsible for biological motion (BM) perception.

BM has been widely studied in ASD, yet the current data is equivocal. The first discrepancy concerns what aspect of this perception is actually impaired in ASD. A number of studies report that the deficit only exists when perceiving *emotional* BM [3–6]. For example, one study found that high-functioning children with ASD only experienced difficulty perceiving point-light emotions. Performance was relatively normal on tasks involving body actions or inanimate movement [7]. Similarly, impairment has been observed when those with autism identify point-light bodily expressions of anger, happiness and disgust [8]. By contrast, there is evidence of the impairment extending to *non-emotional* stimuli too [9–11]. Blake *et al.*, asked children with autism to state whether a brief point-light animation represented a body or not. Such task was relatively unemotional, and should have evoked a normal performance. This was not the case however; those with autism still made many more errors compared to the control group [12]. These findings were later replicated by Annaz *et al.*, [13] and Nackaerts *et al.*, [14], further suggesting that all elements of BM perception is weakened in ASD.

The second discrepancy regards data which conversely report intact BM mechanisms in ASD. One study presented participants with point-light displays (walking figures, translating triangles, or translating unfamiliar shapes) embedded in noise and asked them to determine the direction of movement. Those with ASD performed similarly to controls across all three tasks [15]. Murphy and colleagues also showed that ASD participants could successfully identify the direction in which a point-light walker (embedded in noise) was moving in. The authors suggest that ASD participants were able to integrate local motion cues to produce a coherent perception of BM [16].

Such findings may reflect an experimental bias caused by testing different age groups. Studies conducted with ASD children consistently report a deficit in BM perception [7,12,17], whereas the adult data is less conclusive. Perhaps such perception improves with chronological age [4,13]. It is possible that older ASD subjects acquire compensatory mechanisms, and thus perform similarly to typically developing subjects on BM tasks. For example, the absence of global processing may force ASD adults to acquire superior processing with local cues [18]. Alternatively, factors such as symptom severity [12] or general intelligence [19] could affect the ability of ASD participants to perceive BM. Indeed, Rutherford and Troje [20] showed that only those ASD individuals with a low IQ had a poor perception of BM.

While the existing data has been highly informative, there is a paucity of research exploring the perception of facial BM. Yet, the face facilitates social interaction by providing both categorical (identity, gender, age) and qualitative (emotions, intentions, thoughts) visual information. If we are to assume that BM deficits are accountable for impairments in social cognition, then it is essential we actually investigate this using facial BM. To our current knowledge, only two research groups have utilized dynamic face stimuli when examining emotion recognition in ASD. Pelphrey *et al.*, [21] and Sato *et al.*, [22] observed functional abnormalities within a number of areas responsible for social perception (e.g., amygdala, fusiform gyrus and superior temporal sulcus) and visual processing, respectively. This constellation of neural abnormalities may therefore cause impairments in facial motion perception [23].

Facial BM perception in ASD is thus beginning to attract the attention of researchers. Much of this cognition however is still left relatively unexplored. We therefore utilized averaged facial motion captures [24] to investigate whether ASD individuals could use facial motion to discriminate between sequences, identify different unfamiliar individuals and categorise genders. Previous studies with typically developing subjects have shown that facial motion cues are sufficient in aiding these discriminations [24–29], but see others for conflicting data [30,31]. It demonstrates that 3D dynamic information provides a better structural depiction of the face, perhaps by increasing and refining view-points or conveying idiosyncratic mannerisms typical to the individual [27,32,33].

Presentations of facial motion varied between upright and inverted stimuli. This allowed us to observe significant differences between the ability of ASD and control participants in their perception of facial motion. Studies conducted with static faces have demonstrated that inverted stimuli affect face recognition by disrupting configural processing and early structural encoding [34,35]. As a result, accuracy on such face perception tasks is significantly reduced. Previous research has not found this effect in ASD [36,37,38], suggesting that subjects fail to utilize configural strategies and instead rely on feature-based processing [39]. Indeed, children with autism have a superior perception of individual facial features and are better at recognising partially obscured faces than controls [40]. Recent reviews however have highlighted inconsistencies surrounding this manipulation in ASD [41]. This may be a consequence of studies implicating the often unrealistic static facial display.

Thus, in the current study we sought to address two questions: (1) are ASD subjects able to perceive facial motion, and use such information when making judgments about sequence, identity or gender and; (2) is the performance of ASD subjects unaffected by inversion paradigms, therefore confirming feature-based processing of faces in ASD. Answering such questions might shed light on whether an impaired perception of facial BM contributes to the social cognitive impairments seen in this disorder.

Method

Ethics Statement

Full ethical approval was obtained from the Brunel University Social Science ethics committee. All participants gave written informed consent prior to the study and received a debriefing document following their participation.

Participants

Adults with ASD were recruited from residential care facilities in the London area for individuals on the autism spectrum. Fourteen high-functioning individuals with ASD (*subtype = Asperger's Syndrome, DSM-IV-TR code: 299.80*) took part (11 male, 3 female, *mean age* = 33. 85 years, *range* = 22–51 years, *Autistic Quotient (AQ) score* = 26.40). All fourteen participants were diagnosed by psychiatrists specializing in developmental disorders. The diagnoses were based on the DSM-IV-TR (APA, 2000) criteria. Eleven participants were right handed, and three were left handed. The highest level of education varied within the ASD group from high school to the first year of a university degree. Fourteen individuals with typical development also took part (7 male, 7 female, *mean age* = 31.14 years, *range* = 21–56 years, *AQ score* = 14.45), and were recruited from Brunel University (London, UK). All participants were right handed and the highest level of education ranged from high school to university degrees (or the equivalent). None of the ASD or control sample had any history of other neurological or psychological conditions and reported normal or corrected-to-normal vision.

Groups were matched on age and scales of non-verbal analytic intelligence (Standard Progressive Matrices) [42]. We used such measures of IQ as ASD participants had already received standard IQ testing within a year prior to the current study. It was therefore necessary to use other measures to avoid practise effects. Both groups of participants were also tested on their ability to perceive static faces [43], which they all completed within the normal range. Any difficulty then experienced during experimental testing would therefore suggest a specific problem in facial motion perception, rather than a generalised impairment in face processing. Characteristics of control and ASD participants are presented in Table 1.

Stimuli

Facial animations were generated by applying the motion captured from 12 actors to a three-dimensional averaged face (see [24]). Each animation was of an 'actor' telling simple question and answer jokes. These jokes elicited natural facial expressions and movements. The animations were all identical and only differed in the way they moved. This allowed the experimenters to measure biological motion independently, without information from audio or other visual cues influencing the responses. An inverted version of each stimulus was generated in Matlab by manipulation and re-encoding of the original stimulus video file. The present study used these stimuli to investigate whether individuals with ASD could perceive and discriminate facial motion.

Procedure

The dynamic face stimuli were presented using an LCD display with resolution 1024×768 and 60 Hz refresh rate. Viewing distance was approximately 60 cm, at which distance the 30 cm×22.5 cm display subtended an angle of 26.6°×20.6°. The height of the average face was approximately 10.5°, and the frame rate of the animation was 30 FPS. Instructions were given verbally and the experimenter recorded participants' verbal responses manually. Each participant took part in all of the experimental conditions.

There were three experimental tasks (sequence, identity and gender discrimination), each with two manipulations (upright and inverted). Each condition had 21 trials, plus 8 attention control trials. The first condition was the *sequence discrimination task*. Participants viewed a single facial animation displayed in the centre of the screen. They then viewed the same animation again, plus a completely different animation, shown side-by-side on the screen. All animations were presented for 5 seconds. Using a two-alternative forced choice procedure, participants had to indicate which stimuli (left or right on the screen) were present in both presentations. A similar format was used for the *identity discrimination task*. A single facial animation was presented, followed by another two animations. One of the test animations was from the same actor telling a different joke (the correct response), and the other was of a second actor telling another different joke. The

Table 1. Characteristics of adults with ASD and the control group.

Variable	Controls	ASD	*P-value*
n	14	14	–
Age, years			
Mean	31.14	33.85	0.570
Range	21–56	22–51	–
SPM*			
Mean	49.00	42.31	0.070
Range	31–56	19–52	–
% score	82	71	–
Benton Facial Recognition*			
Mean	47.79	45.79	0.287
Range	45–54	36–52	–
% score	89	85	–
AQ*			
Mean	14.45	26.40	0.001
Range	12–20	21–36	–

*Maximum possible scores for the Standard Progressive Matrices (SPM) = 60; for the Benton Facial Recognition test = 54; scores between 11 and 22 on the Autistic Quotient (AQ) scale were considered average.

gender discrimination test required participants to view a single animation, and respond whether it was male or female. Conditions were randomised to avoid familiarity effects. Please see supporting information for example PowerPoint files demonstrating the procedure for each task (PowerPoint S1–S3).

All conditions included attention-control trials. On every fourth trial, the correct responses were indicated with a blue arrow placed above the animation. The arrow was present at the beginning of the trial, and remained on the screen until the participant made their response. Participants were aware that the arrow indicated the correct answer. The responses to these trials were not included in any subsequent analysis. The purpose of these trials was to be able to eliminate from consideration any data provided by a participant in a given condition who did not show full attention to the task. All control and ASD subjects completed the attention control trials without error. Consequently no data was discarded. It is common practice in the psychological literature of developmental disorders to match participants in experimental and control groups by chronological age and verbal mental age. Such measures are insufficient to ensure that the only difference in responses from participants is due to the perceptual factors under investigation. Observer responses can be influenced by fatigue, boredom or intermittent confusion, for example, and the use of attention-control trials can be used as a conservative criterion for rejecting any data where there is a possibility of non-perceptual factors influencing responses [44].

Results

Figure 1 shows the proportion of correct responses made by ASD and control subjects for each task. One-sampled t-tests were used to compare the performance in each condition with the chance response rate of 10.5 (50%). For the ASD group, performance was not significantly above chance level of 0.05 (Bonferroni corrected) in the (1) inverted identity discrimination; (2) upright gender discrimination; and (3) inverted gender discrimination tasks. The control group did not perform above chance on the inverted gender discrimination task.

A mixed design ANOVA indicated a significant three-way interaction between *task type* (sequence, identity, gender) *orientation* (upright, inverted) and *group* (ASD, controls) ($F_{(2,\ 52)} = 9.965$, $p < .001$). We observed a further significant interaction between *orientation* and *group* on the facial motion sequence ($F_{(1,\ 26)} = 5.236$, $p = .030$), identity ($F_{(1,\ 26)} = 4.826$, $p = .037$), and gender ($F_{(1,\ 26)} = 9.071$, $p = .006$) discrimination tasks.

A follow up one-way ANOVA revealed a significant difference between the performance of the ASD and control group on both the *upright sequence* ($F_{(1,\ 26)} = 7.73$, $p = 0.01$) and *upright identity* $F_{(1,\ 26)} = 9.16$, $p < 0.01$) discrimination tasks. Compared to control participants, the ASD sample made more errors during these tasks. Further, there were no significant differences between ASD and control participants on the *upright gender* discrimination task ($p > 0.05$). However, the difficulty of this task was such that

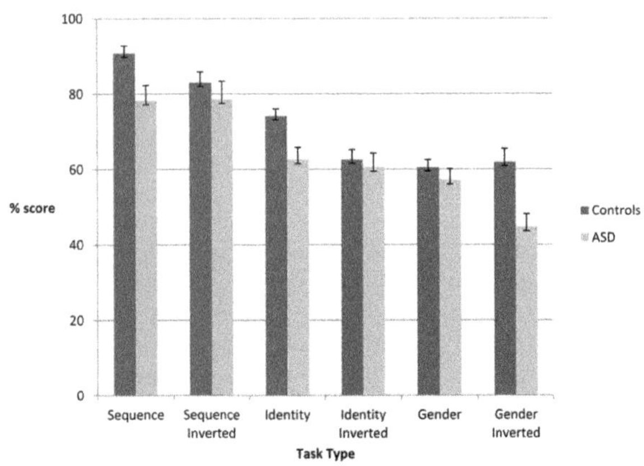

Figure 1. Proportion of correct responses on each task for the control and ASD subjects.

performance was above chance only for the control group in the upright condition.

The same analysis was applied to data from inverted conditions (Table 2). There were no significant differences between the ASD and control group for *inverted sequence* ($F_{(1, 26)} = 0.90$, $p>0.05$) and *inverted identity* discrimination tasks ($F_{(1, 26)} = 0.19$, $p>0.05$). Inverted facial motion affected the controls, decreasing their correct response rate. For those with ASD, there was no difference in performance on upright and inverted conditions. Inverting the stimuli during *gender discrimination* tasks did however produce a significant difference between the control and ASD group ($F_{(1, 27)} = 11.89$, $p = 0.002$). This finding may be discounted though by the below chance performance evident in both groups.

Discussion

Impairments in perceiving BM has been suggested to underlie the social cognitive deficits in ASD [30,31]. We extended such investigations to facial motion perception, examining whether ASD subjects could use these cues to make certain categorizations. Participants therefore engaged in sequence, identity and gender discrimination tasks.

Our findings indicate that although the current ASD sample were able to recognise static faces from the Benton's test, they were still poor on tasks requiring them to discriminate between upright sequences of facial motion. They were also unable to use upright facial motion as a cue for identity. An inability to recognise a number of different individuals from basic motion patterns may significantly impact social cognition in ASD. Moreover, unlike the control group, ASD subjects did not show an inversion effect in either task even though facial motion appears to be processed by a system tuned to upright faces [24]. It would appear then that the neural mechanisms responsible for facial motion perception are weakened in ASD. This finding is comparable to other investigations which have utilized point-light body motion stimuli [4,7,8,10,12,14].

We are disinclined to suggest poor attentional abilities are at the root of the problem as all participants scored correctly on the attention-control trials in each experimental condition. Incompetent cognitive skills can also be dismissed; all participants passed the Standard Progressive Matrices test within the typical range and understood the tasks well. Perhaps the impairment in facial BM perception arises from problems in configural processing [12]. Individuals with ASD may focus heavily on a particular and perhaps trivial feature, at the expense of global motion [45]. There is some evidence to support this view. Van Boxtel and Lu [18] measured accuracy on a central counting paradigm while task-irrelevant biological movements were presented in the periphery of participants with low and high autistic traits. Stimuli were either intact or spatially scrambled. Subjects with fewer autistic traits were found to involuntarily process global aspects of BM even when it negatively affected their central task performance. Individuals with high autistic traits however did not show this attentional distraction, performing identically on the central task in the scrambled and intact conditions. An absence in configural (or global) processing would certainly support the indifference to orientation present in our current ASD sample. Engaging more in featural or local processing would by-pass the disruption caused by inverted motion [38,40].

The impairment could also lie within low-level visual mechanisms, specifically in the transmission of information from primary visual areas to substrates involved in social cognition [46]. This may explain why the superior temporal sulcus -a structure known for its involvement in BM processing- is often hypo-activated in ASD individuals compared to typical controls [47–50]. It is not unreasonable to suggest a deficit in integrating or transmitting complex perceptual information, rather than a dysfunction of a specialised social structure *per se*. Studies of motion perception in ASD have shown the etiology of such deficit to lie within weakened integration mechanisms and/or faulty visual (dorsal) pathways [51–55]. Abnormal connectivity between key substrates could also lead to deficits in the perception of biological movements. For example, Sato *et al.*, [22] observed decreases in the bi-directional connectivity between the primary visual cortex, middle temporal gyrus and the inferior frontal gyrus when ASD subjects viewed dynamic displays of facial emotion. Such neural impairments may therefore underlie the facial motion deficits seen in the current study.

Further, control and ASD participants did not differ in their performance on *upright gender* discrimination tasks. This result is discussed in reference to the stimuli set. Some of the facial motion captures appeared to be somewhat impassive or expressionless. As Berry [26] states, female faces are typically more animated during interaction than are male faces. For the control group, a higher percentage of animations may have therefore been incorrectly judged as male. This larger proportion of incorrect answers would then be more comparable with ASD participants, who seemed to completely guess answers as indicated by a below chance performance. The ASD participants also showed an inversion effect during this task. We are uncertain that this is a genuine effect though due to their below chance performance here.

It is possible that we are running into a floor effect on gender discrimination tasks. However, a similar study which looked at discriminating genders from facial motion found that healthy controls could only do this for 68% of the trials [26]. Such result is

Table 2. Mean scores (Standard Deviations) and results from a one-way ANOVA.

Variable	Mean (SD)		Differences between groups (One-way ANOVA)		
	ASD	*Controls*	*F*	*df*	*P-value*
Sequence	16.43 (3.18)	19.07 (1.59)	7.73	1, 26	0.010
Sequence Inverted	16.50 (2.93)	17.43 (2.21)	0.90	1, 26	0.352
Identity	13.14 (2.63)	15.57 (1.45)	9.16	1, 26	0.006
Identity Inverted	12.71* (3.05)	13.14 (2.14)	0.19	1, 26	0.671
Gender	12.00* (2.35)	12.71 (1.59)	0.89	1, 26	0.355
Gender Inverted	9.36* (2.74)	13.00* (2.68)	11.89	1, 26	0.002

*Indicates any result not above chance.

comparable to the 61% found in the current study. Hill and Johnston [24] also report a just above chance performance on gender discrimination tasks in typically developing individuals. These findings demonstrate that perhaps accurate gender identification relies on the presence of both facial motion and characteristic structural form cues. As the current study did not include stimuli which differed in appearance, we cannot comment on this but encourage future investigations to clarify this issue.

Conclusion

Our data indicates that those with ASD have an impaired perception of facial motion, and are unable to use such cues when making categorical discriminations. This result is discussed in terms of faulty configural mechanisms and/or a dysfunction within visual pathways leading to key BM processing substrates. Such impairment could then contribute to the socio-emotional impairments seen within this disorder. Future studies may wish to elaborate on these results by correlating symptom severity with facial motion perception or examining abnormalities within such networks during facial motion categorisations.

Supporting Information

PowerPoint S1 Example of the sequence discrimination trials.

PowerPoint S2 Example of the identity discrimination trials.

PowerPoint S3 Example of the gender discrimination trials.

Acknowledgments

We are very grateful to all the individuals who volunteered their precious time to take part in this research.

Author Contributions

Conceived and designed the experiments: JS JOB HH AJ. Performed the experiments: JS JOB CG. Analyzed the data: JS JOB CG HH. Contributed reagents/materials/analysis tools: HH AJ. Wrote the paper: JOB JS CG.

References

1. Gepner B, Deruelle C, Grynfeltt S (2001) Motion and emotion: a novel approach to the study of face processing by young autistic children. J Autism Dev Disord 31(1): 37–45.
2. Koldewyn K, Whitney D, Rivera SM (2011) Neural correlates of coherent and biological motion perception in autism. Dev Sci 14 (5): 1075–1088.
3. Hadjikhani N, Joseph RM, Manoach DS, Naik P, Snyder J, et al (2009) Body expressions of emotion do not trigger fear contagion in autism spectrum disorder. Soc Cogn Affect Neurosci 4(1): 70–8. doi:10.1093/scan/nsn038.
4. Hubert B, Wicker B, Moore DG, Monfardini E, Duverger H, et al (2007) Brief report: recognition of emotional and non-emotional biological motion in individuals with autistic spectrum disorders. J Autism Dev Disord 37(7): 1386–92. doi:10.1007/s10803-006-0275-y.
5. Moore D, Hobson RP, Lee A (1997) Components of person perception: An investigation with autistic, non-autistic retarded and typically developing children and adolescents. Br J Dev Psychol 15: 401–423.
6. Swettenham J, Remington A, Laing K, Coleman M, Gomez JC (2013) Perception of pointing from biological motion point-light displays in typically developing children and children with autism spectrum disorder. J Autism Dev Disord 43 (6): 1437–46. doi:10.1007/s10803-012-1699-1.
7. Parron C, Da Fonseca D, Santos A, Moore DG, Monfardini E, et al (2008) Recognition of biological motion in children with autistic spectrum disorders. Autism 12(3): 261–74. doi:10.1177/1362361307089520.
8. Atkinson AP (2009) Impaired recognition of emotions from body movements is associated with elevated motion coherence thresholds in autism spectrum disorders. Neuropsychologia 47(13): 3023–9. doi:10.1016/j.neuropsychologia.2009.05.019.
9. Cook J, Saygin AP, Swain R, Blakemore SJ (2009) Reduced sensitivity to minimum-jerk biological motion in autism spectrum conditions. Neuropsychologia 47: 3275–78.
10. Cook JL, Blakemore SJ, Press C (2013) Atypical basis movement kinematics in autism spectrum conditions. Brain 136: 2816–2824.
11. Koldewyn K, Whitney D, Rivera SM (2010) The psychophysics of visual motion and global form processing in autism. Brain 13: 599–610.
12. Blake R, Turner LM, Smoski MJ, Pozdol SL, Stone WL (2003) Visual recognition of biological motion is impaired in children with autism. Psychol Sci 14(2): 151–7.
13. Annaz D, Remington A, Milne E, Coleman M, Campbell R, et al (2010) Development of motion processing in children with autism. Dev Sci, 13 (6): 826–38. doi:10.1111/j.1467-7687.2009.00939.x.
14. Nackaerts E, Wagemans J, Helsen W, Swinnen SP, Wenderoth N, et al (2012) Recognizing biological motion and emotions from point-light displays in autism spectrum disorders. PLoS One 7(9): e44473. doi:10.1371/journal.pone.0044473.
15. Saygin AP, Cook J, Blakemore SJ (2010) Unaffected perceptual thresholds for biological and non-biological form-from-motion perception in autism spectrum conditions. PLoS One 5(10): e13491. doi:10.1371/journal.pone.0013491.
16. Murphy P, Brady N, Fitzgerald M, Troje NF (2009) No evidence for impaired perception of biological motion in adults with autistic spectrum disorders. Neuropsychologia 47: 3225–35.
17. Klin A, Lin DJ, Gorrindo P, Ramsay G, Jones W (2009) Two-year-olds with autism orient to non-social contingencies rather than biological motion. Nature 459 (7244): 257–61. doi:10.1038/nature07868.
18. Van Boxtel JJA, Lu H (2013) Impaired global and compensatory local, biological motion processing in people with high levels of autistic traits. Front Psychol 4 (209): 1–10. doi:10.3389/fpsyg.2013.00209.
19. Jones CRG, Swettenham J, Charman T, Marsden AJS, Tregay J, et al (2011) No evidence for a fundamental visual motion processing deficit in adolescents with autism spectrum disorders. Autism Res 4(5): 347–57. doi:10.1002/aur.209.
20. Rutherford MD, Troje NF (2012) IQ predicts biological motion perception in autism spectrum disorders. J Autism Dev Disord 42(4): 557–65. doi:10.1007/s10803-011-1267-0.
21. Pelphrey KA, Morris JP, McCarthy G, Labar KS (2007) Perception of dynamic changes in facial affect and identity in autism. Soc Cogn Affect Neurosci 2(2): 140–9. doi:10.1093/scan/nsm010.
22. Sato W, Toichi M, Uono S, Kochiyama T (2012) Impaired social brain network for processing dynamic facial expressions in autism spectrum disorders. BMC Neurosci 13: 99. doi:10.1186/1471-2202-13-99.
23. Sato W, Uono S, Toichi M (2013) Atypical recognition of dynamic changes in facial expressions in autism spectrum disorders. Res in Autism Spectr Disord 7: 906–912. doi: 10.1016/j.rasd.2013.04.008.
24. Hill H, Johnston A (2001) Categorizing sex and identity from the biological motion of faces. Curr Biol 11(11): 880–5.
25. Thornton IM, Kourtzi Z (2002) A matching advantage for dynamic human faces. Perception 31: 113–32.
26. Berry DS (1991) Child and adult sensitivity to gender information in patterns of facial motion. Ecol Psychol 3: 349–36.
27. O'Toole AJ, Roark DA, Abdi H (2002) Recognizing moving faces: Psychological and neural synthesis. Trends Cogn Sci 6(6): 261–266.
28. Pilz KS, Thornton IM, Bülthoff HH (2006) A search advantage for faces learned in motion. Exp Brain Res 171: 436–447. doi:10.1007/s00221-005-0283-8.
29. Thornton IM, Mullins E, Banahan K (2011) Motion can amplify the face-inversion effect. Psihologija 44: 5–22. doi:10.2298/PSI1101005T.
30. Christie F, Bruce V (1998) The role of dynamic information in the recognition of unfamiliar faces. Mem Cognit 26: 780–90.
31. Lander K, Chuang L (2005) Why are moving faces easier to recognize? Vis Cogn 12(3): 429–442. doi:10.1080/13506280444000382.
32. Watson T, Johnston A, Hill H, Troje N (2005) Motion as a cue for viewpoint invariance. Vis Cogn 12(7): 1291–1308. doi:10.1080/13506280444000526.
33. Knight B, Johnston A (1997) The role of movement in face recognition. Vis Cogn 4: 265–273.
34. Valentine T (1998) Upside-down faces: A review of the effect of inversion on face recognition. Br J Psychol 79: 471–491.
35. Itier RJ, Taylor MJ (2002) Inversion and contrast polarity reversal affect both encoding and recognition processes of unfamiliar faces: a repetition study using ERPs. NeuroImage 15(2): 353–72. doi:10.1006/nimg.2001.0982.
36. Webb SJ, Merkle K, Murias M, Richards T, Aylward E, et al (2012) ERP responses differentiate inverted but not upright face processing in adults with ASD. Soc Cogn Affect Neurosci 7(5): 578–87. doi:10.1093/scan/nsp002.
37. Langdell T (1978) Recognition of faces: An approach to the study of autism. J Child Psychol Psychiatry 19: 255–268.

38. Hobson RP, Ouston J, Lee A (1988) Emotion recognition in autism: coordinating faces and voices. Psychol Med 18: 911–23.
39. Spezio ML, Adolphs R, Hurley RSE, Piven J (2007) Analysis of face gaze in autism using 'Bubbles'. Neuropsychologia 45: 144–151.
40. Tantam D, Monoghan L, Nicholson H, Stirling J (1989) Autistic children's ability to interpret faces: A research note. J Child Psychol Psychiatry 30: 623–630.
41. Weigelt S, Koldewyn K, Kanwisher N (2012) Face identity recognition in autism spectrum disorders: a review of behavioral studies. Neurosci Biobehav Rev 36(3): 1060–84. doi:10.1016/j.neubiorev.2011.12.008.
42. Raven J, Raven JC, Court JH (2003, updated 2004) Manual for Raven's Progressive Matrices and Vocabulary Scales. San Antonio, TX: Harcourt Assessment.
43. Benton AL, Sivan AB, Hamsher K, Varney NR, Spreen O (1983) Contribution to neuropsychological assessment. NY: Oxford University Press.
44. Spencer JV, O'Brien JMD (2006) Visual form-processing deficits in autism. Perception 35(8): 1047–1055. doi:10.1068/p5328.
45. Behrmann M, Thomas C, Humphreys K (2006) Seeing it differently: visual processing in autism. Trends Cogni Sci 10: 258–264.
46. Zilbovicius M, Meresse I, Chabane N, Brunelle F, Samson Y, et al (2006) Autism, the superior temporal sulcus and social perception. Trends Neurosci 29(7): 359–66. doi:10.1016/j.tins.2006.06.004.
47. Herrington J, Baron-Cohen S, Wheelwright S, Singh K, Bullmore E, et al (2007) The role of MT+/V5 during biological motion perception in Asperger's Syndrome: An fMRI study. Res Autism Spectr Disord 1(1): 14–27. doi:10.1016/j.rasd.2006.07.002.
48. Freitag CM, Konrad C, Häberlen M, Kleser C, von Gontard A, et al (2008) Perception of biological motion in autism spectrum disorders. Neuropsychologia 46(5): 1480–94. doi:10.1016/j.neuropsychologia.2007.12.025.
49. McKay LS, Simmons DR, McAleer P, Marjoram D, Piggot J, et al (2012) Do distinct atypical cortical networks process biological motion information in adults with Autism Spectrum Disorders? NeuroImage 59(2): 1524–33. doi:10.1016/j.neuroimage.2011.08.033.
50. Shih P, Keehn B, Oram JK, Leyden KM, Keown CL, et al (2011) Functional differentiation of posterior superior temporal sulcus in autism: A functional connectivity magnetic resonance imaging study. Biol Psychiatry 70(3): 270–277. doi:10.1016/j.biopsych.2011.03.040.
51. Spencer J, O'Brien JMD, Riggs K, Braddick OJ, Atkinson J, et al (2000) Dorsal Stream Deficit in Autism. NeuroReport 11: 2765–2767.
52. Pellicano E, Gibson L, Maybery M, Durkin K, Badcock DR (2005) Abnormal global processing along the dorsal visual pathway in autism: a possible mechanism for weak visuospatial coherence? Neuropsychologia 43(7): 1044–53. doi:10.1016/j.neuropsychologia.2004.10.003.
53. Robertson CE, Martin A, Baker CI, Baron-Cohen S (2012) Atypical integration of motion signals in Autism Spectrum Conditions. PloS one 7(11): e48173. doi:10.1371/journal.pone.0048173.
54. Braddick O, Atkinson J, Wattam-Bell J (2003) Normal and anomalous development of visual motion processing: Motion coherence and 'dorsal-stream vulnerability'. Neuropsychologia 41: 1769–1784.
55. Brieber S, Herpertz-Dahlmann B, Fink GR, Kamp-Becker I, Remschmidt H, et al (2010) Coherent motion processing in autism spectrum disorder (ASD): an fMRI study. Neuropsychologia 48(6): 1644–51. doi:10.1016/j.neuropsychologia.2010.02.007.

Permissions

All chapters in this book were first published in PLOS ONE, by The Public Library of Science; hereby published with permission under the Creative Commons Attribution License or equivalent. Every chapter published in this book has been scrutinized by our experts. Their significance has been extensively debated. The topics covered herein carry significant findings which will fuel the growth of the discipline. They may even be implemented as practical applications or may be referred to as a beginning point for another development.

The contributors of this book come from diverse backgrounds, making this book a truly international effort. This book will bring forth new frontiers with its revolutionizing research information and detailed analysis of the nascent developments around the world.

We would like to thank all the contributing authors for lending their expertise to make the book truly unique. They have played a crucial role in the development of this book. Without their invaluable contributions this book wouldn't have been possible. They have made vital efforts to compile up to date information on the varied aspects of this subject to make this book a valuable addition to the collection of many professionals and students.

This book was conceptualized with the vision of imparting up-to-date information and advanced data in this field. To ensure the same, a matchless editorial board was set up. Every individual on the board went through rigorous rounds of assessment to prove their worth. After which they invested a large part of their time researching and compiling the most relevant data for our readers.

The editorial board has been involved in producing this book since its inception. They have spent rigorous hours researching and exploring the diverse topics which have resulted in the successful publishing of this book. They have passed on their knowledge of decades through this book. To expedite this challenging task, the publisher supported the team at every step. A small team of assistant editors was also appointed to further simplify the editing procedure and attain best results for the readers.

Apart from the editorial board, the designing team has also invested a significant amount of their time in understanding the subject and creating the most relevant covers. They scrutinized every image to scout for the most suitable representation of the subject and create an appropriate cover for the book.

The publishing team has been an ardent support to the editorial, designing and production team. Their endless efforts to recruit the best for this project, has resulted in the accomplishment of this book. They are a veteran in the field of academics and their pool of knowledge is as vast as their experience in printing. Their expertise and guidance has proved useful at every step. Their uncompromising quality standards have made this book an exceptional effort. Their encouragement from time to time has been an inspiration for everyone.

The publisher and the editorial board hope that this book will prove to be a valuable piece of knowledge for researchers, students, practitioners and scholars across the globe.

List of Contributors

Drew W. R. Halliday and James W. Tanaka
University of Victoria, Victoria, British Columbia, Canada
The Centre for Autism Research, Technology and Education, Victoria, British Columbia, Canada

Stuart W. S. MacDonald
University of Victoria, Victoria, British Columbia, Canada

Suzanne K. Sherf
The Pennsylvania State University, State College, Pennsylvania, United States of America

Doug Hyun Han
Department of Psychiatry, Chung Ang University Hospital, Seoul, South Korea

Hee Jeong Yoo
Department of Psychiatry, Seoul National Bundang Hospital, Seoul, South Korea

Bung Nyun Kim
Department of Psychiatry, Seoul National Hospital, Seoul, South Korea

William McMahon
Department of Psychiatry, University of Utah, Salt Lake City, Utah, United States of America

Perry F. Renshaw
The Brain Institute, University of Utah, Salt Lake City, Utah, United States of America

Sophie van Rijn and Hanna Swaab
Clinical Child and Adolescent Studies, Leiden University, Leiden, The Netherlands
Leiden Institute for Brain and Cognition, Leiden, The Netherlands

Marjolein Barendse
Clinical Child and Adolescent Studies, Leiden University, Leiden, The Netherlands

Stephanie van Goozen
Clinical Child and Adolescent Studies, Leiden University, Leiden, The Netherlands
School of Psychology, Cardiff University, Cardiff, United Kingdom

Michiko Koizumi
Graduate School of Education, Hokkaido University, Sapporo, Japan
Japan Society for the Promotion of Science, Tokyo, Japan

Haruto Takagishi
Tamagawa University Brain Science Institute, Tokyo, Japan

Susanne Bejerot and Jonna M. Eriksson
Department of Clinical Neuroscience, Karolinska Institutet, Stockholm, Sweden
Tetsushi Sadakata
Advanced Scientific Research Leaders Development Unit, Gunma University, Maebashi, Gunma, Japan
JST/CREST, Kawaguchi, Saitama, Japan

Wataru Kakegawa and Michisuke Yuzaki
Department of Physiology, School of Medicine, Keio University, Tokyo, Japan

Yo Shinoda and Teiichi Furuichi
JST/CREST, Kawaguchi, Saitama, Japan
Department of Applied Biological Science, Tokyo University of Science, Noda, Chiba, Japan

Mayu Hosono
Advanced Scientific Research Leaders Development Unit, Gunma University, Maebashi, Gunma, Japan

Ritsuko Katoh-Semba, Yukiko Sekine, Yumi Sato and Chihiro Saruta
Department of Applied Biological Science, Tokyo University of Science, Noda, Chiba, Japan

Yasuki Ishizaki
Department of Molecular and Cellular Neurobiology, Gunma University Graduate School of Medicine, Maebashi, Gunma, Japan

Masami Kojima
JST/CREST, Kawaguchi, Saitama, Japan
Biointerface Research group, Health Research Institute, National Institute of Advanced Industrial Science and Technology (AIST), Ikeda, Osaka, Japan

Catherine Clumeck
Laboratoire de Cartographie fonctionnelle du Cerveau, UNI - ULB Neuroscience Institute, Universitélibre de Bruxelles (ULB), Brussels, Belgium
Laboratoire de Recherches Psychiatriques, UNI - ULB Neuroscience Institute, Universitélibre de Bruxelles (ULB), Brussels, Belgium

Sarah Suarez Garcia, Mathieu Bourguignon, Vincent Wens, Marc Op de Beeck, Patrick Van Bogaert, Xavier De Tiège, Brice Marty and Serge Goldman
Laboratoire de Cartographie fonctionnelle du Cerveau, UNI - ULB Neuroscience Institute, Universitélibre de Bruxelles (ULB), Brussels, Belgium

Nicolas Deconinck and Marie-Vincianne Soncarrieu
Centre de référence des troubles envahissants du développement et des troubles autistiques, Hôpital Universitaire des Enfants Reine Fabiola (HUDERF), Brussels, Belgium

Veikko Jousmäki
Brain Research Unit, O.V. Lounasmaa Laboratory and MEG Core, Aalto NeuroImaging, Aalto University, Espoo, Finland

Jiyeon Choi, Myka R. Ababon, Mai Soliman and Paul G. Matteson
Center for Advanced Biotechnology and Medicine, Piscataway, New Jersey, United States of America

Yong Lin
Cancer Institute of New Jersey, Piscataway, New Jersey, United States of America

Linda M. Brzustowicz
Department of Genetics, Rutgers University, Piscataway, New Jersey, United States of America

James H. Millonig
Center for Advanced Biotechnology and Medicine, Piscataway, New Jersey, United States of America
Department of Neuroscience and Cell Biology, Robert Wood Johnson Medical School, Piscataway, New Jersey, United States of America
Department of Genetics, Rutgers University, Piscataway, New Jersey, United States of America

Sina Kohl, Carolin Wolters, Joachim Klosterkötter and Jens Kuhn
Department for Psychiatry and Psychotherapy, University Hospital of Cologne, Cologne, North Rhine-Westphalia, Germany

Theo O. J. Gruendler
Department for Psychiatry and Psychotherapy, University Hospital of Cologne, Cologne, North Rhine-Westphalia, Germany
Department of Economics, Otto-von-Guericke-University, Magdeburg, Saxony-Anhalt, Germany
Center for Behavioral Brain Sciences, Magdeburg, Saxony-Anhalt, Germany

Kai Vogeley
Department for Psychiatry and Psychotherapy, University Hospital of Cologne, Cologne, North Rhine-Westphalia, Germany
Institute for Neuroscience and Medicine - Cognitive Neuroscience (INM3), Research Center Juelich, Juelich, North Rhine-Westphalia, Germany

Hikaru Takeuchi
Smart Ageing International Research Center, Institute of Development, Aging and Cancer, Tohoku University, Sendai, Japan

Yasuyuki Taki, Yuko Sassa and Hiroshi Hashizume
Division of Developmental Cognitive Neuroscience, Institute of Development, Aging and Cancer, Tohoku University, Sendai, Japan

Atsushi Sekiguchi and Ai Fukushima
Department of Functional Brain Imaging, Institute of Development, Aging and Cancer, Tohoku University, Sendai, Japan

Ryuta Kawashima
Smart Ageing International Research Center, Institute of Development, Aging and Cancer, Tohoku University, Sendai, Japan
Division of Developmental Cognitive Neuroscience, Institute of Development, Aging and Cancer, Tohoku University, Sendai, Japan
Department of Functional Brain Imaging, Institute of Development, Aging and Cancer, Tohoku University, Sendai, Japan
Frances Caulfield, Louise Ewing, Nichola Burton, Eleni Avard and Gillian Rhodes
Australian Research Council Centre of Excellence in Cognition and its Disorders, School of Psychology, University of Western Australia, Perth, Western Australia, Australia

Maggie Brett and Ene-Choo Tan
KK Research Centre, KK Women's & Children's Hospital, Singapore, Singapore

John McPherson and Steve Rozen
Duke-NUS Graduate Medical School, Singapore, Singapore

Zhi Jiang Zang
National Cancer Centre, Singapore, Singapore

Angeline Lai, Ee-Shien Tan, Ivy Ng and Breana Cham
Genetic Services, KK Women's & Children's Hospital, Singapore, Singapore

Lai-Choo Ong
Universiti Malaya Medical Centre, Petaling Jaya, Malaysia

Patrick Tan
Duke-NUS Graduate Medical School, Singapore, Singapore
National Cancer Centre, Singapore, Singapore

Alessandro Tavano
Institute of Psychology, University of Leipzig, Leipzig, Germany
Scientific Institute "E.Medea", San Vito al Tagliamento (Pordenone), Italy

Anna Pesarin
Department of Computer Science, University of Verona, Verona, Italy

Vittorio Murino
Italian Institute of Technology (IIT), Genova, Italy

Marco Cristani
Department of Computer Science, University of Verona, Verona, Italy
Italian Institute of Technology (IIT), Genova, Italy

Timo Lorenz and Kathrin Heinitz
Department of Psychology, Freie Universität Berlin, Berlin, Germany

Guillaume Huguet, Nathalie Lemière and Elodie Ey
Human Genetics and Cognitive Functions, Institut Pasteur, Paris, France
CNRS URA 2182 'Genes, synapses and cognitioń, Institut Pasteur, Paris, France
University Denis Diderot Paris 7, Paris, France

Etienne Patin and Guillaume Laval
Unit of Human Evolutionary Genetics, Institut Pasteur, Paris, France

Marion Leboyer
INSERM, U955, Psychiatry Genetic team, Creteil, France
Fondation FondaMental, Créteil, France
Caroline Nava
INSERM, U975—CRICM, Institut du cerveau et de la moelle épiniére (ICM), Hôpital Pitié-Salpêtrière, Paris, France
CNRS 7225—CRICM, Hôpital Pitié-Salpêtrière, Paris, France
Université Pierre et Marie Curie-Paris-6 (UPMC), UMR_S 975, Paris, France,
Département de Génétique et de Cytogénétique, Unité fonctionnelle de génétique clinique, AP-HP, Hôpital Pitié-Salpêtrière, Paris, France

Alexis Brice and Christel Depienne
INSERM, U975—CRICM, Institut du cerveau et de la moelle épiniére (ICM), Hôpital Pitié-Salpêtrière, Paris, France
CNRS 7225—CRICM, Hôpital Pitié-Salpêtrière, Paris, France
Université Pierre et Marie Curie-Paris-6 (UPMC), UMR_S 975, Paris, France,
Département de Génétique et de Cytogénétique, Unité fonctionnelle de neurogénétique moléculaire et cellulaire, AP-HP, Hôpital Pitié-Salpêtrière, Paris, France

Pierre Szepetowski
INSERM, UMR_S901, Marseille, France
Aix-Marseille University, Marseille, France
Mediterranean Institute of Neurobiology (INMED), Marseille, France

Christopher Gillberg
Gillberg Neuropsychiatry Centre, University of Gothenburg, Göteborg, Sweden
Institute of Neuroscience and Physiology, Department of Pharmacology, Gothenburg University, Gothenburg, Sweden
Institute of Child Health, University College London, London, United Kingdom

Richard Delorme
Human Genetics and Cognitive Functions, Institut Pasteur, Paris, France
CNRS URA 2182 'Genes, synapses and cognitioń, Institut Pasteur, Paris, France

Fondation FondaMental, Créteil, France
Assistance Publique-Hôpitaux de Paris, Robert Debré Hospital, Department of Child and Adolescent Psychiatry, Paris, France

Thomas Bourgeron
Human Genetics and Cognitive Functions, Institut Pasteur, Paris, France
CNRS URA 2182 'Genes, synapses and cognitioń, Institut Pasteur, Paris, France
University Denis Diderot Paris 7, Paris, France
Fondation FondaMental, Créteil, France

Cara J. Westmark
Department of Neurology, University of Wisconsin, Madison, Wisconsin, United States of America
Vincent A. Fusaro, Todd F. DeLuca, Olivia D'Angelo, Jenna Tamburello and James Maniscalco
Center for Biomedical Informatics, Harvard Medical School, Boston, Massachusetts, United States of America
Jena Daniels and Marlena Duda
Center for Biomedical Informatics, Harvard Medical School, Boston, Massachusetts, United States of America
Department of Pediatrics, Division of Systems Medicine, Stanford University, Stanford, California, United States of America

Dennis P. Wall
Center for Biomedical Informatics, Harvard Medical School, Boston, Massachusetts, United States of America
Department of Pathology, Beth Israel Deaconess Medical Center, Boston, Massachusetts, United States of America
Department of Pediatrics, Division of Systems Medicine, Stanford University, Stanford, California, United States of America

Daniel Radeloff, Angela Ciaramidaro, Michael Siniatchkin, Daniela Hainz, Sabine Schlitt, Fritz Poustka and Christine Margarete Freitag
Department of Child and Adolescent Psychiatry, Psychosomatics and Psychotherapy, Johann Wolfgang Goethe-Universität, Frankfurt/Main, Frankfurt/Main,Germany

Bernhard Weber
Department of Psychiatry, Psychosomatics and Psychotherapy, Johann Wolfgang Goethe Universität Frankfurt/Main, Frankfurt/Main, Germany
Psychiatric University Clinics, University of Basel, Basel, Switzerland

Sven Bölte
Department of Child and Adolescent Psychiatry, Psychosomatics and Psychotherapy, Johann Wolfgang Goethe-Universität, Frankfurt/Main, Frankfurt/Main,Germany
Department of Women's and Children's Health, Center of Neurodevelopmental Disorders at Karolinska Institutet (KIND), Stockholm, Sweden

Henrik Walter
Department of Psychiatry, Psychosomatics and Psychotherapy, Johann Wolfgang Goethe Universität Frankfurt/Main, Frankfurt/Main, Germany
Division of Mind and Brain Research, Department of Psychiatry and Psychotherapy, Charité-Universitätsmedizin Berlin, Berlin, Germany

Simon Baron-Cohen
Autism Research Centre, Department of Psychiatry, University of Cambridge, Cambridgeshire, United Kingdom
CLASS Clinic, Cambridgeshire and Peterborough NHS Foundation Trust (CPFT), Cambridgeshire, United Kingdom

Laura Murphy, Uma Mallya, Silvia Lakatošová, Sally Wheelwright, Carrie Allison and Varun Warrier
Autism Research Centre, Department of Psychiatry, University of Cambridge, Cambridgeshire, United Kingdom

Bhismadev Chakrabarti
Autism Research Centre, Department of Psychiatry, University of Cambridge, Cambridgeshire, United Kingdom
School of Psychology and Clinical Language Sciences, Centre for Integrative Neuroscience and Neurodynamics, University of Reading, Reading, United Kingdom

Ian Craig
MRC Centre for Social, Genetic and Developmental Psychiatry, King's College London, Institute of Psychiatry, London, United Kingdom

Karola Rehnstrom and Leena Peltonen
The Wellcome Trust Sanger Institute, Hinxton, Cambridgeshire, United Kingdom

Simon E. Fisher
Max Planck Institute for Psycholinguistics, 6500 AH Nijmegen, The Netherlands

Donders Institute for Brain, Cognition and Behaviour, Radboud University Nijmegen, Nijmegen, The Netherlands

Junko Matsuzaki and Fumiyo Nagatani
Molecular Research Center for Children's Mental Development, United Graduate School of Child Development, Osaka University Graduate School of Medicine, Osaka, Japan

Kuriko Kagitani-Shimono and Koji Tominaga
United Graduate School of Child Development, Osaka University Graduate School of Medicine, Osaka, Japan
Department of Pediatrics, Osaka University Graduate School of Medicine, Osaka, Japan

Hisato Sugata and Masayuki Hirata
Department of Neurosurgery, Osaka University Graduate School of Medicine, Osaka, Japan

Ryuzo Hanaie
United Graduate School of Child Development, Osaka University Graduate School of Medicine, Osaka, Japan

Masaya Tachibana, Ikuko Mohri and Masako Taniike
Molecular Research Center for Children's Mental Development, United Graduate School of Child Development, Osaka University Graduate School of Medicine, Osaka, Japan
United Graduate School of Child Development, Osaka University Graduate School of Medicine, Osaka, Japan
Department of Pediatrics, Osaka University Graduate School of Medicine, Osaka, Japan

Tamás Spisák, Sándor A. Kis, Gábor Opposits, Csaba Aranyi and Miklós Emri1
Department of Nuclear Medicine, Medical and Health Science Centre, University of Debrecen, Debrecen, Hungary

András Jakab
Department of Radiology, Medical University of Vienna, Vienna, Austria

Ervin Berényi
Department of Biomedical Laboratory and Imaging Science, Medical and Health Science Center, University of Debrecen, Debrecen, Hungary

Tiziana Zalla and Francesca Ervas
Institut Jean Nicod, CNRS, UMR 8129, Institut d'Etude de la Cognition, Ecole Normale Supérieure, Paris, France

Frederique Amsellem, Pauline Chaste and Marion Leboyer
INSERM U 955, IMRB & University Paris Est Creteil, AP-HP, Henri Mondor-Albert Chenevier Hospitals, Department of Psychiatry, Fondation FondaMental, French National Science Foundation, Creteil, France

Maud Champagne-Lavau
Aix-Marseille University, CNRS, LPL UMR 7309, 13100 Aix-en-Provence, France

Chiara Horlin and Richard Parsons
School of Occupational Therapy & Social Work, CHIRI, Curtin University, Perth, Australia

Marita Falkmer
School of Occupational Therapy & Social Work, CHIRI, Curtin University, Perth, Australia
School of Education and Communication, CHILD Programme, Institute of Disability Research, Jönköping University, Jönköping, Sweden

Matthew A. Albrecht
School of Psychology, CHIRI, Curtin University, Perth, Australia

Torbjorn Falkmer
School of Occupational Therapy & Social Work, CHIRI, Curtin University, Perth, Australia
Rehabilitation Medicine, Department of Medicine and Health Sciences (IMH), Faculty of Health Sciences, Linköping University & Pain and Rehabilitation Centre, Linköping, Sweden
School of Occupational Therapy, La Trobe University, Melbourne, VIC, Australia

Ingrid C. Y. Xuan
Department of Pharmaceutical Sciences, Leslie Dan Faculty of Pharmacy, University of Toronto, Toronto, Canada

David R. Hampson
Department of Pharmaceutical Sciences, Leslie Dan Faculty of Pharmacy, University of Toronto, Toronto, Canada
Department of Pharmacology and Toxicology, Faculty of Medicine, University of Toronto, Toronto, Canada

Carolina Cappi, Juliana Belo Diniz, Aderbal R. T. Silva, Viviane N. S. Reis, Euripedes C. Miguel and Helena Brentani
Institute and Department of Psychiatry, São Paulo University Medical School, São Paulo, Brazil

Ana Gabriela Hounie
Institute and Department of Psychiatry, São Paulo University Medical School, São Paulo, Brazil
Federal University of São Paulo-UPIA-UNIFESP, São Paulo, Brazil

Daniel B. Mariani
Inter-institutional Grad Program on Bioinformatics, Institute of Mathematics and Statistics, São Paulo University, São Paulo, Brazil

Ariane F. Busso, Amanda Gonçalves Silva, Ana C. Krepischi and Felipe Fidalgo
International Research Center, AC Camargo Cancer Center, São Paulo, Brazil

Silvia Regina Rogatto
School of Medicine, São Paulo State University, Botucatu, São Paulo, Brazil

Justin O'Brien, Janine Spencer and Christine Girges
Centre for Research in Infant Behaviour, Department of Psychology, Brunel University, Uxbridge, United Kingdom

Alan Johnston
Cognitive, Perceptual and Brain Sciences, Psychology and Language Sciences, University College London, London, United Kingdom

Harold Hill
School of Psychology, University of Wollongong, Wollongong, New South Wales, Australia

Index